Learning Disabilities Toward Inclusion

SIXTH EDITION

Edited by

Helen L. Atherton BSc(Hons) PhD RNLD

Lecturer in Nursing, School of Healthcare, University of Leeds, Leeds, UK

Debbie J. Crickmore BSc(Hons) MSc RNLD

Lecturer in Learning Disability, Faculty of Health and Social Care, University of Hull, Hull, UK

Forewords by

Jonathan Evans

Self Advocate, Speakup Self Advocacy, Rotherham, UK

Eamon Shanley BA(Hons) MSc MCounsel PhD RNID RMN CPN

Mental Health Nurse/Counsellor, Limestone Coast Division of General Practice, Mount Gambier, SA, Australia

CHURCHILL LIVINGSTONE

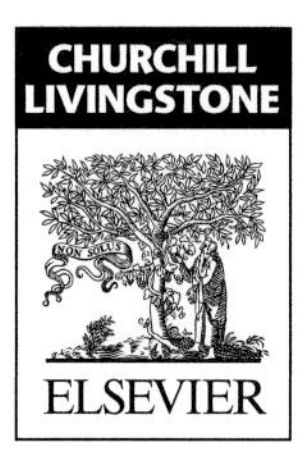

CHURCHILL
LIVINGSTONE
ELSEVIER

ISBN 978-0-7020-4285-0

British Library Cataloguing in Publication Data
A catalogue record for this book is available from the British Library

Library of Congress Cataloging in Publication Data
A catalog record for this book is available from the Library of Congress

Notices
Knowledge and best practice in this field are constantly changing. As new research and experience broaden our understanding, changes in research methods, professional practices, or medical treatment may become necessary.

Practitioners and researchers must always rely on their own experience and knowledge in evaluating and using any information, methods, compounds, or experiments described herein. In using such information or methods they should be mindful of their own safety and the safety of others, including parties for whom they have a professional responsibility.

With respect to any drug or pharmaceutical products identified, readers are advised to check the most current information provided (i) on procedures featured or (ii) by the manufacturer of each product to be administered, to verify the recommended dose or formula, the method and duration of administration, and contraindications. It is the responsibility of practitioners, relying on their own experience and knowledge of their patients, to make diagnoses, to determine dosages and the best treatment for each individual patient, and to take all appropriate safety precautions.

To the fullest extent of the law, neither the Publisher nor the authors, contributors, or editors, assume any liability for any injury and/or damage to persons or property as a matter of products liability, negligence or otherwise, or from any use or operation of any methods, products, instructions, or ideas contained in the material herein.

Printed in China

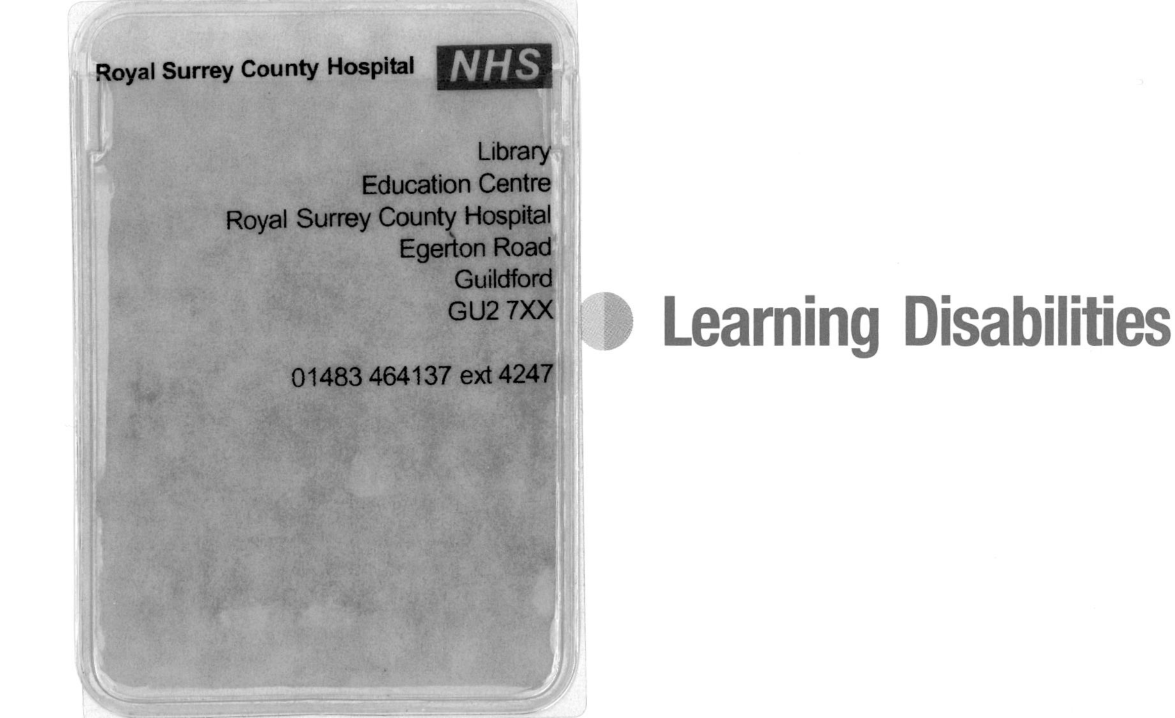

Learning Disabilities

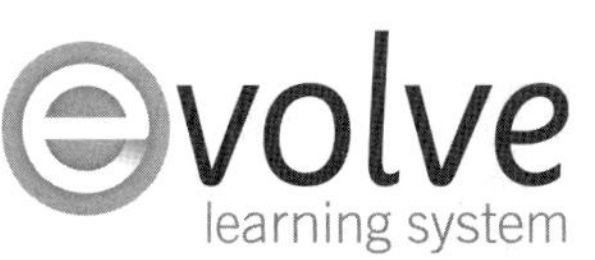

Evolve Learning Resources for Students and Lecturers.

See the instructions and PIN code panel on the inside cover for access to the web site.

Think outside the book...evolve

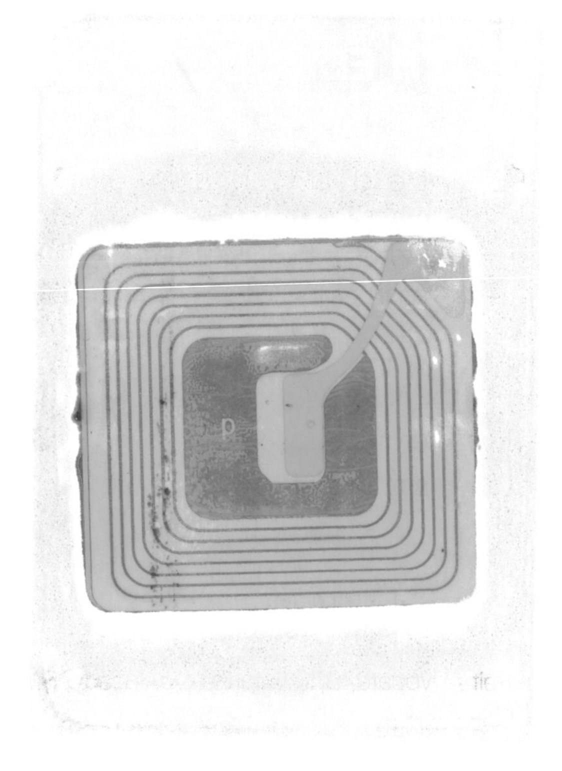

For Elsevier

Commissioning Editor: *Ninette Premdas*
Development Editor: *Sheila Black*
Project Manager: *Vinod Kumar Iyyappan*
Designer: *Charles Gray*
Illustration Manager: *Gillian Richards*
Illustrator: *Ethan Danielson*

Contents

Contributors

Andy Alaszewski BA MA PhD HonMFPHM
Professor of Health Studies, Centre for Health Services Studies, University of Kent, Canterbury, UK

Helen Alaszewski BA RGN
Research Associate, Centre for Health Services Studies, University of Kent, Canterbury, UK

Helen L. Atherton BSc(Hons) PhD RNLD
Lecturer in Nursing, University of Leeds, Leeds, UK

Lisa Belshaw DipOccTher
Occupational Therapist, ESPA Ltd, Ashbrooke, UK

Tom Berney MBChB DPM FRCPsych FRCPCH
Honorary Consultant in Developmental Psychiatry, Northumberland Tyne & Wear NHS Trust, Sunderland, UK

Karen Bunning PhD HPCReg MRCSLT
Reader in Speech and Language Therapy (Intellectual Disability), School of Allied Health Professions, University of East Anglia, Norwich, UK

Maria Caples MSc HDipGerontology RNID
Lecturer, Catherine McCauley School of Nursing and Midwifery, University College Cork, Cork, Ireland

Debbie J. Crickmore BSc(Hons) RNLD
Lecturer in Learning Disability, Faculty of Health and Social Care, University of Hull, Hull, UK

Ros Davies BM MRCGP
General Practitioner, New Hall Surgery, Hull, UK

Mary Dearing BSc(Hons) MSc RNLD
Lecturer in Learning Disability, Faculty of Health and Social Care, University of Hull, Hull, UK

Tony Dennison BA(Hons) MA PGCE RNLD RNMH
Senior Lecturer/Programme Leader, University of Cumbria, Lancaster, UK

Simon Duffy MA PhD DMS
Director, The Centre for Welfare Reform, Sheffield, UK

Julia Fitzpatrick MA(Hons) FCIH
Independent Consultant, Edinburgh, UK

Ruth Garbutt BA(Hons) MA PhD PGDip DipSW
Researcher Training and Development Officer
Staff and Departmental Development Unit (SDDU)
University of Leeds, Leeds, UK

Matthew Godsell PhD RNT RNLD
Senior Lecturer Learning Disabilities, Faculty of Health and Social Care, University of the West of England, Bristol, UK

Heather Gregory RMNH, Prof. Epilepsy Diploma
Epilepsy Specialist Nurse Learning Disability, Aysgarth House, Hull, UK

Susan Hunter BA(Hons) PGDipSocPol PGDipSocWk CQSW
Former Senior Lecturer, Honorary Fellow in Social Work, Department of Social Work, School of Social and Political Science, University of Edinburgh, Edinburgh, UK

Neil James BSc(Hons) PGCE RNLD
Senior Lecturer, Unit for Development in Intellectual Disability, Faculty of Health, Sport and Science, University of Glamorgan, Pontypridd, UK

Rob Jenkins MSc CertEd(FE) DipSocStudies RNLD
Divisional Head of Learning Disability, Unit for the Development in Intellectual Disabilities, Faculty of Health, Sport & Science, University of Glamorgan, Pontypridd, UK

Liane Kirk RNMH
Person Centred Planning Team Leader, East Riding of Yorkshire Council, Beverley, UK

Jo Lay BSc(Hons)Nursing (Learning Disabilities) PGCLTHE RNLD
School of Healthcare, University of Leeds, Leeds, UK

Anna Marriott BA(Hons) MSc
Research Associate, Norah Fry Research Centre, University of Bristol, Bristol, UK

Lynne Marsh RNID BSc MSc PGDTLHE RNID
Branch Leader & College Lecturer, Intellectual Disability Nursing, Catherine McCauley School of Nursing and Midwifery, University College Cork, Cork, Ireland

Roy McConkey BA PhD
Professor of Learning Disability, School of Nursing, University of Ulster, Newtownabbey, UK

Steve Mee BA(Hons) PhD RNLD
Senior Lecturer, Social Work & Applied Behavioural Studies, University of Cumbria, Lancaster, UK

Ruth Northway MSc(Econ) PhD CertEd(FE) RNLD FRCN
Professor of Learning Disability Nursing, Department of Care Sciences, Faculty of Health, Sport and Science, University of Glamorgan, Pontypridd, UK

Karl Nunkoosing BA EdD
Principal Lecturer, Department of Psychology, University of Portsmouth, Portsmouth, UK

Peter Oakes BA(Hons) DipClinPsy DPsy CPsychol AFBPsS
Consultant Clinical Psychologist, Department of Clinical Psychology, University of Hull, Hull, UK

Caroline Dalton O'Connor BNS MSc RNID
University Lecturer, College of Medicine and Health, University College Cork, Cork, Ireland

Sue Read MA PhD CertEdFE CertBerStudies RNMH
Reader in Learning Disability Nursing, School of Nursing and Midwifery, Keele University, Keele, UK

Malcolm Richardson BEd(Hons) PhD CertEd DipNursing (London) RNLD
Principal Lecturer (Learning Disabilities), Department of Nursing and Midwifery, Faculty of Health and Wellbeing, Sheffield Hallam University, Sheffield, UK

Julie Ridley BA(Hons) PhD
Senior Research Fellow, School of Social Work, University of Central Lancashire, Preston, UK

Kim Scarborough BSc(Hons) MSc(PMLD) PGCHE PGC(PSM) RNLD
Faculty Lead – Service User and Carer Involvement; Senior Lecturer (Academic in Practice – National Teaching Fellow), University of the West of England, Bristol, UK

Marion Steff PhD (EdPsych)
Disability Specialist, Center for Disability Studies and Services, State University Sunan Kalijaga, Yogyakarta, Indonesia

David S. Stewart OBE BA(Hons) MEd D.Litt.h.c.
Headteacher, Oak Field School and Sports College, Nottingham, UK

Laurence Taggart BSc(Hons) PhD RNLD PGCEN
Lecturer, Institute of Nursing Research, School of Nursing, University of Ulster, Coleraine, UK

Jenny Talbot MBA
Programme Manager, Learning Disabilities and Difficulties in Prison, Prison Reform Trust, London, UK

Debbie Watson MSc PGDip CertEd RNLD
Lecturer, Learning Disabilities, Department of Health Sciences, University of York, York, UK

Caroline White BSc(Hons) MA DipSW
Research Associate, Centre for Applied Research and Evaluation, Department of Social Sciences, University of Hull, Hull, UK

Val Williams BA(Hons) MEd PhD
Reader in Disability Policy and Practice, Norah Fry Centre, University of Bristol, Bristol, UK

Michael Wolverson BA(HONS) BSc(HONS) MSC PGC RNMH
Lecturer in Learning Disabilities, Department of Health Sciences, University of York, York, UK

Foreword by Jonathan Evans

My name is Jonathan Evans and I have been asked to write a foreword for this new edition of *Learning Disabilities: Toward Inclusion*, a book about how professionals should work with people who have learning disabilities or, as we prefer to say, learning difficulties. I work for a self-advocacy organisation, Speakup Self Advocacy, with people who have learning difficulties. I myself have Asperger's.

It is worth noting that Mencap (http://www.mencap.org.uk) tells us that there are 1.5 million people in the UK with a learning difficulty. The people I know who have learning difficulties face many issues when dealing with professionals and the front-line staff in service organisations. These issues are particularly around communication and understanding. In addition, they also have problems with getting the right, and good quality, services, with obtaining decent housing, getting a mortgage and meaningful employment. Another major issue that people with learning difficulties face on a day-to-day basis is gaining and keeping good relationships. This is largely due to people not getting the right support to make and maintain these relationships.

It is important that those working with a person who has a learning difficulty should have a good understanding of their needs, and who to contact if they are not in a position to help.

When I say people, I mean professionals such as learning disability nurses, occupational therapists, advocates or anyone who is a carer. It is important that people take a holistic/person-centred approach when working with people who have learning difficulties. This will have to happen more as we now have the personalisation agenda, direct payments and individual budgets. Rather than people with a learning difficulty having to fit around a service, services should fit around the people. This means people are offered the chance to choose.

Busy professionals sometimes forget that people are individuals; people with learning difficulties should not all be put in one group with one label. We all need to be supported differently but effectively. That is why it is so important that professionals have a good understanding of people with learning difficulties, their individual problems and their needs.

This is not about treating everyone equally, but discriminating in a positive way. People with learning difficulties will have extra support needs because of their difficulties.

Sometimes professionals and specialists get wrapped up in their specialisms and maybe don't see the bigger picture.

Foreword by Eamon Shanley

Since 1986, when I edited the first edition of this book, I have noted the growth in types of courses and changes in philosophy associated with helping people with intellectual disability. Mental health nurses of my generation who were trained in the 60s and 70s were hard pressed to find books such as this that gave a comprehensive, relevant and humanistic perspective in relating to people with learning disabilities.

I wrote the original book to emphasise the practical means of improving the quality of life of those people experiencing learning disabilities. I feel reassured that there remains this developmental thread that is present in the first edition: a focus on the reality of practice. In addition, this latest edition offers to a much wider national and international audience an understanding of the nature of learning disabilities, a holistic framework and a lifespan approach.

I would like to congratulate Helen Atherton and Debbie Crickmore on bringing together in one volume such a comprehensive and coherent collection of significant contributions. The production of such a large and integrative volume no doubt required considerable collaboration, for which I can only offer my admiration. I have also been impressed by the range of eminent authors and the quality of their contributions. This book truly warrants its description of being one of the leading text books in the field of learning disabilities.

Preface

Welcome to the sixth edition of *Learning Disabilities: Toward Inclusion*. As its new editors, we would like to take this opportunity to thank the departing editor, Professor Bob Gates, for the time and effort he invested in developing a text fit for contemporary learning disability practice over the last three editions. As the next set of editors endowed with this mantle, we felt it timely to reflect on the evolution of this text as it moves into its 25th year. Indeed, we were interested to know how, in the face of an increasingly competitive publishing market, it has maintained its status as one of the leading textbooks in the field of learning disabilities.

In considering its survival, the words evolution and change seem pertinent. This text has weathered the test of time by achieving a sense of freshness with each edition. The changes in editorship have served to invigorate its content through the introduction of new authors and hence different perspectives on key issues affecting the lives of people with learning disabilities and their families. Indeed, over the course of the last five editions, an array of eminent professionals from the field of learning disabilities have contributed their expertise toward ensuring a contemporary focus, with the sixth edition being no exception. The popularity of the book would also appear to lie with its ability to reflect current practice developments including the impact of changing policy and legislation on the nature and configuration of service delivery. Earlier editions focused on the United Kingdom, with a move toward a more international perspective evident in the fourth and fifth editions. Understanding the experiences of other countries can inform development of services and practice and an international feel has been maintained in this new edition, not least by involvement of authors from a range of countries.

The changes in title alone illustrate the journey this text has taken, being initially conceived in the first and second editions as *Mental Handicap: A Handbook of Care*, *Learning Disabilities* in the third and *Learning Disabilities: Toward Inclusion* in the fourth, fifth and now sixth editions. Changes in attitudes and beliefs about people with learning disabilities and the care and support that should be offered to them are evident during this time. In 1986, at the time of the first edition, the philosophy of community care was still in its infancy and it was to be a few more years before the further impetus provided by legislation. Significant numbers of people with learning disabilities were still living in large, long-stay institutions. As the book moved into its third edition in 1997, hospital closures were in full swing, but cracks were appearing in the façade of achieving an ordinary life. While community presence had been achieved, by and large, for a significant majority, real community participation remained elusive. Difficulties experienced by mainstream services in meeting the health needs of people with learning disabilities were also emerging with the publication of Mencap's *Prescription for Change* in 1997. By the fourth edition, published in 2003 under the title *Learning Disabilities: Toward Inclusion*, the devolved administrations of the UK had published a range of policy documents that sought to shift the balance of control from services to the individual. Traditional power relations between service providers and service users became the subject of challenge with more person-centred approaches paving the way for a new style of service delivery. Limitations in key principles of normalisation were also becoming evident and the social model of disability was becoming influential in driving the inclusion agenda.

Since the publication of the fifth edition of the text in 2007, a number of key events have succeeded in driving on the human rights agenda for people with learning disabilities. In 2006 and 2007, widespread institutional abuse was revealed in two NHS trusts in England. In 2007, Mencap published *Death by Indifference* highlighting fundamental inadequacies in mainstream hospital provision that led directly and indirectly to the deaths of six individuals with learning disabilities. The subsequent independent inquiry (Michael 2008) and the Ombudsmen's (2009) report *Six Lives* illustrated how services were failing to meet the needs of people with learning disabilities and provide a level of care that was equal to that enjoyed by the general population. This has guided our intention to widen the target audience of this text to the full range of health, social and personal supporters of people with learning disabilities. Chapter authors represent a wealth of professional backgrounds and roles, including learning disability nursing, education, psychology, therapies, social work, medicine and psychiatry within statutory, private, voluntary and independent practice.

Inclusion in all aspects of life for people with learning disabilities, from the provision of health care and education to the development of personal relationships and friendships, remains a considerable challenge for individuals and those supporting them. With this in mind, we have chosen to retain the title *Learning Disabilities: Toward Inclusion* in the sixth edition as a reflection on a work in progress towards achieving this goal. Use of the term 'learning disabilities' throughout flows from this and is not intended to disregard any preferences expressed by individuals or groups, rather to offer consistency to the reader across the text.

The nature and consequences of the events described above have significantly influenced the content and direction of the sixth edition. While some material from the fifth edition has been refreshed as it continues to have relevance in the second decade of the 21st century, new chapters reflecting important issues for people with learning disabilities and their families are introduced. As ever, the book is designed so that it can be read in part or in its entirety. This flexibility was important as it was understood that people would use it in different ways and for different purposes, for essay writing or the development of aspects of the support they provide to people with learning disabilities.

There are 30 chapters arranged within four main sections with six key themes running concurrently. All authors were asked to embed person-centredness, values, the reality of practice, the range of ability, the range of services and national and international perspectives within their chapters, to draw diverse material into an integrated whole. Where relevant, readers are given cross-references to other chapters to minimise repetition and overtly connect content. To further enhance readers' engagement with topics, case illustrations and reader activities appear throughout the text and within an accompanying electronic resource, a new departure for this text and unique among contemporary learning disability texts.

In furthering our understanding of the nature of learning disabilities, we have chosen to open the book, and the first section, with a thought-provoking chapter on social constructionism, as this theory serves to challenge the knowledge we take for granted about who people with learning disabilities are and the nature of the service provision they require. We have also included a chapter that clearly articulates a values base for the delivery of care and support. Chapters on causes of learning disabilities, eugenics and ethics complete the first section of the book, providing a firm underpinning for development within subsequent sections.

In the second section, we offer a toolbox of approaches that uphold the values outlined in the first section. This includes the introduction of several new chapters – advocacy, personal narrative and life story, inclusive research, risk and safeguarding – to complement communication and person-centred approaches to planning.

Section 3 focuses on health, opening with a new chapter offering a holistic framework for the chapters that follow. While subsequent chapters in this section explore different situations relevant to people with learning disabilities, we recognise they are not mutually exclusive. New chapters are included on sensory awareness and epilepsy.

The fourth and final section of this sixth edition adopts a lifespan approach, beginning with families and children and travelling to older age. Along the way, important aspects of life are explored, including education, leisure and friendships, and housing. Employment is given its own chapter and sexual health is a welcome addition to the sexuality and personal relationships chapter. The section, and the book, closes appropriately with a new chapter reflecting on end of life care.

We hope the care we have taken in editing is matched by the enjoyment and use you are able to derive from the sixth edition of *Learning Disability: Toward Inclusion*. We thank friends and colleagues for their patience and amazing contributions to what we hope is a comprehensive representation of learning disability practice in 2011.

Helen L. Atherton
Debbie J. Crickmore
Yorkshire, 2011

Section 1

Living with learning disabilities

The social construction of learning disability

1

Karl Nunkoosing

CHAPTER CONTENTS

KEY ISSUES

- Social constructionism is a critical theory about how we construct knowledge of learning disabilities
- Language is an important source of understanding how learning disabilities and people with learning disabilities are constructed
- Our knowledge of learning disabilities is negotiated in social practices which until recently did not give a role to the self-advocacy movement
- We construct knowledge practice to serve the purposes of services, service providers and professionals
- Experiencing learning disabilities is not imaginary, but becoming a person with learning disabilities is a social practice
- The social model of disability, while not the same as social constructionism, calls for the development of new relationships between people with learning disabilities and those who claim professional or academic expertise about their lives and those of their supporters

Introduction

This chapter starts by exploring some of the general ideas about how a social constructionist perspective might inform the gaze on that aspect of life we call 'learning disability'. One of the central ideas here is that disability does not exist in people but in social transactions and social arrangements. The various professions and academic disciplines with a stake in the lives of people with learning disabilities are part of such social arrangements.

In addition to the various professions in health and social care and education who are involved in the lives of people with learning disabilities, there are also several academic disciplines that contribute knowledge of, and understanding about, learning disabilities: academic disciplines such as anthropology, psychology, medicine, sociology, cultural studies, disability studies, law, philosophy, the art and humanities to name just a few. These disciplines share some knowledge about learning disabilities and they also differ in their methods of creating knowledge, in their authorities and practices. A consequence of so many academic interests in learning disabilities is the existence of several theories of learning disabilities. Such abundance of theories inevitably leads to competition between theories.

The social constructionist perspective sees these different and differing theoretical views as an asset rather than an impediment to our knowledge of something as complex as the human situation. There is no one way to know. Consider autism for example. During the 1960s autism was a psychiatric condition that affected a few people; currently more and more people are claiming the autistic identity. Autism is even a media event with films and documentaries about the person with autism. In the 1960s it was thought that autism was caused by cold, unresponsive mothering (Bettleheim 1967) – mother blaming was in vogue at the time – now we discourse autism as a neurobiological condition. As our knowledge developed it has moved from the one condition called autism to a variety of signs and a range of impairments called autistic spectrum disorders or conditions (ASDs or ASCs) and the specific Asperger's syndrome. The disability rights and the self-advocacy movements have played significant roles in our thinking of an autistic community (Bagatell 2010).

The autistic community has turned the table on the medical model by labelling those without autism as 'neurotypical' or NT. And they don't mean this in a nice way. They see many professionals as oppressors and allies in the biomedical construction of autism. They are perplexed about our obsession with social interactions. We have here two polarised ways of knowing about autism and autistic people. Either extreme has the potential to be unhelpful to some people with autism, but either understanding has something to contribute to how we do our work with and for people with the label 'autistic'.

This short introductory remark gives you the flavour of the critical and sometimes challenging nature of the social constructionist view. Part of this critical stance is about asking questions. The next section of this chapter starts with some of the questions that the social constructionist might ask about learning disabilities, the lives of people with learning disabilities and of our thinking and actions with people with learning disabilities. The later sections examine ideas and actions we take for granted; the changing nature of knowledge across culture and over time and how it affects our practice; and the relationship between social construction and the social model of disability.

A social constructionist perspective

Social constructionism is a wide-ranging movement that offers 'radical and critical alternatives in psychology and social psychology, as well as other disciplines in the social sciences and humanities' (Burr 2003:1). The social part of social constructionism is that personal status and identity are constructed in human relationships and interactions. It is people who label other people. And in this project, language inevitable plays a very important role.

The power of language

One of the central ideas of the social constructionist perspective is that language is used to serve different purposes and the purposes of different vested interests. Language and knowledge are closely related, therefore knowledge also serves different vested interests. Consider how in the last decade we have been engaged in a constant search for new language about our work supporting men and women with learning disabilities and the actions that we take. We speak of challenging behaviour, holistic care, evidence-based practice, person-centred planning, quality of life, cost-effectiveness, community, individuality, independence, control, social and health care, community learning disability team, the prevalence and incidence of learning disability, inclusion and many other words to inform our actions with people with learning disabilities. In fact we even have many words to speak about learning disability, words such as intellectual disability, learning difficulties, special needs, developmental delay and many words we do not use any more, words such as mental handicap and mental retardation. The language we use to speak and write about learning disability is not neutral. Why do we not use the term 'people with learning difficulties' as advised by the self-advocacy movement? I am often told that this is to do with government policies that refer to learning disability as if the policy also tells us to discount the voices of self-advocacy. We are also told that 'learning disability' is an exact term that refers to people's ability, social skills and the age of the person when the disability started. The language we use informs us about what we do as much as it tells people what we think and the nature of our relationship with the people we talk or write about. What does the language that we use about learning disability tell us about how we think of people with the label 'learning disabilities'?

See Reader activity 1.1 on the Evolve website.

Much of our ways of knowing about learning disability do not come from the experiences of people with the label 'learning disabilities'. What passes as theory about learning disability has privileged the knowledge of professionals and academics. The knowledge of people who experience learning disability and its consequences has been largely ignored. It is not that there is no text written by men and women with this label or that there is an absence of literature about people's experiences, it is just that we have a tendency to privilege the authority of professionals and academics over the authority to know of individuals with learning disabilities and their families and friends. The social constructionist asks 'who can know about the nature of experiencing learning disabilities?'

These questions, and many others that the social constructionist asks, tell you something about this perspective. Social constructionism is a critical discipline. Critical in the sense that it is not comfortable with ideas, concepts and theories that appear to reflect the things that we all know about learning disabilities and the men and women who have been given that label. The stance of being critical is not simply about criticising, it is about the idea that what we know as knowledge is constantly changing. Progress in any aspect of human work is unlikely to be sustained when we stop asking questions and/or when we close our mind to critics and take the authority of what we read for granted. There was a time when we thought that there was nothing odd or wrong about people with learning disabilities being taken from their families and communities and placed in institutions. Note how these places are now referred to as 'campuses' (Hartnett et al 2008, McConkey et al 2005, Owen et al 2008). The discourse 'campus' is used to distract our attention but it cannot replace our memories of the bad things that happened and continued to occur until recently in the institutions. This is simply the most recent example of how language is used to influence how we think. The languages that we use have consequences for people because they influence how we act towards people, things and ideas. A critical perspective is about understanding the consequences of our ideas and concepts for people with learning disabilities and for ourselves. So does it matter that we use people-first language, such as people with learning disabilities instead of learning disabled people?

The social constructionist perspective is about asking questions about the things that we take for granted about the human state that we call learning disability, about the way that we construct knowledge about learning disability and about how disablement is caused by social practices. It is not simply about asking questions, it is about asking questions in new ways. Such as, what is the nature of the human relationship between the man or woman with learning disabilities and the people who are paid to support his or her community inclusion? Professionals who support people with learning disabilities embrace the theories and ideologies of their own professions and these theories are not known to the people who depend on their services (Dowling 2006). What is being asked of helpers and professionals when one's disability is about one's ability to learn? What kind of services are we going to provide for people when we think of them as unfortunate victims of circumstances?

The social constructionist perspective is part of a wider movement concerned with ideas in the social sciences. Its roots lie in philosophy, art, architecture and literary criticism, among others. In the social sciences this movement has a long history. However a convenient starting point is Berger & Luckman (1967:19–20) *The Social Construction of Reality*:

> The world of everyday life is not only taken for granted as reality by the ordinary members of society in the subjectively meaningful conduct of their lives. It is a world that originates in their thoughts and actions, and is maintained as real by these.

Much of what we know and do in our relationships with people who experience learning disabilities is based on 'taken for granted' assumptions which assume that learning disability is something that exists inside the person. When we go along with this assumption, we are likely to engage in a range of social actions such as measuring the degree of the disability, seeking its causes in the genes, cognition, physiology or anatomy of the person. Along with these actions comes the idea that a learning disability exists as a deficit in the person. There is something not quite right with his or her ability to think, to solve problems, to use language and so on. Social construction guides us to take an alternative understanding about learning disability. That is, learning and learning disabilities exist in social and cultural practices rather than in the heads of labelled individuals (Gergen 1990).

When we say things like 'what is wrong with Krishnan, he is not doing what he should for his age?', we situate the problem in Krishnan. Before long, we take him to doctors and psychologists and he gets tested and investigated and we find out that he is developmentally delayed. He has special educational needs. I remember once having a conversation with a woman from India who told me that in India, her daughter was just her daughter, and when she came to England, her daughter became the girl with special needs. I am not saying that there is anything wrong in itself to test a child's intelligence, but there is something wrong in a society that, as a result of an intelligence test, a child is sent to a segregated (often called special) school where he or she does not learn and play, eat or experience the world alongside other children of his or her own age. The social constructionist approach does not simply ask why we do that, it also asks why we continue to defend the existence of such places. How can schools learn how to attend to the learning needs of all children if they are not exposed to all children? So rather than asking what is wrong with the person, I suggest that we ask what is wrong with a culture that tolerates the exclusion of some of its children and adults simply because they are deemed to be (dis)abled in their intellectual capacity?

Rather than defining learning disability as something that resides inside the person in terms of his or her IQ, and his or her social skills, we could consider defining learning disability in societal terms. Rather than defining learning disabilities in terms of what a person can or cannot do, the radical and critical constructionist might suggest that we redefine this human state in terms of the kind of actions that we need to take to effectively support the person. We know that the disability is stigmatising, so what is needed is an advanced level of social acceptance. By definition, a learning disability calls for highly developed teaching methods and educational practices to make learning easier. We also know that some people will need effective and individually developed, and sometimes lifelong, support services for housing, work, leisure and health care. His or her rights will need to be safeguarded and defended. I am seeking here to challenge the idea that we look at the intellectual or social deficit of the man or woman with learning disability and turn the gaze on the deficit of the organisations that create learning disabilities; not to do so is to engage in victim blaming (Duckett 2000, Wright 1993). An example of this idea of victim blaming is the idea that some people with learning disability engage in what is termed 'attention-seeking behaviour'. We all seek and need attention and it is only in the context of services that this is a problem for staff. Logically, people seek attention when they are ignored, when they have little control over the actions of those who care for them. The person needs to be acknowledged, needs the attention of the staff, and when he or she does not get this acknowledgement, he or she has two options – he or she can withdraw into his or her own world or escalate his/her demand for attention. The really frustrating thing is that both his/her withdrawal and attention seeking are constructed as pathologies that originate from his/her learning disability rather than the social organisation of 'care' that sees him or her as demanding. Social construction asks that we are aware of how learning disability is not located inside people with labels but in their relationships with people, organisations, procedures, practices, events, places and ideas where the concept of the 'learning disabled' is constructed. Thus, for the man or woman with a learning disability, this is an identity that he or she acquires. The identity of learning disabled, like any other identity, is a product of interactions between people, ideas, things, places and activities. I imagine that you are reading this book because you are interested in the lives of people with learning disabilities and that confers on you an identity as a scholar of disability studies. How does your identity relate to the situations of men and women with learning disabilities? I feel the need to explain why I use the words 'men and women'. I do so because we often write about learning disability as if the people with this label are genderless. Gender is an important part of our identity.

You simply can't be a person with a learning disability on your own. You do not create this identity by yourself; it is an identity that is imposed in social transactions. Once a boy or a girl or a man or a woman is given this identity, all his actions are explained in the context of this all-defining label. Some labels are so powerful that they mask all the other ways that we can see the person. The power of a label is socially agreed, it is not something inside the person. This is what is meant by the idea that the person with learning disabilities is disabled by the organisations and social relationships he or she is in. Being dependent on services can be a stigmatising, discrediting label. Here are some examples of how the social element of life for either a man or a woman, who depends on the support of a service for people with learning disabilities, can be disabling. This can be by:

- services misunderstanding or misapplying policies. One example of this is staff misunderstanding their 'duty of care' to justify controlling and regulating people.

- carers' negative values and attitudes about him or her such as believing that he or she can't learn and change or benefit from actions to improve his or her life. Sometimes this can take the form of resentment against the person who experiences learning disabilities.
- carers not taking the time to explain things in a language that he or she can understand.
- services lacking concern for his or her future.
- workers' incompetence, intolerance and ignorance.
- environments and practices that exclude him or her from their communities and from experiencing an ordinary life. For example, when they go out for an evening they have to be back in time for the staff shift change.
- people who work closely with him or her not taking the time to reflect on how their ideas and actions affect both the worker and the man or woman with a learning disability.

I am sure that you can add to this list.

The point that I am seeking to make here is that the society that is often invoked as not caring about people with learning disabilities is not out there; the people with the most contact with people with learning disabilities are also members of society. Workers are members of society and they bring into their work the values of their communities. Imagine we turn the gaze from people who depend on services to the people in society. You could consider the characters we see in soap operas, for example. In that gaze we can highlight people who experience problems with alcohol consumption, people who have problems with their relationships, people who are manipulative and spiteful, people whose lifestyles are unhealthy, people who have not learned to live within their means and so on. We do not call them people with a challenging lifestyle, because they are not under the same surveillance as the person with a learning disability who depends on support services.

Some key ideas about social constructioninism

Kenneth Gergen (1985) is a central figure in theorising, and in his seminal paper about the constructionist movement in psychology he identified the following four aspects to the social constructionist perspective:

1. A critical stance towards taken for granted knowledge.
2. Historical and cultural specificity of knowledge.
3. Knowledge is sustained by social process.
4. Knowledge and social action go together.

A critical stance towards taken for granted knowledge

I have already mentioned this aspect of the constructionist view. Here I will extend this somewhat. The critical stance starts by asking two questions:

1. What is the purpose of this knowledge?
2. Whose purpose does this knowledge serve?

Consider the following taken for granted knowledge about learning disability:

> We know that some people are considered to have disabilities (and experience learning disabilities), that this disability is observable (as poor social behaviour and low attainments of developmental milestones) and measurable (as low IQ). We have an objective definition of learning disability, which takes into account the age of the person when these observations and measurements were first made. If a person has this thing called a learning disability, we can reasonably predict how he or she will need special procedures to enable him or her to learn, or how he or she might be vulnerable and need protecting from others who might abuse his or her vulnerability. These differences make the person have special educational needs and either health care or social care needs, which in turn require the people who attend to these needs to possess professional qualifications in education, health or social care or combinations of the three.

All these aspects of 'learning disability' are 'true'. True in the sense that we can observe practices that are based on these ideas. Some textbooks about learning disability are populated with these ideas. Our own practices, our places of work, our authority, our identity and job title are products of these knowledge claims. It is therefore in our interest to behave as if these things are facts. But facts don't have to be right. In an advert on television, it is a fact that 90% of the people who were asked prefer product A. But we will need to know a lot more about the people who were asked before we can go along with the conclusion that 90% of all people prefer product A.

In the above statement about learning disability, these things are true according to the vantage point from which we consider them. However there are likely to be other vantage points that make different knowledge practice claims about learning disability.

In defending our own particular claim, we often discredit the alternatives. Earlier I suggested that we often subscribe to the idea that disability exists inside the person. However the constructionist perspective does not see theories as simply either/or explanations. Each theory can add something to our understanding. In a study about staff explanation of challenging behaviour, Wilcox et al (2006) found that staff constructed their understanding of challenging behaviour as caused both by individual pathology and the social circumstance.

Historical and cultural specificity of knowledge

This refers to the idea that our knowledge of learning disability is specific to time and places and different cultures also have different explanations of learning disability. Culture itself changes over time; the culture of contemporary Britain is in many respects different from the cultures of the 1960s. Arokiasamy (1987) suggests that, over time, there have been four main historical conceptualisations of disability:

1. Disability is caused by supernatural forces.
2. Disability is attributed to medical causes.
3. Disability is attributed to natural causes.
4. People with disabilities constitute an oppressed minority.

These theories and related practices are products of their time and culture. Currently, in the Western world, one would be hard pressed to continue to defend the notion that learning disability is caused by supernatural forces. There was a time in certain parts of Europe when disabled babies were thought to have been 'changelings'. It was suggested that the real baby had been abducted by either demons or fairies or elves and replaced by the disabled child and that the mother has to take good care of the 'changeling' otherwise her real baby would be harmed (Haffter 1968). Note how this explanation also helps the mother to care for the baby in a society when most people lived in poverty and were hostile to people with disabilities. Consider how both the parents and other people might have behaved towards a baby who was thought of as belonging to the devil. We may not continue to believe in the changeling myth, but some parents and staff still attribute the disability to supernatural events.

The issue of historical specificity is not that straightforward in the context of learning disability. I do not think that one idea necessarily just replaces another one. The idea that disabled people constitute an oppressed minority is the most recent way of thinking about disability that comes from the disability movement. Without this activism of disabled people themselves this would not have happened; they argue that medical and natural causes refer to impairment. Impairment happens to the body; disability is a social and oppressive consequence of impairment. These ideas have not been replaced. They are in a sense all competing for our attention. What is interesting from a constructionist perspective is the purpose of each of these ideas and whose purpose is served by each explanation. Each explanation produces its own discourses and consequently its own mode of social actions and professional interventions. Each explanation is the consequence of viewing the world from a different vantage point. Thus the self-advocacy movement is the social action that originates from people with learning disabilities becoming conscious of their oppression.

The eugenicists were convinced that they were serving the best interests of society by their actions (see Ch. 3). We may not subscribe to the eugenics idea of segregating men from women with mild learning disabilities, congregating them in single-sex institutions so that they did not produce more disabled children, yet it would be a mistake to think that the eugenics discourse has disappeared (see also Ch. 3). Consider how in current discourse the death of unborn children with disabilities is legitimised (Aspie 2001, Sooben 2004). The argument is often about the issue that if these children are born, they will constitute a burden to their families or the state and they will have poor 'quality of life'. Social problems are socially constructed from the claims of those who are legitimised by society, such as professionals, policy makers and academics, to make such claims, often as labels and definitions. The person seen as a burden becomes a member of an 'out group' and such 'out groups' are often despised. Therefore we sometimes accept the reasoning that by aborting a baby with a disability, we are saving both the baby and his or her parents from future pains.

It would also be a mistake to assume that our current understanding of learning disability is the definitive knowledge. Our current ideas about learning disability are infused with an ableist discourse (Hehir 2007). Ableism here is based on the belief that people who do not experience intellectual difficulties are somehow superior to people with learning disabilities. It is from this belief that patronising and disrespectful practices stem. Contemporary ideas

Reader activity 1.2

One significant change that has taken place in our concept of learning disability is the shift from thinking of a learning disability as a 'deficiency' to thinking of the persons with learning disabilities as simply different, in the way that being tall, black, talented or gay is different.

Consider these two ways of thinking. Make a list of the actions that might arise from thinking of people with deficient cognition and a separate list of actions that might originate from thinking of learning disabilities as different. Discuss these with your co-students and colleagues.

Compare your list with mine. There is no right or wrong answer to this activity; it is aimed at enabling you to think and to understand your observations of your work.

1. Disability as 'deficient':
   - The person can't learn in the usual way – he or she will need to be protected. A consequence of protective practices is to isolate the 'vulnerable' person from his or her social and cultural environment. This leads to exclusion.
   - The person is seen as not 'whole' or less with the consequence that it is assumed that he or she does not know any difference. This can lead to less emphasis on quality.
   - Seeing disability as 'deficiency' leads to practices that are dehumanising and 'special' in negative ways that accentuate the person as less than his or her peers.
   - Since the 'deficiency' is in the person, workers engage in practices that are aimed at fixing the person rather than the disabling social environments.
   - Workers see themselves as technicians for implementing policies, plans and programmes. The focus is on process, with a tendency to have long lists of boxes to tick. There is little concern about the development of relationship and friendship.
2. Disability as 'difference':
   - There is an emphasis on inclusion so that both the person and his or her culture learn about each other and about tolerance of difference.
   - There is the same concern for and application of quality as there would be for any other citizen.
   - Seeing the person as simply different rather than less implies attention to the ordinary, that is ordinary homes, ordinary work, leisure, worship and so on.
   - Practices seek to enable the person to learn from his experiences, also creating access to wide-ranging experiences.
   - The focus of the service is the development of relationships that are mutual and respectful.

in disability studies are clear about the problems of sexism and racism, but are still relatively silent about ableism. It is a fact that most institutions have been closed down, but it is also a fact that the project of social inclusion continues to be an illusion because most of what we do is geared towards the containment of people with learning disabilities. Nowhere is this more prevalent than in schools (Connor & Ferri 2007, Slee 2008). We construct meanings and create the possibility for change when we engage in talk about an issue. It seems to me timely that we start talking about how we make a fetish of ability and the consequences of our ablelist discourse for ourselves and for people with learning disabilities. To extend the discussion that learning disability is not inside but in our social interactions, this ableist way of thinking is not something that is just out there in society; supporters of people with learning disabilities are also members of the same society. We have a duty to ourselves to raise our consciousness to counter this ablelist attitude whereever it is found, including within our co-workers.

Knowledge is sustained by social process

Our knowledge of learning disability is not necessarily derived from the nature of learning disability itself. People with interest in this thing called learning disability construct this knowledge between themselves. The self-advocacy movement also has a stake in this action. They want to be referred to as 'people with learning difficulties' and we generally ignore this. This has to do with the exercise of power. We do this knowledge construction through the medium of language rather than through objective observations, measurement, assessment and the other rituals of professionals. Gergen (1985:6) refers to this idea thus:

> The degree to which a given form of understanding prevails or is sustained across time is not directly dependent upon the empirical validity of the perspective in question, but upon the vicissitude of social processes.

There was a time when what we now term 'challenging behaviour' was called 'severe problem behaviour'.

Reader activity 1.3

Read the following text of a referral (not an actual referral) to a community learning disability team (CLDT):

> *Viv Reed refuses to go on holiday with the other clients, saying that he prefers to go to his favourite ceramics workshop and literacy class at college. He does not want to understand that the college is shut for the summer. Every morning he waits for the bus which of course does not come and then he goes to his room and sulks all day. He is making himself and all the other residents unhappy and the staff have tried everything to get him to change his mind and get him involved in the activities of the house. Could a member of your team make him see sense as he won't listen to any of us and his key worker is on sick leave?*

Think about this text and consider 'what is going on' in this short account. Do you see/read anything that tells you about this man and his paid for supporters? Have a go at rewriting the same text.

I would start by looking at the hidden discourse in the text. "A discourse refers to a set of meanings, metaphors, representations, images, stories, statements and so on that in some way together produce a particular version of events." (Burr 2003:64).

The hidden discourses in the text include the following:

- Mr Reed has an identity and he is more than a source of problem for the staff and the people he lives with. He may not have chosen to live with these people. Does it matter that he is referred to as Viv and not Mr Reed? It could: 'Viv' could indicate a friendly first-name term relationship between the person who wrote the referral and Mr Reed. Or it could be a way of not acknowledging his status as a man and a citizen. Should we care about his age, which is missing; could it mean that he is too old to want to be a student?
- Note how this text seeks to blame Mr Reed: he 'does not want to understand'; he sulks and if he is of the right age, he might get described by the current ageist discourse of 'grumpy old man'; a source of unhappiness for himself and the people he shares his accommodation with.
- So he is unreasonable and his sense is compromised to the extent that the experts of the CLDT are called for. So he may have a close relationship with his absent key worker: the service still has responsibilities for his wellbeing.
- What exactly is he a client of? What service is he a user of? When I go to Lidl or Waitrose, I am not a user of retail services, I am simply a customer.

There is more that a deep, discursive analysis of how and what we write about people can reveal. Consider a rewrite of this referral:

> *Mr Vivian Reed is 56 years old and we have found it difficult to explain to him that his further education college is shut for the summer vacation and that we are all going on holiday in a week's time. We did not prepare him for the summer closure of the college that he attends 3 days a week. He loves meeting his friends there, he enjoys hanging out with them in the college canteen or around the pool table when he is not in class. He misses college so much that he waits for the bus that does not come and then he gets upset. It is possible that as well as missing the activities and social interactions he loves so much, he also thinks that the holiday is instead of the college. The problem is that he was not involved in planning and choosing the holiday. Had this been done we might have been able to prepare him for the summer closure of the college and that it is usual to have a holiday break in the summer. This is a lesson that we have learnt for the future, and we will consider involving his college tutor in this preparation in the future.*
>
> *Understandably he is upset that he can't go to the college that he loves so much and tends to shut himself in his room, which is quite mature of him as he does not want his unhappiness to affect others. The fuss that we make around his waiting for the bus that does not come diverts attention from his co-residents who need staff to explain to them what is going on.*
>
> *I discussed our concern at the last house meeting, which Mr Reed did not attend, and we think that Mr Reed, the staff team and the people who live here need help to resolve this issue.*

(OK this is a longer text, but it does not blame anybody and presents Mr Reed as rational and that one of his assets is that people want to help him. It also shows the culture of the house as collegial and, importantly, as a learning organisation.)

Two social processes led to this change: first, the need to define objective measurements about the severity/intensity, duration, the environment that sustains the behaviour came with the behaviourism. Second, the ideology of normalisation, the 'people first' movement and deinstitutionalisation contributed to the new discourse of 'challenging behaviour'. People with the same severe problem behaviours were considered to be challenging to services to find appropriate means of enabling these individuals to live ordinary lives. Now the word 'challenging' has found its way into everyday language to mean difficult. We also commonly speak of people with 'challenging needs' to refer to people who require intensive and complex support.

A study by Shaw (2009) demonstrates how learning disability nurses construct stories of people with learning disabilities as problems to themselves and to society and where the nurse has the resources, skills and knowledge to manage these problems. This knowledge is both the product of the nurses' experiences and health and social care policies. The issue is not that the nurses were wrong, it is simply that knowledge is created in context, in situations and the context of the institution makes possible these ways of thinking. Shaw points to an alternative position where consciousness of the way that both the worker and the people with learning disabilities who depend on the workers are trapped in the same structure of power that serves to maintain control and social order (Foucault 1991). In this alternative, nurses understand and challenge privileges of power and make common cause with people with learning disabilities to share power. This new social action, where the person with a learning disability and the nurse are partners, will require new knowledge of theory and practice. Although this study is about nurses, the lesson is for all workers who make their living supporting people with learning disabilities. We all know how to do things to people; we have to create new knowledge about how to work with people, and in this endeavour men and women with learning disabilities will have a prominent role. The best example of this is to be found in the self-advocacy movement and in participatory research (see Atkinson 2005, Brookes & Davis 2008).

Knowledge and social action go together

Paid supporters of men and women with disabilities have a vested interest in thinking about and talking about people with learning disabilities as different from other people, as experiencing problems with living and learning. Just think about the stories that workers in these services tell about their work. The problem is that if people with learning disabilities are ordinary people then what is the point of employing these expensive professionals? Workers and service providers are engaged in discoursing the complexity of their work, and the skills that they possess to ask for more money from funders of services. This discourse of complexity creates on the one hand people with learning disabilities as odd, and on the other hand as rationale for their exclusion.

When we discourse learning disability as something that makes people different and odd and not the same as us, we justify all the practices that were part of the institutional model as described by Brigham et al (2001). New ways of working and thinking include a rejection of the punitive, patronising, controlling and authoritarian ways of the past, which were themselves products of the institutional model of residential service. The hospitals, now referred to as campuses, were in turn based on the punitive model of the workhouses. The consideration that people's behaviours challenge services to provide environments that support alternative behaviours has to reject the older explanations of learning disability as well as explanations of how to relate to persons said to have learning disabilities. This new perspective leads to new discourse and consequently to new social actions. When deinstitutionalisation and community care were proposed during the 1980s, it was said that people with learning disabilities would not be able to live in the community. When the people started to demonstrate that they were capable of living better lives outside the institutions, defenders of the institutional model said that community-based services were suitable only for people with mild or moderate levels of disabilities. When people who need intensive support made successful lives in the community, it was said that people with severe problem behaviours have needs that are best met by the medical model of health care.

Ways of knowing about learning disability and the consequences of this knowledge for people with learning disabilities

Social construction of learning disability is about what we know and how we know about people who have been labelled thus. There are at least two perspectives from which we can know about learning disability:

1. Knowledge of professionals and academics.
2. Knowledge of the lived experiences of the person with a learning disability.

We can think of these two ways of knowing as two different but related paradigms. A paradigm refers to a shared worldview of a given community. It relates to the shared values, beliefs, knowledge, practices, technology and assumptions of a community. Students of learning disability studies constitute one such community alongside others such as social scientists, policy makers, the self-advocacy movements, families and friends of children and adults with learning disabilities, service providers and the various professions engaged in the lives of persons with learning disabilities. Paradigms provide us with the models to make sense of the world of learning disabilities as well as structuring what is and what is not knowable.

A range of processes sustains a dominant paradigm. The community of professionals concerned with learning disability is linked through their education and training experiences that draw on the same technical and ideological literature. Changes occur when anomalies that run counter to the dominant paradigm emerge. An anomaly is a finding or observation that is either not predictable or explainable by the existing paradigm. There are two such paradigms that inform our work and thinking about learning disabilities: positivism and interpretative social science.

Positivism and learning disability

Positivism is a philosophical orientation which holds that experimentation and objective observations are the only true source of knowledge. A consequence of this orientation is that reality is external to the individual and this reality is measurable and predictable. And what is true of one individual is also true of all other persons. From this perspective, the ability and disability of the individual can be measured and diagnosed. For example, we can measure the mobility of an individual by the number of steps he or she can take unaided. In the context of learning disability, intelligence is measurable and the intellect of an individual can be assessed. A specific score in an assessment of intelligence means the same for all individuals with this score. Thus the intellectual functioning of persons with an IQ of 75 is likely to be similar.

The positivist paradigm conceptualises disability as a deficit that is both observable and measurable. In the context of learning disability, the two most widely used measurements are of intelligence and adaptive/social behaviours. Both of these have been shown to be anomalous. Intelligence tests have been strongly criticised in the past for ethnic and class bias, as well as for providing the theoretical rationale for the educational segregation of children with learning disabilities. Measurement of intelligence also led to the invention of the classification of 'feeble minded' (Gould 1996, Trent 1994) (see also Ch. 3). Positivists may agree about such criticisms but are likely to say that the tests themselves are reliable and valid measures of intelligence and that these criticisms relate to the misuse of these tests. A person's adaptive behaviour refers to his or her capacity for the independent social functioning expected for his or her age and culture. Adaptive behaviour is concerned with the person's day-to-day functioning rather than his or her maximum level of performance.

Because the positivist paradigm operates on the assumption that disability is a deficit in the individual who is in need of rehabilitation, often the purpose of rehabilitation is to overcome these deficits. Viewing the person as carrier of a list of deficits does little for his or her identity as a man or woman. Such categorisations are meant to show the person as not like me, but as 'other'.

The positivist orientation has important direct consequences for the social actions and role of the supporter of a person with learning disabilities. Here the deficit resides in the person and the deficit is objectively measured and quantified. The supporter has to seek means of making the person change to remedy the deficit. Such actions might include seeking to treat the person's disability by placing the person in special programmes, searching for effective learning strategies and discovering underlying cognitive and behavioural aspects of learning. It might consider the person with learning disabilities as having low self-esteem as a consequence of his or her learning disabilities. Measurement of progress is via scientific testing. For example, in this paradigm, the debate about inclusive education has to be resolved scientifically. There has to be demonstrable/measurable changes in the attainments and behaviours of the child in inclusive settings that are superior to the attainments of a similar child in a segregated school. The fact that the policy to create such schools in the first place was based on debatable premises is ignored. That children should be educated alongside their peers has no currency as a moral argument when we privilege the values of science.

Interpretative social science and learning disability

I suggest above that one kind of action that is indicated in defining new ways of forming relationships with men and women with learning disabilities is to give up knowledge and practices derived from the medical model of disability. The interpretative social science paradigm seeks understanding of learning disability by focusing on the meaning and purpose of social action and as such stands as the opposite of positivist ways of knowing. Here, the human state we call 'learning disabled' has no universal meaning. The meaning of learning disability is socially negotiated. The person achieves that devalued status of 'learning disabled'. This achieved status does not have to characterise the person in all circumstances. Thus a child may be considered disabled while at school and an ordinary son or daughter, brother or sister after school hours. The interpretative paradigm accepts that people have multiple roles in society. The person cannot be said to have a disability; rather he or she has a status that is renegotiated in different circumstances.

In this paradigm, we are interested in the ramification of the acquired status 'man or woman with learning disability' for the person and his or her supporters. For most of us who are involved in the life situations of people with learning disabilities, the interpretative paradigm requires us to consider how we have come to develop our social actions, rituals and relationships. My guesses are that some of these social actions, rituals and relationships have served to marginalise the voices of people with the status of learning disability and at times some of what we do can actually suppress the voices of people with this devalued status. I suggested earlier how the stories that professionals tell about their work contribute to the devaluation of men and women with learning disabilities.

The interpretative paradigm asks us to seek other ways of describing our social actions, rituals and relationships with people who are said to have learning disabilities. We can understand disability by the stories that we tell about people and about ourselves (see Ch. 8). One type of story populates our learned journals above all other stories that can be told about learning disability. This is the story of the authors, the academics and the professionals, as heroes who find new ways of fixing the deficit of learning disability. These stories are rarely about the triumph of people with learning disabilities.

Everybody has aspects of their lives that are assets and other aspects that are sources of problems to the person. It does not make any human sense to think of people with learning disabilities only in terms of what may or may not be missing and of what they can't do. That is sometimes referred to as the pathological gaze (Foucault 1973). The 'gaze' is not simply about seeing; it refers to a system of medical knowledge behind the act of looking. An alternative is the strengths-based perspective where there is an emphasis on strengths rather than what the person cannot do, and a focus on interventions that are proactive, solution focused and aimed at prevention. In essence, this is about believing that the person with a learning disability can change, can learn, can benefit from participatory actions with supporters. In social work, the strengths perspective is associated with the name of Dennis Saleebey (1992, 1996).

It is worth noting that there was a time when not being very clever did not constitute a disability. There was a time when an intellectual impairment was just another way of being. Our task is to consider at what point in history did an intellectual impairment lead to the state we now refer to as learning disability. I have to make one thing clear here. I am not suggesting that people do not have different intellectual abilities. I am however questioning at what point in history a low intellect became morally discrediting? What led to this new negotiated status? What sustains this gaze about learning disability in the 21st century?

Individual or personal tragedy and social models of disability

Another way of distinguishing between the positivist and the interpretative model is to pay attention to the scholarship of the disability movement, critical disability studies, where the voice of disabled people is paramount. It is true that until recently this movement did not directly refer to people said to have learning disability. However it has much to teach us about what we think, how we think about people with learning disabilities, about learning disability itself and about our relationships and social actions with people who are said to have learning disabilities. Michael Oliver (1990, 1995), who has been in the forefront of this movement, coined the phrases 'individual model' of disability and the 'social model of disability'.

The individual model of learning disability

The individual or personal tragedy or medical model of disability is closely aligned to the positivist framework which locates disability and learning disability within the individual with a learning impairment. Being considered a person with a learning disability makes the person 'in need' of care and under the control of professionals who intervene to help the person adjust to his or her environment. Here disability is considered as a personal tragedy for the person. Learning disability is an individual pathology that renders the person dependent and obliged to live his or her life according to society's expectations. Thus the person and his or her multiplicity of possible roles are given one all-encompassing role that serves to define his or her life. We have expectations about how the person who carries the label 'learning disabled' should behave and what he or she can reasonably expect.

This role includes being passive, being in need of care and guidance, being weak and vulnerable, being unable to benefit from inclusive education, not being capable of work, being odd in behaviour, manners, speech or dress among other things. The dominant discourse of learning disability has constructed the person with this identity as lacking many of the positive attributes of personhood. The person is primarily considered in negative ways; he or she lacks self-determination, has low self-esteem. Just using the rhetoric of learning disability/difficulty rather than 'intellectual disability' or 'mental handicap' has not prevented the person being discoursed as impaired, inadequate or deficient. When the disability movement speaks of the oppression of disabled people, it is referring to the social actions that accompany this discourse. Viewing a person as impaired, inadequate or deficient has serious consequences for both the perceiver and the perceived. One of the most serious consequences is that the knowledge of professionals is often derived from this personal tragedy or individual model of disability (Morris 1991, Oliver 1990).

The social model of learning disability

Here the main focus of understanding is about the ways that society disables the person with impairment. However, an impairment does not have to result in a disabled role for the person. Note that I am not denying that the intellectual impairment exists; I am however posing the question 'what is the consequence of this impairment for the person?' I am also proposing that these consequences have nothing to do with the nature of the intellectual impairment itself. A disability does not have to be the inevitable consequence of impairment. It has to do with the social, cultural, economic and political climate and how these lead to the exclusion, discrimination and stigmatisation of people who are said to have learning disabilities. It is difficult for services and the people who provide services to remove these barriers to an ordinary life for the person with a learning disability, since services are themselves part of these social, cultural, economic and political structures. This is possibly the main reason why professionals usually operate from the individual model of disability, which attempts to fix the individual's impairment.

Whereas the individual or medical model of disability is concerned with individuals' dependency, personal pathology and limitations, the social model is concerned with the interdependency of individuals and with the social creation of problems for people. Here it is not the person with a learning disability who has to adjust to his or her environment as it is the business of society to restructure its environment to make ordinary living possible. If you consider yourself an agent of society you will take on social actions that are radically different from those of an agent of people with learning disabilities.

Notions like independence need to be reconsidered. It is my view that nobody is independent. Humans are interdependent; we rely on each other. The social model of disability calls for a more critical understanding of how service workers are themselves dependent on people who need support. In a sense, both the professional and the disabled person has to relinquish their prescribed discourse of learning disability. When the professional is able to practise from this alternative discourse of learning disability, he or she will also understand how services can contribute to the continued oppression of people. This for me is the starting point of being and doing that can make common cause with people who are at risk of being made less, being turned into 'the other'. This change can only take place when people with learning disabilities acquire a central role in their own emancipation. The shift in focus has to be about what people can do rather than what they cannot do. We have to ask; what will it take for this person to do this or that, to be this or that person? The social model calls for new relationships between people; it calls for new skills.

Reader activity 1.4

Some disability activists and researchers have suggested that common understanding of the concept of care presents people with learning disabilities as passive and dependent so that the notion of care and empowerment and independence are contradictory.

This activity is aimed at enabling you to think about your work as 'caring'.

As a supporter of a person with learning disabilities, make a list of what you understand the word care to mean. It is important that you make a long list of at least 10 items: more is better.

Now look at your list and consider the items that refer to WORK and those that refer to EMOTIONS. Caring is physically and mentally demanding work, but is it care without the emotional bond between the carer and the cared for?

In what ways are you the paid worker and the person with learning disabilities you are working with interdependent? Make a list of what you depend on him/her for and what he/she depends on you for.

Conclusions

So far I have been trying to demonstrate that there are different paradigms of disability and how each paradigm makes different assumptions, leads to different models of disability and calls for different social practices towards disabled people. The social constructionist position is that these different models serve different purposes to different vested interests. All paradigms and their related modes serve some vested interests at the expense of one or more other vested interests. It is up to you to think critically about what kind of relationship you want to create in your work with people with learning disabilities. Are you going to make common cause with the people who depend on the services that you provide or are you going to make common cause with the people who provide services? This is not an easy thing to do. The organisation that employs you has power over both you and the people it serves.

I am not looking to any particular answer to these questions. I do however want to pose the question seriously enough. It is important to be critical and evaluative of the things that we take for granted. For example, we take it for granted that our profession or our practices serve the interest of people with learning disability. I am not sure that this is always the case. There are instances when professionals put the interest of their profession above the interests of the people they serve. We will consider this issue in greater detail in, for example, Chapters 7 (Advocacy) and 8 (Personal Narrative and Life Story) as empowerment. You have to decide on whose side you are on.

While social construction is essentially theoretical, that does not mean that it is simply a commodity for writing essays and for discussions. It allows you to ask questions about the actions that you take, the ideas that inform these actions. Social construction does not tell you how to do things; it makes you think about what you do does for people with learning disabilities and for yourself.

References

Arokiasamy, C., 1987. Cited in: Hershenson, D.B., 1992. Conception of disability: implications for rehabilitation. Rehabilitation Counseling Bulletin 35 (3), 154–160.

Aspie, S., 2001. Disability and the 1967 Abortion Act. RCM Midwives J. 4 (10), 338.

Atkinson, D., 2005. Research as social work: participatory research in learning disability. British Journal of Social Work 35 (4), 425–434.

Bagatell, N., 2010. From cure to community: transforming notions of autism. Ethos: Journal of the Society for Psychological Anthropology 38 (1), 33–55.

Berger, P., Luckman, T., 1967. The social construction of reality. Harmondsworth, Penguin.

Bettleheim, B., 1967. The empty fortress: infantile autism and the birth of the self. Free press, New York.

Brigham, L., Atkinson, D., Johnson, M. et al., (Eds.), 2001. Crossing boundaries: change and continuity in the history of learning disabilities. British Institute of Learning Disabilities, Kidderminster.

Brookes, M., Davis, S., 2008. Pathway to participatory research in developing a tool to measure feelings. Br. J. Learn. Disabilities 36 (2), 128–133.

Burr, V., 2003. Social constructionism, second ed. Routledge, Hove.

Connor, D.J., Ferri, B.A., 2007. The conflict within: resistance to inclusion and other paradoxes in special education. Disability & Society 22 (1), 63–77.

Dowling, M., 2006. Translating theory into practice? The implications for practitioners and users and carers. Practice 18 (1), 17–30.

Duckett, P.S., 2000. Disabling employment interviews: warfare to work. Disability and Society 15 (7), 1019–1039.

Foucault, M., 1973. The birth of the clinic: an archaeology of medical perception. Tavistock, London.

Foucault, M., 1991. Discipline and punish. Harmondsworth, Penguin.

Gergen, K.J., 1985. The social constructionist movement in modern psychology. Am. Psychol. 40, 266–275.

Gergen, K.J., 1990. Social understanding and the inscription of self. In: Sigler, J.W., Shweder, R.A., Herdt, G. (Eds.), Cultural psychology: essays on comparative human development. Cambridge University Press, New York, pp. 569–606.

Gould, S.J., 1996. The mismeasure of man. W W Norton, London.

Haffter, C., 1968. The changeling: history and psychodynamics of attitudes to handicapped children in European folklore. J. Hist. Behav. Sci. 4, 55–61.

Hartnett, E., Gallager, P., Kiernan, G., et al., 2008. Day service programme for people with severe intellectual disability and quality of life: parent and staff perspectives. J. Intellect. Disabil. 12 (2), 153–172.

Hehir, T., 2007. Confronting ableism. Educational Leadership 64 (5), 8–14.

McConkey, R., Walsh-Gallagher, D., Sinclair, M., 2005. Social inclusion of people with intellectual disabilities: the impact of place of residence. Irish Journal of Psychological Medicine 22 (1), 10–14.

Morris, J., 1991. Pride against prejudice: transforming attitudes to disability. The Women's Press, London.

Oliver, M., 1990. The politics of disablement. Macmillan, Basingstoke.

Oliver, M., 1995. Understanding disability: from theory to practice. Macmillan, Basingstoke.

Owen, K., Hubert, J., Hollins, S., 2008. Moving home: the experiences of women with severe intellectual disabilities in transition from a locked ward. Br. J. Learn. Disabilities 36 (4), 220–226.

Saleebey, D., 1992. The strengths perspective in social work practice. Longman, New York.

Saleebey, D., 1996. The strengths perspective in social work practice: extensions and cautions. Soc. Work 41, 296–305.

Shaw, S., 2009. Problems, problems: you are such a problem! J. Intellect. Disabil. 13 (2), 99–112.

Slee, R., 2008. Beyond special and regular schooling? An inclusive education reform agenda. International Studies in Sociology of Education 18 (2), 99–116.

Sooben, R.D., 2004. Valuing people with learning disabilities in the context of the Human Fertilisation and Embryology Act 1990: social policy and legislative incompatibility. J. Intellect. Disabil. 8 (2), 107–112.

Trent, J.W., 1994. Inventing the feeble minded: a history of mental retardation in the United States. University of California Press, Berkley.

Wilcox, E., Finlay, W.M., Edmonds, J., 2006. His brain is totally different: analysis of care-staff explanations of aggressive challenging behaviour and the impact of gendered discourse. Br. J. Soc. Psychol. 45, 197–215.

Wright, S.E., 1993. Blaming the victim, blaming society, or blaming the discipline: fixing responsibility for poverty and homelessness. The Sociology Quarterly 34 (1), 1–16.

Further reading

Anyon, Y., 2009. Sociological theories of learning disability: understanding racial disproportionality in special education. Journal of Human Behavior in the Social Environment 19 (1), 44–57.

Burton, M., Sanderson, H., 1998. Paradigms in intellectual disability: compared, contrasted, combined. J. Appl. Res. Intellect. Disabil. 11 (10), 44–59.

Gergen, K.J., 2009. An invitation to social construction, second ed. Sage, Thousand Oaks.

Woodhill, G., 1994. The social semiotics of disability. In: Rioux, M.H., Bach, M. (Eds.), Disability is not measles: new research paradigm in disability. Roher Institute, Ontario.

Useful addresses

Understanding Intellectual Disability & Health, http://www.intellectualdisability.info/.

The Taos Institute, http://www.taosinstitute.net/.

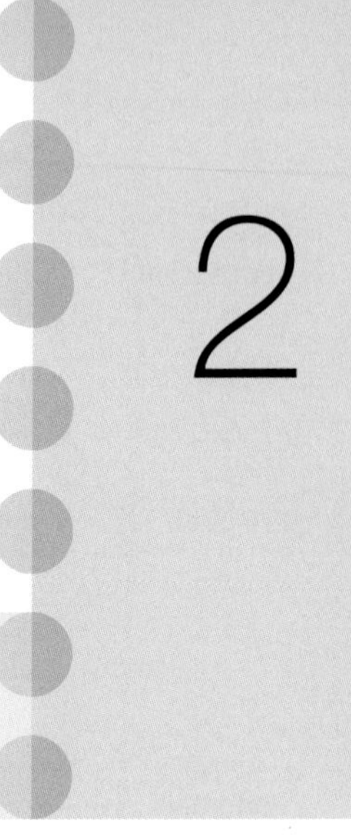

Causes of learning disability

Debbie Watson

CHAPTER CONTENTS

KEY ISSUES

- The term learning disability could be described as an umbrella term under which all affected individuals are described as having varying degrees of impairment of intellectual and social functioning
- There are numerous environmental and genetic factors that may contribute towards the person being described as having a learning disability
- There are four distinct time periods when environmental or genetic factors are more prevalent: preconceptual, prenatal, perinatal and postnatal
- There are a number of screening and diagnostic tests that can contribute towards a diagnosis of learning disabilities

Introduction

In the previous chapter there has been a comprehensive exploration of the concept of learning disability and what it means for individuals who are labelled or described as having a learning disability. This chapter will attempt to further clarify our understanding by identifying why it is important to have an awareness of the major causes of learning disabilities and the methods that are used within the diagnostic process.

The causes of learning disabilities are many and diverse and it is this diversity that can make it difficult when attempting to make a diagnosis during

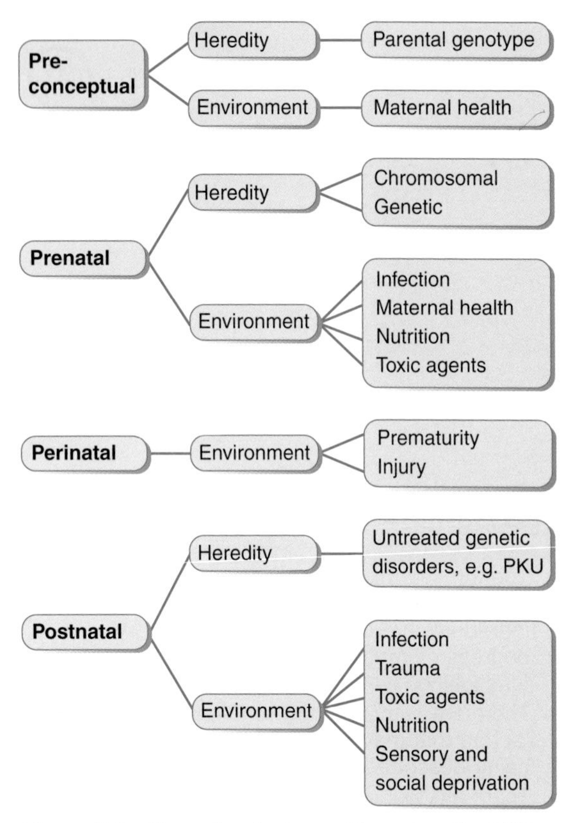

Figure 2.1 • Causative factors of learning disabilities by time

the different stages of the developmental process (Fig. 2.1). Since the beginning of history, assumptions have been made about the causation of learning disabilities: for example, in medieval times many people believed that learning disabilities were the result of supernatural forces (Stratford 1996). In the 1700s, the American psychologist Henry H Goddard postulated that 'feeble-mindedness' was caused by a single recessive gene. Goddard's work also contributed towards the rising eugenics movement and the Darwinian Theory and belief in natural selection and the deterioration of intelligence. More recently, our understanding of the human genome has increased giving rise to a developing understanding of some of the genetic causes of learning disabilities.

So why is it important to identify the causes of learning disabilities and how will it benefit the individual? In the first instance, having an idea of what caused or contributed towards the learning disability could help parents and carers when they are trying to come to terms with the initial diagnosis. Having an understanding also allows carers and professionals to develop, in partnership with individuals, appropriate person-centred care that takes into consideration any specific health-related issues that may impact upon the individual's daily and future life. However, it must be emphasised that labelling someone with a particular condition can have a negative effect. Simply slotting people into categories that inform treatment or aid prognosis should be avoided if we are truly to work with people in an individual and holistic manner. As human beings it is important that we should all treat one another as unique.

It is difficult to estimate the precise number of people who have learning disabilities, however it has been recognised that numbers are set to rise as individuals are living longer due to advances and support in health and social care and more children and young people with complex and multiple disabilities are surviving into adulthood (Department of Health (DH) 2001, 2007, Emerson 2009). An understanding of the potential causes and presentations of learning disabilities is essential for professionals who wish to work holistically with such individuals.

The preconceptual period is an important period of time in which prospective parents can prepare themselves for the conception of a child. This may involve looking at the general health status of both parents or considering any genetic issues.

The prenatal period is the 38–40 week period of time from conception to birth. During this time there are a number of causal factors of learning disabilities including genetic conditions, maternal infections and other environmental issues. This is also the time period when a number of diagnostic tests are carried out to monitor the health and wellbeing of both the mother and the developing child.

The perinatal period of time includes the events surrounding the birth and up to the first 7 days of life (Fraser & Cooper 2009). Learning disabilities can occur during this period due to prematurity of the baby (between 20 and 37 weeks' gestation) or difficult or prolonged labour resulting in lack of oxygen and pressure on the brain and central nervous system.

The postnatal period is the period following the birth when routine screening is carried out. For example, in the first week after birth, newborn blood spot screening, also known as the Guthrie test, can identify metabolic disorders such as phenylketonuria (PKU) and congenital hypothyroidism (National Health Service (NHS) 2007; see later section on newborn blood screening). However, some learning disabilities may only become apparent when the child displays delayed development or is subject to accidents and infections as they grow (more information can be found in Ch. 23).

Before we look in more detail at the different time periods, we should explore the concept of genetics and genetic counselling.

Genetics and inheritance

Variation between individuals is a biological rule, resulting in the variety of the human species. Genetics could be described as the branch of science that is concerned with the study of heredity, that is the passing on of characteristics from parents to offspring (a glossary of terms can be found at the end of the chapter).

Every human being originates as the result of the union of two gametes, one from each parent, the ovum (female) and the sperm (male). The genetic information from the union results in a unique genotype or 'blueprint' for the growth and development of the embryo. The resultant individual will have their own phenotype with observable traits, such as height, eye colour and blood type.

Chromosomes

Each human cell contains 23 pairs of chromosomes (46 chromosomes), each pair consisting of one chromosome from each parent. During mitosis the cell replicates, ensuring that the same chromosomal pattern is achieved in each new daughter cell. The exception to this is in the gametes where, as a result of meiosis, only one set of 23 chromosomes, one from each original pair, is represented. These will join to make up 23 pairs of chromosomes in the newly formed embryo.

Every chromosome is divided into loci, which contain the particular gene substance that determines the individual's inherited characteristics. Dutton (1975) has likened the relationship between chromosomes and genes to that of a string of beads, with the string being the chromosome and the individual beads representing genes.

Of the 23 pairs of chromosomes, pairs 1–22 can be matched and are described as autosomes. Pair 23 is known as the sex chromosomes. In the female these are matched and referred to as XX. In the male they are not matched and are referred to as XY.

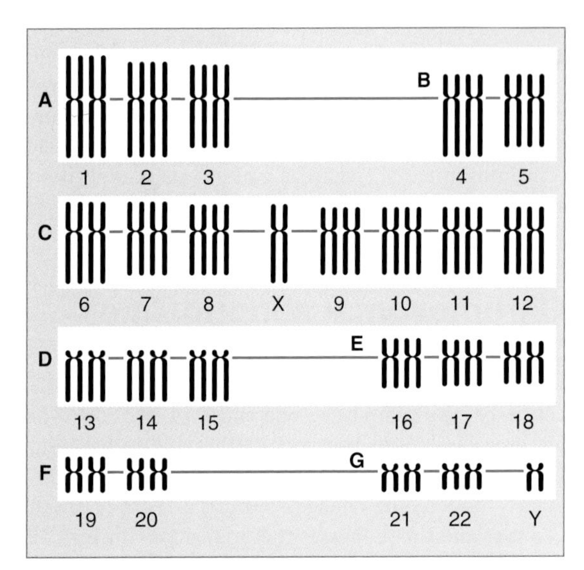

Figure 2.2 • Chromosomes of the human male

The chromosomes are numbered from 1 to 23 according to the Denver system, with the largest pair being number 1 and the smallest being number 22 (Fig. 2.2). Another method of organising chromosomes is to place them in one of seven groups labelled A–G according to size and shape. This enables the description of normal and abnormal karyotypes.

Genes

The human genome contains about 20 000–25 000 genes (Turnpenny & Ellard 2007). Genes are the units of heredity; they reside upon the chromosome and are responsible for many different phenotypical traits, such as hair and eye colour. Like chromosomes they are matched (for the most part), and matched genes that are on the same area or locus of matched chromosomes are called alleles. Therefore, when an individual inherits from each parent the same allelic form of a particular gene, they are described as homozygous for that gene locus. However, if different alleles are present, they are described as heterozygous. When a particular allele present in the heterozygote gives rise to an obvious physical characteristic, it is described as dominant. However, if the particular characteristic only appears in individuals when they are homozygous for the gene, it is described as recessive.

The individual's hereditary characteristics may be described as chromosomal if they can be linked to one or more of the 23 pairs of identified chromosomes, and genetic if they are determined by one or more of the genes that reside upon those chromosomes. For example, an individual's sex is determined by a chromosomal hereditary characteristic (chromosome 23), whereas eye colour is identified as being caused by one or more genes and is referred to as genetic.

Chromosomal abnormalities

Chromosomal abnormalities are estimated to be the cause of approximately one-third of the 50% of learning disabilities that are attributable to heredity (Mueller & Young 2001). However, this figure is constantly undergoing change as more is learned about genetics and the processes that may occur during cell development and division. An example of this can be seen in research conducted by Knight et al (1999) who identified that subtle chromosomal rearrangements were present in children with previously unexplained moderate to severe learning disabilities.

Autosomal

The incidence of autosomal abnormalities has been calculated and is reproduced in Table 2.1.

Autosomal abnormalities may be subdivided into three main categories:

1. Abnormality of number. Here there may be a loss (or more commonly a gain) of one or more chromosomes, for example Down syndrome, or trisomy 21, where there is an extra chromosome in pair 21, or Edwards' syndrome, which has an extra chromosome present in pair 18, or Patau's syndrome, which has an extra chromosome present in pair 13.
2. Abnormality of structure. Here there may be a loss of part of a chromosome (deletion) or a rearrangement (translocation) of the chromosomal material. For example, Cri-du-chat syndrome results from deletion of the short arm of chromosome 5. In translocation Down syndrome, an extra segment of a chromosome may have been rearranged and attached to one of the following pairs: 13, 15, 21 or 22.
3. Mosaicism. Here individuals have cells containing different numbers of chromosomes. This may occur as a result of non-disjunction, or the accidental loss of a particular chromosome, usually during the first few cell divisions following fertilisation. Mosaicisms for autosomes do occur, but are encountered more frequently on sex chromosomes. Examples of mosaicism can occur in people with Down syndrome and Klinefelter syndrome.

Table 2.2 summarises these manifestations of chromosomal abnormalities.

Table 2.1 Incidence of autosomal abnormalities in the newborn

Abnormality	Incidence per 10 000 births
Trisomy 13	2
Trisomy 18	3
Trisomy 21	15

(Turnpenny & Ellard 2007)

Sex chromosomal

As with autosomes, additions and deletions to the sex chromosomes may occur. Primary non-disjunction, if it occurs during the formation of the ova or the spermatozoa, gives rise to a gamete with an extra X or Y chromosome. Sex chromosome abnormalities can be divided into four main conditions:

XO: Turner syndrome.

XXX: Triple X syndrome.

XXY: Klinefelter syndrome.

XYY: syndrome.

The incidence of sex chromosome abnormalities in the newborn has been calculated and is reproduced in Table 2.3.

Gene abnormalities

It may be helpful to group abnormalities of the genes as autosomal dominant (Fig. 2.3), autosomal recessive (Fig. 2.4), sex-linked (Fig 2.5) and polygenetic.

Autosomal dominant inheritance

There are at least 1000 human traits that are known to have their genetic basis in dominant genes located on autosomes. Dimples and freckles are two examples of

Table 2.2 Manifestations of chromosomal abnormalities

Condition/syndrome	Affected chromosome	Physical manifestation of condition/syndrome
Down syndrome	Extra chromosome on pair 21 (trisomy 21). There are three types of the syndrome: • Abnormality of the number of chromosomes. • Abnormality of the structure of the chromosome. • Mosaicism.	There are a large number of characteristics associated with Down syndrome. with the most common being the following: • Muscle tone: reduced muscle tone in the newborn (hypotonia). • Facial features: small, round head (brachycephalic). Hair has a tendency to be dry and very fine with possible focal alopecia in adulthood. Flat face, with small ears. The eyes are usually upward- and outward-slanting, often with an epicanthic fold on the inner aspect of the upper eyelid. Eye conditions such as cataract, strabismus and nystagmus are common. Due to a lack of the enzyme lysozyme in tears which acts as an antibiotic, conjunctivitis and blepharitis are common. Brushfield spots (white flecks) can be found throughout the iris. The mouth is often small with a high narrow palate. The tongue is large with distinctive horizontal fissures on the surface. As a result of this particular anatomy, the mouth tends to be held open with the tongue protruding. There is delayed development of the teeth, with an abnormality in their size, shape and alignment. Mouth breathing increases the risk of respiratory tract infections. • Limbs are relatively short, making the adult height relatively short. • Hands and feet are distinctive, with the hands having a square palm with palmar crease, and a wide gap between the thumb and second finger. Fingers are short and stubby. Toes are shorter than average and there may be a wide gap between the big toe and the second toe. • Genitalia in the male may be underdeveloped and there may be reduced fertility. (Turnpenny & Ellard 2007, Contact a Family 2010a.) See Box 2.1 for more information or visit the Down Syndrome Association website (address at the end of the chapter) for information and positive real-life stories.
Edwards' syndrome	Extra chromosome on pair 18 (trisomy 18). There are three types of the syndrome: • Full form (severe) – in this, every cell in the body has three chromosome 18s instead of two. • Mosaic form (less severe) – in this, some cells have two chromosome 18s while others have three. • Partial form – in some cases, there may be an extra copy of part of chromosome 18. This is referred to as partial trisomy 18. The effects of this may be milder and would require further medical advice (Turnpenny & Ellard 2007, Contact a Family 2010b).	Characteristics and physical manifestations include the following: • Children with all their cells affected do not normally survive beyond infancy. Those affected by the mosaic and partial forms may survive to adulthood. • Features include growth deficiency, low-set and malformed ears, clenched hands, bone abnormalities, hernias, skin mottling, heart defects, feeding and breathing problems in infancy and learning disability (Turnpenny & Ellard 2007, Contact a Family 2010b).

Continued

Table 2.2 Manifestations of chromosomal abnormalities—cont'd

Condition/syndrome	Affected chromosome	Physical manifestation of condition/syndrome
Patou's syndrome	Extra chromosome on pair 13.	Characteristics and physical manifestations include the following: • Babies are of low birth weight • Facial features include scalp defects, structural eye defects, low-set ears, cleft lip and/or palate. • There are extra digits, overlapping of fingers over thumb and abnormal palmar crease patterns. • There are heart defects, meningomyelocele (a spinal defect), omphalocele (abdominal defect) and abnormal genitalia. • Between 80% and 90% of babies do not survive infancy, and in those that do survive, learning disability is present. (Turnpenny & Ellard 2007, Contact a Family 2010c.)
Cri-du-chat	Deletion of the short arm of chromosome 5.	Characteristics and physical manifestations include the following: • The condition is characterised by a distinctive high-pitched cat cry, believed to be caused by the underdevelopment of the larynx. • Babies tend to be of low birth weight and show marked hypotonia. Feeding difficulties are common and the associated failure to thrive may be the initial clinical presentation. Some infants may require enteral feeding • Facial and head abnormalities include microcephaly, rounded face, hypertelorism (wide space between the eyes), low-set ears, broad nasal ridge and short neck. (Turnpenny & Ellard 2007, Contact a Family 2010d).

Table 2.3 Incidence of sex chromosome abnormalities in the newborn

	Abnormality	Incidence per 10 000 births
Female births	45, XO (Turner syndrome)	1–2
	47, XXX (Triple X syndrome)	10
Male births	47, XXY (Klinefelter syndrome)	10
	47, XYY (XYY syndrome)	10

(Turnpenny & Ellard 2007)

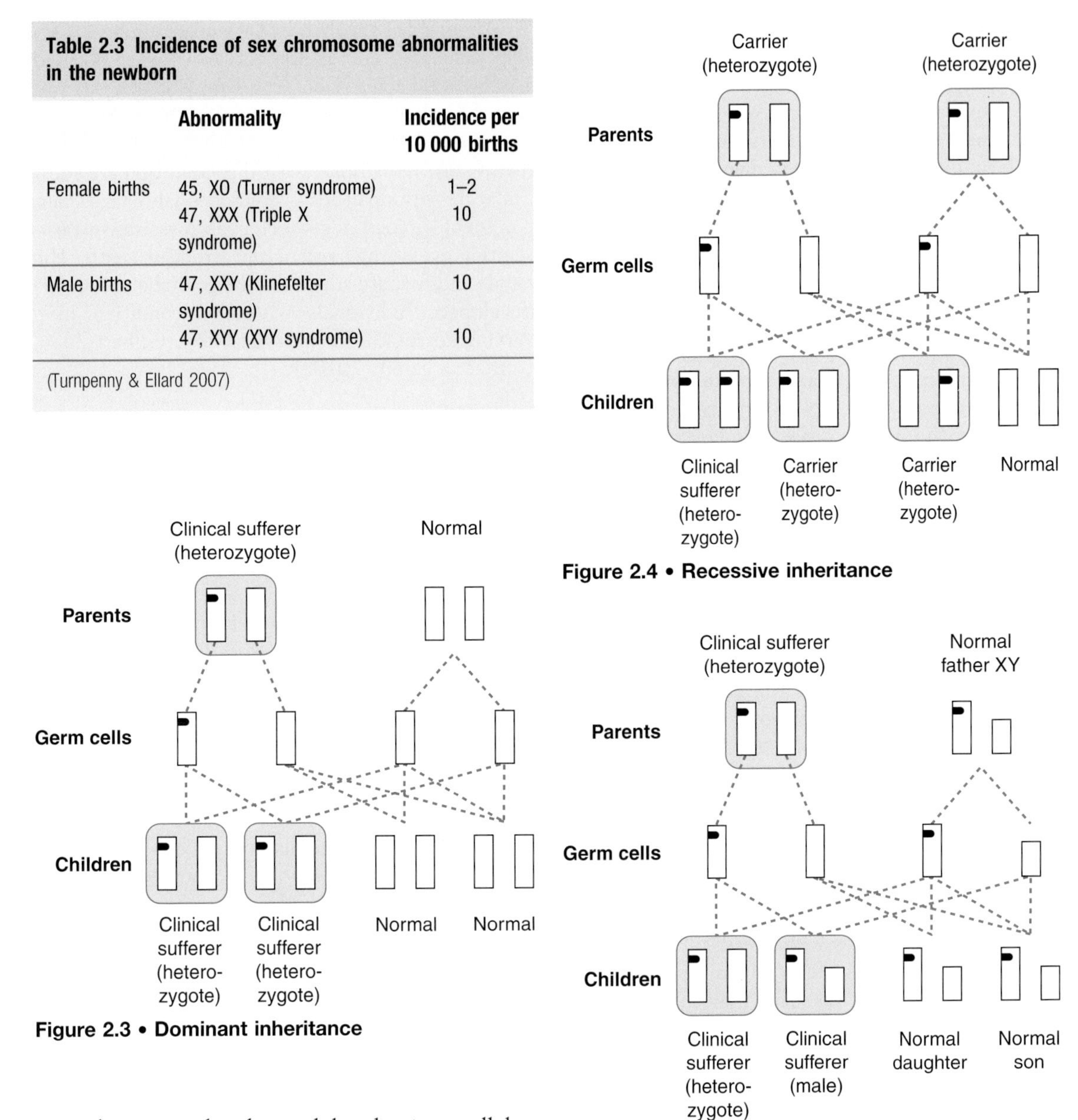

Figure 2.3 • Dominant inheritance

Figure 2.4 • Recessive inheritance

Figure 2.5 • Sex-linked inheritance

traits known to be dictated by dominant alleles. Genetic disorders caused by dominant genes are fairly uncommon as lethal dominant genes are almost always expressed, resulting in the death of the developing embryo, fetus or child. There are, however, some conditions that are less severe, allowing the affected individual enough time to reproduce and pass on the affected gene. Tuberous sclerosis, for example, causes growths in different organs of the body (brain, heart, eyes, skin, kidneys, lungs) and individuals may have epilepsy, learning disabilities, autism spectrum conditions and kidney problems (Tuberous Sclerosis Association 2010).

Autosomal recessive inheritance

There are at least 600 human traits that are known to have an autosomal recessive pattern of inheritance. Many genetic disorders are inherited as simple recessive traits, for example phenylketonuria and Tay–Sachs disease. To be affected, individuals must receive the gene for a particular condition from both parents. Carriers of disorders do not express the disease themselves, but can pass it on to their offspring. Children from consanguineous relationships (between close relatives, such as siblings and first cousins) have a greater chance of inheriting two identical recessive genes and thus expressing the disease. Advice from a genetic counselling service may be of use for relatives of people with genetic disorders, enabling them to discuss the chances of their being a carrier, or of having an affected child.

Sex-linked inheritance

The Y chromosome, which contains the genes for determining maleness, is only one-third the size of the X chromosome and lacks many of the genes present on the X that code for non-sexual characteristics. For example, the gene involved in the production of certain blood clotting factors is only found on the X chromosome. Genes found only on the X chromosome are described as being X-linked. Haemophilia is a classic example of a sex-linked disorder. If a male inherits an X-linked recessive allele (from his mother), its expression is not masked because there is no corresponding allele on his Y chromosome (inherited from his father), which results in the recessive gene being expressed. In contrast, a female must have two X-linked recessive alleles to express the disease.

An example of an X-linked recessive condition is Hunter syndrome. Hunter syndrome is one of the mucopolysaccharide diseases and is also known as MPS Type II. Hunter disease takes its name from Professor Charles Hunter in Canada, who first described two brothers with the disorder in 1917. The incompletely broken down mucopolysaccharides (long chains of sugar molecules that are found throughout the body, often in mucus and in fluid around the joints) remain stored in cells in the body causing progressive damage. Babies may show little sign of the disease but, as more and more cells become damaged, symptoms including learning disabilities start to appear (The Irish Society for Mucopolysaccharide Diseases 2010).

Polygenetic inheritance

Polygenetic inheritance occurs when a number of genes act together, causing complex traits. The estimated risk of inheritance is much less than in single gene inheritance, but the risk does increase with the number of first-degree relatives who have the condition.

Cornelia de Lange syndrome is an example of polygenic inheritance. It affects between 1 in 15 000 and 1 in 50 000 babies (Contact a Family 2010e). It was first described in 1933 by the Dutch paediatrician Cornelia de Lange (it is also known as Amsterdam dwarfism). Individuals with this condition are short in stature with small heads (microcephaly), facial hair, confluent (joined together) eyebrows, downward-slanting eyes, small palate and irregular teeth. The hands and feet are small and the genitalia are underdeveloped. Individuals with this condition have varying degrees of learning disability (Gilbert 2000, Contact a Family 2010e).

Genetic counselling

Genetic counselling and screening has developed significantly within recent times. The first British clinic was set up in 1946 at Great Ormond Street Hospital, London. The aim of genetic counselling is to support the individual or family and give accurate information about the specific condition they have or may develop and to consider the potential risk of passing the condition on to any children.

For the majority of individuals who are planning a pregnancy, genetic counselling is not necessary, however if either parent has a history of an inherited disease or birth defect within their family or if there is a history of previous miscarriages or children that have died in infancy, then genetic counselling may be recommended.

The process of genetic counselling begins with a diagnosis. This is based on the collection of information, taking a full medical history of the individual and their family. An examination of the genetic material and any existing medical conditions comes next. This information is then examined to confirm or refute the diagnosis. This process needs to be undertaken in a sensitive and supportive manner that allows the individual(s) to understand what they have been told about the condition and its associated risks and to reach an informed decision about any subsequent courses of action.

One of the most recent scientific developments that has increased our knowledge and understanding to support genetic counselling is The Human Genome Project. This was an international collaboration undertaken between 1990 and 2003 and involved thousands of scientists worldwide undertaking the task of sequencing the 3 billion bases of genetic information that reside in every human cell.

This information has given us a greater understanding of a range of genetic conditions and diseases.

As we have previously seen, genetic counselling may be appropriate for some individuals to help them establish the level of risk involved in passing on a genetic condition to their children. Communication is a key element within this process and the counsellor's role is to provide support and information necessary for the individual(s) to make their own informed decision about the options and choices open to them.

Turnpenny & Ellard (2007), when talking about the process of genetic counselling, suggest the following key principles are adhered to:

- The counsellor adopts a non-directive approach.
- The problem and its implications are diagnosed in relation to a prognosis and possible treatment.
- The mode of inheritance and the risk of developing or transmitting the disorder are identified.
- There is discussion around the available options and choices.
- Support is offered so that fully informed decisions can be made.

It is at this point that support groups may be of assistance allowing the person(s) to hear the experiences of others who are in a similar position (a list of useful addresses can be found at the end of the chapter).

Environmental and genetic causes of learning disability by time

Preconceptual

There are numerous environmental factors (e.g. physical health, existing medical conditions, lifestyle) that should be considered prior to conception, however pregnancies are often unplanned and the opportunity to prepare is missed (Barrowclough 2009, DH 2004a, Korenbrot et al 2002). There are numerous organisations that now offer preconceptual care and advice, such as the organisation Foresight and The Association for the Promotion of Pre-Conceptual Care. They produce a range of information for men and women prior to conception. More information can be found at their Internet website, details of which can be found at the end of this chapter.

Pre-existing medical disorders should be considered as they may have an adverse effect upon the mother and fetus and require monitoring prior to conception (Barrowclough 2009). For example, a woman who was treated for phenylketonuria as a child but has now ceased her low phenylalanine diet would have high levels of phenylalanine during pregnancy. These high levels of phenylalanine are associated with abortion, intrauterine growth retardation, congenital heart defects, microcephaly and learning disabilities; returning to a low phenylalanine diet would reduce the levels of phenylalanine during pregnancy (Koch et al 2003, Rouse et al 2000).

Nutrition is important at any stage in the lifecycle, and any nutritional deficiencies may take many months to correct. Prospective parents should be encouraged to maintain a healthy balanced diet, not only during pregnancy but also in preparation for conception. Children conceived during periods of poor nutrition, such as in Holland in the 'Hunger Winter' (October 1944 to May 1945), were found to have a high perinatal mortality rate. In those infants who survived, there was found to be an increased incidence of congenital malformation. In addition to a healthy diet, vitamin supplements such as folic acid (a water-soluble vitamin belonging to the B complex) are advised prior to conception and up until the 12th week of pregnancy, to aid in the prevention of neural tube defects (DH 2004a). Foods naturally rich in folic acid include dark green vegetables, potatoes, fruit and fruit juices, beans and yeast extract. Foods such as bread and breakfast cereal can also be fortified with folic acid which is easier for the body to absorb. In some countries (USA, Canada and South Africa) there has been a reported reduction in the number of children born with neural tube defects since the introduction of mandatory fortification of foods with folic acid (Bille et al 2007).

Other lifestyle factors such as smoking, alcohol and drug use are all issues that need to be considered prior to conception. Smoking in itself may not be a direct cause of learning disability, however it can affect fertility in both the male and female making it more difficult to become pregnant. Smoking also increases the risk of having a low birth weight baby

> **Reader activity 2.1**
>
> There are genetic advisory services throughout the United Kingdom. Do you know where your local service is and the type of services they offer?

or a baby with fetal malformations. The National Institute for Clinical Excellence (NICE 2008) recommends that smoking cessation interventions are offered as part of antenatal care.

Prenatal

Heredity and environmental screening

As previously mentioned, there are a number of known conditions caused by genetic factors operating during the developmental cycle. Mothers falling into high-risk categories by virtue of age or known family incidence that have not considered or received preconceptual care and advice should be offered support, counselling and access to appropriate diagnostic tests, such as amniocentesis and chorionic villus sampling, should they require them (such tests are discussed more fully in the next section).

There are also numerous environmental influences that may affect the mother and the unborn child. Appropriate health education and antenatal care may go a long way in ensuring a greater understanding of the potential risk factors.

The NHS in the UK has an antenatal and newborn screening programme (NHS 2007) that considers both genetic and environmental risk factors and it is offered to all pregnant women and newborn children. Women are encouraged to participate within the screening programme, however it is not mandatory. Information regarding the screening needs to be given so that the woman can make an informed choice regarding participation and any decisions that may need to be taken as a result of screening.

A number of the screening tests offered may help predict the possibility of having a child with learning disabilities.

Screening blood test for infectious diseases

This blood test is one of the first tests carried out when pregnancy is confirmed but it can be undertaken at any time during the pregnancy. In addition to syphilis and screening for rubella antibodies, the test also looks for hepatitis B and HIV.

Rubella antibodies help to protect the child against rubella (German measles) if the woman becomes infected during pregnancy. If there are no antibodies, the mumps, measles and rubella (MMR) vaccine will be offered to the woman once the baby has been born. This will protect future pregnancies. If rubella (an airborne virus) is contracted during the first 12 weeks of pregnancy and the mother does not have rubella antibodies, the child has a very high risk of becoming infected and developing congenital rubella syndrome (CRS). If rubella is contracted within the first 3 months of the pregnancy, it can cause damage in 90% of unborn babies, including heart, eye and hearing problems as well as learning disabilities (NHS Choices 2010, Nurse 2009).

Syphilis (a sexually transmitted disease) is fortunately less common today than it was in the past, however it can seriously complicate pregnancy. Improvements in general health education, antenatal care and the use of antibiotics have reduced the number of cases. If syphilis is undetected within the mother and passed onto the child, the child will fail to thrive and develop physically resulting in growth restriction (Medforth et al 2006). Other physical characteristics may include a saddleback nose, peg-shaped teeth, and opacities of the cornea, strabismus and nystagmus (see Ch. 15). The central nervous system is affected to various degrees and epilepsy may also be present. Antibiotics will treat both the mother and the fetus during the pregnancy. Following the birth, the child will be given antibiotics to ensure that they are free of the infection.

Screening for blood group and Rhesus antibodies

Again, this is one of the first tests carried out once the pregnancy has been confirmed. Blood typing, including Rhesus (Rh) factor, is investigated to detect possible blood type incompatibilities. Rhesus factor incompatibility (kernicterus) occurs when a rhesus-negative mother is carrying a fetus that is rhesus positive (inherited from the father). The first child is usually unaffected, but in subsequent pregnancies the number of maternal antibodies increases. The antibodies then pass through the placental barrier and destroy the rhesus-positive blood of the fetus. An exchange transfusion can be given in utero if the blood is being destroyed, or immediately following the birth. At birth, an affected child will be jaundiced, and if no action is taken brain damage will occur. Anti-D gamma globulin, if administered by injection to the rhesus-negative woman within 48 hours of the delivery of the first child, will prevent the formation of the dangerous antibodies.

Early blood test for Down syndrome

In the UK, all pregnant women are now offered the test for Down syndrome (NHS 2007) undertaken at 10–14 weeks. In the UK, the incidence of Down syndrome is approximately 1 in 1000 with approximately 60% of all cases detected prenatally (Turnpenny & Ellard 2007).

Nuchal translucency ultrasound scan

This ultrasound test undertaken at 11–13 weeks measures the thickness of the fluid that gathers at the back of the fetal neck. Thickening of the fluid may indicate that there are chromosomal abnormalities and genetic disorders. This information would then be considered along with other risk factors such as the early blood test and the mother's age to help identify the risk of Down syndrome (Sullivan & Kirk 2009). Anyone can have a baby with Down syndrome, however the risk increases with maternal age. For example, the chance of having a child at the age of 20 is 1 in 1500, at the age of 30 it rises to 1 in 900 and at age 40 it is 1 in 100 (NHS 2007, Turnpenny & Ellard 2007).

Both the early blood test and Nuchal translucency ultrasound scan are screening tests and as such only offer an approximate risk; they cannot confirm that the child has Down syndrome. It is at this stage that the parent(s) should be offered impartial and comprehensive information to help them consider the available options: have no further tests and carry on with the pregnancy; have further screening to further assess the risk of having a child with Down syndrome; have a diagnostic test that carries a risk of miscarriage such as amniocentesis or chorionic villus sampling; or consider a termination.

Combined screening for Down syndrome

This integrated test consists of the early blood results, a late blood test taken at 15–20 weeks and a nuchal translucency ultrasound scan. A computer program then uses the information to calculate the risk of having a child with Down syndrome. If the estimated risk is high then a diagnostic test that can identify if the child has Down syndrome would be offered (see Box 2.1).

Box 2.1

Down syndrome

Down syndrome is often referred to as the best-known chromosomal abnormality. It was first described in 1866 by Dr Langdon Down, from whom the name is derived, however the chromosomal basis of Down syndrome was not established until 1959, when Lejeune and colleagues discovered that people with Down syndrome have 47 chromosomes, the extra chromosome residing with autosome 21 (trisomy 21). The incidence of Down syndrome is 1 in 1000 births and in the UK approximately 600 babies are born each year with Down syndrome (Down's Syndrome Association 2010).

There are a number of physical characteristics associated with Down syndrome (see Table 2.2), however it must be emphasised that not all babies and children will exhibit all of the characteristics and each child must be treated as a unique individual.

Prenatal screening may have prepared the parents and the extended family for the arrival of their child with Down syndrome, however if screening was declined or did not happen then the physical characteristics present at birth can help with a preliminary diagnosis. This would then be followed by a chromosome test that would confirm or refute the initial diagnosis.
It is important that any information given to parents is given in a sensitive and supportive manner that encourages the parent–child bonding process and reduces anxiety.

There are a number of medical conditions that are more common in people with Down syndrome:

- 40–50% of babies with Down syndrome are born with heart problems, half of which require heart surgery.
- A significant number of people with Down syndrome will have hearing and sight problems.
- Thyroid disorder.
- Poor immune system.
- Respiratory problems.
- Obstructed gastrointestinal tract.
- There is a risk of developing dementia and, in particular, Alzheimer's disease.

Again, not everyone with Down syndrome will have or develop the medical conditions identified above. As with the rest of the population, lifestyle, including diet, exercise and environment, impact upon our health and wellbeing. What is important is that we have an understanding of the potential health and social care needs for the individual across the lifespan. Person-centred planning and health action planning are two important tools that can assist the individual in achieving the lifestyle that they want. By having an understanding of the potential medical conditions that the person has or may develop, action can be taken to avoid the condition or reduce the impact it may have. For example, knowing that people with Down syndrome may have hearing and sight problems should prompt regular planned screening appointments to monitor any changes and provide glasses or hearing aids if they are required.

Detailed ultrasound scan to detect any fetal anomalies

The purpose of this scan undertaken at 18–21 weeks is to look for any fetal abnormalities, for example spina bifida (a series of birth defects that affect the development of the spine and nervous system), hydrocephalus and microcephaly. Hydrocephalus arises from a blockage of cerebrospinal fluid (CSF) in the ventricular spaces within the brain. It can be treated with the insertion of a ventriculoperitoneal shunt that drains the fluid from the ventricles of the brain into the abdominal cavity, relieving pressure inside the skull. The shunt will need to be monitored for blockages and replaced as the child grows. If the condition is left untreated or the shunt becomes blocked then the pressure can cause damage and impairment of intellectual functioning and, in severe cases, death (Nurse 2009, Turner & Simpson 2009). Microcephaly is where the head is below normal size. The small head may be the result of an infection such as rubella during pregnancy, fetal alcohol syndrome or part of a chromosomal abnormality. Most babies will have learning disabilities (Turner & Simpson 2009).

Diagnostic tests

Chorionic villus sampling and amniocentesis will be offered if a high risk has been identified following screening. Both tests will be able to confirm if the child has Down syndrome, however they both have a risk of miscarriage following the procedure. For chorionic villus sampling, it is estimated that for every 100 women who have the procedure, 1 or 2 will miscarry; for every 100 women who have the amniocentesis, 1 will miscarry (NHS 2007).

Chorionic villus sampling

This can be undertaken from as early as week 11 of the pregnancy. In the procedure, an ultrasound scanner is used to guide a fine needle through the abdomen or vagina into the placenta to obtain a tissue sample. The cells obtained from the sample are fetal, not maternal, therefore they can be analysed to obtain a complete genetic picture of the fetus (Nurse 2009).

Amniocentesis

This can be undertaken from week 16 of the pregnancy. The procedure commences with an ultrasound scan to check the position of the baby. A fine needle is then inserted through the abdomen into the womb where a sample of amniotic fluid can be taken. The fluid can then be examined to confirm or refute the diagnosis.

Cordocentesis

This can be undertaken from week 18 of the pregnancy. A sample of fetal blood is taken by inserting a fine needle into the fetal umbilical cord. The test can be undertaken to confirm fetal infection, mosaicism, single gene disorders and Fragile X (Evans 2008).

Fragile X is the most common known cause of inherited learning disabilities (Fragile X Society 2010). The term derives from the unusual appearance at the end of the long arm of the X chromosome, which shows a fragile site. The degree of learning disability varies from severe to borderline (Gilbert 2000).

Whichever screening or diagnostic test is offered, information must be given using a non-directive supportive approach allowing the parent(s) to reach fully informed decisions about the options, choices and possible consequences (Turnpenny & Ellard 2007). There are many legal and ethical questions about the use of genetic testing that are now being raised by people with learning disabilities. Groups such as Inclusion International are raising questions about the implications of the developments in genetic understanding and in particular about the eugenic overtones that are associated with prenatal testing. Predictive tests, such as amniocentesis and chorionic villus sampling, may have severe implications for the individual and the family, therefore, as previously stated, the rationale for undertaking predictive tests should be clearly identified and discussed outlining all possible outcomes and not merely as a method of predicting abortion.

Maternal health during pregnancy

Maternal nutrition and health are known to be linked to fetal development. The supply of essential nutrients and oxygen to the fetus is totally dependent upon the mother, and any interruption of this process will affect the fetus. Good health for the pregnant mother should be thought of in the widest possible context, both on a physical and a psychological level, to maximise the development of a healthy pregnancy.

Infections

As we have already seen, there are a number of maternal infections that can, if contracted during pregnancy, cause problems for the developing fetus, for example rubella. In addition to the infections that can be screened for, there are a number of other infections that, if contracted especially during the first few months of pregnancy, may result in a learning disability. These include cytomegalovirus, varicella-zoster (chicken pox) and toxoplasmosis.

Cytomegalovirus is a 'large cell virus' belonging to the herpes family. It is a common infection that usually has brief, flu-like or no symptoms. Without realising it, by middle age most people will have been infected. The most frequent times for contracting the virus are in early childhood and between 20 and 35 years. It is estimated that 4 out of every 1000 women who are pregnant become infected and approximately half pass on the virus to the fetus, resulting in 10% of the infected babies having malformations (Gilbert 2000, Griffiths 2001) The principal malformations seen in cytomegalovirus are microcephaly, deafness, blindness and learning disabilities (Sadler 2010).

Toxoplasmosis is caused by the parasite *Toxoplasma gondii*, which is found in raw meat and cat faeces. If it is contracted during pregnancy, it can lead to fetal infection resulting in a range of problems for the child including, blindness, deafness, epilepsy and learning disabilities (Medforth et al 2006).

Toxic agents

There are a number of known toxic agents that can injure the developing fetus in some way. Smoking, alcohol, drugs and environmental pollutants have all been identified as associated factors in the causation of learning disabilities.

Smoking during pregnancy carries the risk of having a low birth weight or premature baby and there may also be intrauterine growth restriction (Blackburn 2003). Although these issues are not a direct cause of learning disabilities, they do pose a preventable hazard to both the mother and the fetus.

Detailed accounts of the effects of alcohol consumption during pregnancy have only recently been described. However, alcohol consumption during pregnancy and particularly during the first trimester has been linked with spontaneous abortion, low birth weight and fetal alcohol spectrum disorders (Blackburn 2003, British Medical Association Board of Science 2007, Fraser & Cooper 2009, Gilbert 2000, Royal College of Obstetricians and Gynecologists 2010) (see Box 2.2).

See Reader activity 2.2 on the Evolve website.

Drugs, including illegal, prescribed and over-the-counter medicines, taken during pregnancy may have a teratogenic or harmful effect upon the developing fetus causing abnormalities in development. Where possible, drugs should be avoided during the first 3 months of pregnancy, however this may not always be possible as it may pose a greater risk for the mother to cease her current therapeutic medication regime, for example medication taken for epilepsy, diabetes or mental health issues (Rutherford 2009). Low birth weight and respiratory problems are some of the complications that can be seen in babies addicted to illegal drugs (Nurse 2009).

Environmental pollutants such as lead and mercury, and chemical agents such as solvents, pesticides, anaesthetic gases and ionising radiation, have all been identified as hazardous to the developing fetus. Lead pollution in the atmosphere is known to cause stillbirth and congenital damage to the brain and central nervous system, resulting in learning disabilities (Foresight 2010, Sadler 2010).

Box 2.2

Fetal alcohol spectrum disorders

The term fetal alcohol spectrum disorders (FASD) is used to describe the following syndromes and disorders caused by alcohol during the prenatal developmental period:

- Fetal alcohol syndrome (FAS).
- Partial fetal alcohol syndrome (PFAS).
- Alcohol-related birth defects (ARBD).
- Alcohol-related neurodevelopmental disorders (ARND).

FAS describes the severest form of the disorder, with PFAS, ARBD and ARND showing some but not all of the features of FAS.

FAS is characterised by learning disabilities, facial deformities including a thin upper lip, smooth philtrum (area between the top lip and the nose) a flat nasal bridge, epicanthic folds and 'railroad track' ears; physical and emotional developmental problems, memory and attention deficits and behavioural problems.

Alcohol consumed during pregnancy passes via the placenta from the mother to the embryo or fetus. The amount and pattern of alcohol consumed, and the stage of pregnancy during which the alcohol is taken are important factors in determining the severity of the damage caused (British Medical Association Board of Science 2007).

Further information can be found by contacting the National Organisation for Fetal Alcohol Syndrome UK; details at the end of the chapter.

Physical factors

Radiation in the form of excessive use of X-rays has been found to cause damage to the developing fetus, especially if exposure occurs during the first 3 months of pregnancy. Pregnant women in Japan who survived the atomic bomb blasts were found to give birth to children with severe birth defects involving the central nervous system (Sadler 2010). Further studies of this group also identified chromosomal abnormalities and gene mutations. Ultrasound screening is a suitably safe alternative for examinations during pregnancy.

Direct violence

Any trauma to the fetus may result in stillbirth, abortion or brain damage. The severity of the condition will depend upon the stage of the pregnancy and the severity and nature of the violent act(s).

Anoxia

Should the brain be robbed of oxygen (anoxia) for a prolonged period of time then this will trigger irreversible changes in the brain. This is especially true for the developing fetus, which can only withstand very brief periods without oxygen before permanent damage occurs. Oxygen deprivation may be caused by a number of factors:

- Maternal illness, resulting in poorly oxygenated blood.
- Reduction in respiration owing to maternal sedation.
- Abnormal or premature detachment of the placenta.

Perinatal

Perinatal causes of learning disability that occur during this time include conditions such as prematurity, birth injury and/or abnormal labour.

Premature babies

The definition of a premature baby is a child born before week 37 of the pregnancy (England 2009, Ball et al 2010). Babies born before week 37 have varying survival rates: babies born before week 26 weighing less than 737 g have a survival rate of approximately 10%, babies born at 27–28 weeks weighing between 737 and 992 g have a survival rate of more than 50%, and babies born after 28 weeks weighing 92 g to 1.21 kg have a 70–90% survival rate (Nurse 2009).

Although prematurity is not in itself a cause of learning disabilities, premature and low birth weight babies experience a significantly greater number of problems during labour and the birth process than do full-term infants. These include breathing difficulties and intraventricular haemorrhage, placing them at risk for subsequent developmental problems.

Birth trauma

Birth is a traumatic event under any circumstances, for both mother and baby, and full-term babies are also at risk from a number of factors operating during labour that can cause birth trauma or injury, including the following.

Asphyxia

Worldwide perinatal asphyxia is a major cause of death and of acquired brain damage in newborns (McGuire 2010). Asphyxiation results in hypoxia, or decreased levels of oxygen and diminished cerebral blood flow. When the cerebral blood flow is diminished, the self-regulation of the brain's blood supply is impaired, leading in turn to brain swelling and haemorrhage.

Perinatal asphyxia may occur in utero, during labour and delivery, or in the immediate postnatal period. There are numerous causes, including placental abruption, cord compression and birth trauma. Postnatal asphyxia can be caused by an obstructed airway, and medication given for pain relief can cause respiratory depression (McGuire 2010).

Trauma

Trauma may be caused by instrumented delivery, for example forceps delivery. Excessive moulding of the head and breech presentation are also possible causes.

Damage or trauma to the brain may result in cerebral palsy, epilepsy or learning disabilities, depending upon the severity of the damage and the location within the brain. Fetal monitoring, that is determining fetal size and presentation prior to and during labour with ultrasound and other monitoring equipment, can alert the attending professional to the signs of fetal distress and reduce the potential danger.

Newborn blood spot screening

In the first week after birth, all babies are offered the newborn blood spot screening test, also known as the Guthrie test. The test screens for phenylketonuria (PKU), congenital hypothyroidism and sickle cell diseases (NHS 2007).

Approximately 1 in 10 000 babies born in the UK has PKU. Babies with this inherited condition are unable to process a protein in their food called phenylalanine. If untreated, they will develop serious, irreversible learning disabilities. Screening during the perinatal period means that babies with the condition can be treated early, preventing the learning disabilities. The treatment consists of a special diet that is low in phenylalanine. If babies are not screened, but are later found to have PKU, it may be too late for the special diet to make a real difference (Medforth et al 2006).

Congenital hypothyroidism has an incidence of approximately 1 in every 4000 babies born in the UK (NHS 2007). It is caused by an absent or small thyroid gland resulting in the reduction of the production of the hormone thyroxine. Treatment is given via a daily dose of thyroxine. If the condition goes untreated, the individual will develop learning disabilities (Medforth et al 2006).

Postnatal and beyond

The postnatal period is a relatively short period of time and consideration must be given beyond this as some learning disabilities only become evident when the child fails to meet developmental milestones. There are a number of factors that operate during the postnatal period and beyond that may result in learning disabilities, for example untreated genetic conditions, childhood infection, trauma, accidents, toxic agents, poor nutrition, sensory and social isolation.

With appropriate health education and health promotion messages, increased awareness of these causative factors may help to reduce the incidence or promote early intervention to limit the severity of the learning disabilities.

Child development

Although a number of learning disabilities are identified during the prenatal, perinatal and postnatal stages of development, there are others that are only detected during the later stages of the child's life when they fail to meet key developmental stages.

The key stages of child development are:

Newborn – from birth to 1 month
Infancy – from 1 to 12 months
Toddler – from 1 to 3 years
Pre-school – from 3 to 6 years
School age – from 6 to 12 years
Adolescence – from 12 to 18 years (Ball et al 2010).

During these time periods the child develops physically, socially and emotionally. There are numerous staged tests designed to monitor development and it is at theses key stages when learning disabilities may be detected (see Ch. 23 for an exploration of these stages).

Heredity

Many of the inherited conditions only become apparent in the postnatal period, for example phenylketonuria. As stated earlier, if this condition is not treated, the child will become affected when the phenylalanine concentration rises above the critical level (Rouse et al 2000, Koch et al 2003).

Environmental

Infection

A number of childhood infections carry the risk of brain damage as a complication, which may result in the affected individual having learning disabilities and/or an associated physical handicap. Encephalitis, meningitis and gastroenteritis are three examples of infections which, if untreated, can lead to learning disabilities.

Trauma

Accidental injuries to the head can be the result of accidental or non-accidental injury. They may be sustained as a result of road traffic or general household accidents, or as a result of oxygen deprivation. They may also be the result of capillary haemorrhage caused by prolonged and severe coughing during whooping cough infection.

Non-accidental injury may involve hitting, shaking, throwing, poisoning or suffocating the child (DH 1999). The resultant physical injuries may include depressed fractures of the skull, haematomas and blood vessel damage. The severity of the injury will determine the degree of learning disabilities sustained. Children who are suspected of being at risk are placed on a child protection register and will be closely monitored (DH 2009a, HM Government 2006, The Children Act 1989).

Toxic agents

As in the prenatal period, toxic agents can damage the developing brain. Lead intoxication was once commonly known as a causative factor, but increased awareness of the potential problem has reduced the use of this damaging substance (Foresight 2010). Environmental pollutants are another cause for concern, and continued investigation to identify potential harmful substances is required. Mercury, copper, manganese and strontium are all seen as detrimental in the developmental period.

Nutrition

Appropriate nutrition is a central element of health and wellbeing. The developing child who is malnourished may experience both physical and intellectual developmental delay (DH 2009b).

Sensory and social deprivation

Children learn and develop by interacting with their surroundings and environmental stimuli. Deprivation caused by impairment to any of the special senses (sight, hearing, touch, taste and smell; see Ch. 15) or social exclusion may have an effect upon the child's physical and intellectual development. Therefore, in order to prevent secondary handicap, professionals should have an understanding of the holistic needs of the developing individual and be able to educate and advise those who are not so well informed or who require assistance (Department for Education and Skills 2003, DH 2004b, 2009b).

Reader activity 2.3

A number of specific learning disabilities have been identified within this chapter, however there has only been a detailed discussion of Down syndrome. Make a list of the other types of learning disability that you are unfamiliar with and consider the type of information that a practitioner needs to broaden understanding of the condition and assist the individual and their family when planning for current and future holistic needs.

Conclusion

There are numerous methods that can assist in the detection and diagnosis of learning disabilities, however it is such a vast and complex condition that it may not always be possible to have a definitive diagnosis.

Having an understanding of the known causes and the screening and diagnostic tests that are available may offer parents and carers an opportunity to explore and conceptualise the ongoing needs of their child and may enhance the quality of the professionals' practice in a number of ways:

- In the provision of appropriate person-centred care.
- As a means of improving the quality of life for the individual.
- By advising parents or carers as to the nature and potential effects of the individual's condition.
- By answering questions or giving information to potential parents.
- By recognising threats to the health of people with learning disabilities caused by a known disorder.

Glossary of terms

Allele Alternative form of a gene that may occupy the same site on homologous chromosomes

Autosome Chromosome other than the sex chromosome

Chromosome Chromophilic body within the cell nucleus, visible as homologous pairs in dividing cells

Dominant trait One which is determined by the presence of a gene in heterozygous form

Gene The unit of inheritance, occupying a specific locus on a chromosome

Genotype An individual's genetic makeup

Heterozygous Having different alleles at a gene locus on each of a pair of homologous chromosomes

Homozygous Having the same allele at a gene locus on each of a pair of homologous chromosomes

Karyotype The chromosome characteristics of an individual arranged in pairs in descending order of size and according to the position of the centromere

Meiosis The formation of ova and sperm by cell division

Mitosis The process of somatic cell division during which the nucleus also divides generating two daughter cells

Mosaicism The presence of more than one cell type in a single individual

Mutation A spontaneous or induced change in a gene or chromosome
Non-disjunction The failure of chromosome pairs to separate properly during cell division
Phenotype The way in which the genotype is expressed in the body
Recessive trait One which is determined by the presence of a gene in homozygous form
Sex chromosomes The pair of chromosomes responsible for sex determination
Sex-linked trait One determined by the presence of a gene on the sex chromosomes (usually X-linked)
Translocation The transfer of a segment of a chromosome to a site on a different chromosome
Trisomy The presence of one chromosome additional to the normal homologous pair

References

Ball, J.W., Binder, R.C., Cowen, K.J., 2010. Child health nursing. Parenting with children and families, second ed. Pearson, USA.

Barrowclough, D., 2009. Preparing for pregnancy. In: Fraser, D.M., Cooper, M.A. (Eds.), Myles textbook for midwives. fifteenth ed. Churchill Livingstone, Edinburgh.

Bille, C., Murray, J.C., Olsen, S.F., 2007. Folic acid and birth malformations. Br. Med. J. 334, 433–434.

Blackburn, S.T., 2003. Maternal, fetal and neonatal physiology: a clinical perspective, second ed. Saunders, USA.

British Medical Association Board of Science, 2007. Fetal alcohol spectrum disorders: a guide for healthcare professionals. British Medical Association, London.

Contact a Family, 2010a. Down syndrome. Available at: http://www.cafamily.org.uk (accessed 12.07.10.).

Contact a Family, 2010b. Edwards' syndrome. Available at: http://www.cafamily.org.uk (accessed 13.07.10.).

Contact a Family, 2010c. Patau's syndrome. Available at: http://www.cafamily.org.uk (accessed 13.07.10.).

Contact a Family, 2010d. Cri-du-chat syndrome. Available at: http://www.cafamily.org.uk (accessed 13.07.10.).

Contact a Family, 2010e. Cornelia de Lange syndrome. Available at: http://www.cafamily.org.uk (accessed 4.07.10.).

Department for Education and Skills, 2003. Every child matters: change for children. HMSO, London.

Department of Health, 1989. The Children Act. HMSO, London.

Department of Health, 1999. Working together to safeguard children: a guide to inter-agency working to safeguard children and promote the welfare of children. HMSO, London.

Department of Health, 2001. Valuing people: a new strategy for learning disability for the 21st century. HMSO, London.

Department of Health, 2004a. Thinking of having a baby: folic acid – an essential ingredient in making babies. HMSO, London.

Department of Health, 2004b. National Service Framework for children, young people and maternity services. HMSO, London.

Department of Health, 2007. Valuing people now: from progress to transformation. HMSO, London.

Department of Health, 2009a. Improving safety, reducing harm: children, young people and domestic violence. HMSO, London.

Department of Health, 2009b. Healthy child programme: pregnancy and the first five years of life. HMSO, London.

Down's Syndrome Association, 2010. Information. Available at: http://www.downs-syndrome.org.uk/information (accessed 27.01.10.).

Dutton, G., 1975. Mental handicap. Butterworths, London.

Emerson, E., 2009. Estimating future numbers of adults with profound multiple learning disabilities in England. Department of Health. (online). Available at: http://www.dh.gov.uk/en/Publicationsandstatistics/Publications/PublicationsPolicyAndGuidance/DH_103201 (accessed 27.01.10.).

England, C., 2009. The healthy low birthweight baby. In: Fraser, D.M., Cooper, M.A. (Eds.), Myles textbook for midwives. fifteenth ed. Churchill Livingstone, Edinburgh.

Evans, J., 2008. Cell biology and genetics, third ed. Mosby, Edinburgh.

Foresight, 2010. Environmental hazards. Available at: http://www.foresight-preconception.org.uk/research/research-home.aspx (accessed 30.01.10.).

Fragile X Society, 2010. What is Fragile X?. Available at: http://fragilex.org.uk.dnnmax.com/FragileX/tabid/57/Default.aspx (accessed 10.04.10.).

Fraser, D.M., Cooper, M.A., (Eds.), 2009. Glossary of selected terms. Myles textbook for midwives, fifteenth ed. Churchill Livingstone, Edinburgh.

Gilbert, P., 2000. A–Z of syndromes and inherited disorders, third ed. Stanley Thornes, Cheltenham.

Griffiths, P.D., 2001. Cytomegalovirus infection in pregnancy. In: MacLean, A., Regan, L., Carrington, D. (Eds.), Infection and pregnancy. RCOG, London.

HM Government, 2006. Working together to safeguard children: a guide to inter-agency working to safeguard and promote the welfare of children. The Stationery Office, London.

Knight, S.J.L., Regan, R., Nicod, A., et al., 1999. Subtle chromosomal rearrangements in children with unexplained mental retardation. Lancet 345 (9191), 1676–1681.

Koch, R., Hanley, W., Levey, H., et al., 2003. The maternal phenylketonuria international study: 1984–2002. Pediatrics 6, 1523–1529.

Korenbrot, C.C., Steinburg, A., Bender, C., et al., 2002. Preconception care: a systematic review. Matern. Child Health. J. 6 (2), 75–88.

McGuire, W., 2010. Perinatal asphyxia. Available at: http://clinicalevidence.bmj.com/ceweb/conditions/chd/0320/0320_background.jsp (accessed 10.03.10.).

Medforth, J., Battersby, S., Evans, M. et al., (Eds.), 2006. Oxford handbook of midwifery. Oxford University Press, Oxford.

Mueller, R.F., Young, I.D., 2001. Emery's elements of medical genetics, eleventh ed. Churchill Livingstone, Edinburgh.

National Health Service, 2007. Antenatal and newborn screening programmes. UK National Screening Committee. Department of Health, London.

National Institute for Clinical Excellence (NICE), 2008. Ante-natal care: routine care for the healthy pregnant woman. Clinical Guideline 62. NICE, London.

NHS Choices, 2010. Rubella. Available at: http://www.nhs.uk/conditions/rubella/Pages/Introduction.aspx (accessed 27.01.10.).

Nurse, S. (Ed.), 2009. Maternal–neonatal care made incredibly easy. Lippincott Williams & Wilkins, Philadelphia.

Rouse, B., Matalon, R., Koch, R., 2000. Maternal phenylketonuria syndrome: congenital heart defects, microcephaly and developmental outcomes. J. Pediatr. 136 (1), 57–61.

Royal College of Obstetricians and Gynaecologists, 2010. Alcohol and pregnancy information for you. Available at: www.rcog.org.uk/womens-health/clinical-guidance/alcohol-and-pregnancy-information-you (accessed 28.01.10.).

Rutherford, J.M., 2009. Pharmacology and childbirth. In: Fraser, D.M., Cooper, M.A. (Eds.), Myles textbook for midwives. fifteenth ed. Churchill Livingstone, Edinburgh.

Sadler, T.W., 2010. Langmans medical embryology, eleventh ed. Lippincott Williams and Wilkins, Philadelphia.

Stratford, B., 1996. In the beginning. In: Stratford, B., Gunn, P. (Eds.), Approaches to Down syndrome. Cassell, London.

Sullivan, A., Kirk, B., 2009. Specialized antinatal investigations. In: Fraser, D.M., Cooper, M.A. (Eds.), Myles textbook for midwives. fifteenth ed. Churchill Livingstone, Edinburgh.

The Irish Society for Mucopolysaccharide Diseases, 2010. Hunter disease. Available at: www.mpssociety.ie/wordpress/?page_id=80 (accessed 12.07.10.).

Tuberous Sclerosis Association UK, 2010. What is tuberous sclerosis complex (TSC)?. Available at: http://www.tuberous-sclerosis.org (accessed 5.07.10.).

Turner, T., Simpson, J., 2009. Congenital abnormalities. In: Fraser, D.M., Cooper, M.A. (Eds.), Myles textbook for midwives. fifteenth ed. Churchill Livingstone, Edinburgh.

Turnpenny, P., Ellard, D., 2007. Emery's elements of medical genetics, thirteenth ed. Churchill Livingstone, Edinburgh.

Further reading

Bradley, A.N., 2005. Utility and limitations of genetic testing and information. Nurs. Stand. 20 (5), 5255.

Department of Health, 2004. National Service Framework for children, young people and maternity services: disabled children and young people and those with complex health needs. HMSO, London.

Evidence in Health and Social Care, http://www.evidence.nhs.uk/default.aspx.

GeneSense, http://www.genesense.org.uk.

Harper, P.S., 2004. Practical genetic counselling, sixth ed. Hodder Arnold, London.

Human Genetics Commission, http://www.hgc.gov.uk/.

Shakespear, T., 1998. Choices and rights: eugenics, genetics and disability equality. Disability & Society 13 (5), 665–681.

The Human Genome, The Wellcome Trust, http://www.wellcome.ac.uk/genome.

Useful addresses

Alzheimer's Society: http://alzheimers.org.uk/.

Antenatal Results and Choices: http://www.arc-uk.org.

Contact a Family: http://www.cafamily.org.uk.

Down Syndrome Association: http://www.downs-syndrome.org.uk/.

Foresight: The Association for the Promotion of Preconceptual Care, 178 Hawthorne Road, Bognor Regis, West Sussex PO21 2UY, http://www.foresight-preconception.org.uk/.

Fragile X Society: http://www.fragilex.org.uk/.

Inclusion International: http://www.inclusion-international.org.

National Organisation on Fetal Alcohol Syndrome UK: http://www.nofas-uk.org/.

National PKU News: http://www.pkunews.org/index.htm.

National Society for Phenylketonuria (UK) Ltd,
PO Box 26642,
London N14 4ZF,
Tel. Helpline 0208 3643010,
http://www.nspku.org.

NHS Evidence in Health and Social Care (genetic conditions): http://www.library.nhs.uk/.

Public Health Genetics Unit: http://www.phgu.org.uk.

Sense for Deaf Blind People: http://www.sense.org.uk/Home.htm.

SHS International: http://www.shs-nutrition.com.

UK Newborn Screening Programme Centre: http://newbornbloodspot.screening.nhs.uk/.

Eugenics: the creation and maintenance of difference

3

Helen Atherton

CHAPTER CONTENTS

KEY ISSUES

- Eugenics is a term used to define the science of improving the physical and intellectual qualities of populations
- Its principles were popular across many Western countries around the end of the 19th and beginning of the 20th centuries
- It aimed to limit procreation among those considered to be feeble-minded through measures such as institutionalisation, involuntary sterilisation and genocide
- Health and social care professionals were instrumental in the delivery of eugenic programmes which often conflicted with their own professional and moral codes
- Contemporary advances in genetic science may herald a return to eugenics
- Health and social care professionals need to be aware of the conflict that may arise between personal and professional values and external organisational demands

Introduction

The commencement of the Human Genome Project in 1990 was to herald the start of what has been a period of significant advancement in the field of genetic science. Over the course of the last 20 years, our understanding of the genetic origins of some common and less common conditions found within contemporary society has significantly increased. For some disabled people, the identification of those genes responsible for conditions such as Huntington's chorea has undoubtedly provided sufferers with a greater understanding of their condition and how it may affect subsequent generations of their own family. For others, however, the discovery of a 'cause' and the potential to eradicate such conditions carries a more sinister meaning which could be construed as essentially denying disabled people the right to 'be' (Ward 2002).

The discovery of a faulty or defective gene more often than not leads on to a discussion about the methods that could be most effectively deployed in its detection and, in some cases, its elimination. Researchers working to identify the genes responsible for autism have identified the benefits of genetic testing as including aiding an early assessment of the susceptibility of an individual to developing a condition, guiding the prescription of drugs for alleviating symptoms and facilitating genetic counselling for families (Ghosh 2010). Such benefits are supported by the White Paper *Our Inheritance, Our Future* published by the Department of Health (DH) in 2003 in which genetic knowledge in health care is regarded as being important in:

> bringing more accurate diagnosis, more personalised prediction of risk, new drugs and therapies, and prevention and treatment better targeted to the disease and tailored according to a person's individual genetic profile. (p. 4)

When employed on a case by case basis, it could indeed be argued that such tests support the fundamental values of choice and informed decision making, something that as human beings we are all entitled to. However, when such tests are being targeted at the level of populations, questions are raised with respect to their true motives. The case of testing for Down syndrome is a prime example of where there has been a gradual and as such quite subtle move from the offering of tests to only those women who were deemed to be in a high risk bracket for bearing children with the condition, to now offering tests to all women as a routine part of antenatal care (National Institute for Clinical Excellence (NICE 2003)). Vassy (2006), in her exploration of the uptake of prenatal testing and screening in France, makes reference to key discourse in which it is asserted that such practices represent a deliberate attempt to eradicate defective fetuses in order to improve the overall quality of a population, and as such constitutes a new form of eugenics.

While it is recommended that an understanding of genetics should form an integral part of the education and training of all pre- and post-qualified health care workers in England (DH 2003), this does not appear to include a knowledge and understanding of the history of eugenics. Indeed, in the White Paper containing this recommendation, eugenics is only prominent by virtue of its very absence. Yet, there is a growing body of evidence to suggest that without knowledge and understanding of eugenics, there is a risk that health care workers will unquestioningly adopt practices that undermine the human rights of those they are charged with protecting, particularly when such practices emanate from state authority (Lerner & Rothman 1995). Including a chapter on eugenics in this book supports the need for all those working with people with learning disabilities to have an awareness of its impact on the delivery of contemporary care and support to this group, not only in terms of genetic advancements but in its other more subtle guises. The chapter utilises the personal stories of four individuals, the course of whose lives were dramatically altered by eugenics. The inclusion of these is important as Park & Radford (1998:324) have asserted that they can enable people to:

> examine what happened when people were brought under the gaze of the medical community and the state and hopefully restore to the history of eugenics a human face.

What is eugenics?

The term eugenics derives from the Greek word 'eugenès' meaning 'well born' and has been defined as the:

> science which deals with all influences that improve the inborn qualities of the race; also those that develop them to the utmost advantage
>
> (Blacker 1950:21)

The idea that humankind could somehow artificially control the quality of its members was first conceived during the Victorian era by a range of prominent scientists that included Sir Francis Galton in England (Hoskins 2005). Galton was a half cousin of Charles Darwin whose own evolutionary theory had served to challenge traditional creationist beliefs as to the origin of mankind (Keynes 2002). Darwin had theorised that the process of natural selection, governed by events that he termed the war of nature, famine and death, would preserve favourable variations in species while rejecting their weaker counterparts (Darwin 1859). While a keen supporter of Darwin's theories, Galton, when applying his cousin's theory to the human race, was less convinced about the innate ability of nature to select those individuals with physical, social and intellectual attributes considered sufficient to meet the new demands of a developing society. Such characteristics were deemed to be: good hereditary composition; sound physical health; good physique; intelligence; social usefulness; freedom from genetic traits; being a member of a large, well-adjusted family and having a fondness of animals (Blacker 1950). Galton believed that, in reality, nature was tending to favour the survival of coarser social groups that spoiled rather than improved the quality of the population (Jones 1998); he therefore reasoned that without artificial intervention in the workings of nature, a social disaster was imminent. This stance was supported by a number of prominent middle class activists that included the fabian Sidney Webb who concluded that:

> No consistent eugenicist can be a 'Laisser Faire' individualist unless he throws up the game in despair: He must interfere, interfere, interfere.
>
> (Leonard 2009:47)

Central to Galton's theory was the belief that human intelligence was innately determined; the consequence of a single unit of inheritance passing unchangingly through generations of the same family upon which the impact of environmental conditions including levels of sanitation, education or indiscriminate charity had little or no bearing (Mazumdar 1998); in short, moral and environmental melioration of the 'unfit' was considered futile (Waller 2001), a view echoed in the words of H G Wells, a staunch eugenic supporter:

> It has become apparent that whole masses of human population are, as a whole, inferior in their claim upon the future ... to give them equality is to sink to their level, to protect and cherish them is to be swamped in their fecundity
>
> (Ridley 1998:45)

It was believed that parents of high intelligence would naturally give birth to children also with high levels of intelligence. Equally, parents of low intellectual vigour would bear offspring equally marred. The problem was also not just confined to the issue of intelligence as an isolated attribute, but its inextricable link to many of society's social problems; problems that writers believed were also pre-ordained in the offspring of affected families and therefore unresponsive to treatment (Waller 2001).

Galton's dismissal of the environment as a causal factor in the creation and maintenance of difference was to undermine the benevolent ethos that had played a significant role in attempting to ameliorate the social conditions of the poor and sickly classes through acts such as the provision of poor law relief, the building of new hospitals and, importantly, educational provision (Galton 2002). Instead Galton proposed two types of social intervention which while diametrically opposed in practice were equivalent in aim; to improve the physical, social and intellectual health of populations. These interventions were termed positive and negative eugenics and have been defined by Garver & Garver (1991:1109) in the following way:

- Positive eugenics – systematic actions, whether decisional or programmatic, that serve to maximise the spread of desirable genes in society.
- Negative eugenics – systematic actions, whether decisional or programmatic, that serve to minimise the spread of deleterious genes in society.

One would assume that, as the central facet of eugenics was one of control over the individual and their destiny, it would endear itself more to societies with autocratic constitutions. In reality, however, it was to become a significant feature of many Western countries, penetrating the thinking and actions of those whose liberal leanings would have suggested more vocal and strident opposition to its basic principles (Dikötter 1998). In this respect, it has been concluded that eugenics cannot be merely considered an isolated form of extremism as it has historically spanned both political divides and sexes (Burleigh 2000). What did somewhat divide countries was the perception of what constituted the 'dangerous' elements of society, whose reproductive activities were deemed to necessitate eugenic control, to some extent divided countries. Race became interwoven with issues of intelligence as illustrated in the range of target groups: in France, the threat was posed by their 'martial eastern neighbours', Germany feared the 'Slavic hordes', while America, the 'penniless eastern and southern Europeans' and 'poor white trash' (Burleigh 2000:345). In the latter, this gave rise to the introduction of robust immigration controls (Carlson 2001). However, it was the problem of the feeble-minded that was to consistently occupy eugenic discourse in all countries.

The problem of the feeble-minded

While there was widespread use of the term 'feeble-minded' across countries during the late 19th and 20th century, the exact nature of the group to which the term applied tended to differ. For example, in Britain, Radford (1991) identifies feeble-minded individuals as mildly mentally handicapped, lacking in physical stigmata and distinct from other types of mental deficiency such as idiocy and imbecility. This distinction was made explicit in the 1913 Mental Deficiency Act that identified four clear diagnostic categories of mental defect of which the feeble-minded were defined as those requiring care to protect themselves. In comparison, however, the term when employed in America was applied more generically to encapsulate three forms of mental defect – the idiot, the imbecile and the moron – although it has been argued that it came to symbolise all forms of deviance (Mostert 2002, Snyder & Mitchell 2002). What was consistent, however, was the belief that this group, in comparison to others also deemed 'unfit' within society such as criminals, paupers, prostitutes and the mentally ill (Radford 1991), represented the single greatest threat to the stability of nations. A significant rationale attributed to this argument was the ability of this group to live, undetected, among ordinary members of society. Contrary to criminals, who Galton believed to have a distinctive 'felon face' (Waller 2001), the feeble-minded were initially thought not to bear any identifiable hallmarks that distinguished them from ordinary members of the population and as such were able to mate with healthy members of the population and spread social ills:

> The danger lies in the fact that these generates mate with healthy members of the community and thereby constantly drag fresh blood into the vortex of disease and lower the general vigour of the nation
>
> (Tredgold 1909:102)

Part of the science of eugenics was therefore cataloguing physical stigmata that could be used in the identification and classification of defectives (Jackson 1995).

Gender differences in terms of perceived levels of threat also existed with females rather than males considered to be more culpable in the spread of degeneracy. In a review of the history of eugenics in New Zealand, Wanhalla (2007) points to women as a key target group for its implementation. In discourse surrounding this issue, deviant women were typically categorised as both predatory and victims, in the first instance being referred to as oversexed, promiscuous, lacking in self control, exhibiting low levels of morality and being unable to control male sexual behaviour, and in the second, vulnerable to the 'lusts of normal men' (p. 173).

It is reasonable to assume that feeble-minded individuals have always been a part of the natural variation within societies, yet not drawing the type of attention that was afforded to them during the eugenic era. It is interesting to consider, therefore, the contextual events that contributed towards this group being singled out as a potential threat to the survival of nations. As with all contemporary scientific developments, eugenics was framed in the social and political context of the time with Burleigh (2000) asserting that is has alternated between hard and soft faces dependent on public climate and national circumstances. Yet even the briefest of glances at its history suggests that it has arisen most prominently in periods of change and instability such as those that characterised many Western countries during the latter half of the 19th and early decades of the 20th centuries. During this time, concerns about the quality of populations were to occupy the thinking of the middle classes with a number of significant events serving to increase their awareness of the burdensome nature of the feeble-minded and their links to the propagation of many of society's social ills.

Reader activity 3.1

During the height of the eugenic era, the spread of feeble-mindedness was likened to the threat of a contagious disease. Try and imagine how this might have felt by casting your mind back to 2009 when countries across the world were caught in the grip of swine flu that threatened the health of nations. Try to remember how the country reacted to the fear, what sort of measures did the government advocate and how were these publicised? How did you feel?

First, the Industrial Revolution (from about 1760), with its demand for technically skilled labour, is said to have brought about the assessment of people by their ability to cope with the new technological and commercial processes (Race 1995). With this came harsher and narrower definitions of normality (Waller 2001). It was reasoned by eugenicists that the predominance of rural, farming-based economies had, up until this time, successfully accommodated the basic skills of the feeble-minded and, in doing so, had effectively hid them from the rest of society (Snyder & Mitchell 2002). However, with the advancement of more urban-based manufacturing industries that required skills over and above the alleged capabilities of the feeble-minded and the inevitable disintegration of traditional kinship-based support, Snyder & Mitchell argued that this resulted in this group being effectively displaced into the public gaze.

Perceived as lacking in both the practical and intellectual competence to sustain themselves or any dependents in a developing society, in Germany, during the 1930s, they came to be known as useless eaters (Ost 2006) and their perceived burden was illustrated in Nazi propaganda posters such as the one featured in Figure 3.1. The burdensome effect of this group also led many to question the appropriateness of welfare measures being employed to support this group, who Pernick (1997) has suggested that, from a eugenicists evolutionary perspective, should strictly have been dead. In Britain, it was concluded that some two-thirds of the feeble-minded population were partially or wholly provided for by the state amounting to between £1000 and £2000 for the lifetime of an individual (Tredgold 1909). Such a situation was further compounded by the effects of the economic depression that swept across many Western countries after the First World War. As Steppe (1992) has concluded, the humanistic treatment of the individual was to be eventually sacrificed in favour of the health of the nation; where an individual could not contribute to society, society had both a right not to care for them and a right to banish them.

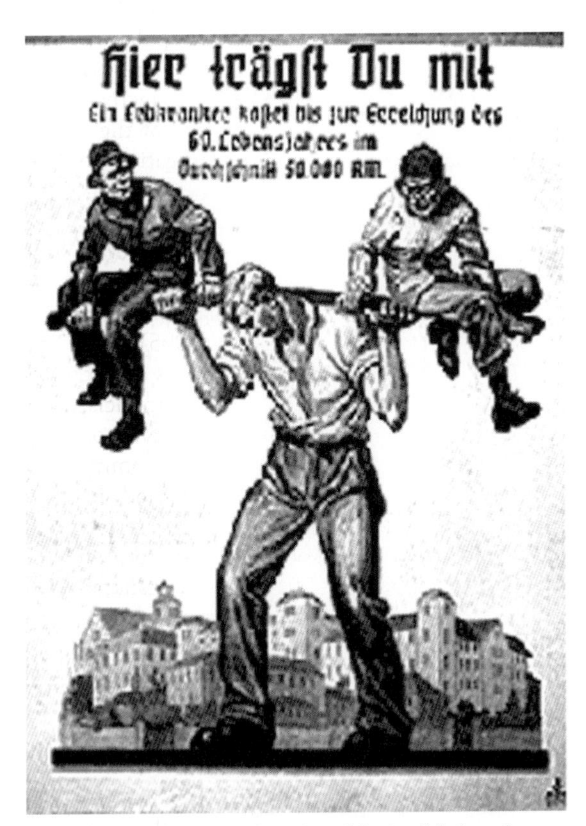

Figure 3.1 • "You are bearing this too" informing the 'German worker' that a hereditarily ill person costs 50 000 RMs to maintain until he or she has reached the age of 60 (Source: Burleigh 1994:188)

Second, events linked to the imperialistic activity that characterised this time led countries across the Western world to specifically consider not only the physical but the intellectual fitness of their populations in gauging their success in impending conflict. In Britain, the embarrassing defeats of British armies at the hands of Dutch farmers and the large number of conscripts rejected as being medically unfit were to focus the attention of the British government on this issue (Alaszewski 1988), while in New Zealand, society mourned the loss of 'virile' young men in the Great War who were essential entities in repairing the race (Wanhalla 2007). Confounding this was also the issue of the declining birth rate among the middle classes thereby reducing the chances of good genes entering the population (Kerr & Shakespeare 2002). Adding weight to the eugenic argument was also the application of notable theories on differential fertility. The concept of differential fertility was first introduced by Malthus (1798) in his *An Essay on the Principle of Population*. Within it, he prophesised that the uncontrolled procreation of the working classes would result in an imbalance between the size of the population and the availability of food supplies, the net result being mass famine (Jones 1998). Such a theory, when applied to the issue of the feeble minded resulted in fears that procreation amongst this group significantly exceeded that occurring amongst the eugenically fit. Research conducted on feeble-minded families, professed to provide hard facts that illustrated the ramifications of allowing this group to continue to reproduce at current levels with leading American eugenicist, Henry H Goddard, concluding that they multiplied at twice the rate of the general population (Goddard 1912). In Britain, Tredgold (1909) drew attention to the significantly higher than average number of offspring borne by this group as compared to the 'normal' population (7.3 as opposed to 4.63).

A key scientific tool in the gathering of data to support such assertions was the pedigree chart. Although its use was gradually superseded in the early part of the 20th century with the growth of statistical testing that supposedly offered more robust measurements of difference within populations (Stubblefield 2007), it had an important function in the presentation of data that could be used as propaganda for generating widespread public support for eugenic practices. Eugenicists used pedigree charts, alongside photographs of 'defective' individuals, to visually illustrate the transmission of feeble-mindedness and associated social problems through generations of the same family (Lombardo 2001). The data upon which such charts were devised were gathered by specially trained field workers (Bix 1997) and deposited in national record centres such as the Eugenics Education Society in England and the Eugenics Records Office at Cold Spring Harbour in America. Using a range of standardised symbols to represent both normal and feeble-minded individuals, and associated conditions such as blindness, epilepsy, pauperism and being physically unsound (Mazumdar 1998), they were used at state fairs in America and public meetings and exhibitions in England to educate, or rather prick the conscience of, societies with respect to the need for careful and considered breeding (Selden 2005). To illustrate the power of such charts, Lombardo (2001) makes reference to the infamous Kallikak Family (Goddard 1912) whose pedigree chart was widely disseminated to illustrate the difference in social consequences of both responsible and irresponsible breeding. This pedigree chart is notable because of its two lineages, both of which originate from Martin Kallikak (see Fig. 3.2), the first illustrating his marriage to a lawful, normal wife that resulted in normal descendents, and in the second, his affair with a feeble-minded girl resulting in generations of paupers, criminals, prostitutes and drunkards which Goddard attributed to the prevalence of feeble-mindedness.

It was widely believed that without proper control, the spread of feeble-mindedness and its associated social ills would have a dysgenic effect on populations characterised by the gradual degeneration of society through the erosion of its physical, intellectual and moral core, culminating in 'volkstadt or 'death of the race' as exemplified in the Nazi propaganda poster shown in Figure 3.3. Countries needed to take control of the problem, work swiftly to stem the tide of degeneracy and rebuild robust societies:

> . . . Society must protect itself; as it claims the right to deprive the murderer of his life, so also it may annihilate the hideous serpent of hopelessly vicious protoplasm. Here is where appropriate legislation will aid in eugenics and in creating a healthier, saner society in the future.
>
> (Charles Davenport 1910 quoted in Mazumdar 1998:25)

What resulted was the introduction of eugenic controls that simultaneously sought to limit the propagation of a degenerate population and increase the numbers of intellectual members of physically sound constitution.

Eugenics in practice

The practice of ridding society of those individuals considered to be either a burden or threat was not borne out of the Victorian era. Indeed, evidence

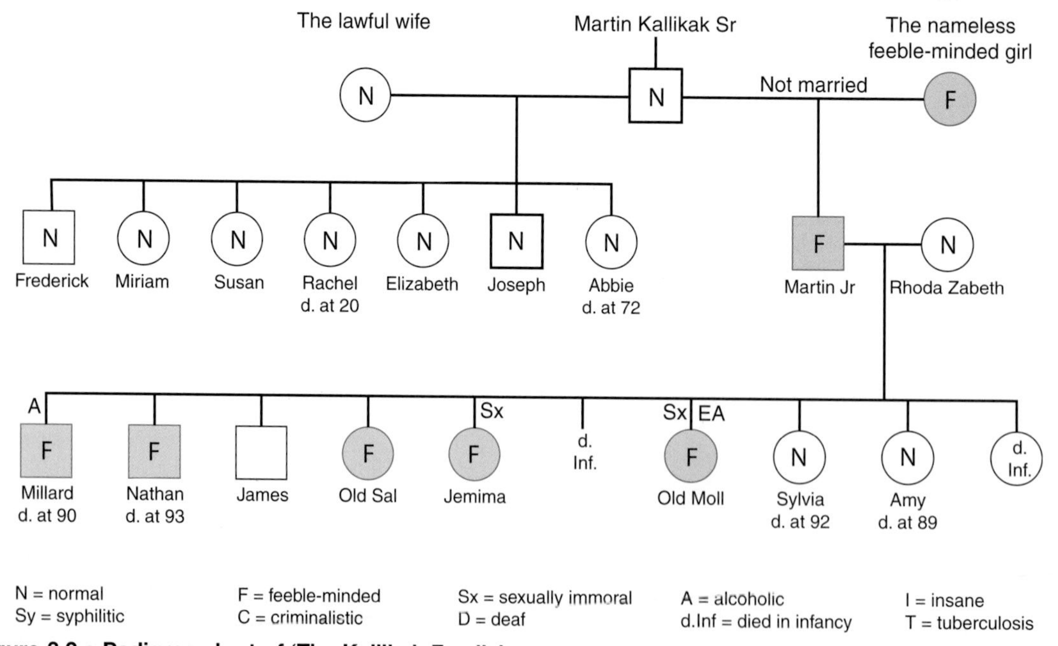

Figure 3.2 • Pedigree chart of 'The Kallikak Family' (Source: Goddard 1912:37)

So würde es enden.
So wird es kommen,
wenn Minderwertige 4 Kinder und Höherwertige 2 Kinder hab

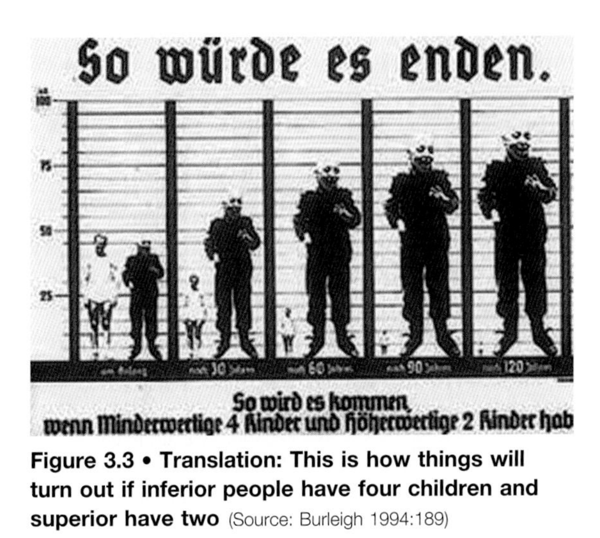

Figure 3.3 • Translation: This is how things will turn out if inferior people have four children and superior have two (Source: Burleigh 1994:189)

suggests that 'eugenic' practices, although not specifically termed as such, can be traced as far back as Spartan times where the parallel practices of rewards for good marriage and infanticide were undertaken in the pursuit of military fitness and defence of a minority race (Roper 1913). Roper also alludes to the writings of Ancient Greek philosophers that suggest that eugenic ideas lay at the very heart of the social and economic programmes deemed necessary for the establishment of civilised societies. While the term eugenics wasn't coined until Galton's 1883 work, *Hereditary Genius*, the foundations for its development were in place in the early decades of the 19th century. Waller (2001) discusses the preoccupation of the medical profession at this time with 'rational' reproduction; drawing upon the principles of stock breeding, individuals were encouraged to make wise marriage choices by scrutinising the hereditary quality of future partners. It was only in later years that the advisory intervention at an individual level was to shift to national programmes of enforced interventions, targeted not only at individuals but entire groups within society, governed by the laws of the land and representing a marked shift from voluntary to coercive measures. As in the case of the target groups selected for eugenic policies, the preferred choice of intervention differed between countries, influenced by the social and political discourse of the time. The range of methods is illustrated in Figure 3.4.

Positive eugenics

Positive eugenic practices sought to optimise the physical and mental qualities of populations and employed what Carlson (2001:9) refers to as 'moral

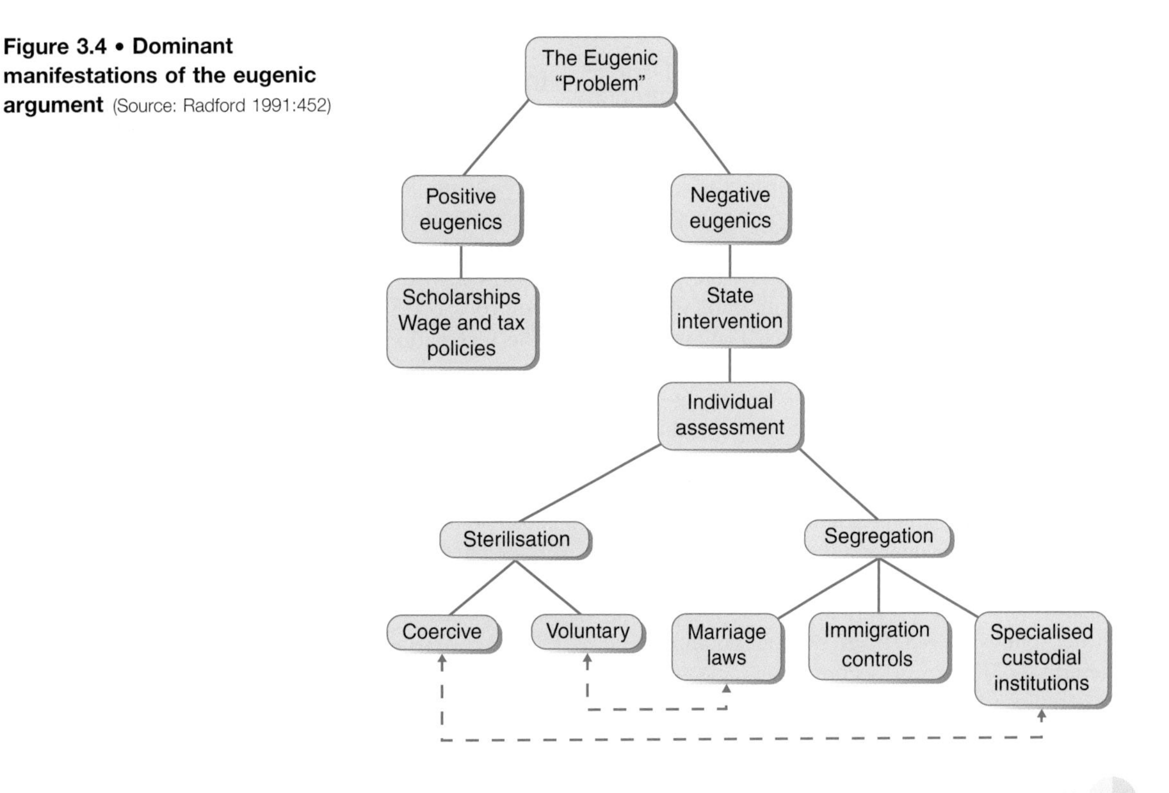

Figure 3.4 • Dominant manifestations of the eugenic argument (Source: Radford 1991:452)

suasion' to encourage the brightest and ablest members of society to have children. In the diagram illustrated in Figure 3.4, Radford (1991) summarises positive eugenic interventions as including school/university scholarships and wage and tax allowances aimed at discouraging the intellectual middle classes from limiting the number of children they bore. Encouraging sensible breeding patterns was also at the heart of positive eugenic policy. As marriage was deemed a vital institution in the subsequent breeding of physically and intellectually healthy individuals, it was given particular attention by eugenicists. Information and guidance relating to responsible marriage and breeding was instilled in populations using a variety of carefully crafted educational strategies, often delivered by women (Wanhalla 2007). In her paper on the employment of positive eugenics in Switzerland, Gerodetti (2006) discusses the development of marriage advice bureaus that provided guidance to individuals and couples on 'healthy' marriages, while Benedict et al (2009) make reference to the 'Lebensborn' programme in Germany through which Aryan children ('Aryan' being deemed the purest race) were purposely bred and rewards given to Aryan women who gave birth to large families. In addition to the use of media such as films and newspapers to instil specific eugenic messages in the psyche of the population, Selden (2005) identifies the use of 'Fitter Families' competitions at state fairs across America. Such competitions involved participants being evaluated in terms of the quality of their hereditary composition, winning individuals and families receiving certificates and trophies such as medals bearing the inscription 'Yea, I have goodly heritage' (p. 205). Yet marriage was also to become a focus of negative eugenic policy. In some countries, Britain being a notable exception, marriage between two hereditarily unfit individuals was outlawed. In France, a marriage law was passed (rather belatedly in 1942) that required individuals wishing to marry to present a certificate of good health that showed that that they were neither severely retarded, syphilitic or an alcoholic (Carlson 2001). In America, marriage between feeble-minded individuals was made illegal in some 30 states before 1914 (Kevles 1995), while in 1935, the National Socialist government in Germany passed the Marriage Health Law that prevented a couple marrying if either one suffered from mental derangement, a hereditary disease or a contagious disease such as tuberculosis (Friedlander 1995). All of these are clear examples of how the values of individual choice and self-determination could be overridden in favour of the more pressing issue of race preservation, however these were to represent the tip of what was to become a much bigger iceberg.

Negative eugenics

In Figure 3.4, Radford (1991) identifies a range of negative eugenic strategies, of which a country's preferred choice would be largely determined by the current social and political context. For some countries, the choice of eugenic intervention was to remain constant; for others, of which Germany is the best illustrative example, a move between different types of method was observed over time. Regardless of the chosen method, however, negative eugenic programmes exhibited many shared features, the most prominent of which was their authoritative and coercive nature and their prohibition of individual choice and right to democracy for their recipients (Cairney 1996). A further common feature was their use of pseudo-religious language in encouraging public acceptance. For example, to comply with eugenic measures was considered a 'duty' of those affected by bad hereditary composition, a situation that was believed by some to be synonymous with the sacrifices being made by healthy members of the population during wartime emergencies (Burleigh 1994).

Institutionalisation

Segregation in specialised institutions for those deemed unfit was a popular method of eugenic control and was implemented across countries. While sometimes used in conjunction with other methods (e.g. sterilisation), in the UK and countries such as Australia, institutionalisation was to remain the dominant method of eugenic control of the feeble-minded. The segregation of this group in this manner was to become enshrined in law in England and Wales with the introduction of the Mental Deficiency Act (1913) and in Australia with the introduction of legislation for the control of mental defectives in individual states starting with Tasmania in 1920, Victoria 1922, Queensland 1938 and New South Wales 1939 (Garton 1994). The Mental Deficiency Act 1913 provided the legal basis upon which to detain four main classes of defectives – idiots, imbeciles, feeble-minded and moral defectives. It was introduced in response to the findings of the Royal Commission on the Care and Control of the Feeble-minded set up in 1904. Interestingly, Thomson (1998) has asserted that the initial driver behind this investigation was not overtly eugenic but was a response to the evident inadequacy of current provision for those needing specialised care and support, for the protection of both themselves and others, particularly after leaving special school. It was the findings on the prevalence of mental deficiency, that had initially fallen outside its remit, that was to fuel eugenic debates with an estimated 138 529 defectives in England and Wales significantly costing society, both money and potential stability (Tredgold 1909). Both in the UK and Australia, segregation in a bid to prevent propagation was deemed vital to thwart future increases in the number of defectives. In the UK, farm and industrial 'colony' style provision, based on the America model of segregation (Radford 1991) was proposed:

> In such institutions the feeble-minded would not only be happy, far happier in fact amid companions like themselves than in the outside world, but they would also contribute to their own support. Society would thus be saved a portion, at least, of the cost of their maintenance, and, more important, it would be secure from their depredations and the danger of their propagation. Colony life would at the same time protect the feeble-minded against a certain section of society and protect society against the feeble-minded.
>
> (Tredgold 1909:104).

While the occurrence of the First World War largely limited progress under the Mental Deficiency Act (1913), the Wood Report (1929) refuelled the need for urgency by suggesting that there had been a marked increase in the number of defectives from 4.6 to 10.49 per 1000 in the population since 1908 (Thomson 1998). It recommended the immediate institutionalisation of 100 000 affected individuals.

The first half of the 20th century was to bear witness to a significant growth in institutionalised provision for mental defectives across countries. In 1926, it was estimated that 27 000 defectives were being legally controlled, rising to 90 000 in 1939 (Tredgold 1952). Such environments were typically characterised by 'strict sexual quarantine' (Radford 1991), which was an obvious active bid to prevent sexual relations that may result in the birth of a defective child. The development and use of life story and narrative work methods, discussed in Chapter 8 of this book, are gradually facilitating the telling of the personal stories of those who lived in such environments and are an important aspect of social history, serving to inject a vital human element into the more academic historical accounts of the period. *The World of Dolly Stainer* (Judge & van Brummelen 2002) is one such example that uses personal narratives to recount both the history of an institution, Kew Cottages in Melbourne, Australia, and one of its residents (see Story 3.1).

See Reader activity 3.2 on the Evolve website.

Sterilisation

In contrast to some other Western countries, England never implemented laws that legalised the sterilisation of those deemed unfit. This did not, however, preclude debate around this issue with the Brock Committee (1934), set up in response to the Wood Report (1929), recommending voluntary sterilisation (Macnicol 1992). Despite its failure to obtain support in England, involuntary sterilisation was a central method of eugenic control in other

Story 3.1

Dolly Stainer

Dolly Stainer was born in Melbourne on 6 September 1910. Her mother, Ceceilia, was a known prostitute and was frequently under arrest for crimes such as 'improper conduct', 'insufficient means', 'offensive behaviour', 'improper conduct in a church' and 'habitual drunkenness'. Classified as a neglected child (which meant you were either ill-treated, under the care of an incompetent person, abandoned or a brothel child), Dolly was removed from her mother and admitted to Kew Idiot Asylum (Melbourne), otherwise known as Kew Cottages, on 15 June 1915 at the age of 4. Labelled as an 'imbecile' at certification, she was described as being 'illiterate with vicious habits, swears volubly and cannot be restrained'. Dolly was institutionalised for 75 years in total although was significantly more capable than her initial diagnosis would suggest. In her adult life, she was a 'working girl', caring for the less able residents, cleaning the nurses' quarters and working in the kitchens and laundry. In the words of a mother whose own child was resident in the cottage:

> *My other clearly-remembered recollection of the first day was wondering about the three middle-aged ladies not in uniform who seemed to be helping in the Cottage, with chores and mothering the babies and toddlers. This was the first time I met Katie Collins, Dolly Stainer and Lorna White ... and to appreciate the role they played in the children's lives.*
>
> (p. 161)
>
> (Judge and van Brummelen, 2002)

Dolly died in 1997 at the age of 86 after having only left Kew Cottages 7 years previously.

Western countries, the most notable of which were the Nordic countries, America and Germany, the latter of which passed the Law for Prevention of Hereditary Diseased Progeny (1933), legalising the compulsory sterilisation of those with hereditary conditions such as schizophrenia, manic depression and epilepsy (Burleigh 1994).

The implementation of eugenic sterilisation programmes in the Nordic countries were fuelled by fears of the effects of immigration and emigration on the quality of populations, lowering birth rates among their desirable members and the simultaneous rise in the number of mental defectives (Kerr & Shakespeare 2002). The true scale of such programmes was to surface in 1997 with the publication of a highly controversial article in the Swedish newspaper *Dagens Nyheter* (Wennerberg 1997). The story created an international storm as the Nordic states had been traditionally viewed as archetypal social democracies with progressive systems of social welfare. What emerged was their employment of both voluntary and involuntary sterilisation to limit propagation among the unfit either because they were perceived as being incapable of looking after children or because their hereditary constitution was thought to present a threat to subsequent generations of a family (Kerr & Shakespeare 2002). Sterilisation laws were passed in Denmark (1929), Norway (1934), Sweden (1935) and Finland (1935), a detailed history of which can found in the work of Broberg & Roll-Hansen (2005). In Sweden alone, it is estimated that 63 000 people, over 90% of whom were women, were sterilised between 1935 and 1975 (Wennerberg 1997), while in Finland, compulsory sterilisation laws targeted mental defectives, the mentally ill and those with epilepsy (Hemminki et al 1997). Sterilisation was also often commonly employed to reduce the burden of provision in institutional care by making it a condition of release back into people's own communities (Kerr & Shakespeare 2002); a common economic solution to the high expense incurred by institutionalising large numbers, not only in the Nordic states, but also America (Block 2000). The effects of compulsory sterilisation were to have lifetime consequences for those individuals affected (see Story 3.2).

Thirty states in America were to pass eugenic sterilisation laws between 1907 and 1931 (Block 2000). The first state to implement such a law was Indiana in 1907 and the last to repeal one was Alabama in 2000. Figures quoted by Sofair & Kaldjian (2000) suggest that somewhere in the region of 40 000 eugenic sterilisations had taken place by 1944 and 22 000 between 1943 and 1963. The multitude of studies pertaining to this period make reference to specific historical milestones, the most significant of which was the court case, Buck vs Bell, that sought to test the constitutional soundness of the Virginia law (Kevles 1995). Carrie Buck, her daughter and her mother had been admitted to the Virginia Colony for the Feeble-minded and Epileptics. It was concluded that all three showed signs of feeble-mindedness and the sterilisation of Carrie was sought and successfully sanctioned through the courts, paving the way for the involuntary sterilisation of some 60 000 feeble-minded and mentally insane people, of which 60% were women (Stubblefield 2007). At the trial in 1927, the presiding judge, Oliver Wendall Holmes, made the now infamous statement "Three generations of imbeciles is enough" (Lombardo 2001:252).

In Germany, experiments carried out on women in the concentration camps were to advance knowledge on the most effective method for mass sterilisation (Benedict & Georges 2006). However, the sterilisation of those deemed unfit was to ultimately constitute the lesser of the evils committed by the Nazi regime in favour of preserving the Aryan race.

Story 3.2

Maria Nordin

In 1943, Maria Nordin, a Swedish national, was identified as having subnormal intelligence after falling behind at school. She was diagnosed by the school doctor as being 'feeble-minded' and 'unable to raise children'. She was subsequently sterilised following an oophorectomy (ovary removal). In actual fact, the educational delay was caused by Maria's near-sightedness which meant that she could not read the blackboard.

> *I'll never forget when I was called into the headmistress's office . . . I was aware of it well before. I hid in the basement bathroom crying all by myself. I was thinking of killing myself, and I have been thinking of it ever since. But I never wanted to give them [the government] the satisfaction of getting rid of me.*

(Hyatt 1998:477)

Genocide

In 1920, Karl Binding and Alfred Hoche published the book *Permission for Destruction of Life Unworthy of Life* in which they questioned the responsibility of

Reader activity 3.3

Think about the human rights laws that exist within your own country and how they seek to protect you as a citizen. How accessible are such laws to people with learning disabilities in informing them of their rights?

the nation for maintaining the lives of those whose 'lives were unworthy of life' ('lebensunwertes leben') or those whose humanity was questionable (Burleigh 1994). While the book failed to generate widespread support, it was a significant milestone in events leading up to the extremist measures to be subsequently employed by the Nazi regime. In 1938, the father of a severely disabled child (family name 'Knauer') appealed directly to Hitler to permit the killing of the child. This incident has frequently been cited as having set the precedent for the systematic killing of those perceived as being of poor physical or intellectual constitution (Friedlander 1995) commencing in August 1939 with the children's euthanasia programme, 'Kinderacktion' (Berghs et al 2007). This programme targeted children (first all those under 3 and then subsequently all those under 16 years) with disabilities including idiocy, Down syndrome, microcephaly, hydrocephalus, spina bifida, all manner of deformities and paralysis (Benedict et al 2009). Such children were admitted to one of 30 special clinics (Kinderfachabteilungen) with the consent of their parents who believed that they would be provided with the most up to date specialist treatment available (Lifton 1988); it was tantamount to nothing more than a death sentence. It has been estimated that around 6000 children were killed under this programme either by starvation, active prescription of drugs such as luminal to suppress breathing or the administration of overdoses of morphine (Burleigh 2000). Certificates of death would indicate fictitious causes such as pneumonia or circulatory disorders (Benedict et al 2009).

In October 1939, the euthanasia programme was extended to incorporate adults and was famously code-named 'Operation T4' after the address of the Berlin Chancellery offices from which the campaign was being run (Friedlander 1995). Patients from institutions were selected for death and then transported to six killing centres based in existing psychiatric hospitals (Benedict & Kuhla 1999). Similarly to the Kinderacktion programme, adults were killed by lethal injection, exposure, sleeping tablets or, more commonly, by gassing with carbon monoxide in specially designed chambers (Lifton 1988). The T4 programme ran publicly until 1941 when it was forced to close due to public and religious opposition, although it was to unofficially continue in what is known as a 'wild or rampant' phase (Lagerwey 1999). T4 personnel were also deployed to continue killing sick and disabled prisoners in the concentration camps, a programme known as Aktion 14f13 (Friedlander 1995). Much attention has been given to the plight of Jewish prisoners in such camps, however in the last decade, attention has also turned to the plight of other groups including those with disabilities (see Story 3.3).

Benedict et al (2009) discuss the significance of the Nazi's employing the term euthanasia; while not a true reflection of the barbaric and untimely deaths of both children and adults, it was important in encouraging public acceptance of the programmes. They discuss the active employment of propaganda in which visibly disabled individuals

Story 3.3

The Ovitz Family

The Ovitz family were Romanian Jews and entertainers whose stage name, 'The Lilliput Troupe', was derived from the fact that 7 out of their 10 members were afflicted with a form of dwarfism known as 'pseudoachondroplasia'. In 1944, they were rounded up in their home village of Rozavela, loaded into cattle trucks and transported to Auschwitz-Birkenau. They survived the selection process; their size and number meant that they were singled out for the purposes of scientific investigation under the auspices of the notorious Dr Josef Mengele. Mengele was fascinated by both issues of hereditary (his studies on twins were infamous) and for 'freaks'. During their time in the camp, the Ovitz's were subjected to sustained and often painful experiments. In the words of Perla, the youngest member of the family:

> *He made never ending comparisons. He drew blood from our older dwarf sisters who were born to another mother, comparing it to ours to see if we were really from the same father. He compared our blood to that of our tall sisters to see in what way it was different – he couldn't stop wondering how such a high quota of dwarfs could be produced from tall mothers and one dwarf family. (p. 100)*
>
> (Koren & Negev 2004)

Undoubtedly the Ovitz family's disability and family lineage enabled their survival, and in January 1945, they were liberated along with thousands of other survivors from the camp.

were portrayed as suffering, encouraging the belief that their death would be merciful. Such beliefs were instrumental in enabling health and social care professionals to partake in activities that would normally be at odds with their personal and professional moral codes.

Role of professional groups

> *One may hang a copy of the Oath of Hippocrates in one's office but nobody pays any attention to it.*
>
> Karl Brandt, Head of the Children's Euthanasia programme (Burleigh 2000:388)

It is now widely acknowledged that the successful implementation of eugenic programmes was reliant on the skill and dedication of a range of professional people at the identification, certification/selection and implementation stages of the process. In addition to general accounts of the history of eugenics, there is a growing body of evidence that specifically seeks to explore the involvement of such individuals and groups. Wanhalla (2007) makes reference to the role of female social workers in New Zealand in the gathering of information with respect to the family, economic and personal histories of the defectives that they came across. In Canada, where the primary method of eugenic control was sterilisation, nurses were involved in the assessment and referral of patients and actual surgical procedures (Mansell & Hibberd 1998), while in America, teachers were charged with detecting feeble-minded children in their classes (Snyder & Mitchell 2002). In England, following the implementation of the Mental Deficiency Act (1913), doctors were responsible for the assessment and certification of mental defectives as a requirement of their institutionalisation (Potts & Fido 1991), while nurses were complicit in securing environments in which people were controlled and not encouraged to develop as individuals (Mitchell & Rafferty 2005). Yet, despite the evidence of professional involvement in countries across the Western world, it is the extremities of the actions of German health care professionals in the so-called 'euthanasia' programmes that have been the subject of significant academic enquiry.

Similarly to other countries, German health professionals were involved in eugenic programmes at all levels. Midwifes and doctors were required to report all children with observable disabilities while independent doctors were involved in the selection of those to be sterilised (Hoskins 2005) and those to be put to death (Benedict et al 2009). Kreuzershreibers, as they were known, marked medical records with a cross for death and a minus for a reprieve (Friedlander 1995). Doctors were also present on the arrival of trains at the concentration camps, selecting those able to work and those who were to go straight to the gas chambers (Lifton 1988). For some, the presence of a man in a white coat was deceiving and served to draw them into a false sense of security, as exemplified in the words of Perla Ovitz on awaiting the arrival Mengele:

> we went numb, then started thinking about the unknown man . . . if this was a graveyard, what was a doctor doing here?
>
> (Koren & Negev 2004:74)

While the actions of Nazi doctors have formed the focus of much academic inquiry (Lifton 1988), more recently attention has switched to the role of nurses in the process. Ost (2006:17) has attributed this surge in interest to the difficulty in fully understanding how a caring profession could become actively involved in processes that were the 'antithesis' of their caring role. Studies into the activities of this group have found that nurses were both directly and indirectly involved in the killing process. They transported patients to the killing centres, helped them undress, escorted them to the gas chambers, sometimes removing their bodies; they sorted through personal possessions of those who had been killed and labelled urns of ashes (Benedict 2003, Friedlander 1995). In other more notable cases, nurses were involved in the actual killing of patients (see Story 3.4). It has been estimated that German nurses were involved in the deaths of 5000 children and 70 000 handicapped adults (Friedlander 1995). Figure 3.5 shows nurses from the Hadamar Psychiatric Hospital that was one of the killing centres based in Germany.

It would be easy and, to some degree, conceptually simpler to purely attribute such actions to innate evilness, but such a conclusion on the one hand serves only to diminish the complexity of the actual decision-making processes behind the involvement of health and social care professionals in the atrocities, and on the other absolves us objective observers of the responsibility of knowing and understanding. Many authors are at pains to conclude that these perpetrators were not, in the main, monsters but ordinary people, yet it has been the tendency of contemporary professionals to view their historical counterparts as totally 'other' (Lagerwey 1999:760). From primary research utilising interviews with the nurses

Story 3.4

Luise E

Luise E was a nurse at the state hospital of Meseritz-Obrawalde (a town within the then Russian province of Pomerania). Initially charged with supervision of patients undertaking work therapy, she began to take part in the killings of patients within the hospitals in either late 1942 or late 1943 and was accused of killing 200 patients.

> *I have mentioned during previous questioning that I myself thought there was a true justification for the killings only in about one-half of the killings ordered. In my opinion, only those patients should have been killed who showed all signs of a very near end of their lives – maybe about three weeks or less until they would die, or other patients who had so many deep bedsores [decubitus ulcers]. They were suffering greatly and there were neither the necessary ointments and bandages nor any medication available for their condition. Or other patients who really were at the end of their human existence such as those who would eat their own faeces and needed continual observation for those and similar acts. I did not approve of killing patients who had totally lucid intervals between their attacks of insanity and those in whom I could see some hope for improvement. These were the cases which caused me the severe conflict that I have talked about*
>
> (Benedict et al 2007:786).

Luise E was acquitted of her crime along with 13 other defendants in March 1965.

(Reproduced with kind permission from Susan Benedict and *Nursing Ethics*)

involved and court testimonies from the Nuremberg trials (Benedict 2003, Benedict et al 2007, Harrison 2008, McFarland-Icke 1999, Steppe 1992), the emerging picture is a complex web of reasoning from which arise a number of consistent themes that have been employed as a framework for analysis, and include:

- obedience
- ideological commitment
- role of religion
- role of nursing education and the nursing professional organisations
- putative duress
- economic factors (Benedict & Kuhla 1999).

McKie (2004) has proffered the concept of duty as one which strongly guided the actions of nurses and can be linked to some of the themes listed above. For example, nurse education had instilled a sense of duty in nurses to be obedient (Benedict 2003). Obedience was an important professional characteristic and one that appeared to be upheld regardless of the nature of the request; in other countries, obedience was seen as synonymous with being a good nurse (Mansell & Hibberd 1998). By doing their duty, some reasoned that they had behaved morally (Berghs et al 2007):

> It never occurred to me not to follow the orders given to me. Just as soldiers on the front line had to do their duty, so did we. To follow orders given by the attending physician absolutely is one of the most important duties of a care giver. For this reason, the proviso that I would also have become a thief if it were ordered is beside the point. The orders given to me were within the field of my work and training.
>
> Margarete T (accused of 150 murders at Meseritz-Obrawalde psychiatric hospital) quoted in Benedict et al 2007:788

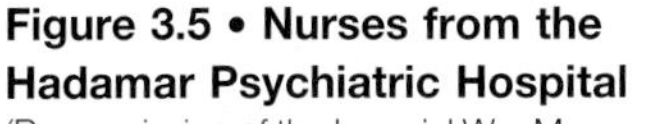

Figure 3.5 • Nurses from the Hadamar Psychiatric Hospital

(By permission of the Imperial War Museum. Image no. EA 621 38.)

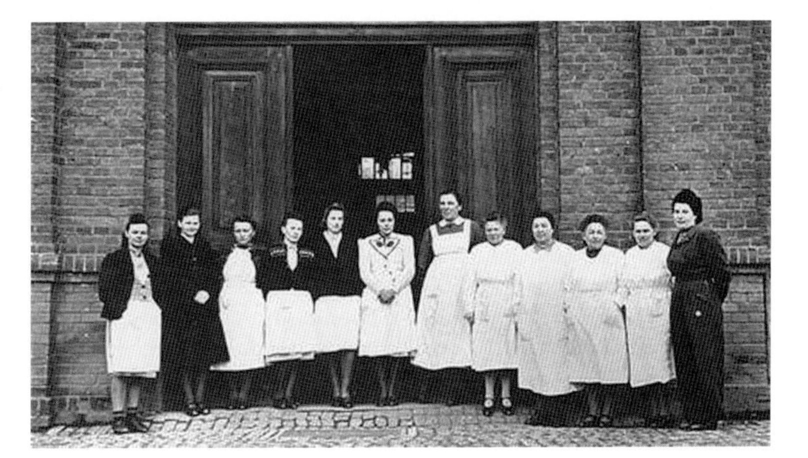

A sense of duty to the Fatherland and a commitment to an ideology that sought to place the needs of the Volk (collective people) over the needs of individuals were also important drivers for nurses involved in such atrocities (Berghs et al 2007). While the euthanasia programmes were never legally sanctioned, by obeying what many thought was the law was an example of a nurse behaving morally:

> Director Grabowski told us we had to help the senior nurses – it was too much for them. We also would have to give the injections. First, I refused and he said that there was no point in it because, being a civil servant of many year's standing, I would perform my duty, especially in times of war . . . I only did my duty, and I did everything on the orders of my superiors. The Director Grabowski always warned us of the Gestapo. He said he would inform the Gestapo if we didn't do what he ordered.
>
> Helene Wieczorek (accused of several hundred killings at Meseritz-Obrawalde Hospital) quoted in Benedict & Kuhla 1999:254–255

While fear of the consequences of not abiding by orders was cited as a reason for obedience, there is little evidence to indicate those resisting came to any harm (Lagerwey 1999). While obedience features significantly in the personal defence of nurses, it has been argued that some accounts suggest that nurses were not purely passive recipients of orders but had a sense of moral responsibility, believing that what they were committing were acts of mercy (Ost 2006):

> Through my daily dealings with them [the mentally ill] I came to the genuine conviction that for many of them life no longer meant anything and that death would be a release for them. I never had the feeling that I had anything to criticize myself for because I had placed myself at the disposal of the euthanasia program.
>
> Pauline Kniessler (accused of murders at Hadamar Psychiatric Hospital) quoted in Harrison 2008:35

For further details on the role of nurses in the euthanasia programme, the reader is directed to the work of Susan Benedict and colleagues (1999, 2003, 2006, 2007).

Eugenics today

Following the Second World War, there was a sharp downturn in the popularity of eugenics across Western countries. The atrocities committed by the Nazis resulted in countries distancing themselves from its legacy while both flaws in the research methods employed by eugenicists and evidence to suggest the deliberate doctoring of results were serving to cast considerable doubt over the legitimacy of previously accepted conclusions about the extent of the actual threat posed by the feeble-minded (Block 2000); conclusions that had undoubtedly led to the institutionalisation, forced sterilisation and murder of this group. Eugenics was beginning to acquire the status of 'pseudo-science' reflecting naked class interests (Macnicol 1992). Moreover, mainline eugenic thinking was starting to give way to more liberal leanings in the form of reform eugenics that recognised the importance of the social and physical environment on the manifestation of a person's physical and intellectual capabilities (Soloway 1998). Yet the desire to pursue eugenics has never gone away, remaining in society, hidden behind more subtle guises and as such termed varyingly as back-door eugenics (Duster 1990) or soft eugenics (Beck-Gernsheim, 1990).

Parallels between the field of contemporary genetics and new eugenics appear to monopolise this debate with researchers citing the significance of developments such as pre-implementation diagnosis (King 1999). The ongoing refinement of prenatal diagnostic methods to reduce the number of false-negative and false-positive results in the case of testing for conditions such as Down syndrome (see NICE 2003) have also come under scrutiny. Contemporary discourse with regard to this issue typically reveals two main threads of argument: first, that the development and implementation of such interventions facilitates choice and informed decision making for individuals (NICE 2008); second, that such developments represent subversive eugenic attempts to eliminate those groups within society that are considered to be undesirable (Vassy 2006).

Important as it may be, the predominance of discourse around new genetics and eugenics precludes debate around other contemporary practices involving people with learning disabilities that could be equally questionable in terms of their true motivations, practices that while clearly contravening the human rights of individuals are slowly becoming the accepted norm because they are being publicised as being in the 'best interests' of individuals. Take, for example, the continuing employment of forced sterilisation of disabled people, or what is beginning to be publicised by Australian opponents as 'sterilisation by stealth' and 'unnecessary and dehumanising violence' (Dowse 2004–2005). In a recent study by Stansfield et al (2007) that explored the sterilisation of men and women with learning disabilities in England and Wales between 1988 and 1999, it was found that compulsory sterilisation was often sanctioned by the courts in the case of individuals where the development of a sexual relationship would be unlikely or the rationale provided would lend itself to less radical interventions. More concerning in the findings of this study is reference to six individuals for whom court agreement for sterilisation was not sought, suggesting that they weren't even afforded their basic rights to protection. Following on from this is the issue of the rights of people with learning disabilities to be or become parents, with some arguing that eugenic beliefs are evident in the literature pertaining to this subject (Woodhouse 1997). To what extent do eugenic beliefs therefore inform the actions of professionals charged with the removal of children from people with learning disabilities on the basis of a diagnostic label (Baum & Burns 2007)?

Another example of where an act of beneficence or malevolence is difficult to discern is in the case of the decisions made by health care professionals not to administer life-saving treatment to children and young people with learning disabilities. In the UK alone, there have been a number of high-profile media cases where the actions of health professionals have been placed under scrutiny such as in the case of David Glass (Day 2004) and Charlotte Wyatt (BBC News 2006). In both cases, do not resuscitate orders were placed on the children and both without the consensual agreement of their families; in the former case, this was subsequently found to have breached Article 8 of the European Convention on Human Rights (1950) (right to respect for one's 'private and family life, his home and his correspondence'), while the latter was the subject of considerable legal dispute. In both these cases, those in charge of the children's care are cited as saying that they were acting in the best interests of the children by not subjecting them to further unnecessary treatment. While this stance is not one that can either be confirmed or disputed, it is undoubtedly the case that such decisions were informed by subjective opinions on the quality of life of the individuals concerned. It could be assumed that in both cases, the doctors regarded the children to not have a life that constituted a life worth living, a belief that legitimised the killings of both children and adults with learning disabilities in Nazi Germany. There is evidence to suggest that this concept is also being applied to children with disabilities that are not considered life-threatening and are in fact ameliorative to treatment such as children with cleft palates being aborted in the late stages of a woman's pregnancy (BBC News 2002).

It remains uncertain as to what extent such decisions are made on the basis of a cost–benefit analysis, in the context of limited health care resources; an argument rather crudely alluded to in the press coverage following the separation of Charlotte Wyatt's parents (Sears & Newling 2006). What is known, however, is that assumptions about the value of the lives of people with learning disabilities in comparison to their non-disabled counterparts is being used to determine the distribution of finite resources such as heart and lung transplants for people with Down syndrome (Lashmar 2000).

Reader activity 3.4

Read the story of the 'Pillow Angel' at http://news.bbc.co.uk/1/hi/world/americas/6229799.stm. Consider the arguments presented for allowing Ashley to undergo such radical and invasive treatment. Do you feel them to be justified? If you were a professional working with this family, what sort of advice or guidance might you be giving them to help protect Ashley's human rights?

The importance of acknowledging and accepting the past

So do contemporary practices such as those discussed above constitute eugenic practices? The fact is that there are no easy answers to this question and any assessment of such would require a full exploration of the social and political context in which they are being employed. What is known, however, is that significant progress has been made in the UK since its initial brush with eugenics to support people with learning disabilities to exercise their human rights in becoming valued members of their communities, to have personal relationships and to become parents; rights that are now enshrined in policy documents guiding service developments in different countries (DH 2001, Department of Health, Social Services and Public Safety 2005, Scottish Executive 2000, Welsh Office 2002). In saying this, Holmes (1996) has argued that contemporary societal conditions that include a general loss of equilibrium, purpose and belonging could precipitate a resurgence of eugenics. O'Mathúna (2006) has specifically alluded to economic pressures within health services that may lead to the types of questions posed in the early 20th century with respect to the resources needed to sustain the lives of certain groups. Historians leading the research into the actions of health and social care professionals at the height of the early eugenic era are united in their belief that those working with vulnerable people today, despite the existence of professional codes, are not immune to changing political demands and may unwittingly or wittingly become involved in acts that contravene personal and professional perspectives on morality (Holmes 1996, Ion & Beer 2003). In order to limit the chance of this occurring, it has been argued that health and social care professionals must be constantly displaying a critical questioning stance to the ethical and moral soundness of what is being asked of them (Berghs et al 2007, McKie 2004). Care delivery should not be seen as a passive response to orders from higher authorities, rather professionals should be fully engaged with the decision-making process (Berghs et al 2007). It is argued that a moral assessment of professional behaviours and interventions can only be achieved with an acceptance and understanding of the past actions of the predecessors of contemporary health and social care professionals in addition to collective support for ethical practice (Lagerwey 1999). In Chapter 5 in this book, Ruth Northway discusses different ethical frameworks that can support this process of assessment. Coupled with this is a responsibility of individual professionals to harness the power of personal reflection to aid in an honest exploration of personal and professional attitudes and values towards people with learning disabilities. Researchers in the field have found that eugenic attitudes prevail among both mainstream health service providers (McConkey & Truesdale 2000), including those charged with delivering genetic advice (Wertz 1998) and providers of specialist services to this group (Atherton 2004). Wolfensberger (1972) believes that such attitudes often exist at an unconscious level and it has been asserted that professionals need support through processes such as clinical supervision to bring such attitudes to a level of self-awareness so that they can be positively managed (Atherton 2004). Finally, O'Mathúna proposes that by recognising the value of inherent human dignity for all will act as ballast in counterbalancing the potential for placing a monetary value on life. The centrality of this value in the provision of care to people with learning disabilities is discussed in Chapter 4.

Conclusion

> *Even if we do not admit an obligation to understand such profound human events, and I believe we ought, we should at least make sense of them in order to create safeguards that will minimise the chances of nurses being complicitous in similar events, now or in the future.*
>
> (Holmes 1996:7)

This chapter has sought to introduce the reader to a historical period when the individual rights of people with learning disabilities were superseded in favour of the overall health of a nation. Eugenics provided a scientific basis upon which to justify a range of extreme interventions that sought to limit the existence of those who were deemed unworthy of life. While traditional eugenics has given way to an egalitarian approach to the lives of people with learning disabilities, which on the surface supports their right to life, marriage and parenthood, new eugenics exists in a much less discernible way. As was the case in the past, health and social care professionals are not immune to social and political demands that may see them revisiting care practices that contravene the basic human rights of those whose care they are responsible for. As such they must be constantly aware and be prepared to sacrifice duty for the protection of others.

References

Alaszweski, A., 1988. From villains to victims. In: Leighton, A. (Ed.), Mental handicap in the community. Woodhead-Faulkner, Cambridge.

Atherton, H.L., 2004. Eugenic attitudes amongst professionals in learning disability services. Hull University, Hull.

Baum, S., Burns, J., 2007. Mothers with learning disabilities: experiences and meanings of losing custody of their children. Tizard Learning Disability Review 12 (3), 3–14.

BBC News, 2002. Police examine 'cleft palate' abortion. Available at: http://news.bbc.co.uk/1/hi/england/2367917.stm (accessed 12.07.10.).

BBC News, 2006. New ruling as Charlotte worsens. Available at:

http://news.bbc.co.uk/1/hi/health/4748008.stm (accessed 12.07.10.).

Beck-Gernsheim, E., 1990. The changing duties of parents: from education to bioengineering? International Social Science Journal 126, 451–463.

Benedict, S., 2003. Killing while caring: the nurses of Hadamar. Issues Ment. Health Nurs. 24, 59–79.

Benedict, S., Georges, J.M., 2006. Nurses and the sterilization experiments of Auschwitz: a postmodernist perspective. Nurs. Inq. 13 (4), 277–288.

Benedict, S., Kuhla, J., 1999. Nurses' participation in the euthanasia programs of Nazi Germany. West J. Nurs. Res. 21 (2), 246–263.

Benedict, S., Caplan, A., LaFrenz Page, T., 2007. Duty and 'euthanasia': the nurses of Meseritz-Obrawalde. Nurs. Ethics 14 (6), 781–794.

Benedict, S., Shields, L., O'Donnell, A.J., 2009. Children's 'euthanasia' in Nazi Germany. J. Pediatr. Nurs. 24 (6), 506–516.

Berghs, M., Dierckx de Casterlé, B., Gastmans, C., 2007. Practices of responsibility and nurses during the euthanasia programs of Nazi Germany: a discussion paper. Int. J. Nurs. Stud. 44, 845–854.

Bix, A.S., 1997. Experiences and voices of eugenics field-workers: 'women's work' in biology. Soc. Stud. Sci. 27, 625–668.

Blacker, C.P., 1950. Eugenics in retrospect and prospect: the Galton Lecture, 1945. The Eugenics Society/Cassell and Company, London.

Block, P., 2000. Sexuality, fertility and danger: twentieth century images of women with cognitive disabilities. Sex. Disabil. 18 (4), 239–254.

Broberg, G., Roll-Hansen, N., 2005. Eugenics and the welfare state: sterilization policy in Denmark, Sweden, Norway and Finland. Michigan State University Press, East Lansing.

Burleigh, M., 1994. Death and deliverance: 'euthanasia in Germany 1900–1945'. Cambridge University Press, Cambridge.

Burleigh, M., 2000. The Third Reich: a new history. Macmillan, London.

Cairney, R., 1996. Democracy was never intended for degenerates: Alberta's flirtation with eugenics comes back to haunt it. Can. Med. Assoc. J. 155 (6), 789–792.

Carlson, E., 2001. The unfit: a history of a bad idea. Cold Spring Harbor Laboratory Press, Cold Spring Harbour, NY.

Darwin, C., 1859. The origin of species. Wordsworth Editions Ltd, Hertfordshire, 1998.

Day, E., 2004. Do not resuscitate and don't bother consulting the family. Available at: http://www.telegraph.co.uk/news/uknews/1456791/Do-Not-Resuscitate-and-dont-bother-consulting-the-family.html (accessed 12.07.10.).

Department of Health, 2001. Valuing people: a new strategy for the 21st century. Department of Health, London.

Department of Health, 2003. Our inheritance, our future: realising the potential of genetics in the NHS. Department of Health, London.

Department of Health, Social Services and Public Safety, 2005. Equal lives. DHSSPS, Belfast.

Dikötter, F., 1998. Race culture: recent perspectives on the history of eugenics. Am. Hist. Rev. 103 (2), 467–479.

Dowse, L., 2005. Sterilising by stealth? Safeguarding the human rights of girls with disabilities in Australia. Australia Health Consumer. Available at: https://www.chf.org.au/pdfs/ahc/ahc-2004-3-sterilising-by-stealth.pdf (accessed 12.07.10.).

Duster, T., 1990. Backdoor to eugenics. Routledge, New York.

Friedlander, H., 1995. The origins of Nazi genocide: from euthanasia to the final solution. University of North Carolina Press, North Carolina.

Galton, D., 2002. Eugenics: the future of human life in the 21st century. Abacus, London.

Garton, S., 1994. Sound minds and healthy bodies: reconsidering eugenics in Australia 1914–1940. Australain Historical Studies 26 (103), 163–181.

Garver, K.L., Garver, B., 1991. Eugenics: past, present and the future. Am. J. Hum. Genet. 49, 1109–1118.

Gerodetti, N., 2006. Eugenic family politics and social democrats: 'positive' eugenics and marriage advice bureaus. The Journal of Historical Sociology 19 (3), 217–244.

Ghosh, P., 2010. Study identifies 'many more' autism genes. Available at: http://news.bbc.co.uk/1/hi/health/10275332.stm (accessed 12.07.10.).

Goddard, H.H., 1912. The Kallikak Family. Macmillan, New York.

Harrison, S.M., 2008. Female killers: nurses and the implementation of the Nazi euthanasia program at Hadamar, 1941–1945. V D M Verlag Dr. Müller, Saarbrücken.

Hemminki, E., Rasimus, A., Forssas, E., 1997. Sterilisation in Finland: from eugenics to contraception. Soc. Sci. Med. 45 (12), 1875–1884.

Holmes, C.A., 1996. Nazism and nursing: a comment on relevance. Int. Hist. Nurs. J. 2 (1), 5–24.

Hoskins, S.A., 2005. Nurses and national socialism – a moral dilemma: one historical example of a route to euthanasia. Nurs. Ethics 12 (1), 79–91.

Hyatt, S., 1998. A shared history of shame: Sweden's four decade policy of forced sterilization and the eugenics movement in the United States. Indiana International & Comparative Law Review 8 (2), 475–503.

Ion, R.M., Beer, M.D., 2003. Valuing the past: the importance of an understanding of the history of psychiatry for healthcare professionals, service users and carers. Int. J. Ment. Health Nurs. 12, 237–242.

Jackson, M., 1995. Images of deviance: visual representations of mental defectives in early twentieth-century medical texts. British Journal of the History of Science 28, 319–337.

Jones, G., 1998. The theoretical foundations of eugenics. In: Peel, R.A. (Ed.), Essays in the history of eugenics. The Galton Institute, London.

Judge, C., van Brummelen, F., 2002. Kew Cottages: the world of Dolly Stainer. Spectrum, Melbourne.

Kerr, A., Shakespeare, T., 2002. Genetic politics: from eugenics to genome. New Clarion Press, Cheltenham.

Kevles, D.J., 1995. In the name of eugenics. Harvard University Press, London.

Keynes, R., 2002. Annie's box: Charles Darwin, his daughter and human evolution. Fourth, London.

King, D.S., 1999. Preimplementation genetic diagnosis and the 'new' eugenics. J. Med. Ethics 25, 176–182.

Koren, Y., Negev, R., 2004. In our hearts we were giants. Carroll & Graf, New York.

Lagerwey, M., 1999. Nursing ethics at Hadamar. Qual. Health Res. 9 (6), 759–772.

Lashmar, P., 2000. Health service accused of ignorance and bias against Down's syndrome sufferers. Available at: http://www.independent.co.uk/life-style/health-and-families/health-news/health-service-accused-of-ignorance-and-bias-against-downs-syndrome-sufferers-698583.html (accessed 19.07.10.).

Leonard, T., 2009. Origins of the myth of Social Darwinism: the ambiguous legacy of Richard Hofstadter's Social Darwinsim in American thought. Journal of Economic Behaviour & Organisation 71 (1), 37–51.

Lerner, B.H., Rothman, D.J., 1995. Medicine and the Holocaust: learning more of the lessons. Ann. Intern. Med. 122 (10), 793–794.

Lifton, R.J., 1988. The Nazi doctors: medical killing and the psychology of genocide. Basic Books, New York.

Lombardo, P.A., 2001. Pedigrees, propaganda, and paranoia: family studies in a historical context. J. Contin. Educ. Health Prof. 21, 247–255.

McConkey, R., Trusedale, M., 2000. Reactions of nurses and therapists in mainstream health services to contact people who have learning disabilities. J. Adv. Nurs. 32 (1), 158–163.

McFarland-Icke, B.R., 1999. Nurses in Nazi Germany: moral choice in history. Princeton University Press, New Jersey.

McKie, A., 2004. 'The Demolition of a Man': Lessons From holocaust literature for the teaching of nursing ethics. Nurs. Ethics 11 (2), 138–149.

Macnicol, J., 1992. The voluntary sterilization campaign in Britain 1918–39. Journal of the History of Sexuality 2 (3), 422–438.

Mansell, D., Hibberd, J., 1998. 'We picked the wrong one to sterilise': the role of nursing in the eugenics movement in Alberta, 1920–1940. Int. Hist. Nurs. J. 3 (4), 4–10.

Mazumdar, P.M.H., 1998. The Galton Lecture 1998 – Eugenics: the pedigree years. In: Peel, R.A. (Ed.), The Galton Institute. Human Pedigree Studies, London.

Mitchell, D., Rafferty, A.M., 2005. I don't think they ever really wanted to know anything about us: oral history interviews with learning disability nurses. Oral History 33 (1), 77–87.

Mostert, M.P., 2002. Useless eaters: disability as a genocidal marker in Nazi Germany. Journal of Special Education 36 (3), 155–168.

National Institute for Clinical Excellence, 2003. Antenatal care: routine care for the healthy pregnant woman. NICE, London.

National Institute for Clinical Excellence, 2008. Antenatal care: routine care for the healthy pregnant woman. NICE, London.

O'Mathúna, D.P., 2006. Human dignity in the Nazi era: implications for contemporary bioethics. BMC Med. Ethics 7 (2) Available at: http://www.biomedcentral.com/1472-6939/7/2 (accessed 19.07.10.).

Ost, S., 2006. Doctors and nurses of death: a case study of eugenically motivated killing under the Nazi 'euthanasia' programme. Liverpool Law Rev. 27, 5–30.

Park, D.C., Radford, J.P., 1998. From the case files: reconstructing a history of involuntary sterilisation. Disability and Society 13 (3), 317–342.

Pernick, M.S., 1997. Eugenics and public health in American history. Am. J. Public Health 87 (11), 1767–1772.

Potts, M., Fido, R., 1991. A fit person to be removed: personal accounts of life in a mental deficiency institution. Northcote House, UK.

Race, D., 1995. Historical development of service provision. In: Malin, N. (Ed.), Services for people with learning disabilities. Routledge, London.

Radford, J.P., 1991. Sterilization versus segregation: control of the 'feebleminded', 1900–1938. Soc. Sci. Med. 33 (4), 449–458.

Ridley, M., 1998. Eugenics and liberty. Prospect 33, 44–47.

Roper, A.G., 1913. Ancient eugenics. B H Blackwell, Oxford.

Scottish Executive, 2000. Same as you? A review of services for people with learning disabilities. Scottish Executive, Edinburgh.

Sears, N., Newling, D., 2006. Baby Charlotte faces foster care as parents can't cope. Available at: http://www.dailymail.co.uk/news/article-410559/Baby-Charlotte-faces-foster-care-parents-cope.html (accessed 12.07.10.).

Selden, S., 2005. Transforming better babies into fitter families: archival resources and the history of the American eugenics movement, 1908–1930. Proc. Am. Philos. Soc. 149 (2), 199–225.

Snyder, S.L., Mitchell, D.T., 2002. Out of the ashes of eugenics: diagnostic regimes in the United States and the making of a disability minority. Patterns of Prejudice 36 (1), 79–103.

Sofair, A.N., Kaldjian, L.C., 2000. Eugenic sterilization and a qualified Nazi analogy: the United States and Germany, 1930–1945. Ann. Intern. Med. 132 (4), 312–319.

Soloway, R.A., 1998. From mainline to reform eugenics – Leonard Darwin and C P Blacker. In: Peel, R.A. (Ed.), Essays in the History of Eugenics. The Galton Institute, London.

Stansfield, A.J., Holland, A.J., Clare, I.C.H., 2007. The sterilisation of people with intellectual disabilities in England and Wales during the period 1988–1999. J. Intellect. Disabil. Res. 51 (8), 569–579.

Steppe, H., 1992. Nursing in Nazi Germany. West J. Nurs. Res. 14 (6), 744–753.

Stubblefield, A., 2007. "Beyond the pale": tainted whiteness, cognitive disability, and eugenic sterilisation. Hypatia 22 (2), 162–181.

Thomson, M., 1998. The problem of mental deficiency. Clarendon Press, Oxford.

Tredgold, A.F., 1909. The feeble-minded – a social danger. Eugen. Rev. 1, 97–104.

Tredgold, A.F., 1952. A textbook on mental deficiency. Baillière Tindall, London.

Vassy, C., 2006. From a genetic innovation to mass health programmes: the diffusion of Down's syndrome prenatal screening and diagnostic techniques in France. Soc. Sci. Med. 63, 2041–2051.

Waller, J.C., 2001. Ideas of hereditary, reproduction and eugenics in Britain, 1800–1875. Stud. Hist. Philos. Biol. Biomed. Sci. 32 (3), 457–489.

Wanhalla, A., 2007. To 'better the breed of men': women and eugenics in New Zealand, 1900–1935. Women's History Review 16 (2), 163–182.

Ward, L., 2002. Whose right to choose? The 'new' genetics, prenatal testing and people with learning difficulties. Critical Public Health 12 (2), 187–200.

Welsh Office, 2002. Fulfilling the promises. Welsh Assembly, Cardiff.

Wennerberg, T., 1997. Sterilization and propaganda. New Left Review 226, 146–153.

Wertz, D.C., 1998. Eugenics is alive and well: a survey of genetic professionals around the world. Science in Context 11 (3–4), 493–510.

Wolfensberger, W., 1972. The principle of normalisation in human management services. National Institute of Mental Retardation, Toronto.

Woodhouse, A.E., 1997. Parents with learning disabilities: does everyone have the right to have children? Journal of Learning Disabilities for Nursing, Health and Social Care 1 (3), 141–146.

Further reading

Ben-Sefer, E., 2006. Lessons from the past for contemporary Australian nursing students: the Nazi euthanasia program. Nurse Educ. Pract. 6, 31–39.

Bryant, M.S., 2005. Confronting the 'Good Death': Nazi Euthanasia on Trial 1945–1953. University Press of Colorado, Colorado.

Evans, S.E., 2004. Forgotten crimes: the Holocaust and people with disabilities. Ivan R Dee, Chicago.

Jones, G., 1992. Eugenics in Ireland: the Belfast Eugenics Society 1911–15. Irish Historical Studies xxviii (109), 81–95.

Koch, L., 2006. Eugenic sterilisation in Scandinavia. The European Legacy 11 (3), 299–309.

Malacrida, C., 2006. Contested memories: efforts of the powerful to silence former inmates' histories of life in an institution for 'mental defectives. Disability and Society 21 (5), 397–410.

Maxwell, A., 2010. Picture Imperfect: Photography and Eugenics 1879–1940. Sussex Academic Press, Sussex.

Mitchell, D., Snyder, S., 2003. The Eugenic Atlantic: race, disability, and the making of an international eugenic science 1800–1945. Disability and Society 18 (7), 843–864.

Rembis, M.A., 2009. (Re) Defining disability in the 'genetic' age': behavioural genetics, 'new' eugenics and the future of impairment. Disability and Society 24 (5), 585–597.

Useful addresses

Image Archive on the American Eugenics Movement, http://www.eugenicsarchive.org/eugenics/.

Memorial and Museum Auschwitz-Birkenau, http://en.auschwitz.org.pl/m/.

Steinhof Hospital, Vienna, http://www.gedenkstaettesteinhof.at/.

Holocaust Education and Archive Research Team, http://www.holocaustresearchproject.org/.

Schloss Hartheim, Alkoven, Upper Austria, http://www.schloss-hartheim.at.

Values-based support

4

Malcolm Richardson

CHAPTER CONTENTS

KEY ISSUES

- A range of values underpin the provision of good-quality support for people with learning disabilities
- Human dignity is the core value from which all other values stem; it is non-negotiable and immutable
- Health care professionals have a duty to facilitate human flourishing and the achievement of self-actualisation
- Promoting citizenship through person-centred approaches is fundamental to good practice
- Working in partnership and forging alliances with people with learning disabilities and their families are key to promoting health and addressing disabling barriers
- Changes in the values afforded to people with learning disabilities have been reflected in the different philosophies that have informed the care and support for this group

Introduction

The respect I bear others or which another can claim from me, is the acknowledgement of the dignity of another man, i.e., a worth that has no price, no equivalent for which the object of value could be exchanged. Judging something to have no worth is contempt.

(Immanuel Kant 1724–1804)

This chapter explores a range of key values that underpin good-quality support to people with learning disabilities. Beginning with the concept of human dignity, it demonstrates how the valuing of human dignity becomes the core value from which all other values stem. It then moves on to specifically consider the individual values of person-centredness, citizenship, partnership and inclusion.

Values rooted in the concept of human dignity have radically altered society's responses to people with learning disabilities, taking it from a world where people perceived to be different were largely excluded from mainstream social, educational and economic opportunities towards one in which the inclusion of disabled people in all aspects of citizenship, social, educational and economic activities is promoted. Such a shift is evident in the different philosophies that have informed the delivery of care and support to this group; this chapter considers both the theory of normalisation and inclusion.

What are values?

The values that support contemporary best practice in relation to people with learning disabilities need to be defined and examined. The *Oxford English Dictionary* (2010 online) offers several definitions of the word *value*. The following example suffices for the purposes of this chapter:

> To consider of worth or importance; to rate high; to esteem; to set store by . . . To commend or praise (to another).

Hence, the values individuals, groups or a society rate highly or esteem are those that are most likely to be implemented and commended for others to share and act accordingly. Therefore, the dominant values held towards people with learning disabilities will determine how most individuals, groups or societies respond to people with learning disabilities. However, any given value or set of values may not necessarily be shared by everyone. For example, people may possess some opposing values such as between members of political parties. Hence, values may be shared or opposed by some few, or by more and sometimes many more people. Additionally, values are not fixed; they may or may not endure the test of time for a whole variety of reasons such as the acquisition of new scientific knowledge, personal life experiences and changes occurring in attitudes, fads or fashionable thinking. Values may therefore change, mutate or simply fade away. That values may be subject to significant changes over time has therefore been the case for some of the values which underpin learning disability support services and the people working within them (Box 4.1).

Reader activity 4.1

Consider the selection of quotations about people with learning disabilities provided in Box 4.1 that relate to people with learning disabilities. What values did or do they represent? Note the changes in terminology–terms such as idiot, feeble-minded, defectives and mentally handicapped were used in the past. Are the messages they attempt to convey evident today?

Box 4.1

Examples of the changing nature of values in relation to people with learning disabilities

Date: 1846

"An idiot is endowed with a moral nature and is influenced by the same things as the rest of the community." (Seguin 1846, cited in Potts & Fido 1991:1)

Date: 1912

"The feeble-minded are a parasitic, predatory class, never capable of self-support or of managing their own affairs. The great majority ultimately become public charges in some form. They cause unutterable sorrow at home and are a menace and danger to the community. Feeble-minded women are almost invariably immoral, and if at large usually become carriers of venereal disease or give birth to children who are as defective as themselves. The feeble-minded woman who marries is twice as prolific as the normal woman."

"Every feeble-minded person, especially the high-grade imbecile, is a potential criminal, needing only the proper environment in which to express such. The unrecognised imbecile is a most dangerous element in the community." (Fernald 1912, cited in Beacock 1992:405).

Date: 1927

"As new institutions will, we hope, be gradually springing up throughout the country, the difficulty of obtaining suitable and trained staff will become a question of ever greater importance than it has been in the past and we have been greatly exercising our minds as to how the difficulty is to be met. The nature of the work is such that unless the candidate has an inborn love of children, and all defectives of whatever age are in reality children, he or she will never be permanently suited to the duties." (Board of Control 1927, cited in Mitchell 1998:47)

Date: 1978

"50 000 citizens of this country are living in hospitals for the mentally handicapped [sic.]. 20 000 of them . . . for 20 years or more . . . Many thousands of them do not need to be in hospital at all. Some look upon the hospital as their home . . . But for others, hospital is a prison without walls . . . where they must remain because there is nowhere else for them to live and nothing for them to do outside the hospital . . ." (Mittler 1978).

Date: 2001

"Nothing about us without us . . . All services should include people with learning difficulties in everything they do. This is not just one person as a token but several people who can support each other . . . This includes: government, health services, employment, social services, housing, housing associations, service purchasers, service providers, inspection, and anyone else!" (Department of Health Strategy User Group 2001)

Continued

Box 4.1

Examples of the changing nature of values in relation to people with learning disabilities—cont'd

Date: 2009

"Our investigation reports illustrate some significant and distressing failures in service across both health and social care, leading to situations in which people with learning disabilities experienced prolonged suffering and inappropriate care. Our investigations found maladministration, service failure and unremedied injustice in relation to a number, but not all, of the NHS bodies and local councils involved. In some cases we concluded that there had been maladministration and service failure for disability related reasons. We also found in some cases that the public bodies concerned had failed to live up to human rights principles, especially those of dignity and equality . . . Our findings contrast markedly with the first principle of the recently published NHS Constitution for England and Wales, which says that 'The NHS provides a comprehensive service, available to all irrespective of gender, race, disability, age, sexual orientation, religion or belief. It has a duty to each and every individual it serves and must respect their human rights'." (Parliamentary and Health Service Ombudsman 2009)

So if values are changeable, what endurable feature or features exist upon which we may set our values, particularly those that are worthwhile when supporting people with learning disabilities? Such a feature would have to forever outlive the fads and fashions that have shaped, sustained and then changed so many of the values that Western societies and organisations have expressed in relation to people with learning disabilities, both now and in the fairly recent past. As will be demonstrated, only one feature has the resilience to withstand this test; human dignity.

Human dignity – the heart of human flourishing

It is an odd-sounding word, dignity; possessing an almost stuffy 'ring'. But there it is: "... the dignity of another man, i.e., a worth that has no price, no equivalent for which the object of value could be exchanged" (Immanuel Kant 1724–1804). In other words, dignity is non-negotiable, the immutable elementary particle of every human being. You and I have it and so does everyone else and in equal measure. So no matter what happens to any of us, human dignity belongs to each of us just as much as if it were imprinted in our genes. And although it is of course possible to deny that a person has dignity, as for example oppressors, murderers and tyrants have attempted throughout the ages, and as occurred during the Nazi Holocaust, we know that the survivors of such atrocities, immensely traumatised as they may be, emerge with all of their dignity intact, regardless of the horrors and atrocities they have endured.

Therefore, if one is to practice within a health or social care context, respect for human dignity, which by definition has no price, no equivalent of exchange, must, I suggest, be the fundamental value from which all other values follow. The Royal College of Nursing (RCN) places dignity at the heart of its activities, and the document *Dignity in Health Care for People with Learning Disabilities* (RCN 2009) contains extensive guidance to which the reader is directed.

Of what then does our human dignity comprise? I do not propose any definitive answer to this question, but rather suggest that our human dignity is the expression of that which makes each of us uniquely human and thus different from every other human being. Hence, when our dignity is being respected, our individual uniqueness can flourish, and this flourishing applies at all points in human life, from the moment of our birth right up to the moment of our death. For even in dying we retain our dignity. These things are evident because throughout our species we are each different and these differences unfold as we begin to develop and progress along our journey through life as biological, psychological and social beings. Abraham Maslow (1943, 1954, 1962) described this as a journey towards self-actualisation, but we self-actualise through the flourishing of our potential all the way along life's journey; not as an end result.

> Through the flourishing of our potential for development we become what our nature and choices allow us to become, and who we become is unique.
>
> (Husted & Husted 2008:58).

Our uniqueness develops in more complex ways reflecting our different circumstances, times and experiences as our life progresses. Hence, each of us has a right to flourish as a human being; to growth and development, to pursue our destiny and realise our full nature (Husted & Husted 2008).

These concepts of human dignity and human flourishing, in Western philosophy, date back at least to the Ancient Greeks and Socrates (Husted & Husted 2008) but equivalent philosophies are probably universal throughout the world and all its continents. For example, in China and some other areas of Asia, Confucius (c. 551 BC) professed a form of respect for human dignity drawing from innate human virtues that warrant the practice of Jen, which is benevolence and humanness towards others, and Xin, honesty and trustworthiness (Peking University 2004/5). Even a cursory reading of Brown's (1971) seminal work on the fairly recent history of the North American Indian is likely to leave its reader humbled by the immense dignity frequently displayed by those peoples in the face of their exterminators and oppressors. The great religions of the world also pay their respects. For example, Siddiqi (undated) explains that within Islam, dignity may be expressed at a personal level by: a lack of arrogance, self-conceit, haughtiness or false pride, and a respect for the nobility and honour of being a person (Karamah and Izzah); respect for the intrinsic value of others and yourself (Qeemah); uniqueness or distinction of each individual (Shraf); and being the best that you can be (Fadilah or virtue).

From a Hindu perspective, Godrej (2005) argues that, despite its caste system, within certain Hindu traditions the notion of human flourishing places important emphasis upon spiritual fulfilment and liberation. The Hindu theory of the Purusharthas suggests that even a life which is spiritually orientated and uncluttered by worldly possessions, without the opportunities for the fulfilment of worldly pleasures, the acquisition of some wealth and the expression of political power, might be somewhat less than a complete or fulfilled life; this notion is visible in Gandhi's political thinking.

So the concept of human dignity has a universal recognition and may be seen to encompass a range of features, yet at the most plain and simple level, when someone says that you are behaving in an undignified way, they are implying that you are doing something that in some way diminishes yourself. That you are not expressing your best attributes, not being quite yourself and not fully expressing that flourishing self that the dignity with which you were born is capable of expressing. Similarly, someone treating a person with a learning disability in an undignified way undermines that person's self so that the person with the learning disability is less able to flourish, direct and control events.

Therefore, although we are all born with an equal and full measure of dignity which remains immutable (i.e. it does not change into something other than dignity), our dignity can potentially be repressed, distorted, compressed or stretched thinly. Sometimes such distortion may be of our own doing, for example when we behave somewhat badly towards ourselves or others, but more serious distortions to one's dignity are likely to result from the direct experience of undignified and oppressive happenings that repress our individual flourishing and thereby diminish true self-expression. The history of people with learning disabilities has, for more than a century, been a history of eugenic oppression which, at its most powerful, sought to extinguish life itself (see Ch. 3). But the resilience of human dignity gives each individual the potential to survive even the most adverse assaults upon it, and to bounce back, as is so eloquently revealed in many life history accounts given by people with learning disabilities who were previously institutionalised (e.g. Edgerton et al 1984, Fido & Potts 1989, Potts & Fido 1991, Richardson 2000, Welshman & Walmsley 2006).

Introducing Mary

Having privileged access to the personal stories of people with learning disabilities can facilitate an understanding of the core issues that have shaped their lives; in effect, what has either repressed or facilitated their human flourishing (see also Ch. 8). The story in Case illustration 4.1 is that of Mary and its inclusion in this chapter is to facilitate the reader's understanding of the impact of key values in the provision of care to someone with learning disabilities. It is expected that you will consider the content of the case illustration and Reader activity 4.2 before moving on.

Three weeks after Mary's father visited the family doctor, another meeting was arranged at the local health centre and attended by the family doctor, the learning disability nurse, the psychologist and Mary's father. Mary was still unwilling to leave her home and so could not have been present at the meeting. Her father had therefore decided that she should stay home with her carer. The family doctor confirmed the purpose of the meeting; to bring together the available information in order to plan further health support with Mary and her family.

The family doctor expressed to the meeting that when she visited Mary, her father and Mary's carer at their home she was concerned about Mary's loss of weight and apparent withdrawal. She had therefore prescribed an enriched nutritional dietary supplement. She had also contacted the learning disability nurse who agreed to monitor Mary's nutritional intake with Mary's home carer to see if the supplement was helping Mary to regain some weight. There was no evidence that Mary was suffering from any underlying physical ailment that could be causing the weight loss, but the doctor wanted to keep an eye on things, and if improvement was not fairly rapid, would wish to organise further tests that potentially might prove distressing to Mary.

The psychologist went on to suggest several possibilities for Mary's symptoms of withdrawal; for example, he explained that the results of his initial assessment were not conclusive as he was still learning from his meetings with Mary, her personal carer and Mary's father about how to understand Mary's communication. Mary's case notes, dating from her time at special school, indicated that Mary was normally sociable, even though she did demonstrate some autistic spectrum behaviours over many years. The psychologist concluded that, clearly, Mary was expressing a significant degree of withdrawal and was possibly suffering a sense of loss and grief following the death of her mother which had created a major gap in her life. The psychologist proposed to begin to address these factors over the next few weeks and went on to describe some initial steps including how Mary, her father, carer, the GP and the learning disability nurse may be able to contribute, and an approximate time line after which to review progress.

Mary's father explained that both Mary's home carer and he were worried about the long hours Mary spent in repetitive behaviours, describing how Mary stared upwards at the ceiling light, flicked her hand over her left eye, banged the piano key board and occasionally poked a finger against the side of her left eye. He wondered how to reduce the extent of this behaviour.

The psychologist had not been able to witness any of this behaviour from Mary as she had been very

Reader activity 4.4

Indentify at least one potential explanation for Mary's apparent withdrawal?

Case illustration 4.1

Mary Ellend is 20 years of age. She was born with significant visual impairment leaving some peripheral vision in her left eye and a complete lack of vision in her right eye. Mary also has some loss of hearing. Each of these impairments became apparent during her infancy and Mary attended a special school until age 19. Mary never developed speech but her communicative repertoire includes vocal sounds that indicate her mood quite well. She will indicate preferences for foods, for example by smiling at its taste, but she does not respond to questions such as "Would Mary like some ravioli or beans?" Sadly Mary's devoted mother died in a traffic accident 6 months ago. Her father, a businessman running his own company, travels abroad frequently and is very devoted to his daughter. He hired a live-in help to support Mary following the death of her mother who previously cared for Mary. Three months ago Mary's father asked his family doctor for help, explaining that since the death of Mary's mother, Mary seemed to have become seriously withdrawn: in her least withdrawn periods, spending long periods of time sitting rocking while banging the piano key board and pushing a finger into her eye. She could not be persuaded to leave the house and also had lost some weight during recent months.

The family doctor arranged, with Mary's father, to visit Mary later that week to undertake an initial medical assessment, and for Mary and her father to be visited by her local learning disability community nurse, as a first step in planning some medium to longer term support to Mary, her father and Mary's home carer. Subsequent to visiting Mary, the family doctor also referred Mary for a psychological assessment.

Reader activity 4.2

As you read through Mary's case illustration and the accompanying commentary, identify some of the ways by which Mary's dignity is supported by the respective parties.

Reader activity 4.3

List the possible reasons why Mary might be losing weight?

Reader activity 4.5

Can you think of a possible explanation for this behaviour by Mary?

withdrawn during his meetings with her, but the learning disability nurse had witnessed this behaviour during the last two of her three visits with Mary. The nurse explained that she felt Mary should not be discouraged from this behaviour, but that it would reduce over time, perhaps, if other, new opportunities to expand Mary's interests and activities could be created. Mary would not then need to spend quite so long at the piano as described above. The learning disability nurse described how she had sat with Mary during such an occasion; 'mirroring' Mary's movements in order to try to 'connect' with her (see Caldwell 2006). While undertaking this 'mirroring' of Mary's behaviour, the learning disability nurse had noticed how, when Mary banged the piano, this, combined with the rocking effect, created a wa-wa sound. Tentatively the nurse went on to speculate that Mary found comfort in the rocking motion. She suggested that Mary might be using the partial vision in her left eye to look at the ceiling light and by flicking her hand across her eye Mary was creating a flickering light effect. Perhaps Mary found the rocking a comfort and was augmenting this by banging the piano and flicking her hand across her line of vision. Pressing her finger against her eye might also create a 'spark' or flash effect, so Mary was perhaps creating her own sound and light disco and quite cleverly maximizing the input from her impaired sensory apparatus. Thus Mary was engaging herself in a meaningful, comforting and rewarding activity which naturally she would repeat whenever she needed. At present, however, Mary's withdrawal was making it difficult to introduce her to other activities that she might also find enjoyable and engaging. Consequently the learning disability nurse wished to plan her nursing support primarily around Mary's nutritional health needs and also to begin formulating a plan to support Mary to broaden her sphere of engagement by gradually introducing her to a range of different activities and opportunities. The learning disability nurse concluded that for this to succeed she would need both Mary's father and her personal carer to be included in the planning as well as the GP and psychologist.

Thinking back to the discussion of dignity above and in relation to how Mary's dignity was supported, consider the following. Mary, like "Everyone of this species, by nature, enjoys an ethical dignity equal to every other ..." (Husted & Husted 2008:57–58). Mary has a right to act according to her unique and independent purposes and desires. Thinking about the people mentioned who were supporting Mary, Husted & Husted go on to say:

> No human being is less or more independent than another. None has a right to override the purposes and desires of others. No one human being, and no collection of human beings, has a right to alienate the self-directedness of another.
>
> (Husted & Husted 2008:57–58).

Therefore, in order to respect Mary's dignity, all of the people trying to support Mary must try to understand her behaviour. It could be possible to mistake some of Mary's behaviour as abnormal or undignified, for example her rocking and eye poking, but actually Mary's behaviour was recognised as a dignified self-expression by which Mary gained some comfort and optimised her impaired auditory and visual senses.

As you considered the questions in Reader activities 4.2–4.5, you probably recognised that Mary was simply doing what we all do, trying to express her unique purposes and desires. She may not fully understand about her mother's death, for example, but she experiences the loss and that loss has affected Mary just as it might any other daughter. Mary expresses that loss in her behaviour.

In relation to Mary, it can be seen that none of her supporters attempted or wished to override Mary's purposes and desires or to alienate (make strange) her behaviour. Mary's father, personal carer, the GP, psychologist and nurse each sought dignified explanations for why Mary acted as she did and therefore Mary's dignity was being supported. This has not always been the case when people intervene in the care of someone like Mary who has a learning disability. For example, some attempts at 'normalisation', which will be considered later in this chapter, sought to manipulate the behaviours of people with learning disabilities, especially if those behaviours might appear 'strange' to other people.

Person-centredness and citizenship

When people recognise and accept your dignity, they are treating you with respect for your person, your self-expression, your autonomy and your personal human flourishing. This person-centredness has become a fundamental value and approach to working with people with learning disabilities and all people using health and social care services. Person-centredness is one of the key values underpinning much of the legislation and policy in the UK regarding support to people with learning disabilities (see Table 4.1), particularly that which

Table 4.1 Examples of policy drivers expressing values that influence services in relation to people with learning disabilities: the following selection are compatible with fundamental valuing for human dignity and human flourishing

Policy driver	Values made explicit	Values common to all
1948 Universal Declaration of Human Rights: heralded the beginnings of the human rights movement	10 December 1948, the General Assembly of the United Nations adopted and proclaimed the Universal Declaration of Human Rights. Following this historic act, the Assembly called upon all member countries to publicise the text of the Declaration and "to cause it to be disseminated, displayed, read and expounded principally in schools and other educational institutions, without distinction based on the political status of countries or territories." Article 1: "All human beings are born free and equal in dignity and rights. They are endowed with reason and conscience and should act towards one another in a spirit of brotherhood." (http://www.un.org/en/documents/udhr/)	Human rights.
United Nations, 1971: Declaration on the Rights of Mentally Retarded [sic.] Persons	In 1971, the General Assembly of the United Nations, in its resolution 2856 (XXVI), proclaimed the Declaration on the Rights of Mentally Retarded Persons: "Bearing in mind the necessity of assisting persons with mental disabilities to develop their full abilities and of promoting their integration, the General Assembly calls for national and international action to ensure that the Declaration is used as a common basis and frame of reference for the protection of their rights." The Declaration establishes that 'mentally retarded persons' have the same rights as other human beings. Specifically, they have the right to: "proper medical care, physical therapy, education, training, rehabilitation and guidance to develop their ability and maximum potential; economic security and decent standards of living; to perform productive work and engage on any meaningful occupation; to live with their own families or foster care, and to participate in community life; a qualified guardian when required to protect their personal well-being and interest . . ." UN (1971 online) (NB: see also United Nations 1975: Declaration on the Rights of Disabled Persons, accessible as above.)	

Continued

Table 4.1 Examples of policy drivers expressing values that influence services in relation to people with learning disabilities: the following selection are compatible with fundamental valuing for human dignity and human flourishing—cont'd

Policy driver	Values made explicit	Values common to all
The Scandinavian Model of Normalisation, 1960s	(Nirje 1969) speaks of "... making available to all mentally retarded people [sic.] (and those with a handicapping [sic.] condition) patterns of life and conditions of everyday living which are as close as possible to the regular circumstances and ways of society ..."	Human rights plus standards by which to judge their effective implementation in relation to people with learning disabilities.
Values Into Action (VIA), 1971 to present	Values Into Action works alongside people with learning disabilities campaigning for equality.	Human rights basis; places the individual at the centre of decision and choice making; supports agenda for an inclusive society, citizenship, distributive justice and its close ally, social justice. Incorporates: equality, fairness, individuality, person-centred approaches with personalisation of supports, empowerment, self-determination, respect, trust, anti-oppression and dignity.
The Disability Discrimination Act (DDA), 1995 and 2005	The Disability Discrimination Act 1995 aims to end the discrimination that many disabled people face. This Act has been significantly extended, including by the Disability Discrimination Act 2005. It now gives disabled people rights in the areas of: • employment • education • access to goods, facilities and services, including larger private clubs and land-based transport services • buying or renting land or property, including making it easier for disabled people to rent property and for tenants to make disability-related adaptations • functions of public bodies, for example issuing of licences. The Act requires public bodies to promote equality of opportunity for disabled people. It also allows the government to set minimum standards so that disabled people can use public transport easily.	
Same as You? A Review of the Services for People with Learning Disabilities (Scottish Executive 2000)	• People with learning disabilities being valued as individuals. • Asked about services and involved in choices about what they want. • Being provided with support that builds upon what they are already able to do. • Being enabled to make effective use of the same local services as everyone else. • Benefiting from specialist social, health or educational services when required. • Services to take account of an individual's age, abilities and other needs.	

Valuing People. A New Strategy for Learning Disability for the 21st Century (Department of Health (DH) 2001)	• **Legal/civil rights**: services to treat as individuals, respect for *dignity*, challenge discrimination, protection of the law when required. • **Independence**: presumed rather than of dependence and support to make full use of services. • **Choice**: expressing preferences and receiving the support when needed to enable those preferences to be expressed and acted upon in daily life. • **Inclusion**: doing ordinary everyday things like most of the rest of society. • **Personalisation**: control and choices over own life and services. Person-centred planning is a key philosophy within *Valuing People* and *Valuing People Now* (see below) by which being human, self-fulfilment, respect for difference, equity, appreciation of personal successes and failures in life, celebrating individuals' uniqueness and personhood are addressed.	Human rights basis; places the individual at the centre of decision and choice making; supports agenda for an inclusive society, citizenship and social justice. Incorporates: equality, fairness, individuality, person-centred approaches with personalisation of supports, empowerment, self-determination, social and economic justice, respect, trust, anti-oppression and dignity.
Fulfilling the Promises, Welsh Assembly, Cardiff. (Welsh Office 2002)	• Comprehensive integrated services. • Effective and effortless movement between services. • Holistic accounting for preferences, hopes, lifestyle. • Ensuring appropriate advocacy. • Accessible information. • Collaborative partnerships. • Well trained, well informed, competent workers. • Completion of National Assembly's programme to resettle people with learning disabilities into the community.	
Equal Lives (DHSSPS 2005)	• Citizenship: individualism, right to equality. • Person-centred: supported for individual needs. • Participation: consultation about services, choices and decisions about their lives. • Interdependence: valued and encouraged to contribute to community life. • Equality: using the same services and having the same entitlements as everyone else.	
Valuing People Now. A New Strategy for People with Learning Disabilities (DH 2009)	After further consultation and review regarding *Valuing People*, the DH placed more emphasis upon the following: **Personalisation**: real choices and control over life and services. **What people do during the day/evenings/weekends**: assistance to be included in communities, obtain paid work. **Better health**: NHS to provide full/equal access to good-quality health care. **Housing access**: to the type that people want and need, home ownership/tenancies whenever possible. **Making sure that change happens**: delivering the policy, making partnership boards more effective.	

directs person-centred planning (see also Ch. 9). This section considers the concept in relation to human flourishing and citizenship.

In relation to human flourishing, numerous approaches to explain, describe or evaluate this aspect of human development have been expounded by a wide range of philosophers. A selection from one approach will be considered here in relation to Mary's scenario (Case illustration 4.1) to help the reader grapple with the concept of human flourishing in some quite specific ways. Nussbaum (2000) identifies 10 capabilities for human flourishing (see Table 4.2).

For Nussbaum, human flourishing is not about how satisfied a person is, or the extent of the resources the person commands. Nussbaum asks in relation to each sphere of functioning: "*is the person capable of this or not?*" Now, at various times and stages in life, each one of us may be more or less capable of one or more of these capabilities and Mary is no different in this respect. Hopefully, at such times, we can anticipate that other people who respect our dignity will therefore support us (and Mary) so that we are not thwarted along our journey of self-actualisation.

Therefore, in relation to Mary, the people supporting her could, potentially, assess the extent to

Table 4.2 Ten capabilities to support human flourishing and citizenship

Capability	Descriptor
Life	"Being able to live to the end of a human life of normal length; not dying prematurely or before one's life is so reduced as to be not worth living."
Bodily health	"... Being able to have good health, including reproductive health; being adequately nourished ...; being able to have adequate shelter"
Bodily integrity	"Being able to move freely from place to place; being able to be secure against violent assault, including sexual assault ...; having opportunities for sexual satisfaction and for choice in matters of reproduction."
Senses, imagination, thought	"Being able to use the senses; being able to imagine, to think, and to reason – and to do these things in ... a way informed and cultivated by an adequate education ...; being able to use imagination and thought in connection with experiencing, and producing expressive works and events of one's own choice ...; being able to use one's mind in ways protected by guarantees of freedom of expression with respect to both political and artistic speech and freedom of religious exercise; being able to have pleasurable experiences and to avoid non-beneficial pain."
Emotions	"Being able to have attachments to things and persons outside ourselves ... in general to love, to grieve, to experience longing, gratitude and justified anger; not having one's emotional developing blighted by fear or anxiety ..."
Practical reason	"Being able to form a conception of the good and to engage in critical reflection about the planning of one's own life. (This entails protection for liberty of conscience.)"
Affiliation	"Being able to live for and in relation to others, to recognise and show concern for other human beings, to engage in various forms of social interaction; being able to imagine the situation of another and to have compassion for that situation; having the capability for both justice and friendship ... Being able to be treated as a dignified being whose worth is equal to that of others."
Other species	"Being able to live with concern for and in relation to animals, plants and the world of nature."
Play	"Being able to laugh, to play, to enjoy recreational activities."
Control over one's environment	"(A) Political: being able to participate effectively in political choices that govern one's life; having the rights of political participation, free speech and freedom of association ... (B) Material: being able to hold property (both land and movable goods); having the right to seek employment on an equal basis with others ..."

Nussbaum (2000): The list includes quotations taken from pp 30–31.

which Mary is capable of expressing herself in each of Nussbaum's domains of capability and, where necessary, support Mary by ensuring that the resources to assist her are brought to bear, correctly placed and working to allow Mary to express herself as fully as possible; that is, they are working in an evidently person-centred way. For example, the most probable explanation for Mary's withdrawal is that Mary is expressing grief at the loss of her mother. As we saw above, the capability for 'emotions' includes Mary being able to have attachments to people and to things, to love, to grieve, to experience longing, gratitude and justified anger. Mary has the capability to express all of these emotions but may need support to cope with them, in her own way, and also to express herself more in some of the other domains that Nussbaum depicts.

As a further example, in relation to the capability, 'Life', the global intention would be to enable Mary to live as normal a length of life as possible, not dying prematurely or allowing her life to be so restricted as to not allow her self-expression. Unfortunately the health care system in the UK was recently found to be endemic with prejudicial attitudes towards people with learning disabilities such that people with learning disabilities are more likely than other people to receive inadequate health support that is clearly not person-centred and that can result in their premature death. You can read more about this in *Death by Indifference* (Mencap 2007) and in *Six Lives: The Provision of Public Services to People with Learning Disabilities* (Parliamentary and Health Service Ombudsman 2009). In such a context, therefore, the importance of supporting Mary's general health in the longer term, and her nutritional health in the short term, acquires an extra dimension.

Drawing from Nussbaum, therefore, the capabilities involved in Mary's, as indeed in all human flourishing, can be listed and, importantly, can serve as a guide and critical stance for the purposes of evaluative and policy planning. This offers a basis for core constitutional principles for citizenship, that citizens have a right to demand from their governments. This has the potential to help ensure that everyone may flourish and enjoy the benefits of citizenship, including the most vulnerable citizens like Mary. Therefore, valuing people with learning disabilities, by virtue of their existence, and promoting their citizenship through working in person-centred ways are fundamental to good-quality practice. To pursue anything less could be deemed unethical (see Ch. 5 for further guidance on ethical values).

Partnership

If, as we have discussed, the values that underpin good-quality support to people with learning disabilities stem, first and foremost, from a respect for human dignity and human flourishing, what other values follow from these?

It has already been said that human flourishing in some areas necessitates the support of others. Working in partnership with service users is therefore probably the first such value that follows from the above question, but extends also to working in partnership and collaboratively with people from other supportive disciplines and including those who most closely support people with learning disabilities in daily life wherever that may take place (Department of Health (DH) 2001, 2009). This value is explored in this section in relation to the social model of disability and quality of life measures.

In recent decades, the disability rights movement has radically influenced the expression of these values within UK national policy (see Table 4.1). In order to appreciate its impact, it is necessary to remind ourselves that until about two decades ago the traditional view of disability was that it equated to a personal tragedy afflicting an individual. This resulted in the medical model of disability by which the 'affliction' was deemed to be located within the individual and so needed medical intervention to 'correct' it; if this proved unfeasible or unsuccessful then charitable and welfare provisions intervened. Barnes et al (1999) explain how, in Western society, a range of assumptions about perceived impairment attributed biological and social inferiority to disabled people in order to legitimise eugenic solutions such as selective abortion, withholding of life-saving treatment, 'mercy killings' and a general hostility towards this group. In relation to people with learning disabilities, therefore, the first half of the 20th century was spent perusing eugenic solutions to prevent people in this group from having children (see Ch. 3). At best, therefore, disabled individuals were deemed to warrant the charity, health care and welfare system approaches that emerged from the 19th century onwards.

Over recent decades, disabled people have developed the social model of disability in order to challenge and overthrow the assumption that it is the presence of an impairment that greatly reduces a person's quality of life and devalues them as human beings; a stance typified by the medical model of disability. Contrary to this, the social model defines disability as being due to social and physical barriers in the built environment and has been described as:

> ... the loss or limitation of opportunities that prevents people who have impairments from taking part in the normal life of the community on an equal level with others due to physical and social barriers.
>
> (Finkelstein & French 1993:28)

The word 'impairment' has been defined as:

> ... The lack of part or all of a limb, organ or mechanism of the body.
>
> (Finkelstein & French 1993:28)

This limitation of opportunities that disabled people face can be traced back to the Industrial Revolution which introduced significant changes in patterns of working, prior to which many disabled people, including people with learning disabilities, worked to earn their living. This exclusion of disabled people led the disabled rights movement to call for political policy changes in order to redress the balance by removing disabling barriers. Therefore, as Oliver (1996:31) points out, because:

> ... disability occurs in structured ways dependent upon the material relations of production ... the problem of adjustment is one for society, not for individuals and that search should be concerned with identifying the ways in which society disabled people rather than the effects on individuals ...

Society therefore needs to make fundamental adjustments to some of its shared values in order to include disabled people. For example, in relation to the medical model of disability described above, consider what value we place on human life. In the UK in 2009, the average working wage is about £24 000 per annum (Office for National Statistics 2010). Over a working lifetime of about 45 years, this would potentially amount to £1.08 million at current prices. Put quite crudely, one might ask "is this then the value that should be placed on an average person's life?" Or, from a medical point of view, if that person becomes ill or injured in the long term, should £1.08 million be the limit that an organisation like the National Health Service should pay out in health support? Of course there are many possible permutations of such questions and other factors that might be included in the equation such as the age of the person and whether the cost of supporting their health might result in that person's return to economic productivity and so on. One way that Western medicine has attempted to grapple with rising demand for expensive and scarce medical interventions is the Quality Adjusted Life Years or QALY (National Institute for Clinical Excellence 2010).

Broadly speaking, QALY draws a range of factors into an equation, such as financial costs of treatment weighted against the probable extension in time of the life in question and the subsequent anticipated quality of that life. The usefulness of the kinds of measure employed in applying QALY has been challenged on a number of grounds, for example on validity and the problematic nature of defining perfect health. The disability rights movement reminds us that within Western societies the attitude prevails that it is better to be dead than disabled. *Death by Indifference* (Mencap 2007) depicted how the lives of six people with learning disabilities were foreshortened and their suffering exacerbated by such negative attitudes. In this context, the QALY holds eugenic overtones and therefore a potential threat to disabled people in general (Davies 1987, Mortimer & Segal 2008).

Over the past two or three decades, professionals working with people with learning disabilities have increasingly adopted the social model approach to disability, working in partnership with the disabled person and their supporters in order to form working alliances. Partnership approaches aim to promote health and address disabling barriers via a person-centred approach to planning, implementing and evaluating outcomes. This approach recognises, for example, that a person with a learning disability has a right to autonomy and to express an independent uniqueness, as shown in Case illustration 4.1. But this approach is not about expecting a person with a learning disability eventually to do everything for him or herself. None of us can do everything for ourselves nor do many of us attempt to be completely self-sufficient. We all rely, for example, upon farmers, builders, economic systems, importers, national and regional utilities and a host of other people far too lengthy to list (Richardson 1997).

Therefore, partnership working with people with learning disabilities to facilitate self-expression, overcome disabling barriers and live full and healthy lives has become integral to the values within learning disability support agencies. While learning disability nurses accept and operate within the social model of disability, they additionally recognise that the health

Reader activity 4.6

In the discussion of Mary's scenario (Case illustration 4.1), the beginnings of a working alliance or partnership approach are depicted and plans are taking shape to support her grieving by broadening her horizon of experiences and engaging her interest and enjoyment in other activities.

1. Can you think of people, not yet included in this partnership, who could be called upon to help realise and develop this plan?
2. Working through each of the Capabilities in Table 4.2, can you identify the support that may be needed to assist Mary to express her citizenship in each of the areas and the range of people who might assist?

support needs of people with learning disabilities need to be addressed because people with learning disabilities are significantly more at risk of suffering adverse health and of receiving a less than adequate service from the health care system (e.g. Mencap 2007, Parliamentary and Health Service Ombudsman 2009). Interprofessional and collaborative working is essential for effective support. Therefore, working alliances that includes people with learning disabilities, their closest supporters, relatives, other services and personnel are mainstream values and practices to ensure that health and social support is accessible and effective (DH 2001, Richardson 1997).

From normalisation to inclusion

This section of the chapter considers how changes in values with respect to people with learning disabilities have influenced the evolution of key philosophies that have shaped the nature of service provision for this group. It starts by looking at the theory of normalisation and ends with inclusion.

Normalisation

During the 1950s and 1960s, humanist concepts of person and being (e.g. Maslow 1943, 1954, 1962, Rogers 1951, 1980) had proven a source of inspiration for a broad spectrum of professionals, as had combining the principles of human value and human rights, particularly after the Nuremberg trials (Beacock 1992). In response to the Holocaust and other atrocities of war, the United Nations (UN) made a universal declaration of human rights, Article 1 stating, *"All human beings are born free and equal in dignity and rights"* (UN 1948). Later, the 1971 UN Declaration on The Rights of Mentally Retarded [sic.] Persons defined specific rights to education, citizenship, health and work (UN 1971). Beacock (1992) identifies how these rights and humanist values were combined within the principles of normalisation (Bank-Mikkelsen 1969, Grunewald 1977, Nirje 1969, O'Brien & Tyne 1981, Wolfensberger 1972, 1983).

There are several versions of the normalisation principle (see Table 4.3), all of which, to some extent, influenced a generation of professionals working with people with learning disabilities from the 1960s onwards (Race 1999). Normalisation originated in the Danish Mental Retardation Act of 1959 where it was defined in terms of the creation of an existence for people with learning disabilities as close to normal living conditions as possible (Bank-Mikkelson 1969). This definition was further expanded in the work of Nirje in the 1960s who took normalisation to mean:

> making available to the mentally retarded [sic.] patterns and conditions of everyday life which are as close as possible to the norms and patterns of the mainstream of society.
>
> (Nirje 1969:181)

This original Scandinavian position advocated the inclusion of people with learning disabilities within mainstream society as a basic human right. Hence, normalisation started from a rights basis in which choices were emphasised, however later versions of normalisation deviated from this path. For example, Grunewald (1977) proposed that by utilising the strengths of people with learning disabilities, any weaknesses became less problematic, but stated that occasional special provision may be necessary. Juul & Linton (1978) emphasised obligations as well as rights, which implied that if people did not behave acceptably, then their participation in mainstream society might be restricted.

The notion that an individual's human rights should be honoured only if that person can meet some obligations would seem, potentially at least, to exclude some people with more severe or profound learning disabilities. For example, to restrict an individual's human right if some obligation has not been met by that individual diminishes the concept of 'human rights' by excluding from those rights any individuals unable to comprehend the social obligations attached to those rights. The consequence

concerned about the real socioeconomic basis of disability, the celebration of difference and tackling discrimination worldwide (Culham & Nind 2003, Oliver 2000).

Normalisation as a leading philosophy has therefore served its time, and many of its purposes, such as hospital closure and community living, have at least, in part, been achieved due to its influence (Culhum & Nind 2003). Normalisation has largely been replaced by a philosophy of inclusion.

Inclusion

Inclusion is human rights based (like Nirje 1969) but, unlike normalisation, inclusion is driven primarily by disabled people and, importantly, people with learning disabilities and their supporters are key to this movement. Inclusion is not a single concept; it addresses values associated with human rights, citizenship, economic and social justice, gender, ethnicity, poverty and sexuality as well as disability. It is also closely aligned to the social model of disability. Inclusion incurs a continuous process of societal adjustment, reconstruction and reform by which society adapts to increase access and participation and decrease exclusion from mainstream settings and communities, regardless of any individual's or group differences (Booth & Ainscow 1998, Culham & Nind 2003).

As such, the inclusion agenda has had a major influence upon UK policy (see Table 4.1) promoting values such as:

- human rights (discussed above)
- citizenship by which individuals are able to participate in democratic and socioeconomic activities
- equality and fairness which aims at distributive justice so that people with learning disabilities can access a decent quality of life both socially (social justice) and economically
- individuality and personalisation (such as person-centred approaches) by which support is tailored according to individual circumstances and controlled by that person
- empowerment and self-determination whereby people with learning disabilities are trusted to have control of what happens to them and the choices they make
- anti-oppression by which, for example, services and information are accessible and support at hand to enable people with learning disabilities to obtain best use of them so that dignity and personal fulfilment are respected.

With the last point in mind, neither normalisation nor inclusive approaches would condone the segregation of people on the grounds of their difference, yet many disabled people draw from the civil rights movement and thereby gain strength and pride from being with other disabled people. In terms of inclusion, therefore, the desire of some people with learning disabilities to live and socialise with their learning disabled peers, with whom they may find much common experience and solidarity, reminds us all that it is the person with the learning disability who should decide and be at the centre of decision-making processes. For people with profound learning disabilities that are also associated with severe physical and sensory impairments, we must consider how best to engage with each individual so that their choices are properly understood and their human flourishing supported and celebrated, as in Mary's scenario presented above. UK policy in the direction of the personalisation of services and supports has the potential to facilitate an inclusive citizenship for the most vulnerable groups and individuals, provided we also evaluate this against measures such as those proposed by Nussbaum (2000) and outlined above.

In summary, the disabled rights movement has resulted in the most radical rethink of disability policy in Western societies. Inclusiveness has largely

Reader activity 4.7

In relation to Mary (Case illustration 4.1), can you identify some opportunities and facilities in your local community that Mary might like to access and how she might be supported to gain full benefit from her participation and inclusion? In addressing these, you might consider how to support Mary in terms of the following:

- Citizenship – participation in democratic and socioeconomic activities.
- Equality and fairness – access to a decent quality of life both socially and economically.
- Individuality and personalisation – tailoring to Mary's circumstances and controlled by Mary.
- Empowerment and self-determination – trusting Mary to have control of what happens and personal choices.
- Anti-oppression – making services and information accessible and support at hand to enable Mary to obtain best use of them.

replaced normalisation. Policy is now steered largely by disabled people themselves and is reflected in the partnership approaches that prevail today. Hence the agendas associated with inclusion are continuing to make headway in partnerships that include people with learning disabilities and, when necessary, their supporters, professionals and other paid staff. Some examples of these alliances are seen in organisations such a Values Into Action (VIA) and in those social enterprise groups either largely or wholly run by people with learning disabilities and those employing people with learning disabilities such as United Response, New Horizons Partnership, Co-Options Community Co-Operative Limited and Equal Works (see USEFUL addresses section). Organisations such as these have emerged over the past 20 years to, among other things, change the culture of services supporting disabled people into one of employment, through the creation of new commercial work opportunities. Of course there are some people with learning disabilities who have profound levels of sensory impairment, often combined with physical impairments, for whom some of these initiatives may hold less direct relevance and where equivalent inclusive opportunities that serve their interests, needs and self expression are much more lacking. However, this chapter has shown that human flourishing can be achieved by all and it is the job of the professional to work in a person-centred way to support this.

See Reader activity 4.8 on the Evolve website.

Conclusion

This exploration of the values that underpin supporting people with learning disabilities began with an exploration of the meanings of dignity and it was seen that dignity is a concept that holds true for all individuals throughout life. It has shown that dignity is best expressed when we are self-actualising or being and becoming what our makeup most suits and that its expression requires physical, social and psychological nurturing. We saw from Mary Elland's story that dignity expresses itself differently for different people and that it is possible to nurture and support an individual's dignity so that human flourishing may take its course.

The values that are eminent today in relation to people with learning disabilities are very different to the eugenic values that prevailed in the first half of the 20th century where their dignity was largely denied. Today's values draw primarily from a human rights basis which places the individual at the centre of decision and choice making and supports an agenda for citizenship within an inclusive society that is reflected at policy level. These values of human rights and inclusion incorporate values such as equality, fairness, individuality, empowerment, self-determination, social and economic justice, respect, trust, personalisation and anti-oppression – all of which stem from the recognition and acknowledgement of one constant and fundamental quality, human dignity.

References

Bank-Mikkelsen, N.E., 1964. The ideological and legal basis of the national service for the mentally retarded. In: Öster, J., Sletved, H. (Eds.), International Copenhagen Congress on the scientific study of mental retardation, Det Berlingske Bogtrykkeri, Copenhagen.

Bank-Mikkelsen, N.E., 1969. A metropolitan area in Denmark – Copenhagen. In: Kugel, R.B., Wolfensberger, W. (Eds.), Changing patterns in residential services for the mentally retarded. Department of Health, Education and Welfare, Washington.

Barnes, C., Mercer, G., Shakespeare, T., 1999. Exploring disability: a sociological introduction. Polity Press, Cambridge.

Beacock, C., 1992. Triggers for change. In: Thompson, T., Mathias, P. (Eds.), Standards and mental handicap: keys to competence. Baillière Tindall, London.

Booth, T., Ainscow, M. (Eds.), 1998. From them to us: an international study of inclusion in education. Routledge, London.

Brown, D., 1971. Bury my heart at wounded knee: an Indian history of the American West. Henry Holt, New York Reprinted 2008.

Caldwell, P., 2006. Finding you finding me: using intensive interaction to get in touch with people whose severe learning disabilities are combined with autistic spectrum disorder. Jessica Kingsley, London.

Chisholm, A., 1993. Quality of care. In: Shanley, E., Starr, A. (Eds.), Learning disabilities: a handbook of care. Churchill Livingstone, London.

Culham, A., Nind, M., 2003. Deconstructing normalisation: clearing the way for inclusion. J. Intellect. Dev. Disabil. 28 (1), 65–78.

Davies, A., 1987. Women with disabilities: abortion or liberation. Disability Handicap and Society 2 (3), 275–284.

Department of Health, 2001. Valuing people. A new strategy for learning disability for the 21st century. Department of Health, London.

Department of Health, 2009. Valuing people now. A new strategy for people with learning disabilities. Department of Health, London.

Department of Health, Social Services and Public Safety (DHSSPS), 2005. Equal lives. DHSSPS, Belfast.

Department of Health Strategy User Group, 2001. Nothing about us without us: report of the National User Group. Department of Health, London.

Edgerton, R.B., Bollinger, M., Hess, B., 1984. The cloak of competence after two decades. Am. J. Ment. Defic. 80, 345–351.

Fido, R., Potts, M., 1989. It's not true what was written down! Experiences of life in a mental handicap institution. Oral History, Autumn, Reminiscence 31–35.

Finkelstein, V., French, S., 1993. Towards a psychology of disability. In: Swain, J., Finkelstein, V., French, S., Oliver, M. (Eds.), Disabling barriers – enabling environments. Sage, London.

Godrej, F., 2005. The 'developed' human life: non-Western approaches to human flourishing and development. Paper presented at the annual meeting of the American Political Science Association, Washington DC 1 Sep 2005 Available at:http://www.allacademic.com//meta/p_mla_apa_research_citation/0/3/9/7/5/pages39756/p39756-1.php (accessed 20.01.10.).

Grunewald, K., 1977. Community living for mentally retarded adults in Sweden. Current, Sweden 159, 1–10.

Husted, J.H., Husted, G.L., 2008. Ethical decision making and health care; the symphonological approach. Springer, New York.

Juul, K.D., Linton, T., 1978. European approaches to the treatment of behaviour disordered children. Behavioural Disorders 3 (4), 232–249.

Kant I., 1724–1804. The metaphysics of morals, part ii: the metaphysical principles of virtue, Ak419-420. In: Kant, I. (Ed.), 1983. Ethical philosophy (J. W. Ellington, Trans.). Hackett, Indiana.

Maslow, A., 1943. A theory of human motivation. Psychol. Rev. 50, 370–396.

Maslow, A., 1954. Motivation and personality. Harper Row, New York.

Maslow, A., 1962. Towards a psychology of being. Van Nostrand, London.

Mencap, 2007. Death by indifference. Mencap, London.

Mezibov, G.B., 1990. Normalisation and its relevance today. J. Autism Dev. Disord. September 379–390.

Mitchell, D., 1998. Learning disability nursing: reflections on history. Journal of Learning Disabilities for Nursing, Health and Social Care 2 (1), 45–49.

Mittler, P., 1978. Helping mentally handicapped people in hospital: a report to the Secretary of State for Social Services by the National Development Group for the Mentally Handicapped. DHSS, London.

Mortimer, D., Segal, L., 2008. Comparing the incomparable? A systematic review of competing techniques for converting descriptive measures of health status into QALY-weights. Med. Decis. Making 28 (1), 66–89.

National Institute for Clinical Excellence, 2010. Measuring effectiveness and cost effectiveness: the QALY. Available at:http://www.nice.org.uk/newsroom/features/measuringeffectiveness andcosteffectivenesstheqaly.jsp (accessed 19.01.10.).

Nirje, B., 1969. The normalization principle and its human management implications. In: Kugel, R.B., Wolfensberger, W. (Eds.), Changing patterns in residential services for the mentally retarded. President's Committee on Mental Retardation, Washington DC.

Nussbaum, M., 2000. Women and human development. Cambridge University Press, New York.

O'Brien, J., 1987. A framework for accomplishment. Responsive Systems Associates, Decatur, USA.

O'Brien, J., Tyne, A., 1981. The principle of normalisation: a foundation for effective services. Campaign for the Mentally Handicapped, London.

Office for National Statistics, 2010. Annual Survey of Hours and Earnings (ASHE). Available at:http://www.statistics.gov.uk/cci/nugget.asp?id=285 (accessed 17.06.10.).

Oliver, M., 1996. A sociology of disability or a disablist sociology? In: Barton, L. (Ed.), Disability and society: emerging issues and insights. Longman Sociology, London.

Oliver, M.J., 2000. Capitalism, disability, and ideology: a materialist critique of the normalization principle. In: Flynn, R.J., Lemay, A.L. (Eds.), A quarter century of normalization and social role valorization: evolution and impact. University of Ottawa Press, Ottawa.

Oxford English Dictionary, 2010. Available at:http://dictionary.oed.com/cgi/entry/50274674?query_type=word&queryword=value &first=1&max_to_show=10&sort_type= alpha&result_place=4&search_id= U1GB-c6qIc6-3800&hilite=50274674 (accessed 21.04.10.).

Parliamentary and Health Service Ombudsman, 2009. Six lives: the provision of public services to people with learning disabilities. HMSO, London.

Peking University, 2004/5. Peking University Centre for the Study of Constitutional and Administrative Law. The idea of human dignity: a reconstruction of Confucianism III. Nanjing University, PR China. Available at:http://www.publiclaw.cn/article/Details.asp?NewsId=1279&Classid=&ClassName= (accessed 20.01.10.).

Potts, M., Fido, R., 1991. A fit person to be removed : personal accounts of life in a mental deficiency institution. Northcote House, Plymouth.

Race, D.G., 1999. Hearts and minds: social role valorization, UK academia and services for people with a learning disability. Disability and Society 14 (4), 519–538.

Richardson, M., 1997. Addressing barriers: disabled rights and the implications for nursing of the social construct of disability. J. Adv. Nurs. 25, 1269–1275.

Richardson, M., 2000. How we live: participatory research with six people with learning difficulties. J. Adv. Nurs. 32 (6), 1383–1395.

Rogers, C., 1951. Client centred therapy. Constable, London.

Rogers, C., 1980. A way of being. Houston Mifflin, Boston.

Royal College of Nursing, 2009. Dignity in health care for people with learning disabilities: RCN guidance. Royal College of Nursing, London.

Scottish Executive, 2000. Same as you? A review of the services for people with leaning disabilities. Scottish Executive, Edinburgh.
Siddiqi, undated. Muslims for human dignity. Dr Muzammil Siddiqi, President of the Fiqh Council of North America. Available at: http://www.asktheschoIar.com/5-194-2–muslims-for-human-dignity-dr-muzammil-siddiqi.aspx (accessed 20.01.10.).
United Nations, 1948. United Nations General Assembly, Universal Declaration of Human Rights, 10 December 1948, 217 A (III). Available at:http://www.unhcr.org/refworld/docid/3ae6b3712c.html (accessed 19.01.10.).
United Nations, 1971. UN General Assembly, Declaration on the Rights of Mentally Retarded Persons, 20 December 1971, A/R ES/2856. Available at:http://www.unhcr.org/refworld/docid/3b00f04e5c.html (accessed 19.01.10.).
Welshman, J., Walmsley, J. (Eds.), 2006. Community care in perspective: care, control and citizenship. Palgrave Macmillan, Basingstoke.
Welsh Office, 2002. Fulfilling the promises. Welsh Assembly, Cardiff.
Wolfensberger, W., 1972. The principle of normalization in human services. National Institute on Mental Retardation, Toronto.
Wolfensberger, W., 1983. Social role valorization: a proposed new term for the principle of normalization. Ment. Retard 21 (6), 234–239.

Further reading

Bates, P., Davis, F.A., 2004. Social capital, social inclusion and services for people with learning disabilities. Disability and Society 19 (3), 195–207.
Carlson, L., 2010. Who's the expert? Rethinking authority in the face of intellectual disability. J. Intellect. Disabil. Res. 54 (1), 58–65.
Royal College of Nursing, 2009. Dignity in health care for people with learning disabilities: RCN guidance. RCN, London.
Sellman, D., 2006. The importance of being trustworthy. Nurs. Ethics 13 (2), 105–115.

Useful addresses

For more information on social enterprise organisations run by people with learning disabilities, the following websites may be of interest.

Cooptions, http://www.cooptions.co.uk.
New Horizons Partnership, http://www.tandtwo.co.uk/social-enterprise.html.
United Response, http://www.unitedresponse.org.uk/what-we-do/supported-employment/social-enterprise.

Ethical issues

5

Ruth Northway

CHAPTER CONTENTS

KEY ISSUES

- Supporting people with learning disabilities can give rise to a number of ethical issues and dilemmas
- These dilemmas can challenge our personal and professional value bases
- Different ethical perspectives enable us to consider situations from alternative standpoints
- Consideration of the ethical principles of autonomy, beneficence, non-maleficence and justice can assist in identifying the key issues within given situations
- A structured approach to resolving ethical dilemmas is recommended

Introduction

> *Working in partnership with people with learning difficulties, whether as a nurse or in any other professional, formal or informal capacity, is a privilege and an extremely rewarding experience. It means enabling this frequently undervalued group of people to realise their potential and take ownership of their lives. However, it is not without its challenges and can be a minefield of ethical and moral dilemmas.*
>
> (Kay 1994:1)

Although written a number of years ago, the above quotation clearly suggests that, no matter what your personal or professional background, if you are involved in supporting people with learning disabilities you are likely to face ethical dilemmas. Why this should be the case is also implied in the quotation. First, as a group, people with learning disabilities are 'frequently undervalued': this places them at risk of being subjected to negative and degrading treatment. Second, it is noted that they need to be supported to 'take ownership' of their lives which suggests that there is a risk that their lives will be inappropriately controlled by others. Seeking to change this situation, however, means challenging existing views and preconceptions, it means challenging poor practices and it means working in person-centred ways to bring about positive changes in the lives of the people we support. Practitioners are thus going to be confronted with ethical dilemmas.

Clearly it is not possible to have thought through every single type of ethical dilemma you may face in advance. Indeed, it might not be viewed as desirable to have done so since it is important to consider the unique nature of each situation which arises and the unique needs of the individuals we support. However, it is possible to develop knowledge and skills which will enable you to approach such situations in a structured and considered manner. The aim of this chapter is, therefore, to assist you to develop your skills in 'thinking ethically'. It will introduce you to some ethical theories and principles, consider their applicability to practice and encourage you to think systematically when confronted with ethical dilemmas. Throughout the chapter you will be encouraged to make direct links between theory and practice. This will be achieved both by using client-based scenarios and reflection on your personal practice. Before reading further, take time to complete Reader activity 5.1.

The nature of ethics

When introducing a topic, it is customary to define key terms. However, Seedhouse (2009) argues that if we are to understand the importance of ethics we must first understand what it is not. He goes on to state that ethics "is not a single body of knowledge about what is right and wrong" (p. 17). Such a view might feel a little frustrating as often we like clear-cut answers as to what is right or wrong in a given situation: there is a sense of security in such a position. In the absence of clear-cut answers, we have to find ways of making sense of a situation, and to assist us in this process it is helpful to have frameworks upon which to draw. This is where ethics and thinking ethically come in.

Ethics is viewed as a complex subject that is not easy to define (Holloway 2007). However, one clue as to the nature of ethics is given in the quotation which opened this chapter (Kay 1994) when it refers to 'ethical and *moral* dilemmas'. Ethics encompasses ways of examining moral life (Beauchamp & Childress 2009). It is concerned with what is morally acceptable and unacceptable, what is right and wrong and what is good and bad. It is concerned with the relative value which is placed upon alternative courses of action. The choice of the word 'relative' is deliberate here since there may not be an absolute answer. For example, what is good and acceptable in one situation may not be good and acceptable in another. Alternatively, there may be two possible courses of action neither of which are positive yet action has to be taken. In such situations, it may be necessary to take the action which is least negative. It is also important to note that what is acceptable at one point in history may not be acceptable at another. Take, for example, the terminology which has been used to refer to people with learning disabilities over the past century, much of which would be viewed as offensive if used today. Ethical thinking also develops over time as exemplified by Seedhouse (2009) who, in the third edition of *Ethics: The Heart of Health Care*, explains how his thinking has progressed over almost 20 years since the first edition. Thus, what we believe to be morally correct at one point in our lives may not be the same at another since our life experiences will shape our thinking.

Of course, morals and morality also operate at a number of different levels. For example, Beauchamp & Childress (2009) refer to what they term the 'common morality' whereby, at the level of society, there is a general level of agreement as to what is right and wrong, what is valued and what is not. For example, it is generally held that we should not kill or steal. Society is, however, comprised of groups and individuals who have their own value base which may, or may not, be shared with wider society. For example, some members of minority cultures may adhere to a set of values which differs in some way(s) from those of the majority culture.

Most professions will also have their own set of values as expressed in codes of conduct. Such values or virtues may encompass qualities such as compassion, discernment, trustworthiness, integrity and conscientiousness (Beauchamp & Childress 2009).

Reader activity 5.1

Take a few minutes to think about your own practice and identify some situations where you feel there was an ethical dilemma. Why did you feel that there was a dilemma? How did you try to resolve the dilemma?

Beauchamp & Childress argue that, for health professionals, additional guidance concerning moral direction comes from public policy. This is also true for many other professional groups. For example, in England, policy relating to provision for people with learning disabilities is firmly rooted in the principles of rights, independence, choice and inclusion (Department of Health 2001). Such principles clearly express the value base for learning disability services, provide direction and guide the decision making of both the individual practitioner and services.

In considering the above discussion concerning values and morals, it can be seen that there is the potential for there to be clashes between the different levels. For example, an individual practitioner may find they are working in a service which has a different value base to their own or find themselves in a situation whereby there is a clash between their personal and professional morals. For example, a nurse may, due to religious reasons, have a strong personal conviction that it is wrong to use contraception. This may lead to a dilemma when a client asks her to support them in obtaining contraception, particularly if they are to uphold the service value base of choice and independence. It is suggested that an awareness of personal values and beliefs is thus necessary for coping with ethical dilemmas (Hessler & Kay 1993). Indeed it is an important first step in the process of recognising such dilemmas. However, while it may be necessary, it is not sufficient, and an understanding of ethical perspectives and principles is also required if such dilemmas are to be resolved.

Reader activity 5.2

Take some time to reflect upon your personal value base. Then, if you are working in a professional capacity, take a look at your professional code of conduct and information concerning the value base of the service in which you work (expressed, for example, in mission statements and policies). Is there agreement between your personal values and your professional values? If there are differences, what are the implications of these? Did you choose your profession because of your personal value base? Have your personal values altered as a result of joining your chosen profession? If you are supporting someone with a learning disability as a family member or friend, consider how your personal value base informs the support you provide. Have your personal values changed as a result of you providing such support?

Ethical perspectives

There are many ethical perspectives or theories which can be referred to when seeking to examine an ethical issue or dilemma. Two such perspectives will be considered here to illustrate how they offer differing understandings of situations which have an ethical dimension.

Deontology

The concept of 'duty' is one which most people working in learning disability services feel familiar with. It is common to speak of being 'on duty' and of having a 'duty of care'. Deontology is concerned with actions which are motivated by duties. Indeed it is viewed as being concerned with people acting as a result of duties regardless of the consequences of such actions (Baggini & Fosl 2007). For example, an individual may believe that they have a duty to tell the truth in all circumstances even if doing so has the potential to cause harm to others. Similarly, another individual may believe that they have a duty to undertake all personal care for an individual even if that individual is capable of performing some tasks unaided. While such an action may be motivated by the desire to do things correctly (that is, out of duty), the consequence may be that independence is undermined.

The idea that individuals act out of a moral duty has its attractions: it is concerned not only with the act itself but also with the motivation for undertaking that act. For example, consider the difference between a student nurse who notices that a client with profound learning disabilities appears to be uncomfortable and who seeks to find the cause of their discomfort because they feel they have a moral duty to promote comfort, and another student nurse who fails to notice the client and who eventually takes action simply because they are told to do so by a senior member of staff. The former is motivated by concern for the comfort and wellbeing of the individual whereas the latter is motivated by the prompting of others. However, deontological theory has also been criticised as being too rigid for use in a health care setting – for example, it is argued that there may be instances where it is justifiable to lie if doing so protects someone from serious harm (Edwards 2009). You may like to reflect upon this suggestion and consider its implications for practice. Also such an approach leads to problems where there are conflicting duties. For example, consider the situation where three people are living together in a group home. One has extremely challenging behaviour and frequently becomes aggressive towards the other residents. The staff are working proactively with the individual to reduce their challenging behaviour. However, this takes up a considerable amount of their time which means that the other two residents receive less attention and undertake fewer activities. Staff have a duty of care to all three individuals but, at present, they feel they have conflicting demands which cannot be reconciled using a deontological approach.

Utilitarianism

Utilitarianism argues that an action is morally right because "... on balance, its consequences offer more good to everyone than harm" (Holloway 2007:71) and that "... the best (most moral) actions are those that produce the most favourable balance of good over bad" (Seedhouse 2009:19). From these definitions, it may be deduced that, in contrast to deontology, it is concerned with the consequences of actions rather than with the motivation: what happens as a result of action or inaction. In considering the balance of good over bad it can be seen that this can operate at the level of the individual (what will bring about the optimum result for the individual?), at a group level (what will bring about the greatest good for the group as a whole?) and even at the level of society (what actions will most enhance societal wellbeing?). To place this in a practice context, let us return to the scenario of the three people living in the group home. Using a utilitarian approach to that situation, it could be argued that working with the individual whose behaviour challenges at the expense of the other residents can be justified in the short term since, if the interventions are successful, they will lead to an improved quality of life for all. To give another example, consider the situation of an individual with mild learning disabilities who also has a mental health problem. They are currently experiencing a period of psychosis and are at risk of self-harm. While the individual concerned has said that they do not wish to be admitted to hospital, and were they to be admitted it would be a traumatic experience for them, a decision is taken to admit them under the provisions of the Mental Health Act 1983. The rationale given is that such an act is justified to prevent greater harm from occurring: the most favourable balance of good over bad (Seedhouse 2009) is achieved.

As with any theory, utilitarianism is not without its critics. One criticism is that this approach can permit a great deal of hardship among a minority of people (Wheat 2009). The example given by Wheat is that of rationing medical treatment such that it prevents anything other than a basic level of care being provided for patients with certain chronic but non-life threatening conditions in order to release resources of a higher standard for the rest of society. The argument here is that the greatest number would benefit but this is at the expense of a minority who could suffer. This example is particularly relevant when the situation of people with learning disabilities is considered, since they are a minority group within society and policies which are designed to achieve the greatest societal good could result in their being disadvantaged. It is also important to consider whether some policies could advantage some groups of people with learning disabilities at the expense of other groups who also have learning disabilities. For example, could people with mild and moderate learning disabilities benefit while those with severe and profound learning disabilities suffer? Could people with learning disabilities from minority ethnic groups be disadvantaged by provision which is aimed generally at people with learning disabilities but which fails to take account of their specific cultural needs?

These two ethical theories have offered two different approaches to understanding moral behaviour. One is concerned with motivations and the other with consequences. In practice, however, it has been suggested that practitioners need to be informed by both perspectives as "it is morally best to consider both consequences and duties since each are relevant to the moral justification of acts" (Edwards 2009:53). In other words, in seeking to address ethical concerns, it is necessary to take account not only of what we do (or don't do) but also to be clear why we do what we do and the likely outcomes.

Reader activity 5.3

Read through Case illustrations 5.1 and 5.2 and try to apply the deontological and utilitarianism theories to the situations. What duties do the various parties in the scenarios have? What actions might these lead them to take? How can the maximum degree of 'good' or benefit be achieved? How do these two theories help you to approach a practice situation from different perspectives?

Case illustration 5.1

Emma and Simon Lewis have three children. Their eldest son, James, has profound learning disabilities and associated physical disabilities. As a result of this he requires a high level of care, and although their home is adapted, meeting these needs takes a considerable amount of Emma and Simon's time. Recently they have begun to worry that this is having a negative impact on their other children. Family life revolves around James' needs which means that sometimes activities have to be cancelled and it is often difficult to do things as a family. However, despite recognising that there is a problem, Emma and Simon feel that they have a duty to care for James without external help as he is their son and this is what parents do. You are the family's key worker and you are aware of their views. However, you are also aware of a local respite care facility which could provide short breaks for James thus allowing Emma and Simon some dedicated time for their other children.

Case illustration 5.2

Christine Hain is 55 years old and for the past 15 years she has lived in a group home with two other women. Christine has, until recently, been very active working on a part-time basis in a local cafe, attending classes in the local leisure centre and going to the local bingo club on a weekly basis. When she was younger she was assessed as having mild learning disabilities, and while she has been able to be independent in many aspects of her life she has also required support in others, hence her living within a group home. In recent months, however, Christine has started to become very confused and has taken to wandering from the house during the night. She has given up all of her activities outside of the home and was asked to leave her job as she was becoming confused and agitated when customers asked her for something. As a result of these changes in behaviour, she was recently assessed by a psychiatrist who diagnosed the early stages of dementia. She has now started to be aggressive towards the other women in the house who, while they understand that Christine is unwell, are becoming afraid of her. Reluctantly the staff in the house have come to the decision that they can no longer support her within that environment since they do not have the resources to provide the level of support she currently requires or the increased level she will require in the future. They feel it would be better for Christine to be moved while she is still able to have some understanding of what is happening. However, Christine is adamant that she does not want to move. In addition, the only place she can move to is a nursing home which caters predominantly for older people.

A principles approach to ethics

Another approach to ethics is what is termed the 'principles' approach. Within this approach, key principles are identified and utilised to analyse a situation. The principles are said to "provide key reference points in commonsense morality" and thus to assist in decision making (Edwards 2009:49). Edwards goes on to argue that a principles-based approach is easily applicable within the context of nursing. However, it would seem that it has wider utility within other professions since it allows a situation to be examined from a variety of perspectives (Edwards 2009).

Perhaps the most commonly quoted principles framework is that offered by Beauchamp & Childress (2009) who identify four key principles:

1. Autonomy.
2. Beneficence.
3. Non-maleficence.
4. Justice.

Each of these will be examined in more detail below. First, however, it is important to note that Beauchamp & Childress give equal weight to the four principles: one does not have more importance than another at a theoretical level. However, in practice, it may be that one principle is more important than another in a given situation. For example, in an emergency situation, the need to prevent harm (non-maleficence) may need to take precedence over respecting the autonomy of an individual. It is also important to acknowledge that in some situations there may be clashes between principles which means that dilemmas arise. In such situations, Beauchamp & Childress argue that "trust, compassion, objective assessment, caring responsiveness, reassurance and the like" (p. 22) need to inform decision making.

Edwards (2009) questions whether there is a need to add a fifth principle, namely 'respect for persons'. This is the respect which is due to individuals by virtue of their being a person. However, he steps back from doing so and in the discussion below it will be seen that respect for persons is inherent in each of the four principles. This is particularly important when considering the situation of people with learning disabilities since at various points within history their personhood and humanity has been questioned and they have been seen as 'less than' human. This has led to negative and often degrading treatment. Even today, people with learning disabilities are at risk of negative and inhuman treatment and practitioners must be alert to this possibility, recognise when it occurs and take action to stop or prevent it. In considering the following four principles, readers are thus encouraged to reflect upon the issue of personhood (see also Ch. 4).

Autonomy

Autonomy is something which is much valued in today's society. It is also something which is fundamental to independence and choice which form key elements of the value base underpinning learning disability services (Department of Health 2001). Edwards (2009) argues that someone is autonomous if they have the ability to make decisions about their life and they are self-governing. Beauchamp & Childress (2009:99) take a similar view, arguing that:

> Personal autonomy encompasses, at a minimum, self rule that is free from both controlling interference by others and from certain limitations such as inadequate understanding that prevents meaningful choice. The autonomous individual acts freely with a self chosen plan . . .

Certain aspects of these definitions need further consideration in relation to people with learning disabilities. First is the suggestion that autonomy requires the individual to be self-governing and to exercise skills such as understanding and decision making. Here it can be seen that such skills are those which people with learning disabilities may find difficult and the question of competence arises. Indeed people with learning disabilities are often assumed to be globally incompetent: because they may lack skills in one area, this is generalised to most or all areas of their lives. Opportunities to make decisions are thus not provided, learning does not take place, and even where views are expressed (through verbal or non-verbal means) these may be overlooked.

It is interesting to note, however, that the Mental Capacity Act 2005 starts from the premise that competence should be assumed unless there is evidence to suggest otherwise. In addition, it recognises that competence is situation specific: an individual may not be competent to make one decision but be able to make another. It is thus not an 'all or nothing' situation. It should also be remembered that competence can be affected by a number of things such as the support an individual is given and manner and format in which information is provided. Finally it should be noted that competence is a developmental process and that our abilities at one stage of our lives will differ from that at another. Therefore, in striving to work ethically, it is important to provide the people we support with opportunities to acquire and extend their competence to enable them to acquire greater control over their own lives.

The second point to consider from the definitions is the suggestion that the individual should be able to make decisions concerning their own life free from 'controlling interference by others'. The history of people with learning disabilities illustrates how they have often been subjected to control exerted by others at both an individual and a group level. For example, in some countries, women with learning disabilities were compulsorily sterilised without their consent, people were forced to live in large congregate settings and decisions were made concerning what was deemed to be in their best interests without reference to their views and wishes (see Ch. 3). Taking a utilitarian view, it was argued that sterilisation of women with learning disabilities was for the greater good of society and incarcerating people in large institutions was both to protect them and to protect society. While none of us is totally autonomous (since there are some areas of our lives where we exercise less control), people with learning disabilities are at greater risk of having their autonomy restricted than other groups within society because of their perceived lack of competence. Seeking to change this situation requires both that we support people with learning disabilities to assume greater control over their own lives and also that we, and others, refrain from taking control unnecessarily away from them.

It must be remembered, however, that exercising control over the lives of people with learning disabilities does not always arise from negative motivations. Indeed, in some instances, it is necessary for others to make decisions in what are deemed to be the best interests of an individual. For example, it may be extremely difficult to determine the views and wishes of an individual with profound and multiple disabilities yet decisions have to be made concerning their lives. This issue will be returned to later

Reader activity 5.4

Think about some of the people with learning disabilities you support. To what extent are they subject to the control of others? How could their control over their lives be enhanced?

in this chapter when paternalism will be explored. Beauchamp & Childress (2009) do, however, argue that respect for the autonomy of others can be expressed in terms of negative and positive obligations. The negative obligation involves not subjecting others to controlling constraints and the positive obligation requires respectful treatment in the disclosure of information and taking action to foster autonomous decision making. These two obligations offer a helpful basis for practice inasmuch as they lead us to question whether we are unnecessarily controlling others and also to consider what actions we could take which would assist the people we support to make decisions. For example, this may involve enabling individuals to receive support from self-advocacy groups or citizen advocates, particularly at times during their lives when key decisions need to be made (see also Ch. 7).

Meininger (2001:242) argues that whatever concept of autonomy is proposed, we always have a moral obligation "to do the utmost to understand the personal language of any person with intellectual disabilities". He expands upon this idea by offering three different conceptions of the 'autos' or self. First, there is the 'autos' as a 'garden'. Here, the self is independent and self-enclosed just as a garden is. Entry within this territory is at the invitation of the owner and hence may be granted or denied. Second, there is the 'autos' as the 'way'. Here, there is a continuing process towards greater self-determination and liberation from the power of others. This perspective might be viewed as particularly relevant to the situation of people with learning disabilities as they seek to acquire greater self-determination and control: it is a developmental process. The third conception of 'autos' is as a 'story'. Here, just as the plot of a story develops, so the individual is involved with others "in the movement towards self-esteem which characterizes human existence" (p. 245). Key to this approach is the relationship of the self with others – "It is about my involvement with others and their involvement with me" (p. 245). Meininger argues that within this conception of autonomy, dependence is not viewed as problematic but rather as an essential characteristic of being human. We all operate in a state of interdependence relying for some things on others just as they rely upon us. Care giving thus becomes a dialogue between the care giver and the care receiver which requires a "process of careful listening and interpreting" (p. 248). Again this is particularly helpful when considering how best to support the autonomy of people with learning disabilities since it directs us not only to listen to what they say but also to observe and interpret what they do. In taking such an approach, we can work towards enhancing choice and promoting self-direction wherever possible.

The importance of relationships between people with learning disabilities and their care givers is also borne out in practice. In a study which focused on what informs ethical practice in learning disability services, Wilson et al (2008:613) found that 'almost all' respondents:

> ... reported that the relationships they had gave them an intimate understanding of the lives of people with intellectual disability and were the vehicles by which they could improve their quality of life.

It is thus the knowledge which arises from our relationships with the people we support that assists us to understand their views, preferences and wishes and hence to respect their personhood and autonomy.

Beneficence

The principle of beneficence requires that we act for the benefit of others (Beauchamp & Childress 2009). It goes beyond simply the prevention of harm and requires that we actively strive to promote good for other people. Beauchamp & Childress (2009) go on to distinguish between what they term 'general beneficence' whereby we have a general responsibility to act for the good of all others, and 'specific beneficence' where we have a particular duty to act for the good of those with whom we have a special relationship. Such relationships include those such as family and friends but also include those we have with the people we support. As has been noted above, relationships with people with learning disabilities are central to ethical practice.

In seeking to work for the benefit of people with learning disabilities, reference can be made to the principles underpinning service provision, namely rights, choice, independence and inclusion (Department of Health 2001). Our actions should thus be aimed at translating these values into practice. However, it is also important to ensure that our practice is person-centred and hence we should also be guided by what matters to individuals, their hopes, dreams and wishes. Person-centred planning (see also Ch. 9) can thus be a tool which enables us to work for the good of the people we support.

Edwards (2009) argues that beneficence is particularly important where an individual lacks autonomy and, as has been seen in the previous section, people with learning disabilities may be at particular risk of not having their autonomy respected. Edwards thus states that actions which place obligations of beneficence above those involved in respecting autonomy can be described as paternalistic. Paternalism involves one person intentionally overriding the wishes of another, justifying such actions by arguing that the action has been taken to benefit the other or preventing harm from occurring to them (Beauchamp & Childress 2009). For example, a member of staff may take the decision to remove some chocolate from an area when a client with diabetes known to like chocolate and to eat it when it is available is present. In supporting people with learning disabilities, however, it may not always be possible to determine their wishes and thus action may be taken in the person's best interests.

Paternalism can be viewed negatively as there is the danger that the wishes of people with learning disabilities could be overridden unnecessarily. Indeed, people with learning disabilities are at particular risk of having their views overridden by other people who either believe that they are acting in their best interests or who do not feel that their wishes should be respected. However, Beauchamp & Childress (2009) argue that paternalism can be justified if there is the risk of significant harm, if the paternalistic action will probably prevent the harm, if the projected benefits outweigh the risks, if there is no reasonable alternative to limiting autonomy and if the least autonomy restrictive alternative is adopted. The onus for justification, however, is seen as lying with the person who seeks to override the autonomy of another (Edwards 2009). In practice, it can thus be seen that it may be necessary to act in the best interests of those we support. However, when we seek to do so we must be clear regarding our motivations, the nature of our actions and the implications of acting in such a way.

Reader activity 5.5

Think of a practice situation where you felt that you acted in the best interests of a person with a learning disability. Did you act paternalistically? Using criteria offered by Beauchamp & Childress (2009), are you able to justify acting paternalistically?

Non-maleficence

According to Beauchamp & Childress (2009), the principle of non-maleficence requires that we do not intentionally harm other people. They go on to argue that it places an obligation to not only refrain from inflicting harm but also to refrain from inflicting risks of harm. In practice, then, it becomes apparent that appropriate risk assessments are important. However, there can be a difficult balancing act here in determining what acceptable and unacceptable risks are. Without an element of risk then lives can become very constrained and, to some extent, we learn by taking calculated risks. Nonetheless, risks have to be proportionate (see also Ch. 11) and it is important that such issues are carefully considered. In some situations, an element of harm may be justified through reference to a greater good which occurs as a consequence. For example, a small amount of pain may be acceptable when taking blood for analysis if it is likely that this will aid diagnosis and facilitate prompt treatment.

It also has to be remembered that harm can arise not only where one takes action but also where one omits to act (Edwards 2009). For example, if a member of staff is supporting a client and observes that they are thirsty but fails to give them a drink then they are causing harm. Harm and abuse can also occur unintentionally. For example, in Sutton and Merton Primary Care Trust (Healthcare Commission 2007), a lack of awareness, lack of specialist knowledge, lack of training and a lack of insight led to abusive treatment of people with learning disabilities. In some instances, unacceptable behaviours were not recognised by staff as such. It would thus appear essential that all those working in learning disability services develop an awareness of harm which can arise and that they take action to eliminate or reduce such harm.

In developing such an awareness, it must be remembered that staff members are not the only potential source of harm to people with learning disabilities. The environments in which they live may be impoverished and thus have a detrimental effect on their quality of life. They may live with people with whom they do not get on and who, in some situations, may be aggressive towards them. As a result they can experience physical danger. They may also experience hostility and abuse from the general public who feel that it is acceptable to call them names or make negative comments about them.

Such behaviours may cause psychological harm and have a negative impact on their wellbeing.

Edwards (2009) argues that while 'don't harm others' would appear to be a simple rule, it can be difficult to interpret and apply since those applying it will have their own conception of harm. For example, while there would be general agreement that it is wrong to physically attack someone, there is likely to be less agreement concerning whether it is wrong to use clients' money to buy staff members a drink when they are accompanying them to the pub. Furthermore, harm has a subjective dimension, and what one person experiences as harmful, another may not be adversely affected by. This is a particular issue in relation to people with learning disabilities who may have had a long history of poor and negative treatment such that they may view such treatment simply as 'how things are'. They may not interpret negative actions as being harmful simply because they have been conditioned into thinking this is normal behaviour. Additionally, even if they do experience something as harmful, they may not be able to express this in a way which other people understand or, if they can express it, others may not listen or respond appropriately. Practitioners may thus be involved in supporting people to recognise when harm has occurred and taking action both to seek redress and prevent future harm from occurring (see also Ch. 12). In addition to developing an awareness of potential sources of harm, non-maleficence demands that practitioners are morally alert and that they have clear ideas as to what is acceptable and unacceptable behaviour. A commitment to a positive value base and an understanding of ethical principles can assist in this process.

Justice

Justice is concerned with issues relating to equality and fairness. It is particularly important in relation to people with learning disabilities given their historical and current experiences of oppression (Northway 1998). Edwards (2009: 86) argues that:

> ... justice is done if equals are treated equally and unequals are treated unequally in proportion to relevant difference between them.

This does, however, give rise to the question of what is to be considered a 'relevant difference' and the dilemma which is associated with labelling. For example, if you take the issue of admission to a general hospital for treatment, it would seem important that the staff team are aware that an individual has a learning disability in order that appropriate support can be provided. However, in such a situation, applying the label 'learning disability' may mean that the individual concerned receives poorer treatment if, for example, the staff team feel they do not have the relevant experience or they believe that other people should provide the support for people with learning disabilities. Indeed we have seen recent examples of situations whereby people with learning disabilities failed to receive appropriate health care despite – or possibly because of – other people being aware that they had learning disabilities (Local Government Ombudsman and Parliamentary and Health Service Ombudsman 2009, Mencap 2007, Michael 2008).

In the reports cited above, there was a failure to take account of relevant differences when planning and delivering appropriate health care. Reasonable adjustments were not made in order to provide care which met the individual needs of the patients with learning disabilities. In short, justice was not done. There is often a misconception that treating people equally means treating them the same. This does, however, mean that account is not taken of relevant differences. Indeed, in the Executive Summary of his report, Michael (2008:7) noted that staff "commonly fail to understand that a right to equal treatment does not mean treatment should be the same". Reasonable adjustments are thus essential if health care is to be delivered in a fair and equitable manner.

Of course it is not just in the arena of health care that the issue of justice needs to be considered. Resources are limited and hence practitioners face and make decisions on a day-to-day basis concerning their allocation. For example, we make decisions concerning how we allocate our time – perhaps spending time with one client as opposed to another. We make decisions concerning access to services – who is and who is not eligible. We can also control access to information, making decisions about what to share with whom. Justice requires that when we make such decisions, we do so taking account of fairness and need rather than acting unconsciously or unfairly. It also demands that we do not unfairly discriminate.

At a broader level, it is also important to note that choice, independence, rights and inclusion (Department of Health 2001) are closely linked to matters of justice. People with learning disabilities are at particular risk of having their rights infringed upon, they may have unnecessary limits placed upon their independence and their choices may be constrained. Furthermore, the support required for inclusion to become a reality may not be forthcoming. Considering these issues as ethical concerns and matters of justice (or injustice) challenge us to take action in order to being about change.

While most of the discussion in this chapter has been concerned directly with people with learning disabilities, in relation to issues of justice it is also important to consider the issue of staff management. Staff will also have individual support needs and wish to be treated in a fair and equitable manner. Indeed, if they feel valued and supported they are more likely to value those whom they support. Developing strategies for positive staff management and support is thus important in the process of achieving real change for people with learning disabilities.

Each of the four ethical principles proposed by Beauchamp & Childress (2009) has now been discussed and it can be seen that, in any given situation, more than one principle may apply. Furthermore, in some situations, two principles may be in conflict with one another. For example, it may be necessary to act beneficently to safeguard an individual from harm but in doing so it is necessary to override their autonomy. This can lead to ethical or moral dilemmas which are discussed in the section below. Nonetheless, consideration of the four principles in such situations can allow us to pose questions which assist us in examining alternative perspectives and potential courses of action. Box 5.1 thus provides some examples of questions which can arise from consideration of the four principles.

Case Illustration 5.3

Jumila Khan is 25 years old. She lives at home with her family who provide her with support. Most of her activities centre on her family but she also attends a local day service for people with learning disabilities 2 days a week. She has severe learning disabilities, but while she only has a limited verbal vocabulary, she understands most of what is said to her so long as simple language is used. Usually she enjoys good health but over the past 2 days she has been reluctant to eat, has appeared to be in pain and has generally been unwell. Her family take her to see her GP but she advises that Jumila should be taken to hospital. At the hospital, appendicitis is diagnosed and she is admitted to a ward in preparation for an operation. The staff on the ward, however, appear reluctant to engage with Jumila and her family. They seem to assume that her family will take care of her with ward staff only undertaking clinical activities such as taking her temperature or blood pressure. As Jumila has not been in hospital before, she has not had these procedures performed on her and thus becomes very agitated when staff approach her. This only serves to reinforce the views of ward staff that they are not trained or equipped to provide care for people with learning disabilities. They also have concerns as to who will provide consent for Jumila to have the operation.

Reader activity 5.6

Read through Case illustration 5.3 and then analyse the scenario using the four ethical principles offered by Beauchamp & Childress (2009). How useful do you find this framework? Were there any clashes between the principles?

Working through ethical dilemmas

As can be seen from the preceding discussion, there can be situations where we are faced with a choice between one or more possible courses of action where both seem necessary but performing both is not possible. Conversely, we may be faced with two alternatives, both of which we feel are negative. We would prefer not to take either course of action but action is required. In such situations, we are faced with an ethical or moral dilemma. For example, a key worker could be involved with a client who wishes to leave home to live in supported living. They wish to support their client in this action and so respect their autonomy. However, they also know that the client's family will object to such a move and will both make it difficult for it to happen and make life difficult for the client at home. Moreover, if the key worker is viewed as supporting the individual rather than the family, this will adversely affect the relationship they have with the family which may, in turn, mean that it will be more difficult for them to see the client.

Another example is where a nurse is in charge of an assessment and treatment unit. As part of his treatment programme, one patient goes out on a daily basis to a day service in order to begin the process of moving back to a community setting. However, to go to the day service, the patient requires the support of a member of staff from the assessment and treatment unit and today it is short staffed. If a member of staff goes with the individual to the day service, the unit will be left understaffed which may put other patients

Box 5.1

Some questions arising from the four ethical principles

Autonomy

- What are the views, preferences and wishes of those concerned?
- Are individuals able to express their views in a manner that other people can understand?
- Are they subjected to unnecessary external control?
- Can support be provided to promote competence and assist decision making?
- How can the views and wishes of others best be respected?

Beneficence

- Who decides what is best/beneficial?
- How can the maximum good/benefit be achieved?
- If acting in the best interests of another, can such actions be justified (particularly if they override the autonomy of an individual)?

Non-maleficence

- Is there risk of harm?
- Can that risk be eliminated?
- If not, how can it be minimised?
- Are support systems in place to deal with potential harm?

Justice

- Is there a danger of infringing upon someone's rights?
- Is there a danger of people being treated unfairly and being discriminated against?
- Are there relevant differences which mean that people should be treated differently in order to promote equality?
- Which actions would promote greater fairness?

Adapted from Beauchamp TL Childress JF 2009 Principles of Biomedical Ethics, 6th Edition, Oxford: Oxford University Press.

at risk. Alternatively, if the individual does not go to the day service then their process of reintroduction to community facilities will be adversely affected.

See Reader Activity 5.7 and Case Illustration 5.4 on the Evolve website.

Rowson (2006) highlights the importance of practitioners developing strategies for resolving ethical dilemmas:

> When ethical demands compete in a professional situation it is part of their job to use their expertise and skills – often in conjunction with clients – to work out a way forward. They cannot just wring their hands in agony; they have an obligation to do something.

Clearly, taking action is a professional responsibility. However, Rowson also suggests that in seeking to find a way forward it is important to work in collaboration with clients. This could perhaps be overlooked if a professional feels under pressure to resolve the situation single handed. In seeking to develop our skills of ethical reasoning we should thus seek, wherever possible, to involve clients who can provide an important perspective.

A number of approaches are available to assist us in working through ethical dilemmas. Professional codes of conduct and ethics are one example of frameworks which act as guides for action. Within such documents, the standards of behaviour required of a practitioner are set out and these standards are a measure against which professional behaviour is assessed. In consulting their code of conduct when faced with an ethical dilemma, the practitioner may find that the required course of action is clear.

When faced with ethical dilemmas, another guide to decision making is the legislative framework within which we work. For example, when faced with a dilemma concerning consent to treatment in England and Wales, the Mental Capacity Act 2005 identifies clear requirements in relation to capacity to consent and actions to be taken where capacity is not demonstrated. Similarly, when faced with a client who is in an acute phase of psychosis and who is threatening self-harm, we have the provisions of the Mental Health Act 1983 which permit compulsory detention of the individual to protect them from harm. This is not to say that we may not still experience some disquiet if, for example, a client becomes very distressed at being compulsorily detained but rather to stress that there is no real dilemma since the appropriate course of action is prescribed in law: ethics and law can have different implications.

Ethical advisory groups can assist practitioners and services with exploring ethical issues (Malin & Wilmot 2000a, 2000b, Malin et al 2000). Malin et al (2000:110) detail one such group which met on a monthly basis "with an aim to offer advice to staff to resolve problems of a broadly ethical nature which they encounter in their day-to-day work covering the care of people with learning disabilities". One reason for establishing the group was that policy directives and guidelines did not cover every practice eventuality. The group was multidisciplinary and included citizens' advocates. Issues discussed were wide ranging but included those relating to the balancing of client autonomy against client protection (Malin & Wilmot 2000a). Paternalism and 'best interests' also featured regularly in the discussions (Malin & Wilmot 2000b). Malin & Wilmot (2000b) conclude that such an ethics groups can assist in the translation of policy into practice and in promoting evidence-based practice.

Multidisciplinary team working and reflective practice are also viewed by practitioners as being helpful when seeking to resolve ethical dilemmas (Holloway 2004). Indeed reflection is viewed as increasing practitioners' self-awareness concerning their personal values and attitudes which they bring to the consideration of ethical issues (Holloway 2007). Nonetheless it is helpful to have a framework for such reflection and consideration and a number of such frameworks are available. Boxes 5.2 and 5.3 provide two such examples.

Box 5.2

Framework for ethical decision making (1)

A six step approach

1. Get the story straight by gathering relevant information.
2. Identify the type of ethical problem.
3. Use ethical theories, approaches or principles to analyse the situation.
4. Explore the practical alternatives which are available.
5. Complete the action.
6. Evaluate the process and the outcome.

(Purtilo 2005)

Box 5.3

Framework for ethical decision making (2)

The DECIDE model

D Define the problem – what are the facts? What are your duties?
E Ethical review – with reference to ethical principles.
C Consider the options – what alternative courses of action are available?
I Investigate the outcomes – what are the probable consequences of the different courses of action.
D Decide on action – set clear objectives.
E Evaluate results – were the goals achieved?

Thompson et al (2006)

In examining the two frameworks for ethical reflection and decision making, it can be seen that there are some similarities between them. First, they both offer a structured approach to consideration of the issue and seeking a resolution. This is important since it means that all aspects are addressed and there is less likelihood of important issues being overlooked or forgotten. Second, both frameworks encourage you to consider a range of perspectives and to use ethical theories and principles such as those discussed in this chapter to inform your analysis and decision making. Both suggest that you explore alternative courses of action and Thompson et al (2006) argue that you should also consider the likely consequences of the alternatives. Finally, both conclude by identifying the need to evaluate the process and the outcomes.

While both frameworks are presented in a linear format, it might be more helpful to think about them in terms of a cyclical approach. Within such an approach, practitioners would reflect upon and evaluate the process and the outcomes of one ethical dilemma before taking forward any learning to the next. They thus engage in a continual process of personal ethical development and their ethical awareness and reasoning skills will develop over time. It is also important to note that these frameworks could also be used by a staff group who are seeking to address an ethical dilemma since they provide a framework for both discussion and action. Indeed, in a group context, they can provide an important guide for teamworking.

Reader activity 5.8

Read through Case illustration 5.5 and then use one of the frameworks for approaching ethical dilemmas to analyse the situation. If you were a member of staff working in the respite care unit, what course of action would you take? Why?

Reader activity 5.9

Look back at the answers you gave to Reader activity 5.1. As a result of reading this chapter and undertaking the activities, would you act differently when faced with a similar dilemma in the future?

Case illustration 5.5

Alex Jones is 24 and has a mild learning disability. He attends the local further education college where he has met Gemma Banks. Gemma is 22 and is said to have a moderate learning disability. At the college, Alex and Gemma have developed a close relationship but their parents are against this and will not let them see each other outside of college. Both Alex and Gemma use a local small-scale respite unit but their parents are adamant that they do not want them to be there at the same time. Indeed, they have each said that they would remove their son or daughter from the unit if they found out that the other was there. Alex, however, has confided in staff within the unit that he would like them both to be there so that he could 'sleep with Gemma'. To date, their stays at the respite care unit have been coordinated such that they have not been there at the same time. Currently, however, Gemma is staying there for a week and the staff have just received an emergency request from Mr and Mrs Jones for Alex to stay in the unit as there has been a family bereavement and they have to go away for a few days. Given the expressed wishes of both sets of parents while also taking account of the fact that Alex and Gemma are both adults who very much want to develop their relationship, the staff are faced with a dilemma.

Conclusion

This chapter has provided an introduction to ethical theories and principles considering each of these in relation to the provision of support for people with learning disabilities. It has been seen that practitioners who support people with learning disabilities are likely to encounter many ethical issues in their day-to-day work. In some instances, they may be faced with ethical dilemmas whereby they are forced to make difficult decisions concerning the appropriate course of action. In such circumstances, it has been argued that it is helpful to have a framework to guide the process of decision making. Seedhouse (2009:27) argues that ultimately ethics is 'a matter of personal deliberation' which emphasises the importance of practitioners being ethically and morally aware. They must be able to recognise ethical issues and provide reasoned responses. In short, they must be able to think ethically. Rowson (2006) thus offers what he terms the FAIR framework for ethical thinking in the professions:

- To treat individuals justly and **F**airly.
- To respect people's **A**utonomy.
- To act with **I**ntegrity.
- To seek the best **R**esults.

Utilising this framework as a basis for practice, both at an individual and service level, should assist us in providing support which is both ethically sound and which enhances quality of life for those whom we support.

References

Baggini, J., Fosl, P.S., 2007. The ethics toolkit. A compendium of ethical concepts and methods. Blackwell, Oxford.

Beauchamp, T.L., Childress, J.F., 2009. Principles of biomedical ethics, sixth ed. Oxford University Press, Oxford.

Department of Health, 2001. Valuing people. The Stationery Office, London.

Edwards, S.D., 2009. Nursing ethics: a principle-based approach, second ed Palgrave Macmillan, Basingstoke.

Healthcare Commission, 2007. Investigation into the service for people with learning disabilities provided by Sutton and Merton Primary Care Trust. Healthcare Commission, London.

Hessler, I., Kay, B., 1993. Ethical issues. In: Shanley, E., Starrs, T.A. (Eds.), Learning disabilities. A handbook of care. Churchill Livingstone, Edinburgh, pp. 293–305.

Holloway, D., 2004. Ethical dilemmas in community learning disabilities nursing: what helps nurses resolve ethical dilemmas that result from choices made by people with learning disabilities? J. Intellect. Disabil. 8 (3), 283–298.

Holloway, D., 2007. Ethical issues in learning disabilities. In: Gates, B. (Ed.), Learning disabilities. Towards inclusion. sixth ed. Churchill Livingstone, Edinburgh, pp. 67–79.

Kay, B., 1994. People with learning difficulties. In: Tschudin, V. (Ed.), Ethics: nursing people with special needs, Part II. Scutari Press, London, pp. 1–43.

Local Government Ombudsman and Parliamentary and Health Service Ombudsman, 2009. Six lives: the provision of public services to people with learning disabilities, Part 1. Overview and summary investigation reports. The Stationery Office, London.

Malin, N., Wilmot, S., 2000a. An ethical advisory group in a learning disability service: what they talk about. J. Intellect. Disabil. 4 (3), 217–226.

Malin, N., Wilmot, S., 2000b. An ethical advisory group in a learning disability service: members' views on outcomes. J. Intellect. Disabil. 4 (4), 333–342.

Malin, N., Wilmot, S., Beswick, J.A., 2000. The use of an ethical advisory group in a learning disability service. J. Intellect. Disabil. 4 (2), 105–114.

Meininger, H.P., 2001. Autonomy and professional responsibility in care for persons with intellectual disabilities. Nurs. Philos. 2, 240–250.

Mencap, 2007. Death by indifference. Mencap, London.

Michael, J., 2008. Healthcare for all. Report of the Independent Inquiry into Access to Healthcare for People with Learning Disabilities. The Stationery Office, London.

Northway, R., 1998. Oppression in the lives of people with learning difficulties: a participatory study. Unpublished PhD Thesis, University of Bristol, Bristol.

Purtilo, R., 2005. Ethical dimensions in the health professions, fourth ed. Elsevier Saunders, Philadelphia.

Rowson, R., 2006. Working ethics. How to be fair in a culturally complex world. Jessica Kingsley, London.

Seedhouse, D., 2009. Ethics: the heart of health care, third ed. Wiley Blackwell, Chichester.

Thompson, I.E., Melia, K.M., Boyd, K.M., Horsbugh, D., 2006. Nursing ethics, fifth ed. Churchill Livingstone, Edinburgh.

Wheat, K., 2009. Applying ethical principles in healthcare practice. Br. J. Nurs. 18 (17), 1062–1063.

Wilson, N., Clegg, J., Hardy, G., 2008. What informs and shapes ethical practice in intellectual disability services? J. Intellect. Disabil. 52 (7), 608–617.

Further reading

Buka, P., 2008. Patients' rights, law and ethics for nurses. A practical guide. Hodder Arnold, London.

Clements, L., Read, J. (Eds.), 2008. Disabled people and the right to life. Routledge, London.

Meininger, H.P., 2005. Narrative ethics in nursing for persons with intellectual disabilities. Nurs. Philos. 6, 106–118.

Useful addresses

The Nursing and Midwifery Council, http://www.nmc-uk.org.

The General Social Care Council, http://www.gscc.org.uk.

The Northern Ireland Social Care Council, http://www.niscc.info.

Care Council for Wales, http://www.ccwales.org.uk/home.

The Scottish Commission for the Regulation of Care, http://www.carecommission.com.

The UK Clinical Ethics Network, http://www.ethics-network.org.uk/.

The British Institute of Learning Disabilities, http://www.bild.org.uk/.

Section 2

Implementing values-based support

Let me speak – facilitating communication

6

Karen Bunning

CHAPTER CONTENTS

KEY ISSUES

- Communication is not a solitary activity – it takes two to make it happen!
- Communication is about two or more people building meanings together
- Communication does not happen in a vacuum – the context is integral to the whole process
- Facilitating the communication of people with learning disabilities means building on existing strengths
- Acceptance of a multi-dimensional view of communication is a good place to start – there are always alternatives to the spoken word!
- Inclusive communication is about establishing an environment that places the least possible restrictions on the people present

Introduction

It is widely acknowledged that communication problems among the population with learning disabilities are common, although reported estimates on prevalence vary (Rondal & Edwards 1997), ranging from 50% (Enderby & Davies 1989) to 78% (Parker & Liddle 1987). Use of different survey methods and operational definitions of what is meant by 'communication difficulty' probably account for disparities in this area. An earlier survey by Blackwell et al (1989) concluded that 33% had some verbal communication difficulty (25% demonstrating marked problems) and 29% were non-verbal, indicating that 62% of the population experience identifiable communication problems. Law & Lester (1991) looked at the communication of people attending a social education centre and found slightly higher levels of need: 81% were considered to require support for their communication skills; 9.5% being non-verbal and 5.9% experiencing low comprehension and/or low expression. No matter the variation in reported prevalence figures, it is clear that there is an increased risk of communication difficulties occurring in people with learning disabilities compared with the general population (Kerr et al 1996).

In order to respond to the communication problems experienced by people with learning disabilities, we need to make sense of the difficulties that occur. However, even before we reach that point we need to establish what it is we are talking about. In other words, what is 'communication'?

What is communication?

There is no doubt about it – communication is a complex business. Take the example of a woman who enters a shoe shop at 5.25 pm. Having ignored the sign on the door that states in bold print – CLOSES AT 5.30 pm – she approaches a nearby assistant and asks cheerfully if the shop is still open. The assistant replies quite politely in the affirmative. The woman, on hearing the response, apologises and leaves the shop rapidly. Now, on the face of it, the exchange is all quite straightforward – the woman asks a question and the assistant provides her with an answer. On hearing that the shop is still open, the woman can set about the task in hand – finding a new pair of shoes – except she leaves. So what has gone on here? If we look more closely at the detail of the exchange, we notice the assistant looking fleetingly at her watch while answering the woman. Furthermore, we hear the tightness in her voice as she gives her 'yes' response. The 'tut' she utters is barely perceptible as she turns her head to look at her colleague, but if we listen closely, it is there. What are the messages being communicated here? The words suggest that the shop is open because there are 5 minutes to go until closing time. The detail communicates quite a different story. "Yes, the shop is still open, but I am not happy with your request. We are about to close." Suddenly realising her mistake, the woman stumbles her apology and flees in embarrassment vowing never to return to that particular shop. So we see that communication is much, much more than just words.

What does this tell us about communication? First, it tells us that it is multi-faceted. It is not just about the exchange of messages through spoken words. For instance, the printed sign on the shop door informed the woman of the closing time. Then of course the tone of voice belies the words spoken by the assistant and conveys, instead, her annoyance at the late request to look at shoes. The way we utter words, the pitch, stress patterns, intonation – all add to the meaning being communicated and are termed paralinguistic phenomena (Box 6.1). Non-verbal behaviours are also integral to communication (Coupe O'Kane & Goldbart 1998) and the shop assistant's fleeting look at her watch and her final 'tut' and turn of the head provide yet more signals of her displeased state. Thus we see that the actions and movements used by a person can bear meaning. For example, the person who stamps their foot in expression of anger; the person who grabs hold of a person's sleeve to attract their attention – these all have the potential to convey meaning. Mehrabian (1971) stressed the importance of non-verbal elements for communicating feelings and attitude, and in particular the prior importance assigned to tone of voice and facial expression when there is a lack of congruence between the words spoken and the non-verbal aspects of an exchange. Now we see how the communication of the shop assistant is more than just words!

> **Box 6.1**
>
> **The different guises of communication**
>
> Here are just some of the different formats we use for communication every day:
>
> - Speech – the strings of words we utter.
> - Prosody – our use of intonation and volume, our use of pause, the rate at which we speak, e.g. high-pitched and rapid speech denoting excitement, slow, languid delivery with a flat intonation revealing our tiredness.
> - Vocal gestures – vocalisations, e.g. gasps to show amazement, screams indicating delight.
> - Body gestures – often referred to as body language, e.g. a shake of the fist to convey inner emotional state, leaning forward showing attentiveness to a subject.
> - Hand/arm gestures – that hold meaning within a culture, e.g. shaking a fist to convey anger, waving to denote departure.
> - Text – the words that we and others write, e.g. in books, on street signs, on websites.
> - Graphemes – the pictorial images and symbols that capture a concept or meaning, e.g. the 'female' symbol on the toilet door indicating 'Ladies', the picture on the food packet denoting its contents.

A categorical view of communication

The second aspect of communication that warrants consideration is how communication takes place. A reductionist view would be to adopt a categorical perspective where one person sends a message to the other person for decoding, before sending back a response. On its own, this more aptly describes the exchanges between two ships using Morse code. Characterised by strict demarcation of turns, there is silence after each message is sent so that the other person can make a response; the 'sender' actively encodes the message which is sent through the noise in the air for the receiver who decodes it. Referred to as the code model, the sender role is seen as active in the communication process and the receiver as passive (see Sperber & Wilson 1995). Now there is nothing particularly wrong with this, after all we saw an exchange of messages between the woman and the shop assistant in the example above. *Except* that it ignores a huge amount of the exchange, for instance the role taken by the listener as an active participant in the construction of meaning and all the non-verbal and paralinguistic phenomena that are critical to the meanings being constructed. As for the code model, it describes only one small part of human communication and neglects some critical components.

It takes two to communicate!

An alternative view is to look at communication as something that involves two or more individuals making contributions to a shared construction of meaning. There is usually the coordination of actions so that each person takes turns in the conversation, but maintains an active role even when it is not their 'speaking' turn. That is, listening to and interpreting what the other person says and does are as important to the meaning as expressing your own ideas in a communication turn. Consideration of the phenomenon of ambiguity is key, whereby it is a given that far from being categorically clear, meanings constructed in interaction are frequently unclear. This is because the intentions behind acts of communication do not map precisely onto the words. The shop assistant's words were probably driven by multiple intentions, not least of which might have been: to perform the role of the courteous shop assistant who perhaps does not want to be reported to her manager; and the shop assistant who does not want to delay getting away from work and therefore wants to let this 'nuisance' of a customer know. Of course, intentions may be conscious and deliberate, but also they may operate at a subconscious level. We just need to be aware that social communication is characterised by multiple intentions and more than one meaning.

All this corresponds very neatly to the inferential model proposed by Grice, Lewis and others (see Sperber & Wilson 1995), which simply means that the act of interpreting a message is as important to the resultant meaning as the act of sending a message. Therefore communication is achieved through *producing* and *interpreting* the evidence. This means that communication is not simply a matter of sending code or words to each other, but the meaning behind those words and the accompanying non-verbal behaviour needs to be extracted. Related to this is the continuous processing model proposed by Fogel (1993), which describes communication as two or more people working together and coordinating their actions in ongoing response to each other and the context (Bunning 2009, Grove et al 1999, Olsson 2004). In this way, two people influence the actions of one another: the shop assistant's communication sends the woman out of the shop vowing never to cross its threshold again, and perhaps the stumbling apology and hasty exit of the woman causes the assistant a moment of regret – or maybe not! This is an important model for thinking about communication with people with learning disabilities because it implies a shared responsibility for building meanings together. The onus for successful exchanges does not rest with just one person, but with the number of people involved in communication at any one time.

Making sense

Because, for most of us, communication is immediate and spontaneous, we take for granted the way two communicators are able to follow a conversational thread and take their turns as the interaction progresses. The other person says something and we interpret the meaning, which triggers our response. However, many factors influence the way we act in social situations and how meanings are established.

Reader activity 6.1

If communication is multi-faceted, think of all the different ways you are able to communicate? Once you have done that, think about a recent conversation you have had with a friend or work colleague. What were the different ways you communicated? What did you do when the other person was talking? How did you let the other person know that you were attending (actively listening) to what they were saying?

The person with whom we are communicating will affect our contributions to the conversation. The way we communicate with a close friend is markedly different to the way we communicate with our boss. Our relationship and experience of the person colours our communicative style. For example, familiarity and closeness with a person enables us to pick up on the little nuances of conversation and shape our responses accordingly. After all, the communication between partners of many years standing will be in marked contrast to the same two people out on a first date! The context in which the communication takes place also plays its part. The degree of informality, the purpose of the context, for example work place, home, classroom; the attributes of the setting, for example using a loud voice to make ourselves heard in a noisy environment, using hushed tones in a quiet environment such as a library (see Box 6.2).

As we have seen, and to repeat my earlier mantra, communication is much more than just words. At this stage it is probably a good idea to put all this into some kind of framework. Bronfenbrenner (1979, 2005) proposed a model to describe human development and functioning in context. Conceived as a series of nested circles which define the different systems in human ecology, the individual is placed at the centre. From here it moves outwards to the immediate and familiar contexts in the person's life, to community settings and finally society. A simplified version of this defines the communication context in three concentric circles around the *Individual* (1) (source: Bunning 2004, Bunning & Grove 2002). The circle that immediately surrounds the individual is called the *Communication Partnership* (2). It comprises the range of communication partners with whom the individual engages on a daily basis. This may include parents, keyworkers, friends and teachers. The next circle is termed the *Communication Environment* (3), which represents the various settings in which the individual works, plays and socialises with the communication partners, for example the classroom in school, the home, the social club and the local shop. Beyond these inner circles is the *Social, Cultural and Political Context* (4), where social, political and cultural aspects are represented. This includes government legislation and social policy, which exert influence over the inner two circles (Fig. 6.1).

The best way to make sense of the communication ecology is to picture a person. Take the example of that most famous of boy wizards – Harry Potter. The first and second circles that surround him contain the significant communication partners in his life and the contexts in which Harry encounters them. For example, there is his foster family comprising mean aunt and uncle, and spoilt cousin Dudley at number 1 Privet Drive and the close friendship circle of Ron Weasley and Hermione Granger at Hogwarts. These different communities and settings correspond to what Bronfenbrenner (1979, 2005) calls 'Microsystems', which have their own "pattern of activities, roles, and interpersonal relations" (Bronfenbrenner 2005:148). So for Harry, the way he communicates will vary across partners and environments. Finally, what are the main political, social and cultural influences operating in Harry's life? Well, there is his membership of both the magical community and the muggle (non-magic) world, two very different cultures and both of which inform his conduct and communication behaviour.

Finally, what do we find to communicate about? Is it simply a case of giving and receiving information? No, of course not! Human beings communicate about a multitude of things and for a variety of reasons.

Box 6.2

Situational factors affecting communication

- Knowledge and experience each person has of the other.
- Cultural identity and personal values.
- Relationship between the two people, whether intimate and highly familiar or else formal and distant.
- Attributes of the physical setting, e.g. ambient noise level, luminescence.
- Purpose of communication, e.g. formal job interview, gossip between two friends.

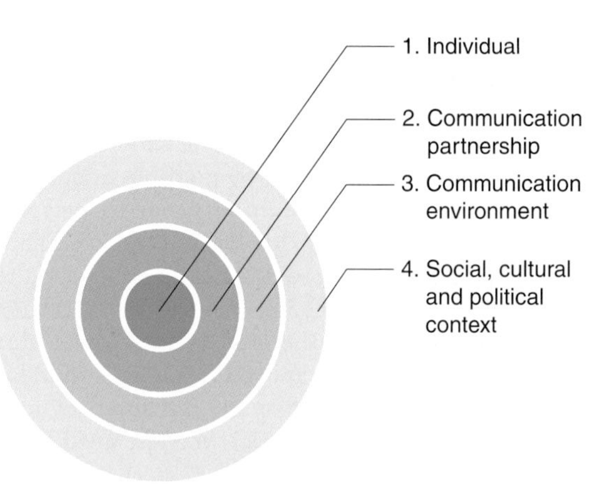

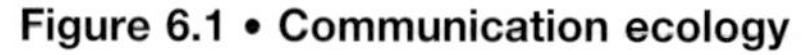

Figure 6.1 • Communication ecology

Reader activity 6.2

There are a number of factors that are critical to communication: the individual – the skills and experiences; the other people – your knowledge and experience of them, the relationship you share; the context – the different settings in which you encounter the various people in your life, the purpose of those settings and your role. Now take a blank piece of paper and draw four large circles, one inside the other (see Fig. 6.1). Write your name inside the circle at the centre. Next reflect on the people with whom you communicate on a daily basis. Write them down in the outer circle. Next, identify the different places or settings where communication happens for you. Finally, tackle the outer circle. What are the key political, social and cultural influences on the communication activities represented in the inner circles? Think about your work, your home life and your leisure outlets. Do the same for someone with a learning disability whom you know or have worked with. How do the circles compare?

We communicate meanings and exchange information; we make propositions and tell jokes; we share our thoughts and ideas; we express our beliefs and inner emotions; we evince attitudes and report facts (Sperber & Wilson 1995). We assert our views, make requests, give instructions, accept some things and reject others, access goods and services – the list goes on!

Challenges in everyday communication

Having a communication difficulty frequently leads to a breakdown in the ability to exchange information and to engage in social interaction. This may take the form of impaired verbal comprehension, difficulties in formulating utterances or speech sounds, or using available skills in different contexts with a range of other people. It also means that opportunities for self-expression and self-determination are likely to be fewer and far between (Bradshaw 2002, Bunning & Grove 2002, Sack & McLean 1997, Scott & Larcher 2002). There are many reasons why this should be the case: person-centred factors interact with factors that are external to the individual – located in the environment (Bunning 2004). A summary of these factors is provided in Box 6.3.

So where does it all go wrong? On the whole, children with learning disabilities seem to receive the same type of parental language input as their typically developing peers (Maurer & Sherrod 1987). However, the language output and communicative behaviour of children are likely to affect the ways parents, and for that matter carers and support staff, respond. For example, an apparent lack of responsiveness in a child may lead to the parent adopting more directive and instructional styles of communication. Rondal & Edwards (1997), among others, suggest that mothers of children with learning disabilities may be more concerned to try to teach language explicitly as a way of addressing the apparent lack of output. Marfo et al (1998), reviewing a series of studies, suggest that we need to look at two parameters affecting communication: (1) the directiveness or the extent to which the adult 'directs' the actions of the child; and (2) the sensitivity to child behaviour or the degree to which the adult is 'tuned in' to the child's response repertoire. Intrusive directiveness combined with a lack of sensitivity seems to inhibit child responsivity. However, directiveness combined with sensitive, contingent responses to child behaviour appears to facilitate development.

Box 6.3

Factors that challenge everyday communication

Person-centred factors

- Compromised or limited communication skills that make it difficult to express ideas and to influence the environment.
- Personal reluctance to challenge those in a position of power because of a fear of failure.
- A lack of confidence in own abilities.
- Individual experience of communication difficulties triggering emotional reactions that protect or sustain self, such as extreme passivity and apathy, defensiveness or aggression.

Factors external to the person

- A predominantly verbal environment that proves inaccessible to the individual.
- Being placed within a 'carer–being cared for' relationship that nurtures dependence and compromises individual autonomy.
- Limited or inappropriate opportunities to use available skills.
- A lack of sensitivity to the subtle ways an individual may communicate, e.g. eye gaze, vocalisation, facial expression.

With regard to adults with learning disabilities, over-estimation of an individual's communication skills is a frequently encountered problem among specialist services (Bartlett & Bunning 1997, McConkey et al 1999, Purcell et al 2000). Conversely, spontaneous contributions to conversations by people with learning disabilities seem to increase when staff adopt a facilitative style, avoiding closed questions and directives, and increasing non-verbal feedback (Mirenda & Donnellan 1986, Money 1997). Purcell et al (2000) found that increased staff responsiveness to clients was associated with increased communication by clients.

See Reader activity 6.3 on the Evolve website.

Communication breakdown

Living with a communication difficulty means that problems with influencing what happens in your immediate environment and affecting the actions of others happen all too often (Bunning 2004, Bradshaw 2000, Bartlett & Bunning 1997). Social connections as part of routine interactions are frequently hard-won and misunderstandings crop up frequently. The trouble starts with the unequal share of communication skills in many communication partnerships (Bunning 2004). Critical differences in the communication skills of the person with a learning disability and the people who provide support, for example carers, teachers, support staff, may lead to an imbalance in what Kagan (1998) refers to as the communication equation. On one side of the equation is the person who is cognitively able and equipped with a full set of linguistic skills for making contributions to the interaction; on the other is the person with a learning disability who has delayed development or restricted cognitive functioning, and impaired communication skills. The chance of something going wrong in an interaction is quite likely.

Case illustration 6.1

Abdullah has a lot to say for himself and shows a great deal of interest in the people around him. He has had a great weekend – he met his sister's new baby for the first time. On Monday morning he greets his tutor at college enthusiastically and starts to tell him about his news. Abdullah's speech is difficult to understand – many of the speech sounds are produced incorrectly. This makes it difficult for the listener to decipher what he is saying. The tutor, who is sorting out the day's work, gives Abdullah only half attention, makes some placatory noises and walks over to some other students. The communication is over and Abdullah's news is unshared and his real competence, i.e. the ability to report an event, remains hidden.

Box 6.4

Chain reaction of communication breakdown

What happens when communication does not succeed? Using Case illustration 6.1 of Abdullah, we can see a chain reaction where there has been:

- A struggle to express ideas or to understand what is being communicated, which may lead to...
- Failure to construct meaning so that communication breaks down, which may lead to...
- Feelings of disempowerment, where the person with a communication difficulty does not participate, which may lead to...
- Feelings of self-doubt and frustration, which may lead to...
- Inappropriate ways of responding, withdrawal or problem behaviour, which may result in...
- Social isolation and exclusion.

(Adapted from Bunning 2004, Bunning & Grove 2002)

Reader activity 6.4

Think about someone with a learning disability. Describe a typical situation where communication struggle takes place, focusing on:

Struggle: What was the communication about and how did you know there was struggle in the communication?

Breakdown: How did the communication break down, e.g. failure to understand, unclear use of speech, signs, etc?

Disempowerment: How balanced was the interaction, e.g. who spoke the most, etc?

Feelings: How did it feel when communication broke down, e.g. experience of dissatisfaction or frustration?

Consequential behaviour: What did the person do at the end of the interaction, e.g. withdraw from situation, get cross, etc?

Outcomes: What were the social implications for the person, e.g. left alone, excluded, etc?

Addressing communication difficulties

So where do we begin to address the problem of living with communication difficulty? The first principle must always be to build on the inherent strengths of the individual. No matter the severity of the learning disability or the extent of the communication problem, there is always a level at which the individual may connect with the people in the immediate environment, whether it is via fleeting eye gaze, vocalisation, gesture, words or other non-verbal behaviour. We need to respond at whatever level the individual is functioning. It is about optimising communicative potential.

Adapting our communication

The art of pitching our communication to the perceived level of the person with a learning disability is easier said than done! There are two main types of communication error that may occur in a communication partnership (Bunning 2004). The first error type involves failure on behalf of the partner to recognise the language and communication skills of the person. This is depicted as a 'cycle of devaluation' in Figure 6.2. In Case illustration 6.2, this would be paramount to not recognising the discriminating nature of Jacqueline's vocal behaviour and the different meanings they convey. This act of masking the person's competence will limit opportunities for social participation, inclusion and personal development. The second error type is attributing skills and competencies to the person that they do not possess. By inflating an individual's communicative competencies and simultaneously making no adjustments to how communication happens, the partner may literally talk 'over the head' of the person, using vocabulary and linguistic structures that cannot be processed. Similar to error type 1, the person's ability to participate is curtailed by the provision of an inaccessible opportunity for social interaction. The risks associated with these two error types are defined in two interlocking cycles: (1) 'inflation or over-estimation' of the person's communication skills and (2) the reverse of this, the 'devaluation or under-estimation'. These are illustrated in Figure 6.2 (adapted source: Bunning 2004:167), which was based on two contrasting models by O'Brien in Tyne (1981) and Bartlett & Bunning (1997). The risk of cycle (1) is that the true needs of the person may be overlooked, essential adaptations to communication neglected and expectations of the individual too high, leading to negative or diminished experiences with a corresponding weakening of self-esteem, for example the person experiences failure in communication too often. The risk of cycle (2) is that the true competencies of the person may go unnoticed and expectations pitched at too low a level, again leading to a negative or diminished experience that is disempowering to the individual. Thus we see the importance of striving for a pitch of communication with which the person can both engage and respond.

Consideration of how to communicate with Jacqueline in Case illustration 6.2 highlights the risks associated with the two cycles depicted in Figure 6.2. If her communication partners think that she has full understanding of language and make no attempt to adapt their communication to suit Jacqueline's needs, there is no opening for Jacqueline to use her skills. The opportunity is inaccessible and her ability to self-determine is overlooked. This is cycle (1). Conversely, if her communication partners believe that she has no ability to convey her pleasure or disapproval, they will make all decisions without recourse to Jacqueline. There is the failure to tune in and recognise Jacqueline's own ways of communicating. This is cycle (2). Thus, in both cycles, Jacqueline is excluded from determining the things that matter to her and she is prevented from affecting change in her environment.

Augmentative and alternative communication

Augmentative and alternative communication (AAC) offers a wide range of approaches, techniques and tactics for supporting communication (Beukelman & Mirenda 1998). The main purpose of intervention is to bring about tangible benefits to the person's existing situation and to provide "... the best opportunities for developing language and communication ..." (Martinsen & von Tetzchner 1996:39). It is the "... hope of a language system that allows one to communicate competently with family, friends, teachers and employers ..." (Yoder 2001:4). AAC is an area of practice whereby "an individual can supplement or replace spoken communication" (Royal College of Speech & Language Therapists 2006:230). von Tetzchner & Martinsen (2000) identified the

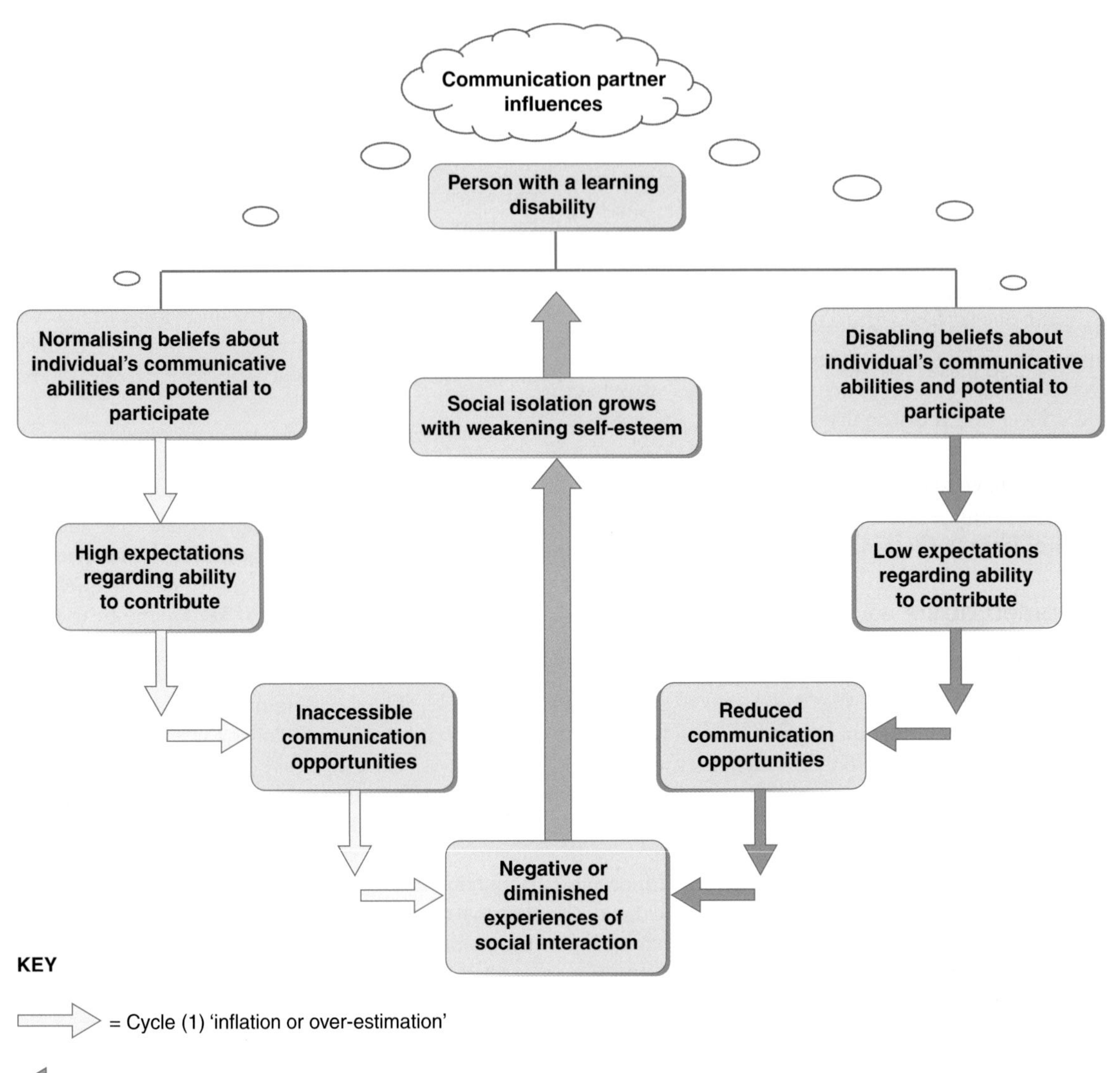

Figure 6.2 • Risks associated with cycles of communication inflation and devaluation

different groups of people who may benefit from some form of AAC:

- Augmented group: those who understand and use spoken language, but need a system as a back up.
- Expressive group: those who have good understanding of spoken language, but need the system for expression.
- Receptive group: those who need a system to understand as well as to express themselves.

So what are the choices in terms of AAC? Briefly, the options fall into one or other of two camps: unaided communication and aided communication. *Unaided* describes typical face-to-face communication where the interactants or the people who are generating utterances use the characteristics of natural communication, for example speech, manual signs, facial expressions and eye gaze. *Aided*, on the other hand, includes all types of communication where the linguistic 'utterances' (letters, words/graphic symbols,

Case illustration 6.2

Jacqueline is 9 years old with severe to profound and multiple learning disabilities. She uses a specialised seating system and is dependent on others for her day-to-day care. She is able to use her left arm to reach and grab for items. Jacqueline is blind in her right eye but retains some vision in her upper left field of vision. Her hearing is unimpaired. Her teacher has told us that she looks at coloured pictures and objects held in her left field of vision – she smiles, vocalises and jerks her body. She vocalises, using back vowels such as 'ah', mainly making a 'happy' sound and a 'cross' or 'fed up' sound. All these things represent starting points with Jacqueline.

objects) have to be selected from a display, for example communication boards, books, electronic aids, sets of objects (Fig. 6.3).

Unaided options

Signing

Signs have been used with people with communication impairments for around 40 years, beginning in the 1960s in the USA and the UK (Cornforth et al 1974). Different from the sign languages of deaf communities, the use of signs with the population with learning disabilities provides a compensatory strategy to support deficiencies in communication, for example verbal comprehension difficulties, expressive language limitations. The signs themselves are usually taken from sign languages, and paired with spoken language. Thus signing becomes not a replacement for speech but a support. Signing therefore follows the grammatical structure of the spoken language, often known as key word signing, where important information-carrying words are signed. You can use one sign or several to support the meanings being communicated. Take the sentence 'What do you want for dinner?' There are a number of options for supporting the key meanings being communicated, which are based on what we know about the communication needs of the person in front of us. In Case illustrations 6.3–6.5, the sign-supported words are in **bold**.

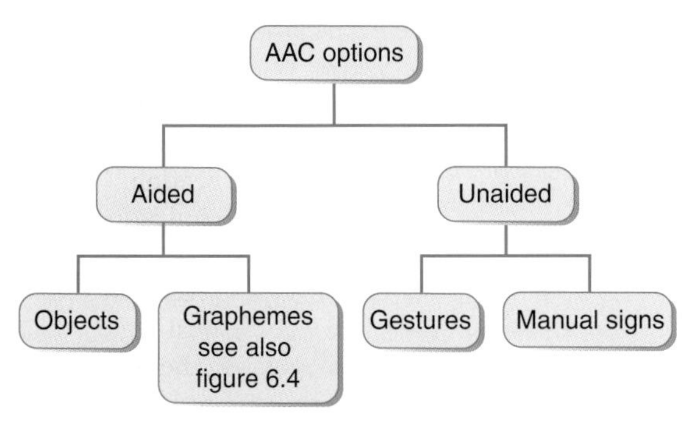

Figure 6.3 • Main options for AAC

Natural gestures

Le Prevost (1993) was concerned with supporting the communication development of very young children but recognised that some parents may find signing somewhat of a threat to the development of speech. She developed an introductory sign teaching resource for parents and children called 'See and Say', which focused on natural gestures and basic meanings, for example wash, brush hair, drink, goodbye, sit, come, go, eat, sleep, read (Le Prevost 1990). This approach builds on studies of early communication showing that infants and toddlers rely equally on gestures and vocalisations/words (Capirci et al 1996). Furthermore, children described as late

Case illustration 6.3

Jadine understands one piece of information at a time. Her attention for speech is fleeting but she responds well to facial expression and body language. Her mother asks Jadine: 'What do you want for **dinner**?' signing **dinner** in a slow and emphatic way lasting for the length of the spoken utterance.

Case illustration 6.4

Alexis is able to understand two key pieces of information in an utterance. His carers are trying to get him to use his language to respond to questions asked of him. His carer asks him: '**What** do you want for **dinner**?'

Case illustration 6.5

Nehemiah understands most of what is said to him when key word signing is used. When he attempts to speak himself, it is very difficult for others to understand what he is saying. The main people who communicate with him at school and at home are trying to encourage him to use signing by exposing him to sign support in his environment. They ask him: '**What** do **you want** for **dinner**?'

talkers and children with Down syndrome have been reported as using gestures more frequently than their age-matched peers with normal expressive language (Franco & Wishart 1996, Thal & Tobias 1992).

Makaton Vocabulary: signs

This is a vocabulary that was developed by Margaret Walker in the early 1970s (see Grove & Walker 1990). It loosely follows the lines of typical vocabulary acquisition in stages. Used internationally, it draws on the lexicon of the indigenous sign language, for example British Sign Language (BSL) in the UK and American Sign Language in the USA. Signs are selected from the range of alternatives available, with some consideration given to ease of production, for example the sign for 'look' is used for both 'look' and 'see'; 'fish' is made with a flat hand in neutral space, rather than being specifically located at chin level with separated fingers as it might be in BSL. There is a core vocabulary of around 350 signs, arranged in stages of around 35 signs per stage, starting with those that are highly functional for both the person with a learning disability and the teacher. Progression of concepts is evident across the stages, as more abstract concepts such as vocabulary associated with time, for example yesterday, before, next, are taught in the later stages. Additional resources are available as a series of topic-based vocabulary sets, for example sexuality; emotions and relationships; early attainment targets of the national curriculum; fire and its hazards (see The Makaton Charity in Useful addresses section).

Signalong

This is an extended lexicon which also uses signs from BSL in a broad developmental sequence. Similar to Makaton, it also follows spoken word order. Signalong content is organised according to major topics and themes, "providing vocabulary for life and learning" (see Signalong Group in the Useful addresses section).

Peer tutors

Signs are taught in workshops run by individuals who have been trained through the Makaton Vocabulary Language Programme (MVLP), in order to maintain some consistency. Peer tutoring in Makaton has been a development taken up by many service organisations (Hooper & Bowler 1991, Hooper & Walker 2002). It involves adults with learning disabilities who are trained as the expert users in particular settings. It has been found to offer an effective way of circumventing the lack of generalised use of signing in day centres. The MVLP provides certificated courses for those wishing to qualify as peer tutors (see The Makaton Charity).

Signing environment

It is vitally important to ensure that your teaching of signing is actively supported by the management team in the setting. Grove & McDougall (1991) found that high signing schools were those which provided regular training, attended by the head teacher, and where signing/AAC use was given a high priority in the curriculum. A vital element in successful training is to ensure that all significant others take part. The commonsense view is that signs are more likely to be used consistently if everyone agrees on a core vocabulary. Spragale & Micucci (1990) used a 'sign of the week' approach to encourage use by staff. Put line drawings up on the wall, and ensure that signs are used in all the main forums where communication takes place, for example in school assembly and at residents' meetings. Teach signs to all the people who share the environment so that they recognise the communication efforts of their peers for whom signing is a critical part of communication.

Why use signs to support language?

There are a number of advantages that signing brings to spoken communication. If we speak a word, it disappears almost in the instant that it leaves our lips. Signs and gestures, however, are produced more slowly allowing for a longer processing time (Buckley

Box 6.5

Tips for a positive signing environment

- Regular training for all workers who communicate – even after initial training, it is important to maintain your skills!
- Prioritise the use of signs in the environment – make a deliberate effort to use signing with other staff members as well as the people who need it.
- Make sure that the head of the service is trained as effectively as the frontline staff.
- Enhance the environment so that it reminds people to use signing, e.g. introduce a new, topical sign each week, display line drawings of signs as aide memoires.
- Capitalise on the main events that happen in a setting and make a deliberate effort to include signing, e.g. person-centred planning meetings, school assembly, self-advocacy meetings.
- Train and employ peer tutors who can help to take signing forward in the setting.

1995). Furthermore, a sign can be held in space as a model for the other person acquiring a sign. This makes it highly suited to the needs of some individuals with learning disabilities.

The visuo-spatial structure of signs provides greater opportunity to forge links between the symbol and what it represents. For example, the sign for 'drink' mimics the action of having a drink. There is a correspondence or similarity between the sign and the real life meaning. This is what we call iconicity, which is the opposite of arbitrariness where the link between sign and meaning is much more random. Iconicity can make a difference to initial learning – iconic signs are learned more quickly than arbitrary signs by individuals with learning disabilities in structured teaching contexts (Doherty 1985). However, remember that iconicity is 'in the eye of the beholder' – the sign for 'milk' (which mimics the action of squeezing the cow's udders for milk) is only iconic if you know how cows are milked; 'house' if you come from a culture which builds dwellings with peaked roofs.

Parents and teachers are often concerned that the introduction of signing may mean that speech will deteriorate or be abandoned. In fact, the use of sign and gesture appears to facilitate speech production (Gompertz 1997, Kouri 1989, Launonnen 1996). Young children with Down syndrome who are taught signs have gone on to develop intelligible speech, at which point their use of signs declines (Kouri 1989, Launonnen 1996, Le Prevost 1993). Launonnen and Grove (2002) report on the case of a boy with Down syndrome who was mute and sign dependent until the age of 12, when he suddenly started to speak, possibly because of hormonal changes to the larynx making initiation of voice easier.

Expressive signing helps to promote communicative success. There is plenty of evidence that the introduction of manual signing and gesture allows individuals to develop functional vocabulary use (Grove & McDougall 1991, Kiernan et al 1982). Signing to the children can help to disambiguate words and meanings receptively, particularly for those with hearing impairments (around 80% of children with Down Syndrome, according to estimates) (Downs 1980, Gompertz 1997). Signing seems to help with speech intelligibility, possibly because it may slow down the rate of speaking slightly and helps to emphasise syllabic structure (Wells 1981). A small study of adults with learning disabilities with very poor and with reasonably intelligible speech found that listeners consistently rated speech which was accompanied by signs as more intelligible than speech alone, even when they could not see the speaker (Powell & Clibbens 1994).

Box 6.6

Principles of a positive communication environment

Van der Gaag (1998) identified a number of core principles considered critical to establishing a positive communication environment:

- The communication needs of the individual are at the heart of all practice.
- The involvement of significant others in the individual's environment is critical.
- The focus is on partnership communication and therefore considers not only communication skills use of service users but also that of significant others.
- The remit of speech and language therapists includes assessment of and planning to meet communication needs while also encouraging others to have a share in communication.
- There is managerial commitment to developments in practice.

Aided communication: objects and graphemes

There is an array of graphic forms and symbol sets designed to support communication. It is perhaps useful to start this section with a look at the hierarchy of aided communication options. Drawn as a pyramid, the options at the base represent the easiest, progressing through more sophisticated alternatives towards the top (Fig. 6.4).

Objects of reference

Starting at the base of the pyramid, objects of reference involves the use of 'objects' to stand for categories of events and things. Just as signs are used to represent meanings, so it is with everyday objects. Objects are selected that provide strong associations with particular events. Unlike spoken or signed communications, which do not hang about in the air once they have been delivered, objects are both permanent and open to manipulation presenting lower demands on cognitive abilities, memory and vision. They require only simple motor responses and can be represented at a number of different levels according to the presenting needs of the person (see Park 1995, 1997, 2002) (Table 6.1).

See Reader activity 6.5 on the Evolve website.

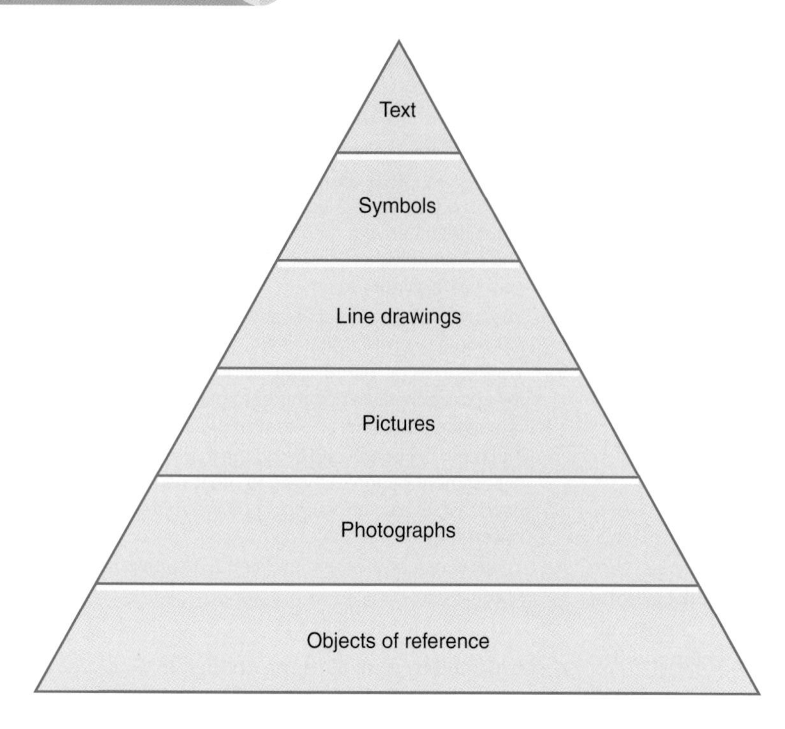

Figure 6.4 • Hierarchy of options for representing words and meanings

Table 6.1 Objects of reference: different levels of representation

Level	Examples
Real objects used in activity – sometimes referred to as 'index' objects	Fazil is being alerted by his teacher to the fact that it is time to go to the domestic science room at school for the cookery lesson. He has an object box in the classroom that contains a selection of key objects for use in different lessons. The teacher takes out a wooden spoon and gives it to Fazil to represent the shift in activity. He takes the spoon to the lesson and uses it when he is stirring the soup.
Objects not used in activity: • Identical objects not used in activity • Non-identical objects not used in activity	Sarah wants to go to the shop to buy a magazine. She gives a small purse containing a few coins to her keyworker who understands that a shopping trip has been requested. He gives Sarah her bag containing the real purse money for her excursion. It is identical to the purse Sarah used to communicate her wish to go shopping. Esme also wants to go shopping. Her object of reference is a green material purse with a zip fastener. The actual purse she uses is a wallet style purse made of red leather that fastens with a popper. Despite these differences, Esme understands that they both symbolise money, which she needs to buy the things she wants.
Associated/partial objects with some corresponding features to real life object	Darren wants to have a bath. He uses a small square of towel to indicate this to his carer. This is a more subtle object of reference, i.e. an item with features (the fabric) relating to the real life object of his bath towel.
Miniature objects providing a smaller and more portable representation of real life object	Frances is going on a bus trip into town with his parents. He loves going on the bus and will frequently point to the red buses that go down his street. His father shows him a toy double decker bus to let him know what they are going to do.
Abstract objects	The big timetable displayed on the wall of Jason's classroom displays all the different lessons for each week day. Objects are attached by fabric hook and loop fastener (e.g. Velcro) and the teacher directs Jason to pull off the silver whistle, which he loves to blow when he is outside doing gardening. The whistle has nothing to do with the actual activity but there is an association for Jason.

Graphic symbols

Sometimes referred to as 'graphemes', these include photographs, pictures, line drawings and symbols before the final level of representing meaning through text. The question of what to use is dependent on the developmental and cognitive level of the individual, language ability, sensory issues (for example vision) and any physical issues. Ultimately, it is a question of trying out the different representations with the individual and noting their responses. No matter what type of grapheme used, it is important to check for prerequisite skills in the areas of attention to pattern (figure–ground discrimination); recognition of representational status of pattern; recognition of specific meaning. Questions to ask yourself are: Can this person select a picture when it is named? What about labelling the picture? Can they match object to object and object to picture?

There are a number of pictorial vocabulary sets such as Picture Communication Symbols (PCS), Rebus and Makaton Symbols, and Bliss Symbolics. Many of them are available in computer software, such as PCS, which was developed in the USA by Mayer Johnson in association with Boardmaker and Writing with Symbols 2000. As well as being used for communication boards and books, these programmes can be used for creating written work along the lines of a specially adapted word processing package. CHANGE Picture Bank is a collection of images or composite line drawings specifically designed by people with learning disabilities to make written information more accessible.

Anyone using pictures to support the communication of an individual needs to be aware of the range and diversity of symbol systems and the variations in usage. Graphic communication forms are used for a number of purposes including to support language development and literacy skills; to represent meanings in a communication book or board; to facilitate access to information; to support the advocacy process. This can make for a somewhat confusing picture across the lifespan of an individual. For example, PCS tends to be used by speech and language therapists, schools frequently opt for Rebus, and adult services, particularly self-advocates, use the CHANGE Picture Bank.

Reader activity 6.6

There is an excellent resource entitled *Augmentative Communication in Practice: An Introduction* available as a free download from the Call Centre at: http://callcentre.education.ed.ac.uk/SCN/Intro_SCA/intro_sca.html.
Go to pages 19–26.

- What are the key differences among PCS, Rebus, Makaton and Bliss?
- Which symbols are most useful to the people you work with and why?
- Which symbols would present the greatest challenges for people with learning disabilities and why?

Picture exchange communication system (PECS)

Commonly referred to as PECS, this approach was developed for young non-speaking students with autistic spectrum conditions, because of concerns about their lack of initiation for communication, poor motor imitation, 'competing hand movements' when attempting to point and a general lack of response to social rewards. For more information the reader is referred to Chapter 20.

Communication books and boards

For some people for whom the physical demands of talking are too much, graphic communication offers an appropriate alternative. Photographs, pictures, symbols and text may be combined to provide the individual with an alternative means of communicating their needs, feeling and ideas. The construction of a book or board is achieved through consideration of the layout of graphemes (how the display will work in terms of arrangement of pictures on a page and arrangement of pages); the representations to be used (what combination of photographs, symbols, pictures and words); the organisation of content (will it be topic based or linguistic based?).

Accessible information

Low levels of literacy among people with learning disabilities means that access to information in text is problematic for many. Strategies for circumventing some of the complexities of printed matter have been devised by Mencap (Mencap 2009). Similar guidelines have also been produced by the European Commission (Freyhoff et al 1998) and CHANGE (2009). Strategies include covering only one idea per sentence, use of active rather than passive verbs, and avoidance of abstract concepts. The business of producing easy to read documentation is growing steadily. The Mencap website contains a number of policy documents that have been rendered as 'easy to read' following adherence to their published guidelines and using their specially designed easy to read font, i.e. FS Mencap. The orientation of text and pictorial support varies according to the language used (Mencap 2009). English text would be located on the right with supporting images on the left, for example Valuing People Now on personalisation; Learning Disability Partnership Board Easy-read policy. Accessible information about health is also available in formats that are advertised as eye catching, use simple words and have photos, symbols and pictures (see Easy Health in the Useful addresses section). Developments in this area by Mencap and the other similar organisations are to be welcomed, for example Working with Words; however, the best test of accessibility is whether or not it gets a clear response from the person thereby indicating their understanding. It is very often the case that simplifying the linguistic content and altering and enhancing the visual presentation of information is not enough in itself. Access to meanings need to be supported by significant others as well.

Talking Mats

Talking Mats is "... an interactive resource that uses three sets of picture symbols – topics, options and a visual scale" (Murphy & Cameron 2002:8). It was developed so that people using some form of alternative communication system were able to express their internal judgements and feelings. It involves an ordinary carpet mat, which is typically used on a table top, upon which graphic symbols are placed. On the back of each picture symbol is the hook side of a material fastener (e.g. Velcro) so that it adheres to the mat when placed. Talking Mats provides support for many different activities, including joint goal planning, planning communication passports (Millar 2003), self-perception of intervention outcomes, developing relationships with others and planning activities. The views expressed range from a personal evaluation of activity preferences to feelings about different forms of transport and life course aspirations, for example choice of occupation after leaving college, etc. Any one topic explored within a mat may be looked at in more detail. These are called sub mats. The use of a video camera is recommended to record the views expressed by the individual and to monitor the veracity of the process. A still photographic image provides a permanent record of each completed Talking Mat for feedback to the individual and their significant others.

Early-stage communication

Individuals with profound and multiple learning disabilities are likely to function at the earliest stages of communication development (Bunning 2009, Coupe O'Kane & Goldbart 1998, Ware 1996). Self-expression is through the use of subtle communication behaviours such as eye gaze, body language, facial expression and vocalisation, all of which may not be immediately recognisable to others (Grove et al 1999, 2001). This is compounded by the emission of behaviour patterns that are unique to that individual, which lack conspicuous features to make them noticed by others as signals bearing communicative meaning (Carter & Iacono 2002, Green & Reid 1996, Iacono et al 1998, Snell 2002) and behavioural states that are highly variable, with levels of alertness and activity changing within short periods (Guess et al 1993). The high prevalence of additional motor and sensory impairments is a further consideration (Iacono et al 1998). All this means that everyday communication is far from straightforward. There is a strong reliance on significant others, for example teacher, carer, teaching assistant, to assume an inferential role; efforts are made to work out the most likely meaning of observed behaviours by drawing on personal experience of the individual and cues from the immediate environment (Bunning 2009). In this way, meaning is constructed via a process of close observation, inference based on best guess and scrutiny of consequential effects on the individual and their environment (Olsson 2004).

A number of tools have been produced to help us make sense of communication with people who are functioning at the earliest stages of communication development.

- The Affective Communication Assessment (see Coupe O'Kane & Goldbart 1998) provides a structure for exploring the responding behaviours and sensory preferences of individuals. The individual is presented with a range of individualised sensory stimuli which have previously been identified in discussion with significant others. The person's responses are noted on an 'observation recording sheet' together with an interpretation of what they mean.
- The Early Communication Assessment (ECA) (Coupe O'Kane & Goldbart 1998) utilises 'communicative landmarks' (p. 59) rather than an exhaustive list of communicative behaviours in checklist format. The ECA provides a format for

capturing information about an individual against an early communication framework with the joint purpose of keying significant others into the individual's communicative level(s) as indicated by their observed behaviours while also highlighting the starting point for establishing communication with the person.

- The Manchester Pragmatics Profile (Coupe O'Kane & Goldbart 1998) is concerned with the social and functional behaviours that are critical to communication. It is a structured format for recording "evidence of skills in communicative intentions, social organisation and presupposition" (p. 93). The idea is to reveal information about successes and difficulties, communication partners and contexts, and relevant factors affecting the individual's performance, e.g. time of day, before developing an intervention that focuses on the individual, communication partners and context.
- See What I Mean' (Grove et al 2000) is a set of guidelines designed to help significant others question, check out or validate accuracy of meanings ascribed to an individual's communication. Its starting point is that uncertainty and ambiguity are a part of everyday communication and therefore the intuitive skills that are used by communication partners should form one thread of the assessment. It comprises a series of steps whereby evidence from the individual's behaviour is gathered to support the different interpretations so that the most likely meaning may be identified.

See Reader activity 6.7 on the Evolve website.

Multi-sensory approaches

Multi-sensory environments (MSE) come in a variety of shapes and forms, offering what Pagliano (1999) refers to as an 'open-minded space' for individuals to engage with available stimuli in a safe and supportive environment. Snoezelen is one such environment. It is a fixed environment that typically comprises a mixture of sensory equipment and materials – some of which are contingent on the activity of the person, for example touching a large Perspex tube sends bubbles and light floating upwards, and some of which occur as part of the general ambience of the environment, for example gentle music may be played as part of the background. In this way the person experiences a range of sensations by means of light, sound, touch, smell and taste (Hulsegge & Verheul 1987). Although primarily devised as a leisure and recreation resource, the therapeutic and educational value of such environments has also been recognised. However, the segregationalist nature of such specialised settings has been called into question. The findings of research are mixed with little evidence of generalised effects on behaviour even immediately after the sensory environment experience (Hogg et al 2001). Vasklamp et al (2003) concluded that an MSE was only as effective as a responsive learning environment while Porter & Miller (2000) question whether users of MSEs wouldn't be equally served by a natural environment with sensory opportunities.

Intensive Interaction

Intensive Interaction offers a practical approach to developing social relationships and communication with people with the most severe and complex learning disabilities (Nind 2009, Nind & Hewett 2005). For further information, the reader is referred to Chapter 20.

Profiling an individual's communication strengths and support needs

Communication Passports

A Communication Passport is a personalised catalogue of information about an individual's communication that is presented in a variety of formats, designed to be accessible and easy to follow. The point of a Communication Passport is to capture the unique and sometimes subtle or idiosyncratic ways an individual communicates and represent this profile to the people who matter to the individual, for example carers, teachers, support staff, GP, etc. They can be used to navigate particular junction points in a person's life, for example transition from primary to secondary education or just moving from one class to another; or to facilitate communication in a variety of community settings, for example a visit to the local medical practice.

Millar (2003) warns that a comprehensive Communication Passport entails a lot of hard work and considered preparation; however, she also points out that the very act of compiling a passport can be an 'enriching process and learning experience' (p. 6) because it brings significant others together around the individual encouraging information pooling and experience sharing. What exactly are Communication Passports? Very often they are small, portable booklets but can be almost any format that is accessible and meaningful to those involved. They can be wallet-sized cards, wall displays and table mats, videos and other more technical forms of rich and multiple media.

New media

Digital video, still photography, sound, graphics and text have been used to construct 'multi-media profiles' for people with learning disabilities. Personal life experiences are stored in the form of video clips (for example preferred activities) and still life images (for example favourite possessions) on a computer for access in planning and review meetings. They help to convey the personal agenda of the person with severe, profound intellectual disability and complex needs, for example physical and sensory impairments (see Acting Up in the Useful addresses section). The Trans-active project, developed by Mencap and the Rix Centre, provides a comprehensive approach to transition planning and inclusive practice in the education setting (see Trans-active). Pupils with learning disabilities are enabled to use multi-media techniques to produce individual web-based passports that capture the individual's self-concept, expressed preferences and personally meaningful choices, which can then be used in transition planning meetings. A key feature of Trans-active is the bringing together of young people with learning disabilities with their typically developing peers of similar age and interests for the purposes of support and friendship. The development of new technologies and applications of rich and multiple media occupy a place in the inclusion debate and in the address of societal marginalisation to which people with learning disabilities may be vulnerable. The defining contribution lies in the forging of links between images and meanings, past and present, school and home, so that the need for conventional linguistic exchange is obviated (Bunning et al 2009). The Rix Centre's mission of 'innovation in learning disability' embraces developments in new media for the enablement and self-advocacy of children and adults with learning disabilities. They manage a learning disability portal that acts as a window to local and national developments in this area (see The Big Tree in the Useful addresses section). They are engaged in action-based research in the development and application of new media technologies with this population.

Inclusive communication

Finally, we come to the over-arching issue of inclusive communication. If inclusion in education translates as learning in the *least restrictive environment* (Millar 2001), so inclusive communication must imply an environment free of constraints. This is an interesting proposition as it places the onus on environmental adaptation. Ultimately inclusive communication is about the person having an equal place in situations where human engagement happens (Kenworthy & Whittaker 2000). The dominant form of communication in Western culture is speech (Flewitt 2006). Users of alternative or non-conventional ways of communicating, for example signing and computer-aided devices, are in a minority.

We have seen earlier in this chapter how it is helpful to view communication from a partnership perspective where mutuality and social coordination are features of the interaction process (Grove et al 1999). It is the person with a full set of skills who has the opportunity to promote, or else cast in doubt, the abilities of the person by virtue of their own communicative behaviour (Kagan 1998). Thus an individual's difficulties with communication are not seen as deriving solely from the primary cognitive deficit, but rather as by-products of the interactional process (Nind et al 2001). Far from being static, the competencies that each person brings to a partnership are underpinned by "a relative and dynamic interpersonal construct" (Light 1989:137), whereby the contributions of one will affect the other, and vice versa.

A responsive environment

So how do we go about establishing a communication environment that is responsive and supportive? One approach is to ensure that the people who provide support to and communicate on a regular basis with people acquire skills and knowledge to help them in their efforts. A range of instructional models for enskilling significant others has been documented, including classroom-based staff training programmes (e.g. McLeod et al 1995, MacMillan et al 2000), where there is an emphasis on knowledge acquisition, skills development and problem solving; staff training that combines classroom-based learning with partnership practice with service user and staff member (e.g. Bjorck-Akesson et al 1996); and an apprenticeship approach whereby individuals are encouraged to reflect on and alter their practice by use of a range of strategies, including video playback, guided observation and verbal feedback (e.g. McConkey et al 1999, Money 1997, Purcell et al 2000). Reported outcomes of such initiatives include an increase in staff knowledge of communication matters (MacMillan et al 2000, Money 2002), heightened awareness of communication and positive changes to staff behaviour during interactions with service users (McConkey et al 1999, Money 1997, Purcell et al 2000) and an increase in spontaneous initiation made by service users during interaction (Mirenda & Donnellan 1986). However, Bjorck-Akesson et al (1996) stress the need to focus on the *process* whereby significant others are able to apply newly acquired knowledge and skills to real life situations, to receive feedback about the application of skills and to problem solve relevant issues as they arise in communication contexts. This approach is evident in the work of Purcell et al (2000) who implemented a work-based training programme that was specifically designed around the assessed needs of people with learning disability and their support staff. It involved video recordings taken before and after the intervention. Post-training evaluation revealed an increase in staff responsiveness that correlated significantly with an increase in client communication acts. The changes were attributed to the fact that the training was work based, client centred, 'mentor guided' with a formal mechanism for sharing positive practice. A comparison of three models of speech and language therapy service delivery revealed that combining staff training and direct work with service user and staff member was more effective than either approach in isolation, although positive outcomes were reported in these as well (Money 1997).

Total Communication

Total Communication (TC) is just one area that has given rise to service developments across the UK. Typically, Total Communication initiatives involve multiple agencies and involve some form of instruction and skills transference to support staff, as well as the development of practical resources to facilitate multi-modal communication (Bradshaw 2000). Despite the magnitude of service activity in this area, evaluation has been largely restricted to internal audit and interview with service users (see Jones 2000). Areas of concern include variable compliance rates among staff and limited address of individuals who are at the earliest stages of communication development (Jones 2000). Jones further comments that, in spite of the training, staff continued to make errors in the judgement of verbal comprehension. Vendetozzi et al (2010) reported on increased knowledge scores of staff participants attending training courses on Total Communication. They state that "referrals are now more specific and the expectations of intervention are more realistic" (p. 24) as an indirect effect of the work. However, such evaluations fall short of any direct measurements of staff–service user communication in the natural environment.

Conclusion

So where does all this leave the establishment of a positive and responsive communication environment? The UK Government has issued documents telling us how important inclusion is (e.g. Department of Health 2001, 2009), but where does communication come in? Although communication was not identified specifically as one of the core principles of the *Valuing People* White Papers, it is generally acknowledged that it is the cornerstone of the four attributes of rights, social inclusion, choice and independence (Jones 2000). So what can each of us do to facilitate inclusive communication? We can start by accepting and supporting the diverse ways of communicating and engaging socially used by people with learning disabilities. This requires that we place equal value on the different ways people communicate in any given setting. Ware (1996:1) uses the term 'responsive environment' and defines it as one in which "... people get responses to their actions, get the opportunity to give responses to the actions of others, and have the opportunity to take the lead in interaction". Enough said!

express their views and feelings. University of Stirling, Scotland.

Nind, M., 2009. Promoting the emotional well-being of people with profound and multiple intellectual disabilities: a holistic approach through intensive interaction. In: Pawlyn, J., Carnaby, S. (Eds.), Profound and multiple intellectual disabilities: nursing complex needs. Blackwell, London, pp. 62–77.

Nind, M., Hewett, D., 2005. Access to communication: developing the basics of communication with people with severe learning difficulties through intensive interaction, second ed. David Fulton, London.

Nind, M., Kellett, M., Hopkins, V., 2001. Teachers' talk styles: communicating with learners with severe and complex learning difficulties. Child Lang. Teach. Ther. 17, 143–159.

Olsson, C., 2004. Dyadic interaction with a child with multiple disabilities: a systems theory perspective on communication. Augment. Altern. Commun. 20, 228–242.

Pagliano, P., 1999. Multisensory environments. David Fulton, London.

Park, K., 1995. Using objects of reference: a review of the literature. European Journal of Special Needs Education 10, 40–46.

Park, K., 1997. How do objects become objects of reference. British Journal of Special Education 24, 108–114.

Park, K., 2002. Objects of reference: promoting early symbolic communication, third ed. Royal National Institute for the Blind, London.

Parker, M., Liddle, K., 1987. The communication needs of the mentally handicapped population in West Berkshire: a survey. RCSLT Bulletin 428, 1–2.

Porter, J., Miller, C., 2000. The use of multisensory environments, First ed. PMLD Link 43–44.

Powell, G., Clibbens, J., 1994. Actions speak louder than words: signing and speech intelligibility in adults with Down syndrome. Downs Syndr. Res. Pract. 2, 127–129.

Purcell, M., Morris, I., McConkey, R., 2000. Staff perceptions of the communicative competence of adult persons with intellectual disabilities. British Journal of Developmental Disabilities 45, 16–25.

Rondal, J., Edwards, S., 1997. Language in mental retardation. Whurr, London.

Royal College of Speech and Language Therapists, 2006. Communicating quality 3. RCSLT, London.

Sack, S.H., McLean, L.A., 1997. Training communication partners: the new challenge for communication disorders professionals supporting persons with severe disabilities. Focus Autism Other Dev. Disabil. 12, 151–158.

Scott, J., Larcher, J., 2002. Advocacy with people with communication difficulties. In: Gray, B., Jackson, R. (Eds.), Advocacy and learning disability. Jessica Kingsley, London, pp. 170–188.

Snell, M.E., 2002. Using dynamic assessment with learners who communicate nonsymbolically. Augment. Altern. Commun. 18, 163–176.

Sperber, D., Wilson, D., 1995. Relevance, communication and cognition, second ed. Blackwell, Oxford.

Spragale, D., Micucci, S., 1990. Signs of the week: a functional approach to manual sign training. Augment. Altern. Commun. 6, 29–37.

Thal, D., Tobias, S., 1992. Communicative gestures in children with delayed onset of expressive vocabulary. J. Speech Hear. Res. 35, 1281–1289.

Tyne, A., 1981. The principle of normalization. Values into Action, London.

Vasklamp, C., de Geeter, K.I., Huijsmans, L.M., Smit, I.H., 2003. Passive activities: the effectiveness of multisensory environments on the level of activity of individuals with profound multiple disabilities. J. Appl. Res. Intellect. Disabil. 16, 135–143.

Vendetozzi, M., Beltran, H., McMillan, F., et al., 2010. Training others to communicate. RCSLT Bulletin 696, 22–24.

von Tetzchner, S., Martinsen, H., 2000. Introduction to augmentative and alternative communication, second ed. Whurr, London.

Ware, J., 1996. Creating a responsive environment for people with profound and multiple learning difficulties. David Fulton, London.

Van der Gaag, A., 1998. Communication skills and adults with learning disabilities: eliminating professional myopia. British Journal of Learning Disabilities 26, 88–93.

Wells, M., 1981. The effects of total communication training versus traditional speech training on word articulation in severely mentally retarded individuals. Appl. Res. Ment. Retard. 2, 323–333.

Yoder, D.E., 2001. Having my say. Augment. Altern. Commun. 17, 2–10.

Further reading

Chinner, S., Hazel, G., Skinner, P., et al., 2001. Developing augmentative and alternative communication policies in schools. Ace Advisory Service, Oxford.

Latham, C., 2004. Developing and using a communication book. Ace Advisory Service, Oxford.

The Call Centre, 2002. Augmentative communication and inclusion: children and adults. Call Centre, University of Edinburgh, Edinburgh.

The Call Centre, 2003. Communicating with pictures and symbols. Call Centre, University of Edinburgh, Edinburgh.

Wilson, A., 2006. Practical solutions to support communication. Call Centre, University of Edinburgh, Edinburgh.

Useful addresses

Ace Centre Advisory Trust, http://www.ace-centre.org.uk.

Acting Up, http://www.acting-up.org.uk.

CHANGE Picture Bank, http://www.changepeople.co.uk.

Easy Health, http://www.easyhealth.org.uk.

Makaton Sign Language Programme, http://www.makaton.org/.

Signalong Group, http://www.signalong.org.uk.

The Big Tree – learning disability portal, http://thebigtree.org/.

The Call Centre, http://callcentre.education.ed.ac.uk/.

Trans-active, http://www.trans-active.org.uk.

Working with Words, http://www.workingwithwords.org/.

7

Advocacy

Ruth Garbutt

CHAPTER CONTENTS

KEY ISSUES

- Advocacy has clear values and principles
- Advocacy requires specific skills, such as communication, providing support to make choices, listening, interviewing, assertiveness, negotiation and recording
- There are different types of advocacy, including self-advocacy, citizen advocacy, collective advocacy, peer advocacy, short-term/crisis advocacy, legal advocacy and professional advocacy
- The roles of the Independent Mental Capacity Advocate and the Independent Mental Health Advocate have been established in recent legislation
- The process of advocacy can be challenging to professionals, but it is an inevitable and necessary development

Introduction

The *Chambers English Dictionary* (2008:22) defines an advocate as:

> an intercessor or defender; one who pleads the cause of another, one who recommends or urges something.

In health and social care settings, 'advocacy' is also referred to in terms of giving people a voice and in talking about the way in which individuals and groups obtain their rights. Brandon (1995 cited in Bateman 2000:17) suggests that advocacy is a

> . . . device to influence the balance of the needs/rights of the group in the favour of needs/rights of individuals, especially those on the social margins.

The notion of advocacy for people with learning disabilities embodies the social model of disability (Oliver 1990, 1996) in that it focuses on the rights of people with learning disabilities and the importance of consulting them on the services that they access. People with learning disabilities are therefore encouraged to speak up for themselves. In this way, people with learning disabilities are able to challenge the way services are run and thereby contribute to challenging the structures of society (Monach & Spriggs 1994). Advocacy is also connected to concepts such as participation, user-empowerment and consultation. Historically, for people with learning disabilities, advocacy has been part of the individual and collective processes of their fight for rights and their need to exercise choice and control in their lives. Advocacy can also be about challenging the power of professionals. Ultimately, it is about treating our fellow human beings with the same respect and dignity that we would like others to treat us.

In 1995 the International League of Societies for Persons with a Mental Handicap (ILSMH, now called Inclusion International) produced a document outlining the beliefs, values and principles of advocacy. These are shown in Box 7.1. These beliefs, values and principles are the keys to developing successful advocacy relationships and they will be referred to throughout this chapter.

This chapter will look at the policy and legislative context of advocacy. It will then look at the two main types of advocacy found in a learning disability context: self-advocacy and citizen advocacy. It will also refer to other types of advocacy, for example collective advocacy, peer advocacy, short-term/crisis advocacy, legal advocacy, professional advocacy and the roles of the Independent Mental Capacity Advocate and Independent Mental Health Advocate. Finally, it will look at the changing ethos and practice of services and advocacy skills for professionals.

Box 7.1

Beliefs, values and principles of advocacy (ILSMH 1995)

Beliefs and values

- Being a person first.
- Being able to make our own decisions.
- Believing in my value as a person.
- Having other people believe in you as a person.

Principles

- Empowerment
- Equal opportunity
- Learning and living together
- Non-labelling

Policy and legislative context of advocacy

The NHS and Community Care reforms in the UK in the 1980s and 1990s saw the beginning of rights-based policy for people with learning disabilities. As a result of community care reforms, many people with learning disabilities moved out of institutions and into the community. This was a challenge for people with learning disabilities themselves, for services and for staff. Dowson (2002) suggests that there were three possible responses to this:

1. To reduce the provision of specialist services for people with learning disabilities because they would now be accessing mainstream services and having the same rights as everyone else.
2. To 'import' ordinary aspects of life into services for people with learning disabilities, through normalisation principles and through schemes such as citizen advocacy (Wolfensberger & Zauha 1973) and circles of support (Beeman et al 1988).
3. To change the way services operate to include systems where service users could have a voice, such as user consultation and participation forums.

The NHS and Community Care Act 1990 stated that people should "live as independently as possible in their own homes or in 'homely' settings in the community . . ." Individuals were to be given "a greater . . . say in how they live their lives and the services they need to help them to do so . . ." (Department of Health (DH) 1989:3–4).

Consultation with service users and carers around community care services became a legislative duty. When a community care plan was being prepared, social services were required to consult with its key stakeholders, including voluntary sector bodies that represented the views of service users. In this way, the services users began to be referred to as 'consumers'. However, research suggested that quite often in practice, consultation would take place with the carers of people with learning disabilities, rather than the individuals themselves (McGrath 1989). It was mainly through the growth of the People First movement in the UK and other advocacy groups that people with learning disabilities themselves began to be consulted. The historic development of the People First movement will be explored more in the next section.

Grant (1992) analysed and evaluated the involvement of service users within community care planning and found the accomplishments and challenges shown

Box 7.2

Accomplishments and challenges of service users within community care planning (Grant 1992:69)

Accomplishments for users

- Development of opportunities for personal growth and development.
- Improved access to services for individuals.
- Better targeting of resources to needs and aspirations of individuals.
- Enhancement of self-esteem through participation in socially valued activities.
- Increased influence for individuals in decision making about service packaging and life choices.
- Cultural shifts in service settings from paternalistic models to systems that promote both participation and calculated risk taking for individuals.
- Opportunities to provide valued services to the community, in partnership with the community.

Challenges for users (and services)

- Uneven territorial development of opportunities for personal development.
- Minority of users with individual plans.
- Surface or tokenistic involvement which is devaluing.
- Involvement restricted to forums which do not hold service providers to account.
- Marginal involvement in forums dominated by parents or other informal carers.
- Exposure to unrealistic expectations about capacities for involvement.
- Ensuring that representatives' views are transmitted in the planning and development of services.

in Box 7.2. In this way, therefore, the community care reforms gave people with learning disabilities confidence, self-esteem and more personal power to have their say. Furthermore, the concept of market forces, value for money, the consumer citizen and an emphasis on consultation and participation in all public services gave a strong policy landscape that was conducive to recognising the views of people with learning disabilities in service planning (Braddock 1994) However, the balance of power still often remained in the hands of the professional.

More recent policy developments have given advocacy a high profile. The government White Paper, *Valuing People* (DH 2001a), set out the government's commitment to improving the life chances of people with learning disabilities. In it, the government gave their commitment to increasing, developing and supporting self-advocacy and citizen advocacy services for people with learning disabilities. This White Paper pledged to have a range of independent advocacy services available in each area so that people with learning disabilities could choose the one which best met their needs.

The ensuing strategy, *Valuing People Now: a new three-year strategy for people with learning disabilities* (DH 2009), sees advocacy as important and shows a commitment to supporting and developing advocacy programmes for people with learning disabilities. It states that one of its objectives is for all people with learning disabilities to be able to speak up and be heard about what they want from their lives, and if they need support, such as an advocate, they should be able to get it.

The *Valuing People* White Paper (DH 2001a) also stated that all people with a learning disability should have a health action plan by June 2005. The Health Action Plan for a person with a learning disability (and usually co-produced by them), outlined the actions needed to maintain and improve the health of that individual and any help needed to accomplish this. As part of this there was a designated role of 'health facilitator', whose task was to be involved in service development work and also to work on a one-to-one basis with the person with learning disabilities to give them information and ensure they achieved the best possible outcomes for their health. The health facilitation role might be undertaken by a health professional, a support worker, an advocate, a friend or a family carer.

Another policy document that had an advocacy element was the Person Centred Planning Guidance (DH 2001b) which was part of the *Valuing People* strategy. This guidance emphasised the importance of using Person Centred Planning, where the person with a learning disability is at the centre of the planning of their lives. This approach was rooted in the principles of shared power and self-determination, which correlated with the values and principles of advocacy. Person Centred Planning, therefore, discovered and acted upon what was important to the person themselves. It involved continual listening and responding to an individual's wishes, capacities and choices. The document stated that:

> Specialist learning disability professionals have a vital role to play in driving forward the shift towards person-centred services and supports. A significant part of this is supporting and responding to the lead from self-advocates and family members . . . But their own practice must also become increasingly person centred . . .
>
> (DH 2001b:43)

The government's Personalisation Agenda also emphasised that every person who received support would have choice and control over the shape of that support in all care settings. This has been outlined in the document *Putting People First* (DH 2007). *Valuing People Now* (DH 2009) states that *Putting People First* makes an explicit commitment to transform services, and make them more personalised to the needs of the individual user. It identified the need to empower citizens to participate in their communities as well as shape their own lives and the support they receive. It set out a vision for transforming social care, supporting local authorities and social care partners to reshape, and in this way, therefore, recent policies around learning disability are emphasising an approach in which advocacy, choice and control are central.

In the UK, the Disabled Persons Act 1986 gave all disabled people the right to a representative (i.e. an 'advocate') if needed. However, this has not been enforced, mainly due to the cost of such provision. But more recent legislation in the UK (e.g. The Disability Discrimination Act 1995; The Mental Capacity Act 2005; The Human Rights Act 1998) brought the issue of the rights of people with a learning disability higher onto the agenda and this has brought the issue under closer scrutiny.

As health and social care professionals, it is our responsibility to be aware of legislation and policy, to provide an accountable service, to be professional and to treat people with learning disabilities with equality, respect and as 'people first'. Quite often, we might find ourselves in positions where we are required to advocate for a service user. We might also find ourselves using the advocacy schemes of other services. It is therefore important to have a good understanding of what advocacy is and the different formats it can take.

The following section outlines the different types of advocacy: self-advocacy; citizen advocacy; collective advocacy; peer advocacy; short-term/crisis advocacy; legal advocacy, professional advocacy and the roles of the Independent Mental Capacity Advocate and Independent Mental Health Advocate.

Self-advocacy

Self-advocacy is:

> ... a process of individual development through which a person comes to have the confidence and ability to express his or her own feelings and wishes.
>
> (Simons 1992:5)

It is therefore a process whereby a person speaks up or acts for himself or herself (Williams & Shoultz 1982). This can be in a group setting or as an individual. It involves such skills as being able to express thoughts and feelings with assertiveness if necessary; being able to make choices and decisions; having clear knowledge of rights; being able to make changes (Clare 1990). Another way of describing advocacy is that it is:

> ... the act of making choices and decisions and bringing about desired change for oneself ... any activity that involves self-determination can be called self-advocacy.
>
> (Crawley 1988:1)

The self-advocacy movement has arisen through a combination of a collective response from people with learning disabilities to the experiences of discrimination, prejudice and institutionalisation and also of a professional/policy response to a need for greater service accountability.

The term 'self-advocacy' is also used to refer to groups of people with learning disabilities who have historically been denied a voice and who work together to make collective changes. Sometimes the people in these groups are referred to (or refer to themselves) as self-advocates. These groups have various labels, including self-advocacy groups, speak-out/up groups, Student Council trainee committees, working groups and People First.

Although disabled people in the UK have been campaigning as a collective group since the 1960s, it is only really since the 1970s that self-advocacy began to be formally recognised. In 1974, the first self-advocacy convention happened in Oregon, USA, when the name 'People First' was adopted. The Campaign for People with Mental Handicaps (CMH) later developed a self-advocacy pack in which they describe the reason for the term 'People First':

> 'People First' is a statement by the members that they are human beings first and that their disabilities are second. People First is a statement that people with disabilities desire to be seen as people who have value and dignity, to be seen as people who can participate and contribute to the community.
>
> (CMH 1986:4)

Self-advocacy in the UK developed as a result of a few people with learning disabilities from the UK attending a People First conference in the USA in 1984 and, on their return, setting up their own People First in London. Since then, numerous People First organisations have sprung up in the UK, though this has been slow and patchy. Even though many People First groups had developed, it wasn't until 1994 that a national People First for England was created.

A number of studies have explored the experience and practice of self-advocacy (e.g. Beart et al 2004, Crawley 1982, 1988, 1990, Dybwad & Bersani 1996, Gilmartin & Slevin 2010, Hampson 1994, Hanna 1978, Mitchell 1997, Shearer 1972, 1973, Shoultz 1997a, b, c, Simons 1992, Sutcliffe & Simons 1993, Williams 1982; Williams & Shoultz 1982; Worrel 1987, 1988). These studies show how people with learning disabilities have developed their own self-advocacy groups and some of the difficulties the self-advocacy movement faces.

Collective campaigning by people with learning disabilities happened in conjunction with an emphasis on *normalisation* principles in the USA (Wolfensberger 1972). Normalisation attempted to promote lifestyles for people with learning disabilities that were as close as possible to everyday living. O'Brien (1987a) promoted normalisation and the empowerment of service users through making sure they had choices, that they were respected and that they were able to participate within their community. The principles of normalisation and of self-advocacy therefore have been closely linked.

Self-advocacy might also be expressed in formal settings, such as Individual Programme Planning (IPP), Person Centred Planning (PCP), Health Action Plan (HAP), the planning of individualised budgets, careers interviews, educational settings, day centres, homes and hospitals. In all these settings, the person with learning disabilities is placed at the centre of the decision-making process and uses advocacy as a method of empowerment in the process. Crawley (1988) describes four models of self-advocacy groups:

The 'autonomous' or 'ideal' model

These groups are independent from professional services and will often employ an independent advisor or coordinator. They benefit from being independent because they can express their concerns and stand up for their rights without worries about recrimination. The advisor/coordinator has no conflicts of interest.

The 'divisional' model

This type of group is formed as a sub-group of an existing organisation. Examples include Speak Up groups within the Mencap service or a self-advocacy group within an established advocacy agency. These groups can benefit from the venues, financial and administrative resources of the organisation. However, there can be a conflict of interest between the self-advocates' requests and the views of the professionals. Another disadvantage is that the group can be subservient to the organisation and the organisation would have power in how much priority to give the group amidst its other priorities.

The 'coalition' model

These groups are usually sub-groups of a wider disability rights organisation, such as Derbyshire Coalition for Inclusive Living (DCIL, see Useful addresses). The advantages here are that people with learning disabilities are able to tap into a wider political campaigning process, they can develop a positive identity as a disabled person, and they can possibly achieve more funding. However, the danger is that people with learning disabilities could be overshadowed by more articulate, politically aware members.

The 'service-system' model

These are groups that are based in a service setting, such as a Student Council in a day centre or a residents group within supported accommodation. The advantages of this model are that it has access to transport, venues and other resources. It is also easy to access people to make up the group. However, disadvantages include the conflict of interest when members of the self-advocacy group challenge the system or structure of the service. In some cases this has been known to stop the group (Shearer 1986). The power of the group can be weak and a token gesture if the system or structure of the service is too powerful.

Reader activity 7.1

You know eight service users who you think would benefit from being in a self-advocacy group. They lived in an institutional setting for 10 years and now live in supported accommodation in the community. Two of them want to get a job, two of them are not happy in their accommodation, two of them miss their friends from the institution and the other two lack confidence in making choices. There is no independent self-advocacy group in the immediate town. As a practitioner, you think it would be a good idea to set up a self-advocacy group. How would you go about it? What model would you use? What advantages and disadvantages can you see of the model you have chosen? How would you address the issues? What would be the purpose of the group? Who would have the authority/power within the group?

How does a self-advocacy group work?

Downer & Ferns (1998) state that a self-advocacy group is defined by the following characteristics:

- Independent of services and workers.
- Has funding without any 'strings' attached.
- Controlled by people with learning difficulties.
- Advised by experienced disabled people and/or non-disabled people skilled in enabling self-advocacy.
- Not shaped by the 'outside' expectations of non-disabled people.
- Given space and time to grow and develop.
- Built on the strength of the group members.
- Taken seriously by services which should not pretend to support self-advocacy when they really do not.
- Has its advice and decisions listened to carefully and acted upon by service workers.
- Has real power and representation in important decisions about services which affect users' lives.
- Becomes a pressure group for positive change in services.
- Empowers group members to change their own lives with the support of other disabled people.

In general, the direction and agenda of most self-advocacy groups is led by the service users. Usually, the group will elect officers to be in the position of chairperson, deputy chairperson, secretary and treasurer. Other people might take on other roles such as helping with refreshments, photocopying the agenda for the meeting, welcoming new people, etc. The minutes and agenda of the meeting would be in an accessible format, such as easy words and pictures. When a group includes people with severe learning disabilities, care has to be taken to make sure their views and wishes are expressed. This could happen by an advocate or trusted friend or professional finding out in the previous week what concerns that person has or comments they may want to make. This could be written down for the chairperson of the group to read out at the meeting so that it could be discussed. Communication aids, the use of Makaton or sign language, pictures or photographs might also be appropriate during the meeting so that a person with a severe learning disability might be involved.

In the 'forming' period of the group, emphasis would be on building friendships and trust, developing skills and gaining an understanding of how groups work. Over time, the members of the group would bring their individual and collective concerns to the group and the group would consider their course of action to address the concerns. Examples of issues a group could address include the following:

- Campaigning to the local council for extensions to the hours a disabled person can use their bus pass.
- Better lockers in the day centre.
- Better choice of food in the residential accommodation.
- Investigating hate crime in the area.
- Inviting speakers (such as police, policy makers, researchers, nurses, etc.) to come and talk about a topic of concern.
- Making contact with another self-advocacy group to exchange ideas and meet together.

As a result of being involved in a self-advocacy group, members find that they can influence things to change. Additionally, members can also develop skills such as confidence, self-esteem, responsibility, sensitivity, assertiveness, a sense of identity, improved social skills, a greater ability to express themselves and communication (Beart et al 2004, Gilmartin & Slevin 2009, Stalker 1997). They also gain knowledge about the advocacy movement, about their own rights, and about local and wider systems and structures.

The role of the advisor of a self-advocacy group

Most self-advocacy groups would have an advisor. Sometimes the advisor would be an independent paid worker. Sometimes the advisor would work in a voluntary capacity. Sometimes the advisor would be an existing member of staff of a service or organisation. The advisor should have some knowledge of the local systems, services and structures and an understanding of the issues involved for people with learning disabilities. Most of all the advisor should uphold the social model of disability and should embody the beliefs, values and principles of self-advocacy.

The advisor's role would include building up the skills of the members of the group and supporting the group in their discussions of possible options and courses of action. The advisor would have a responsibility and commitment to the group and would be there to be utilised in the way in which the members required. Essentially the advisor can be seen as a resource for the group.

Reader activity 7.2

A group of service users want to set up a self-advocacy group. They want someone else (i.e. an 'advisor') to help them. Think about the issues involved if the person who helps them is:

- a community nurse
- a teacher
- a care worker
- a parent
- an independent person
- a volunteer.

You might like to consider, for example, issues around conflict of interest, resources, power, independence, knowledge and payment.

Reader activity 7.3

Is there a self-advocacy group and/or a People First group in your area? Is it an independent group or a group within a mainstream organisation? How does it operate? Is it consulted by mainstream services? Does it have a good relationship with mainstream services?

Self-advocacy is not just about self-advocacy groups. The recent policies around Person Centred Planning and Health Action Planning, for example, put the person with the learning disability at the centre of their own lives, with a conscious commitment from professionals towards shared power and shared decision making. The focus in these policies is around discovering what is important to the individual and supporting them to make their own choices and have their voice heard. They are policies in which professionals provide more of a signposting role rather than as an advisor. This necessitates a shift in thinking for the professional and the service. In this way, therefore, the person with a learning disability acts as their own self-advocate, to determine their own future. The challenge is for professionals to work closely with individuals to find out how they communicate and enable them to express their needs and wants. Crawley (1988:1) suggests that self-advocacy is "the act of making choices and decisions and bringing about desired change for oneself . . .". This act of self-determination, therefore does not have to be from a self-advocacy group situation. It could also be from an individual who has developed their own skills and confidence to express their needs.

Citizen advocacy

Citizen advocacy was originally conceived by Wolfensberger & Zauha (1973) and supports the notion of attempting to 'import' ordinary aspects of life into services for people with learning disabilities. In the citizen advocacy model, a volunteer trained worker (a citizen advocate) is partnered with an individual who finds it difficult to speak up for themselves (in our case, a person with a learning disability), with the objective that the advocate will promote and defend the interests of the 'partner'. The role of the citizen advocate is defined by John O'Brien in the following way:

> a valued citizen who is unpaid and independent of human services creates a relationship with a person who is at risk of social exclusion and chooses one or several of many ways to understand, respond and represent that person's interests as if they were the advocate's own, thus bringing their partner's gifts and concerns into the circles of ordinary life.
>
> (O'Brien 1987b, cited in Bateman 2000:24)

A citizen advocate may do many everyday things with the person with a learning disability, such as helping that person to deal with personal issues, representing that person at a case conference, helping to press for changes in a person's living arrangements, helping a couple get married despite opposition from parents. The Commission on the Status of People with Disabilities (1996:106) suggests that citizen advocacy may involve:

> . . . helping to express the individual's concerns and aspirations, obtaining day-to-day social, recreational, health and related services, and providing other practical and emotional support to him or her.

The strength of citizen advocacy is in the appointment of an *independent* person from outside a service, who acts on behalf of another person. It is also widely accepted as a way of making sure that those people, who find spoken words difficult, are still heard. In citizen advocacy schemes, advocates might act on behalf of an older person, someone with a mental illness, someone with a physical disability or someone with a learning disability, for example. The citizen advocacy model would help to re-establish the links between an individual and the community they live in, through a long-term relationship that emphasises choice and personal commitment. The citizen advocate would assist the individual in making their own choices and, if needed, would speak up for that person within meetings and decision-making processes (after exploring the options and finding out that person's wishes). This can be seen as similar to the role of a sign language interpreter for a person who is deaf – the interpreter does not necessarily give advice, but rather translates complex information into a more manageable form and also provides a voice for a person who communicates in a different way. Most citizen advocacy schemes operate outside mainstream services, within the voluntary and community sector. This has its difficulties due to lack of sustainable funding streams.

Citizen advocacy is well developed in the US (O'Brien 1987b, Ward 1986, Wolfensberger & Zauha 1973), Netherlands and Scandinavia (Cambridge & Ernst 2006, Health Equality Europe 2006) and has been slower to develop in the UK and other parts of Europe (Ledger & Tilley 2006, Traustadottir 2006). Funding has been deemed to be a problem in the UK. Sometimes, social services departments might provide funding for citizen advocate schemes, but this can cause a conflict of interest because a citizen advocate might be assisting a service user to push for some change in care/health/housing provision from social services. The citizen advocate is then in a difficult position, needing to represent the service user, but not wanting to cause too much conflict to the extent that social services withdraws the funding for the whole scheme.

People with profound and severe learning disabilities, who may not be able to express their own wishes and preferences, can benefit from having an independent citizen advocate appointed to them to help them uphold their rights and represent their views:

> Citizen advocacy is needed for people with severe learning disabilities because their access to services and other facilities may depend on their having someone to speak up on their behalf . . . citizen advocates are needed because others involved in the lives of people with learning disabilities are likely to have pressures on them which prevent them from being independent and objective.
>
> (Brooke & Harris 2000)

Reader activity 7.4

Is there a citizen advocacy scheme in your area? Are the people who provide the scheme volunteers? Paid? Independent? Do you know service users who would benefit from being linked into a scheme?

Although the People First movement in the UK has greatly improved the sense of choice and control for many people with learning disabilities, sometimes this change has not been apparent for people with profound and multiple disabilities.

Other types of advocacy

Other types of advocacy include the following: collective advocacy; peer advocacy; short-term/crisis advocacy; legal advocacy; professional advocacy; and the roles of Independent Mental Capacity Advocates and Independent Mental Health Advocates who have duties under the Mental Capacity Act 2005 and Mental Health Act 2007 respectively. These will be discussed below.

Collective advocacy

'Collective advocacy' is similar to self-advocacy, but it is a term used to describe more the way in which self-advocacy groups or user-led organisations raise public awareness, lobby policy makers, become involved in the wider disability movement, have political and economic power and campaign for better treatment and services. Examples might include tenants' associations, trade unions, mental health campaigning organisations such as MIND and parents' groups which challenge school governors. Collective advocacy for people with learning disabilities brings together people with a learning disability to have a shared voice in improving rights and working to change the structures of society. In this way, collective advocacy addresses the social model of disability and the disabling environments and attitudes that people with learning disabilities face.

Peer advocacy

'Peer advocacy' is a model where people speak up on behalf of their peers, that is people with learning disabilities speaking up on behalf of other people with learning disabilities. Quite often this can be people with learning disabilities who have gained confidence, skills and assertiveness who can speak up for others. Sometimes it could be older people with learning disabilities speaking up for younger people with learning disabilities.

Bristol and South Gloucestershire People First, for example, offers a peer support advocacy service for people with learning disabilities by people with learning disabilities, called 'Side by Side'. In this service, a peer supporter might accompany another person with a learning disability to a meeting. After a while, the person with a learning disability might eventually gain the confidence to attend the meeting themselves without their peer supporter.

What would you see as the advantages and disadvantages of peer advocacy?

Short-term or crisis advocacy

'Short-term or crisis advocacy' is where an advocate would be brought in to help to stand up for a person who has a particularly pressing or crisis issue, such as having to move house without much warning or a serious medical issue. It is useful if the advocate is someone who has built up a trusting relationship with the service user in the past so that the service user is confident that their views will be represented.

What would you see as the advantages and disadvantages of short term or crisis advocacy?

Legal advocacy

'Legal advocacy' is the process of representing clients before courts and tribunals, speaking in court and examining witnesses as part of a professional duty and legal system. Legal advocacy involves debating complex points of law and requires considerable legal training. Legal advocacy is also typically based on a contractual or financial relationship, which does not usually happen in advocacy within health and social care professions.

Professional advocacy

Social workers, nurses, care workers, community development workers and others may often be required to play an advocacy role, for example:

> Strategies of change ... might sometimes need to be directed, not at the client, but at dysfunctional elements in the client's environment
>
> (Davies 1994, cited in Bateman 2000:33)

This can be referred to as 'professional advocacy'. Nurses, for example, may be expected to act as an advocate in their role (Nursing and Midwifery Council (NMC) 2008) with vulnerability being seen as the main reason why this is needed (Malik 1997, Wheeler 2000). In fact, nurses can be well placed to act as advocates because they are available, they generally have a longer term relationship with service users and they have a knowledge of the health care system. Advocacy is a tool that can be used to empower and protect a service user. Carpenter (1988:26) suggests that:

> Advocacy is an important part of the role of the registered nurse ... being prepared to act as an advocate if required is part of the duty of any nurse ... advocacy aims to facilitate outcomes which the patient would have wished for had he been in a position to make his own decisions.

Cahill (1994:371) reiterates this by saying:

> ... the parallel definition of advocacy is the act of 'informing the patient of his rights in a particular situation, making sure that he has all the necessary information to make an informed decision, supporting him in the decision he makes and protecting and safeguarding interests' ...

It is important when acting as an advocate in a professional capacity to be aware of possible conflicts of interest to the service and to the needs of the service user. There is also a power relation between the professional and the service user. The professional in this case cannot claim to be 'independent'. However, they can provide a level of advocacy that may be appropriate in certain contexts. In situations of abuse, for example, there is a clear expectation for a nurse to advocate on behalf of a service user (NMC 2008). There will also often be situations where an independent citizen advocate would not be available because there is no citizen advocacy scheme in the area.

Bateman (2000:63) suggests that a practitioner in health and social care undertaking an advocacy role should hold the following principles within their work:

1. Act in the client's best interests.
2. Act in accordance with the client's wishes and instructions.
3. Keep the client properly informed.
4. Carry out instructions with diligence and competence.
5. Act impartially and offer frank, independent advice.
6. Maintain rules of confidentiality.

Reader activity 7.5

You have set up a planning meeting for a service user with multiple and profound disabilities. Would you invite the service user to the meeting? (Think about the arguments for valuing that person in a meaningful way using a person-centred approach, but also think about the need to make sure it is not a token gesture.) If you invite the person, how would you ensure that his/her wishes are represented?

Reader activity 7.6

Sometimes, professionals who work in health and social care services claim to act as advocates for service users. It is important in advocacy to have a genuine commitment to represent the person's interests as if they were your own (Tyne 1991). However, sometimes a practitioner has their own views on what is best for the individual that might clash with the views of the service user. How would you deal with this?

Independent Mental Capacity Advocate

Under the Mental Capacity Act 2005, a person with a learning disability is entitled to an Independent Mental Capacity Advocate (IMCA) to speak up for them, provide support and ascertain their wishes, when decisions are required that the individual lacks the capacity to make. This is a new, professional role that is independent of any other organisation. The IMCA must follow the Code of Practice that supports the legal framework of the Mental Capacity Act. The role of the IMCA is particularly useful for people with complex needs who are unable to express their wishes and who might not have appropriate support from family or friends. The IMCA might play a role in ascertaining the wishes of an individual in relation to a decision about serious medical treatment or about moving to a different hospital or care home, for example. IMCA currently applies in England and Wales. In Scotland, there is similar legislation called the Adults with Incapacity (Scotland) Act 2000.

Independent Mental Health Advocate

From April 2009, the amendments to the Mental Health Act 2007 came into force. These amendments required the provision of independent mental health advocates (IMHAs). An IMHA is a specialist type of mental health advocate who is granted specific roles and responsibilities under the Mental Health Act. IMHAs help qualifying patients understand the legal provisions to which they are subject under the Mental Health Act and the rights and safeguards to which they are entitled. They also ensure that the patient's voice is heard, help patients to get information, support patients in exploring options and making better-informed decisions. The IMHA has a statutory advocacy role. This can involve certain roles that other advocates would not be able to do, for example, in order to support people and *with their consent*, the IMHA will be also be able to:

- visit and talk to them in private
- visit and interview anyone concerned with their medical treatment (e.g. nurses or consultants)
- request relevant medical and social services records.

The Mental Health Act 2007 describes patients who are eligible for IMHA services as 'qualifying patients'. A qualifying patient is a patient who is one of the following:

- A detainee under the Mental Health Act 1983 (even if they are currently on leave of absence from hospital).
- A conditionally discharged restricted patient.
- Subject to guardianship.
- A supervised community treatment patient.

In addition, informal (voluntary) patients qualify for an IMHA service if they are either:

- being considered for a Section 57 treatment
- under 18 years of age and being considered for a Section 58A treatment.

IMHA currently applies in England and Wales.

The changing ethos and practice of services

As a result of a greater focus on advocacy, services have begun to address their own values and methods of practice. Some of the general ways in which services can change to have a commitment to effective advocacy can include the following:

- "Make a public commitment to self-advocacy and ... recognise that it is an important way of empowering service users

- Take positive steps to make sure self-advocacy happens in residential and day care establishments
- ... set up systems for talking to self-advocacy groups and take their views seriously ...
- ... get resources to support and develop self-advocacy
- Make sure that self-advocacy is put into practice in all areas of daily living
- Help people set up self-advocacy groups without taking them over and making them part of services ...
- ... make sure that self-advocates are given real power in decision-making services
- Provide people with the necessary assistance to attend self-advocacy groups, such as transport
- If a person wishes to attend a self-advocacy group, look on this as very important ...
- Train workers to develop skills to help disabled people take more part in everyday living tasks, choices and decisions ..."

(Downer & Ferns 1998:147–148)

Downer & Ferns (1998) also emphasise the need to make sure that advocacy is proactive in including black people with learning disabilities. People with learning disabilities from black and minority ethnic (BME) communities may be subjected to 'dual discrimination' (Baxter et al 1990). There is also a concern that people with learning disabilities from BME communities are under-represented in learning disability services and under-use the services. Some under-representation can occur as a result of services stereotyping BME families as having large extended families and internal support networks and therefore not in need of services (e.g. Gunaratnam 1993). Downer & Ferns (1998) suggest that in order to improve services, providers could encourage black communities to see the value of self-advocacy; support black people to use the service; find independent black advisors for self-advocacy groups; provide training to staff about race issues; and help black people be more involved in training staff. Other suggestions could be to provide translators for people whose first language is not English. It is important to not assume that everyone who has a learning disability has the same needs.

When involving people with learning disabilities more in services, this means that staff need to think about shifting their thinking in terms of the balance of power. This can be difficult for some staff that might see it as a watering down of professional culture. If a service is to embrace the beliefs, values and principles of advocacy, then this would not just be through enabling people with learning disabilities to have their own choices; it would be a key part of the way in which the service runs. Box 7.3 lists some of the ways in which a service could embrace a higher level of participation for service users.

Box 7.3

Ideas to increase participation of service users

- When recruiting staff, people with learning disabilities could contribute by being equal partners on the interview panel.
- When developing strategies, people with learning disabilities, or their self-advocacy groups, could participate in the planning and setting of priorities.
- People with learning disabilities could participate in focus groups to discuss their ideas for services.
- Self-advocacy groups could develop peer support projects to assist other people with learning disabilities to have their voice heard.
- People with learning disabilities should have choices in their day-to-day lives and their care packages.
- Complaints procedures should be made accessible so that people with learning disabilities have the same right to complain as anyone else.
- People with learning disabilities could be involved in the monitoring and review of services.
- People with learning disabilities should be encouraged to access mainstream services within their communities.
- Staff who work in specialist services should therefore see individuals in their wider context of family, friends and community. People with learning disabilities could be encouraged to join a Circle of Support. Circles of Support are schemes where a small group of individuals agree to meet regularly to help an individual person with a learning disability achieve his/her goals. These could be friends, family, people from the local community or significant others.

Reader activity 7.7

A 30-year-old Muslim man with multiple and profound learning disabilities and a visual impairment has arrived at a residential unit. How would you get to know him, find out about his background, interests and culture? How would you go about making sure his preferences are taken into account?

Advocacy skills for professionals

As health and social care professionals, we may have to take on a role that involves advocacy, or we might come across forms of advocacy that we can signpost to service users. The main way in which an advocate would work is by their beliefs, values and principles. In addition, certain skills should be in place. The following discusses some of the skills needed by citizen advocates, by advisors to self-advocacy groups and by professionals taking on an advocate role. The following skills will be addressed: communication, providing support to make choices, listening, interviewing, assertiveness, negotiation and recording.

Communication

Good communication is an essential skill for anyone in an advocate role. It is only through communication that a service user builds up trust and confidence in the advocate. The service user needs to believe that his/her views have been understood and will be acted on. Communication tools such as Makaton, Rebus symbols (Phoenix NHS Trust 1993) or an electronic communication device might be of benefit (see Ch. 6 for more detailed information).

Accessible information is critical. If people with learning disabilities are to have their own choices and control over their lives, there is a need for information to be presented/explained to them in an accessible format. This could involve easy words and pictures or symbols. Makaton symbols can be imported into a document through a software package such as Widgit. However, it is important to be aware that many people with learning disabilities have not been taught these symbols so, for many, the symbols are as hard to understand as words. A more effective way of using pictures is by having bespoke pictures to represent words/phrases. The national organisation, CHANGE, based in Leeds, creates 'Picture Banks' of professionally drawn pictures, based on different themes, for example health and housing, that can be purchased from their website (see Useful addresses). They always consult people with learning disabilities when creating the pictures and then endeavour to include 'real'-looking people (i.e. not perfectly slim, stylised people), with disabilities and from different cultural backgrounds. Other ways of communicating include British Sign Language, photographs, music, drama and mime. The aforementioned organisation, CHANGE has used drama extensively in its practice. A recent action research project led by CHANGE (2010) used drama and mime to find out about the views and experiences of young people with learning disabilities around relationships and sexuality. The young people acted out scenes that explored their experiences and feelings. This method was particularly effective for those young people who found it difficult to express themselves verbally. It was also an appropriate method to use for such a sensitive subject area, where talking about sex and relationships can be embarrassing for young people.

Again, the importance of using accessible information and accessible processes in meetings cannot be emphasised enough. If people with learning disabilities are going to participate in a meaningful way, then systems, structures and processes need to be looked at so that participation can really happen. For example, extra time needs to be given, and papers for meetings need preparation in advance so that a person with a learning disability has a chance (maybe with assistance from a support worker) to fully understand the agenda and purpose of the meeting. People with learning disabilities should be paid fairly for their time, in the same way that anyone else would be. There should be appropriate breaks in meetings so that no-one gets too tired. People with learning disabilities should be appropriately supported or represented so that their voice is heard.

Providing support to make choices

One of the advocate's main skills is to provide support to an individual to help them to make their own choices. In this way, service users are able to express their individuality and personal freedom. An advocate needs to present information in a clear and concise way, explaining the options without influencing the service user to choose one particular course of action.

A Person Centred Planning approach would be preferable with all people with learning disabilities, and especially those with profound and multiple disabilities. This approach involves looking at two main areas:

1. Who are you and who are we in your life?
2. What can we do together to achieve a better life for you now and in the future?

This Person Centred Planning approach takes a long period of time, where staff begin to learn more about the service user's background, what they like/dislike, what is important to them, what their lifestyle is like and what choices they want to make (Sanderson et al 1997). In this way, the values of the service change from providing a general service that all service users have to fit into, to a service focused on the needs and preferences of individuals. The notion here is to value people, rather than seeing them as passive, inactive people with no personality or individuality. The focus is more on improving a person's quality of life rather than assessing a person's deficits. This is in contrast to normalisation therefore. Normalisation attempted to create a person's environment and lifestyle as near to 'normal' as other people, leading to independence and integration. Independence and integration are important values but the Person Centred Planning approach does not fit all individuals into the same 'box' or the same stereotype of 'normal'. It focuses specifically on the individual as an individual and responds to their own needs and preferences (Ch. 9 provides a review of person-centred approaches to planning).

The importance of working in this way means that people with learning disabilities can participate in their plans more. The information gathered might focus on a person's communication patterns, or the person's history or their aspirations. Sometimes it is difficult to work out the preferences of an individual, but the best possible outcome should be achieved through collecting information, finding out from significant people their experiences of the person and by getting to know that individual.

Different ways of identifying a person's identity and working with it include the following:

- Collecting together objects that relate to a person's past, e.g. pebbles from a beach; an object that creates a noise the person likes; a religious symbol.
- Collecting photographs/pictures of significant people/events.
- Visiting places of significance to that person, e.g. a school they went to; a mosque; a street.
- Videoing/recording people/voices/music/scenes.
- Collecting together stories/memories from other people.
- Spending social/leisure/activity time with that person to get to know them.
- 'Dreaming in' about what that person aspires to by talking to significant people in their lives.

Again, this involves finding out the best style for the individual. Some people, for example, like to handle objects and have others around them, while others respond more to sounds or other sensory information.

Once information is gathered, and a clear picture built up, the advocate needs to then provide support to help that person understand the options and give their views and preferences. For someone with a profound and multiple disability, this may take some time.

Reader activity 7.8

You know a young man with a learning disability who wants to live independently. His care worker doesn't think he should because he doesn't know how to cook. The local advocacy forum that used to run various citizen advocacy schemes has closed because of lack of funding. How would you go about trying to make sure that the young man had his voice heard within the decision-making processes?

Listening

Listening is a very important skill in advocacy, because the advocate must be clear about the wishes and views of the service user. The advocate needs to gather facts and show empathy. Active listening involves hearing the information an individual is telling you, reflecting back to make sure that you have heard them correctly and not being judgemental about the information you have heard. The interview situation needs to be prepared so that it is conducive to effective listening, for example with no interruptions or distractions. The interviewee needs to be alert and focused. When listening, non-verbal communication is important. For example, it is not advisable to cross your arms or legs or to sit behind a desk as these actions represent a defensive pose. It is also important to not rush to advise the service user or to solve their problems. There needs to be a clear boundary between the listening stage and the discussing of options stage. It is also important to keep focused and to bring the service user back to the purpose of the interview if they go off on a tangent. There also needs to be a comfortable physical space between the interviewer and the service user and eye contact should be maintained. Nodding and smiling are also useful ways to show that you are actively listening.

Interviewing

Interviewing is a key skill required of advocates. An initial interview with a service user is usually required to find out what the issue is and to work out the best ways of moving forward. The following can be a guideline of the important aspects of carrying out an interview:

1. At the beginning of the interview, state how much time the interview will take.
2. Start where the service user is and explain to them why the interview is taking place and what role you are playing.
3. Try to have sympathy for the service user even if it is a situation in which you do not feel very sympathetic.
4. See the situation through the service user's eyes, that is, have empathy.
5. Do not be judgemental or condemning – be accepting and tolerant.
6. Smile.
7. Don't ask closed questions (those that can only be answered 'yes' or 'no').
8. Do not ask leading questions (those that seem to be leading the interviewee into a certain answer).
9. Do not probe too deeply unless there is a reason for doing so.
10. Don't be afraid of silences but don't prolong silences if it is uncomfortable for the interviewee.

(Adapted from Jamieson 1978)

The interview should involve active listening, verbal and non-verbal communication, reflecting back, questioning and sensitivity.

Assertiveness

Effective advocates need to be assertive. Their role usually requires them to stand up for other people and to obtain a satisfactory outcome. Assertiveness involves expressing yourself in a direct, honest, non-manipulative way. Sometimes this may involve an element of force when trying to defend or secure a person's rights. Advocates need to not be intimidated by someone getting defensive when they are being challenged. This situation arises frequently when standing up for others – it is almost inevitable that there will be some resistance. To be assertive, an advocate needs to be prepared with all the facts of the case. They need to be clear in their objectives and principles. They need to believe in their case. They need to have practised their arguments for their case and to have thought through any counter arguments they might come across. They need to have confidence, and to put forward their case without being manipulative or confusing. The advocate also needs support and supervision from their seniors. One way of being assertive is to repeat your request clearly and calmly, without getting drawn in to the opposing side's excuses. You need to be as objective as possible and use emotion sparingly.

Negotiation

Negotiation in an advocacy situation is about getting the best result for the service user. Sometimes negotiation will be used when there is no other available approach. Negotiation can be used when there is no clear system or structure for resolving a problem. When using negotiation as a strategy, you need to have collected all the important information and identified the relevant facts. The goals and interests of the service user need to be identified. The strengths and weaknesses of the service user's position and of the other side's position need to be identified. The options and the possible responses need to be thought through. The following may be a good way forward in the negotiating interview:

1. Obtain information through questioning.
2. Separate the people from the problem:
   - listen to the other side
   - confirm understanding of the other side's problem
   - allow the other party to let off steam.
3. Focus on interests not positions:
   - describe the problem in terms of the impact on the client
   - encourage the other side to explain the client's interests and goals
   - explain your own client's interests and goals
   - identify shared interests and goals
   - focus on present and future concerns, not past grievances.
4. Ascertain scope of other party's authority.
5. Develop and discuss alternative settlement options.
6. Make offers that are justified by objective criteria.

7. Insist on and probe for objective criteria based on law, precedents, facts or evidence.
8. Be open to reason, closed to threats.
9. Make a note of agreements and concessions as they occur.

(Summarised from Dye 2010:1–9)

Recording

It is important to record your advocacy interactions with the service user. You will need to record important facts, and you will have records available if another advocate has to take over your case, or to provide information for future research. It is important to make sure you adhere to the confidentiality arrangements of your profession/organisation. This also means that you will be accountable to other professionals. You may also need to consider the Freedom of Information Act (2000) and to write your remarks in a factual, non-judgemental way in case your client wishes to see them at any point. You may need to keep copies of any letters/e-mails written or any reports that you have written on behalf of the service user. Recording must also be concise and to the point.

Conclusion

Advocacy has a powerful role to play in terms of challenging the historic marginalisation of people with learning disabilities:

> The advocacy process itself, for a group like disabled people who have historically been excluded from public life, combats exclusion.
>
> (Gooding 1994:44)

Advocacy can take various forms, but the main aim of advocacy is for the service user to have a voice in the way they live their life. This chapter has discussed self-advocacy, citizen advocacy, collective advocacy, peer advocacy, short-term/crisis advocacy, legal advocacy and professional advocacy. Quite often health and social care professionals will be called upon to undertake an advocacy role for service users. It is important that professionals do not undertake this role lightly and give due consideration to any conflict of interests and power dynamics that might effect a successful outcome. They need to be aware of other advocacy options that might be available in their area. When undertaking an advocacy role, they need to work from the beliefs, principles and values that underpin advocacy and they need to develop sophisticated skills to achieve a good advocacy relationship. They also need to be aware of the legislation and policies around disability rights that might affect the way they work. Finally, they need to reflect on the working policies and practices of the organisation in which they work in order to make any changes to increase the level of accessibility and participation for their service users.

The social model of disability states that it is the structures and attitudes of society that create difficulties for disabled people, rather than their impairment. Advocacy is one way in which people with disabilities can stand up for their rights, assert their choices and challenge the structures and systems of which they find themselves a part. Health and social care professionals have the opportunity to embrace these changes in attitudes and practices and welcome a new era in which people with learning disabilities are treated with dignity and respect. Professionals need to become part of the system that empowers people with learning disabilities to have a real voice, political power and social equality. The process of advocacy can be challenging to professionals, but it is an inevitable and necessary development as a result of the historic campaigning of people with learning disabilities, anti-discrimination laws and changes in a market economy, where all customers have a right to a good service.

References

Bateman, N., 2000. Advocacy skills for health and social care professionals, second ed. Jessica Kingsley, London.

Baxter, C., Poonia, K., Nadirshaw, Z., 1990. Double discrimination. King's Fund, London.

Beart, S., Hardy, G., Buchan, L., 2004. Changing selves: a grounded theory account of belonging to a self-advocacy group for people with intellectual disabilities. J. Appl. Res. Intellect. Disabil. 17, 91–100.

Beeman, P., Ducharme, G., Mount, B., 1988. What are we learning about circles of support?. Communitas, Manchester, CT.

Braddock, D., 1994. Presidential Address 1994. New frontiers in mental retardation. Ment. Retard. 32 (6), 434–443.

Brandon, D., 1995. Advocacy power to people with disabilities. Venture Press, Birmingham.

Brooke, J., Harris, J., 2000. Pathways to citizen advocacy. British Institute of Learning Disabilities, Kidderminster.

Cahill, J., 1994. Are you prepared to be their advocate? Prof. Nurse 9 (6), 371–375.

Cambridge, P., Ernst, A., 2006. Comparing local and national service systems in social care Europe: framework and findings from the STEPS anti-discrimination learning disability project. European Journal of Social Work 9 (3), 279–303.

Campaign for People with Mental Handicaps, 1986. Self-advocacy pack. The Campaign for People with Mental Handicaps, London.

Carpenter, D., 1988. Advocacy. Nurs. Times, Open Learning Programme, Module P9, 24 June and 1 July, 26 and 27.

Chambers, 2008. Chambers English Dictionary. Chambers Harrap, UK.

CHANGE, 2010. Talking about sex and relationships: the views of young people with learning disabilities. CHANGE, Leeds.

Clare, M., 1990. Developing self-advocacy skills. Further Education Unit, London.

Commission on the Status of People with Disabilities, 1996. A strategy for equality. Report of the Commission on the Status of People with Disabilities. The Stationery Office, Dublin.

Crawley, B., 1982. The feasibility of trainee committees as a means of self-advocacy in adult training centres in England and Wales. Unpublished PhD. Manchester.

Crawley, B., 1988. The growing voice: a survey of self-advocacy groups in adult training centres and hospitals in Great Britain. Values into Action, London.

Crawley, B., 1990. Advocacy as a threat or ally in professional practice. In: Brown, S., Wistow, G. (Eds.), The roles and tasks of community mental handicap teams. Avebury, Aldershot.

Davies, M., 1994. The essential social worker. Arena, Aldershot.

Department of Health, 1989. Caring for people – community care in the next decade and beyond. Cm.849. HMSO, London.

Department of Health, 2001a. Valuing people: a new strategy for learning disabilities for the 21st century. Department of Health, London.

Department of Health, 2001b. Valuing people: a new strategy for learning disabilities for the 21st century. towards person-centred approaches: planning with people. Department of Health, London.

Department of Health, 2007. Putting people first: a shared vision and commitment to the transformation of adult social care. Department of Health, London.

Department of Health, 2009. Valuing people now: a new three-year strategy for learning disabilities. Department of Health, London.

Downer, J., Ferns, P., 1998. Self-advocacy by black people with learning difficulties. In: Ward, L. (Ed.), Innovations in advocacy and empowerment. Lisieux Hall, Lancashire.

Dowson, S., 2002. Empowerment within services: a comfortable delusion. In: Ramcharan, P., Roberts, G., Grant, G., Borland, J. (Eds.), Empowerment in everyday life: learning disability. Jessica Kingsley, London.

Dybwad, G., Bersani, H. (Eds.), 1996. New voices: self-advocacy by people with disabilities. Brookline Books, Cambridge MA.

Dye, T.A., 2010. Winning the settlement – keys to negotiation strategy. In: ABA Section of Litigation Corporate Counsel CLE Seminar, February 11–14, Florida, USA.

Gilmartin, A., Slevin, E., 2010. Being a member of a self-advocacy group: experiences of intellectually disabled people. British Journal of Learning Disabilities 38 (3), 152–159.

Gooding, C., 1994. Disabling laws, enabling acts: disability rights in Britain and America. Pluto Press, London.

Grant, G., 1992. Researching user and carer involvement in mental handicap services. In: Barnes, M., Wistow, G. (Eds.), Researching user involvement. Nuffield Institute for Health, University of Leeds, Leeds.

Gunaratnam, Y., 1993. Breaking the silence: Asian carers in Britain. In: Bornat, J., Pereira, C., Pilgrim, D., Williams, F. (Eds.), Community care: a reader. Macmillan/Open University, London.

Hampson, Y., 1994. Self-advocacy and people with learning difficulties. Unpublished MEd, University of Sheffield, Sheffield.

Hanna, J., 1978. Advisor's roles in self-advocacy groups. Am. Rehabil. 4 (2), 31–32.

Health Equality Europe, 2006. Challenges facing the health advocacy community–a Europe-wide survey of health campaigners. Health Equality Europe.

International League of Societies for Persons with a Mental Handicap (ILSMH), 1995. The beliefs, values and principles of self-advocacy. Brookline Books, Cambridge, MA.

Jamieson, J., 1978. What is an interview? Community Care. 8 February 1978, cited in Davies M. Op cit.

Ledger, S., Tilley, L., 2006. The history of self-advocacy for people with learning difficulties: international comparisons. British Journal of Learning Disabilities 34, 129–130.

McGrath, M., 1989. Consumer participation in service planning – the AWS experience. J. Soc. Policy 18 (1), 67–89.

Malik, M., 1997. Advocacy in nursing – a review of the literature. J. Adv. Nurs. 25, 130–138.

Mitchell, P., 1997. The impact of self-advocacy on families. Disability and Society 12 (1), 43–56.

Monach, J., Spriggs, L., 1994. The consumer role. In: Malin, N. (Ed.), Implementing community care. Open University Press, Milton Keynes, pp. 138–153.

Nursing and Midwifery Council, 2008. The code: standards of conduct, performance and ethics for nurses and midwives. NMC, London.

O'Brien, J., 1987a. A guide to lifestyle planning: using the activities catalogue to integrate services and natural support systems. In: Wilson, B.W., Bellamy, G.T. (Eds.), The activities catalogue: an alternative curriculum for youth and adults with severe disabilities. Brookes, Baltimore.

O'Brien, J., 1987b. Learning from citizen advocacy programmes. Advocacy Office, Atlanta, GA.

Oliver, M., 1990. The politics of disablement. Macmillan, Basingstoke.

Oliver, M., 1996. Understanding disability: from theory to practice. Macmillan, Basingstoke.

Phoenix NHS Trust, 1993. A guide to using symbols. Connect, Bristol.

Sanderson, H., Kennedy, J., Ritchie, P., Goodwin, G., 1997. People, plans and possibilities – exploring person-centred planning. Scottish Human Services, Edinburgh.

Shearer, A., 1972. Our life. CMH/VIA, London.

Shearer, A., 1973. Listen. CMH/ VIA, London.

Shearer, A., 1986. Building community with people with mental handicaps, their families and friends. CMH/ King's Fund, London.

Shoultz, B., 1997a. More thoughts on self-advocacy: the movement, the group and the individual. Article from Internet homepage of the Centre on Human Policy, Syracuse University, New York. http://soeweb.syr.edu/.

Shoultz, B., 1997b. The self-advocacy movement. Article from Internet homepage of the Centre on Human Policy, Syracuse University, New York. http://soeweb.syr.edu/.

Shoultz, B., 1997c. The self-advocacy movement: opportunities for everyone. Article from Internet homepage of the Centre on Human Policy, Syracuse University, New York. http://soeweb.syr.edu/.

Simons, K., 1992. 'Sticking up for yourself': self-advocacy and people with learning difficulties. Community Care publication in association with the Joseph Rowntree Foundation.

Stalker, K., 1997. Choices and voices: a case study of a self-advocacy group. Health and Social Care in the Community 5, 246–254.

Sutcliffe, J., Simons, K., 1993. Self-advocacy and adults with learning difficulties: contexts and debates. National Institute of Adult Continuing Education, Leicester.

Traustadottir, R., 2006. Learning about self-advocacy from life history: a case study from the United States. British Journal of Learning Disabilities 34, 175–180.

Tyne, A., 1991. A report on an evaluation of Sheffield Citizen Advocacy. National Development Team, Manchester.

Ward, J., 1986. A point of view: citizen advocacy: its legal context. J. Intellect. Dev. Disabil. 12 (2), 91–96.

Wheeler, P., 2000. Is advocacy at the heart of professional practice? Nurs. Stand. 14, 39–41.

Williams, P., 1982. Participation and self-advocacy. CMH Newsletter 20 (Spring), 3–4.

Williams, P., Shoultz, B., 1982. We can speak for ourselves. Souvenir Press, London.

Wolfensberger, W., 1972. Normalisation: the principle of normalisation in human services. Leonard Crainford, Toronto.

Wolfensberger, W., Zauha, H., 1973. Citizen advocacy and protective services for the impaired and handicapped. National Institute on Mental Retardation, Toronto.

Worrell, B., 1987. Walking the fine line: the people first advisor. Entourage 2 (2), 30–35.

Worrell, B., 1988. People first: advice for advisors. National People First Project, Ontario.

Useful addresses

About Learning Disabilities: http://www.aboutlearningdisabilities.co.uk.

British Institute of Learning Disabilities: http://www.bild.org.uk.

CHANGE: http://www.changepeople.co.uk.

Department of Health: http://valuingpeople.gov.uk.

Derbyshire Coalition for Inclusive Living: http://www.dcil.org.uk.

Equality and Human Rights Commission: http://www.equalityhumanrights.com.

People First: http://www.peoplefirstltd.com.

The Foundation for People with Learning Disabilities: http://www.learningdisabilities.org.uk.

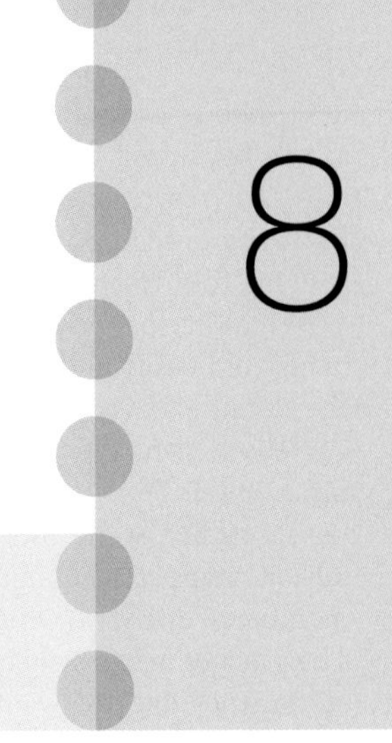

Personal narrative and life story

Tony Dennison Steve Mee

CHAPTER CONTENTS

KEY ISSUES

- The voice of people with a learning disability has typically been unheard in the past
- Engaging with oral histories can enable professionals to develop an empathic understanding of the world of the people they support
- Truly listening to individual narrative should underpin person-centred planning
- People with a learning disability are empowered by telling their own story
- People with a learning disability can be perceived more positively when acting as storyteller

Introduction

This chapter considers the gathering of oral histories, narratives and the use of life story work with people who have a learning disability. There is consideration of the ways in which these tasks can be carried out and consideration of some of the common ethical problems which may be encountered along the way.

The increasing popularity of this type of work is also considered, along with some evaluation of the work, both from the point of view of a person with a learning disability and from the point of view of a person learning from the material.

> Steve: The first time you ever went to Royal Albert
> Geoffrey: It was when the war was on
> Steve: Were you a boy?
> Geoffrey: A little boy
> Steve: Do you know why you went to the Albert?
> Geoffrey: I didn't know that
> Steve: You don't know why you went?
> Geoffrey: No
> Steve: How did you get there?
> Geoffrey: My mother put me there

The above is a piece of narrative which may be viewed at *Unlocking the Past: a Royal Albert Hospital Archive* (see Useful addresses). Why can it be described as a piece of narrative? It can be described as this because it is a record of something being narrated (no matter how informally this is being done). In this case, an important instant from someone's life is being told to another person.

We all have stories about ourselves to tell; some being told easily and freely. We probably will adapt the detail and vocabulary for the audience we find ourselves with. We may tell the same story several times in our life, each time a little differently, refining it, adding some bits, dropping others. We may inherit stories from our parents and other family members, many of which will be about ourselves. There is not necessarily one true story. We are aware of the meaning we want to convey and utilise the story as a vehicle to achieve this. Usually our stories will have a point such as to amuse, to show ourselves in a good light or to illustrate empathy with regard to a point made by someone else who has just taken a turn in a conversation. We may not recall exactly who we have told which stories to, but tell them we have, and this contributes to a sense of having a history, both to ourselves and those we have met and spent time with. This is an important part of being for everyone (Thompson & Westwood 2008).

In most respects, the same can be said of people with a learning disability. They have stories to tell. They will tailor what they tell and to whom. Is the listener looking interested? Will they get in trouble if they say this or that? Should they aim for a punchline in order to amuse? Will it be okay for them to be seen as the hero of the story? For some, this is not a problem. They have the social skills and social networks to have been able to develop the confidence to speak about themselves. For others, it is less straightforward. Some may not have the ear of a person to listen. Some may not have the ability to tell their story unaided. Others may find it impossible to tell stories of the horrendous things that they have seen and perhaps taken part in. Some may feel powerless in the presence of more articulate people and not like to risk offending.

It may be noted that even Goffman's *Asylums* (Goffman 1961), while a master work on the workings of institutions, made no reference to learning disability. Within their incomplete history, the voice of people with a learning disability has largely been absent (Atkinson & Walmsley 2000). The point being that people with a learning disability have generally either had a low profile, or been totally invisible from historical accounts of learning disability policy and practice. Generally, this has also been the case for them in society in general (Allen 2009, Atkinson 2005, Jukes 2009, Ryan & Thomas 1981).

What are oral histories, narratives and life stories?

Knowledgeable first-person accounts, set in either the distant or recent past, whether brief or prolonged stories about ourselves, if recorded, may amount or contribute to an autobiography. Unless actually writing an autobiography, most people are unlikely to write down or otherwise record these stories. This is an unlikely occurrence for most, as publishing houses will be reluctant to commission work that does not promise large sales. Other forms of autobiographical account may be accessible for more people – for instance web-based local history accounts and also audio recordings of oral histories. Whether, and to what extent, other web-based media such as Twitter, Facebook and blogs amount to autobiographical accounts is yet to be fully debated.

Thompson (1988) suggested that life histories had the ability to be a vehicle for the transformation of historical understanding and analysis. Thompson also considered it significant that life stories gave a person their history back. It may be that oral history is simply the spoken account of people's memories. Such individual perspectives provide nuanced understanding of the past. Oral history is essentially the voice of people who experienced that history. In the context of this chapter, it is the voice of people with a learning disability telling their stories, including some happy tales of good times, but also some unhappy tales of experiencing disenfranchised lives, experiencing prolonged subjugation. Positive results of this telling include the empowerment of the individual, the step towards self-advocacy, the feeling of worth.

In even plainer terms, an oral history is a series of stories told by someone and recorded verbatim. This can be an audio recording, a video recording or written down. Until it is recorded, it is a story – another word for this being a narrative. Narratives can be grouped together (for example, more than one narrative by one individual; or more than one narrative with a shared focus, by a number of individuals) to form an oral history. To some extent it can be argued that oral histories can be shaped by both the teller and by the historian. They may mediate (i.e. the story is told through them) and constitute meaning. The teller is clearly influential in this as they recount the history from their perspective. The historian is also instrumental as, without them, there may not be a prompt to uncover the history in the first place, and it is they who piece together stories and other evidence to create or construct the history (Moses & Knutsen 2007). Hamilton & Atkinson (2009) indicate that this work is also useful in that it makes epistemological connections, constructing a version of history for the reader to engage with.

It may be the case that people with a learning disability have not told their stories – very few have had them written down or otherwise recorded to enable them to be accessible to a broader public. Well known instances among the few exceptions to this generalisation include Joey Deacon (Deacon 1974), whose story sold as a book and was also televised. Mabel Cooper's own story is a further example of this genre (Cooper 1997). Other important examples of the voice of people with a learning disability in oral history include Atkinson & Williams (1990), Booth & Booth (1994), Braginsky & Braginsky (1971), Edgerton (1967), Fido & Potts (1989) and Hunt (1967).

Case Illustration 8.1 and Reader Activity 8.1 will give you the opportunity to consider the nature of a narrative version of events, compared to a third-party written version of events. They are clearly very different.

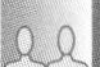

Case illustration 8.1

In the early 1940s, it was considered appropriate for some people with a learning disability to live in long-stay institutions. Indeed a large percentage of people with a learning disability did live in these institutions. Some people stayed in the institutions for most of their lives and had very little control in their lives. In the 1980s, the resettlement programme started and, over the following 20 years, most people left the institutions to live in the community.

These bald facts tell us something about the historical context.

Reader activity 8.1

Now watch the video which includes this transcript from 2 minutes 23 seconds to 3 minutes at *Unlocking the Past: a Royal Albert Hospital Archive* (see Useful addresses).

- Can you distinguish between the type of information offered at the start of this chapter and the type offered by Geoffrey himself? As writers on this topic, we would be writing fiction if we were to offer you something as powerful as what Geoffrey offers to you.
- How is your response to the two forms of knowledge different?

The data from such a website can be interrogated and the findings may show the person negatively or positively. Learning may well take place: 'Ah, so that is what it was like to be a person with a learning disability in that place'.

Case illustration 8.2

This is a transcript from a video which may be viewed at *Unlocking the Past: A Royal Albert Hospital Archive* (see Useful addresses). Geoffrey is talking to Steve about his experience of witnessing 'low grades' (using the terminology of the time) being abused.

> *Steve: what did they (staff) used to do to them?*
> *Geoffrey: They used to thump them.*
> *Steve: Did they?*
> *Geoffrey: They used to drag them.*

Steve had heard many times of people being thumped but had never heard mention of being 'dragged'. This image hit Steve in the moment and stayed with him after the interview. It caused the recall of a long forgotten memory of when he worked in a hospital and someone was being dragged along the floor screaming. Somehow this image felt worse than thumping. Being 'thumped' is bad enough but it is possible for people to thump each other as equals but being dragged vividly portrays an extreme power difference. Animals are dragged by a leash. A person being dragged is being forcibly taken somewhere they have no wish to go. This is an extreme example of the frequently repeated lack of power reported by people who lived in the institutions. People with a learning disability may not be literally dragged to places today but Steve does know of people who end up going to college courses that are of no interest and living in houses with people they do not like.

> *Stories appeal to our own positions in life resonating as another's story collides with our own.*
>
> (Goodley 1996:336)

Reader activity 8.2

Take time to look at the oral history website *Unlocking the Past: a Royal Albert Hospital Archive* (see Useful addresses) and look at oral transcripts or listen to recordings of peoples' accounts. Wait for something to 'hit you' as the image of being dragged hit Steve (see also Case illustration 8.2).

- Why did this comment strike you?
- What image does it evoke?
- What does it tell you about the broader experience of having a learning disability?
- Does this theme appear in the life of someone you know now, albeit in a less extreme form?

Goodley (1996:335) makes a salient point when discussing how narratives work on the listener:

> Reinforcing the insider's subjective understandings of their own position prompts readers to challenge their own (often generalised) understandings of the tellers. In short, our own 'truths' are quickly challenged by the personal narrative.

The perspective of the person who lived a particular history is an essential dimension of that history but it can also be argued that oral history might also be seen as 'anti-history' in that it challenges formal histories (Atkinson & Walmsley 2000). For example, Geoffrey describes others being 'thumped' and 'dragged' (see Case illustration 8.2 for context of this comment). The hospital policies and formal records would have listed specialist services, training and behavioural therapies offered to people who lived at the institution, but would have made no reference to abuse. Geoffrey's account paints a very different picture. They present very different narratives.

Why is this approach gaining popularity?

Sources such as Ancestry (see Useful addresses), television programmes such as *Who Do You Think You Are?* and the BBC's World War II archive of people's own stories (see Useful addresses) illustrate the broader popularity of first-hand accounts. More pertinent to this chapter, there is also a drive to establish their own histories by people with a learning disability themselves. A further catalyst here is the arrival of purposeful person-centred approaches, resulting in staff striving to get to know a person as meaningfully and comprehensively as possible. Often, as indicated by Atkinson (2005:10), the individual can enjoy this process, finding 'positive affirmation of identity'. However, in some instances, there can be limits to this, as was found by one of the authors of this chapter (see below). It is clear in some stories that have been recorded by people with a learning disability that talking through the events helps them to find a context for what happened and, in doing this, they may build resilience – they may see what they have come through and are stronger, hardier, more resilient for it (this is not to suggest that being oppressed and ignored is a desirable state to experience).

Some authors would situate the rise in popularity of oral history even earlier. For example, Gilbert (2009) felt that its development was facilitated by reconfiguration of the political and social context stemming from those changes to social policy in the late 1980s which led to the promotion of user involvement and consumerism promoted by such vehicles as the NHS and Community Care Act of 1990. In the same decade, choice and participation came to be fundamental to some variations and developments of normalisation (Gilbert 2009).

What about life stories?

The authors of this chapter view life stories and life story work as different in focus to more general work with narratives and oral histories. Therefore, as you will have noticed, in this chapter we will not use the terms interchangeably. We view life story work as essentially something engaged in by a professional with a person with a learning disability as a therapeutic intervention. Hussain & Raczka (1997) provide an excellent overview of this therapeutic work. This matter is covered more fully below. Wider in her definition is Kwiatek (2009) who writes of compiling a life story as what is done to gather insights to inform the construction of a person-centred plan, mentioning some benefits for health care professionals of compilation of a life story of a particular person with a learning disability. She also mentions benefits for the individual with a learning disability such as empowerment, participation and increasing self-identity.

Building and exploring the context for narratives and oral histories

Call them what you will ... Why do they matter? What do they do? Obviously there are many answers to these questions and, in answering them, further questions are raised. We do not aim to answer all the questions here – space does not permit this. However, what we do aim to achieve is for the reader to be able to reflect on and explore possible answers to the questions in a manner that is helpful to their future work with people who have a learning disability.

Let us begin by offering some superficial responses to the questions raised so far, including questions along the lines of 'Why does this matter?' It probably matters because they are part of people with a learning disability having a voice. A voice that is worth hearing – they are experts on their own lives. The individual knows what it was like to live in location X with person Z. They know what it is like to live where they are now, supported in their daily lives by staff members A, B and C. They know what they like, what they don't like. They have a sense of humour, a sense of justice and injustice, they are complete human beings – complete with strengths along with faults.

Telling the story creates a history – often one that was previously unheard. Perhaps not only unheard, but hidden. These histories can assist in the development and maintenance of a sense of identity for the teller – and sometimes this can also be applied for the listener. Both the authors of this chapter have featured in stories told by people with a learning disability. This has enabled them to reflect on and better understand how the part they played in a person's life was received by that person. Often it is the case that the histories of people with a learning disability are lost (some may say stolen) formally in the professional records created in their name, and formally and informally lodged in the memories of people they have no further contact with (Thompson & Westwood 2008).

Enabling people to tell their stories and listening effectively to them, undoubtedly encourages reflexivity in thinking, for the teller, the listener and those accessing the accounts second hand. This reflexivity, as indicated above, can in turn inform action. It can also help to develop a sense of historical awareness – an insight into what a person has experienced and how this has been instrumental in shaping them into the person they now are – socialisation in action. Part of the process of helping to generate and gathering a story moves this socialisation process on. Often it is the case that the story is of how things were not very pleasant – perhaps the person's point of view was not valid or respected. The process of oral history generation can be a process of secondary socialisation in that the views and memories of the person are valid and the historian is interested in them. The person moves from thinking of themselves as someone whose thoughts do not matter, to someone whose thoughts do matter. This is not only the case for people with a learning disability, but also for many other minorities who had their histories hidden or subsumed by the mainstream. Atkinson (2005:9) suggests that this has been the case for other groups including women, mental health survivors and black people. Johnson (1998) presents the stories from elderly women who had been institutionalised. 'Elderly' is arguably a further group of excluded people. Within those largely forgotten accounts, women's accounts have been under-represented. Women who have a learning disability have the dual exclusion resulting from belonging to two groups of excluded people; women and people with a learning disability (Traustadottir & Johnson 2000). Vernon (1999) describes the negative impact of dual stigmatisation.

The official histories tell official stories and the participants, as suggested above, are hidden or silent. Official histories are not their histories, they are the histories of officialdom. For example, documents from long-stay institutions lodged in record offices tend to include items such as management board meeting minutes, newspaper articles of open days and so forth, and audited accounts. The individual people with a learning disability who lived there are more often than not missing from these accounts. Documentary sources of history focus on the powerful events which are meaningful to those who compiled them. Earlier in this chapter, we mentioned an example of how oral history could be perceived as anti-history. Geoffrey had provided a narrative of others being 'thumped' and seeing people being 'dragged'.

A recent example of this exclusion from their own history can be found in the chapter of a book called *Learning Disability Nursing Practice* which relates the story of an institution through its official records, press releases and the like (Allen 2009), and the subsequent chapter, through selected interviews with a few ex-members of staff, constructs a one-sided image of everyday live in the same institution (Jukes 2009). Both are very good, well informed and well constructed chapters, but the voices of the people with a learning disability who lived there are completely missing from each of them.

Gathering a narrative or oral history

What should you do if you want to gather a narrative or an oral history from someone? This section will provide you with some practical tips and also share some experiences to help you on your way.

The person may be aware that others will hear their words. They may be aware that perhaps their interview will be uploaded to a website. However, for example, do they appreciate (could any of us fully appreciate?) what learning may take place as a result of students accessing the website, listening to the interview and using that information to address

Case illustration 8.3

A video was being made for the *Unlocking the Past: A Royal Albert Hospital Project* website (see Useful addresses). During the making of the film, Steve recorded a conversation with Gill which took over an hour. He sat out of camera shot for the whole time. A video camera was left running for the duration of this interview. He left the room twice, once in the middle of the interview and the second time at the end of the interview. When subsequently editing the video, he found two comments from Gill during these two absences. She had apparently forgotten the video camera was recording. In the first out take, Gill said:

> *Come on* ... *I want to go* home! *(The emphasis is how Gill expressed these words. She was looking at her watch and sounding annoyed.)*

At Steve's second absence, the following happened:

> *Gill rummaged in her handbag and watched me leave the room. As the door clicks shut she says "Talking about the Royal Albert". Following an 8-second gap, she says "Talking about the Royal Albert gets me all upset". Her tone suggests that she is upset.*

At a subsequent meeting, Steve asked Gill:

- Would she like to exclude herself from the oral history project?
- Could the out-takes be used in a conference presentation?

At first Gill said "Yes, finished with the Royal Albert", giving a sweep of her hand which conveyed finality to me. While acknowledging that Gill could do exactly as she pleased, the supporting staff member suggested that when Gill had done an oral history session she was always pleased that she had done it. Gill replied "Yes that's right I do". Furthermore, when Steve sought permission to use the out-takes at a conference, Gill said "I will be able to come to that". She appeared to be ambivalent; she wanted to go to the conference but also did not want anything more to do with the project. Steve explained that his purpose in using the out-takes was to help people like him, doing work with people who were telling their story to do it in a way that might be less upsetting. She readily agreed to this. Having presented at conference, Gill clearly understands the concept.

Reader activity 8.3

- Should people with a learning disability be asked to give their account if they become upset?
- Can meaningful consent be given when the person seeking the consent is an academic or professional? Can the power ever be appropriately apportioned?
- Can someone who has never written or read an article (or indeed cannot read or write) ever give meaningful consent to their words being published?
- Consider the person-centred plan for someone you work with. Can they give meaningful consent to their words being written down? Do they understand the permanence of written records? Are their words written exactly as spoken or are they mediated (and even sanitised) by a professional?

questions and challenges put to them by a lecturer? Such learning may well be powerful, but is by its very nature difficult to quantify. A significant question to ask of oral history work is whether there is benefit to the people who are telling their stories. It is critical that this issue is explored when those who are telling their story have histories which may prove distressing and where those organising the work have the relative power of 'professional' or 'academic'. There are claims made for advantages in oral history work for the person who is telling the story. An initial benefit of telling one's own story is that it offers a means of making sense of one's life. (Coleman 1986).

Traustadottir & Johnson (2000:22) suggest three ways in which this coming together of the academic/historian and the person with a learning disability is problematic.

1. Othering. The process of collecting an oral history is, of itself, an objectifying process. The people telling their story are made 'other' simply because they are being differentiated as a group.
2. Ownership. Are the academics/professionals involved 'colonising' the world of the people whose story it is? How different is their role to that of an anthropologist observing a tribe?
3. Accessibility. The academic/historian takes the stories and produces them in a way that is suitable for an academic medium, or even a chapter in a book such as this. Presented in such a way, the stories become inaccessible to many people with a learning disability almost by definition.

Atkinson argues that people with a learning disability who are involved in oral history projects find empowerment through the process (Atkinson 2004). This includes making sense of one's life, being seen as 'expert witness' (Birren & Deutchman 1991), role reversal where the story-teller becomes 'hero' and collaboratively re-telling stories and sharing the meaning as an act of survival or defiance. Atkinson (2004:700) goes as far as saying:

> The research on which this paper is based may be seen as part of a 'resistance movement' (Gillman et al 1997) where people with learning difficulties have co-constructed their personal and shared histories.

Helping someone to tell and record their life story, or aspects of it, can be termed life story work. This can be a liberating or self-affirming experience, or it can have significant therapeutic worth.

Practical points

First of all you will need time. A problem faced by many people with a learning disability is that they are not familiar with speaking up or being listened to. The experience of the authors is that some people who have lived in long-stay hospitals might be reluctant to speak up when doing so might have resulted in 'getting into trouble' in the past. How will this person know that speaking up is safe? Of course, one thing you will need to be clear about is what you will do if the person who is telling their story talks about abuse. The obvious professional answer is that you will report it but there may be a cost to the person who has shared the story; they may well experience the fall-out as 'getting into trouble'. You will also need to consider what you will do with any accounts of less direct abuse such as 'the staff are rude to me'.

It is possible that the person may become upset if there were unhappy times in the past. Subjects such as being removed from one's family as a small child, being bullied, being hit by staff or being scared may obviously cause the storyteller to become distressed. How will you support that person at the time and afterwards? One of the ongoing issues raised for the authors is that some individuals often become angry or unhappy and yet they repeatedly agree to attend the oral history group. It appears that many people with a learning disability who have been subject to services learn to keep out of trouble and one aspect of this is to give the answer that the powerful other (staff) seems to want.

It can be very difficult to overcome lack of skill and lack of motivation to speak up that has resulted from a lifetime of not being heard. It is probable that a one-off meeting would be of limited use. It would be more typical for trust to have to build over a period of time. Within each session there may be long silences. It can sometimes happen that some stories become 'favourites' and get discussed time after time. This is similar to a group of friends who might meet in the pub and have a stock of favourite topics and opinions. When asking questions, it is important to use language which is clear, unambiguous and appropriate to the level of language development for the person with a learning disability. For example, Booth & Booth (1994) avoided the requirement for numeracy in an answer. The authors have found it more useful to ask, for example, "Were you a small boy or a man when you went to the hospital?" rather than "When did you go to the hospital?" or "How old were you when you went to the hospital?"

One excellent method of helping people to know where to start with a story is to share pictures or objects. The following pictures have all helped to prompt discussion in the Royal Albert Project (see Useful addresses)

- The recreational hall.
- The communal dining hall.
- Dormitories.
- The front of the hospital.
- Sports teams.
- Senior members of staff.
- Recreational activities.
- Work activities.

Possibly other visual and tactile items are required to not only trigger the memory, but to be presented in order to recreate that memory whenever the topic is revisited. It may be the case that the person requires the use of augmentative communication aids such as Talking Mats or digital technology (Kwiatek 2009).

It is important to consider the physical environment. How will you arrange the seating to reduce positional distancing? In whose environment will the recording take place? Will there be drink and food available?

It is important to be conscious of power when working with a person's account of their life. Control of the agenda has clear power issues. As professionals, we are used to having information that we wish to obtain and we run the risk of taking the practice model into the process. The authors have found that the accounts which offer some of the most vivid insights emerge when the story takes on a life of its own. A picture of a dormitory may well start discussion of staff, or jobs allocated, or fear of the dark or something that seems to have no relationship. Go with it. Ordinary conversation is unplanned and free flowing and this is how vivid stories may emerge.

There are three main ways of recording the narrative. It is possible to take notes but this has two down sides. The first is that as practitioners we may be used to assessment procedures and pro-formas and this may inhibit the unconscious practice model adopted when following a line of enquiry. This might seem threatening, particularly if the person telling their story cannot read. The person with a learning disability may associate note taking with assessment processes and this may inhibit free flow of the narrative. Some people may have very negative associations with note taking and find the process unpleasant. The second down side of note taking is that the person telling their story should have one's close attention. A true dialogue helps and encourages the storyteller.

An audio recording is an excellent way of collecting the story. Once the machine is running, the storyteller and listener can forget about it. It has been the author's experience that people very quickly forget about the recording. It will be necessary to satisfy the ethical requirements of the organisation and seek consent from the storyteller for the story to be recorded. Having a permanent record can be critical for accuracy. As described above, stories change in constant re-telling and so a permanent record offers a more reliable account. Also, the authors have found that listening to past recordings is an excellent way of prompting further discussion, particularly with people who may have difficulties with memory and recall. The potential ethical issues in this process are discussed below.

Transcribing the recording can take 6 hours for every 1 hour of narrative. It will be necessary to decide how completely the story is to be transcribed. Will the 'umms' and 'ahhs' need to be transcribed? The best policy is to record as completely as possible. A good alternative is to complete a written list of what was discussed in each recording. This will allow easier access where a particular issue is being researched at some future date.

The most illuminating way of recording the narrative is on video. Standing back and watching the process can offer many rich insights. For example, the storyteller might give an anxious glance to any support staff, they may smile, they may display some agitation or unhappiness. It can also be sobering for the interviewer/facilitator to observe their own performance.

The ultimate aim should be for the people who own the stories to control the process of collecting the narrative. Atkinson (2004) gives an interesting account of such a project.

Life story work

Life story work with people who have a learning disability can be traced back many years. A seminal paper on the topic was by Hussain & Raczka (1997). Here they explored the ways that Life story work helped to effectively minimise the stress felt during transition from a long-stay institution to ordinary homes in an ordinary community. Life story work here was viewed as a therapeutic person-centred approach, focusing on particular aspects of the individual's life. Not only was this important in facilitating coping (or even resilience) in the face of transition and change, but the work for many also assisted in dealing with the loss of a previous way of life and the people associated with the way of life. It achieved this by allowing the person to focus on matters of concern to them on a very practical level. This is an important point highlighted by Hussain & Raczka (1997) – the fact that the individual's perception of what is important to them is invaluable, but rarely articulated or recorded. Thirteen years later, perhaps this is not so frequently the case as it was. Meininger (2006) suggests that this positive approach encourages self-advocacy and enables the person to feel good about themselves. The lack of feeling good about oneself is something often overlooked in service assessment and provision. Hamilton & Atkinson (2009) acknowledge this positive message in their work, viewing the actual process of telling a life story as being empowering for a person with a learning disability, as it may include recording and acknowledging examples of resilience and struggle against discrimination and subjugation.

At its most straightforward, life story work involves gathering information about an individual's life. All aspects are included – feelings, thoughts, history – the aim being not so much to gather and record a complete and detailed history, but to be in a position to guide an improved understanding of the individual and highlight certain aspects that are important to them.

Life story work had its inception in children's services (Hussain & Raczka 1997), in particular with children who were fostered or adopted. The past of these children could have been lost of forgotten. Life story work helped to gather and record these histories, and aided the children to accept their loss, work through their grief at the loss of their old lives and move towards adjustment and acceptance. Similar work has been carried out with people who have a learning disability. This work has aimed to enable the person to develop a sense of security in the present, this being important where the past has been insecure. Alongside this has been the development of a sense of identity, principally by being able to speak meaningfully about their memories, ideas and thoughts.

Life story work has also been successfully employed to help from a bereavement perspective for a person with a learning disability. In such cases, photos of the person who has died, special memories such as holidays and other events can be gathered together to form a memory book (if indeed a book is the most appropriate medium for storage; see below).

Hussain & Raczka (1997) suggest that there is no particularly rigorous order to be followed if engaging in life story work. Usually the start is with the present day context rather than delving immediately into the past. Initially the worker would probably merely spend time with the person, establishing rapport, developing an understanding of the context and seeking clarifications to avoid misunderstandings later. Questions and prompts would be open enough to allow and encourage freedom of response and direction, but there would probably be some closed questions, in order to avoid becoming too abstract or detached.

As with narrative or oral history work, visual and auditory prompts may be useful. Videos, photographs, letters, news clippings and objects have all been employed successfully.

The actual life story can be constructed in a variety of ways. It is important to ensure accessibility. It may be a book, or a folder or box file may be useful as they could include a greater range of artefacts. This may be known as a memory box, containing artefacts such as photographs, postcards and other memorable objects. A well produced poster can be a welcome item. The integration of video and audio items is often in the finished product, and so are photographs. Increasingly it is common for these to be also stored digitally on a memory stick or DVD and accessed by means of laptops or simply a digital photo frame.

Ethical considerations

It is clear that there are significant ethical issues to be considered and addressed when people with a learning disability are facilitated to find their voice. These should not be minimised or ignored. They include:

- causing distress to those recalling their past which may, for example, include abuse
- issues of consent and capacity when presenting information in the public domain
- the relative power of people with a learning disability as compared to professionals and academics
- the matter of whose agenda is served by publishing first-hand accounts.

Working with vulnerable people on oral histories or life story work is inevitably fraught with ethical difficulties. These are referred to throughout this chapter and woven into the discussion. Some of the suggested activities explore these issues. However, we offer a brief summary of the main points.

Ellem et al (2008) suggest four aspects of ethics which should be applied to life story work. These are integrity, justice, respect for persons and beneficence.

Integrity

Ellem et al (2008) argue that the fact that the person's contribution is treated with respect is an indication of the integrity of those collecting the information.

Over time, the person collecting the story may become part of the story, a process described by Atkinson as 'reverse commodification' (Atkinson 2005). There will also be problems of compromise of professional relationships. When professionals work with a 'client' they are bound by confidentiality. If any of the work we do is to be published then they are working in the domain of 'researcher'. At the same time, the person with a learning disability may have difficulties distinguishing between the two roles and relationships they imply.

Justice

A frequent theme in narratives from vulnerable people is injustice. It can be argued that giving voice to an injustice is, in itself, an act that promotes justice.

What should one do if the person telling the story makes contradictory statements or states something that is objectively wrong? For example, a person with a learning disability may have problems using numbers and as a consequence offer an inaccurate date for an event.

Beauchamp & Childress (2001) argue that the benefits of involvement in research must outweight the costs. Our experience is that involvement in the process often causes participants distress. Memories of abuse and oppression often causes anger and tears for the people telling the story.

Respect for the person

The participants do agree to take part but how valid is agreement from people who may have learnt the survival strategy of agreeing to things in order to 'stay out of trouble'? However, the experience of the authors is that people who experience these narratives often find that their attitudes to people with a learning disability change; they see people in more positive roles such as *expert* or *survivor*. Capacity for consent is important and consent, or lack of it, must be respected.

Beneficence

The essence of beneficence is doing good to others (Beauchamp & Childress 2001), for example change in professional practice, respect for the individuals, understanding challenging behaviour.

In brief, is it possible that the person with a learning disability could be being used? They are being encouraged to participate to achieve a service target of having person-centred plans, or they are a tool for the achievement of work and prestige for oral historians and other academics?

Consider the closeness of contact of the researcher and the researched, as illustrated in Atkinson's (2005:6) mention of the danger of 'reverse commodification', above. Such close working over a period of time can leave a sense of loss when the researcher withdraws and writes their final piece.

If consent is given for the information to be used in a person centred-plan, to guide necessary support and activities, this becomes one possible use for the person's words. However, they may change their mind. They may revise their story. The past is no guarantee of the future. Therefore, while such sources of information are often a good starting point, it should be borne in mind that life story work as is the case with person-centred planning, is not a once and for all task. It is more a matter of continual listening and learning; readjusting and refining as and when necessary (Kwiatek 2009, Sanderson 2007).

Case illustration 8.4

In the video which may be viewed at *Unlocking the Past: A Royal Albert Hospital Archive* (see Useful addresses) Geoffrey gives the following account to Steve of how men were not allowed to dance with the women in the institution:

Geoffrey: No you're not to dance with girls
Steve: How did Matron used to say it?
Geoffrey: You can't sit here, it's for the girls! (in a comic falsetto)
Steve: And what would happen if you did dance with the girls?
Geoffrey: She'd poke her bloody nose in (laughing)
Steve: What would she do then?
Geoffrey: I said shut your bloody trap! (laughing)
Steve: What did she say to you?
Geoffrey: Any more and you'll go to Welch home! (laughing)
Steve: And what was Welch home?
Geoffrey: For bad people

In this scenario, Geoffrey stands up to Matron and swears at her. She in turn threatens him with the lock-up ward. He is laughing at her and at his response to her. He does not appear passive here; more like the character Mac in *One Flew Over the Cuckoo's Nest* (the 1975 film adapted from Ken Kesey's 1962 novel). At another point in the video he describes telling them "in the office" that some people were being abused.

Reader activity 8.4

We have no way of knowing whether Geoffrey's account is 'true' at any level. The authors would argue that this does not matter but the reader can decide what is learnt about:

- the image Geoffrey wants to convey
- power in the institution
- institutional attitudes to sexuality and normal development.

For those readers familiar with current learning disability support services there is then a supplementary question:

- What account might a person with a learning disability give of their current experiences in these three areas?

Practical examples

Working with people who have a mild learning disability

Andy is a 17-year-old who lives with his family. He has a learning disability, autism and cerebral palsy. He offered to take part in resilience research, and over an hour he talked about his life. He was on a mechanics course and described his experience with others in the group:

> Just calling me names like spastic and retard and all that for no reason. Just because they think it's fun to do it. I said to them 'I find that word very offensive so don't use that word again'. That's when I started threatening to hit them.

He had completed the course but was deemed unsuitable to go on to the workshop experience. He did not understand why he could not go on to the further course. He then went on to describe a life in which he was harassed and bullied in education and socially in the local town. He said that he did not do much other than stay at home with his XBox.

The interview was transcribed verbatim. One hour's talk took 5 hours to transcribe. Andy allowed the family to read his account; they were shocked. However well they thought they knew him, some of the detail had never been fully described. Mum said:

> Andy's story was a reality check for me . . . he was isolated at home, talking to himself and immersed in a fantasy world, fearful of going out. It was there written in black and white, it was a true reflection of Andy's life at that time.

Andy now had his story on paper and he chose to present it at meetings. It helped him to speak, giving a full account of his life. His support and care was radically changed.

What had started out as a transcript of a research interview became a powerful tool which enabled a man with learning disability to gain personal power and ultimately shape his life. The transcript allowed a man who struggled to tell his story 'in the moment' to get his views across to professionals.

Case illustration 8.5

Consider the last person-centred plan with which you were involved. Now tackle Reader activity 8.5.

Reader activity 8.5

- How much of the personal account was in the person's own words and how much was mediated by others? If the first person was used, could you describe this as genuinely their own words? Can you justify the use of the first person if that person had never said those things?
- Consider the time used to create the person's own story in the example of Andy given in the text (1 hour interview and 5 hours transcribing). How long was dedicated to obtain the person's story in the person-centred plan?
- Was the person whose plan you are considering given 'free reign' to talk about whatever they wished or did they answer a series of questions from a pro-forma?

Working with individuals who have a profound learning disability

One of the authors worked with a service introducing person-centred planning for some individuals (a total of six) who have a profound learning disability and also a number of physical impairments. Only one of these people used speech to communicate. The others were more limited in their communication, some using communication aids, others being more reliant on those close to them to understand and interpret their communication.

Clearly the one person who used speech was a vital source of information about himself. There were occasional barriers to overcome – in the first instance, trust and familiarity had to be established. A rather literal, concrete frame of reference was evident and, in gathering the information, account had to be taken of this. The person also had a very limited concept of time and was not able to sequence past events temporally.

In order to reach a position where person-centred plans could be developed, much more information had to be gathered about all the people. Staff employed by the service who were working closely with the people concerned were one source, as were the people themselves. Also included were parents and siblings, along with as many significant people from the person's past as possible.

A history was gathered and written. Typically, parents had clear and detailed memories of early years; of the birth; when problems first became evident; how a diagnosis was arrived at; treatments and interventions tried; and battles with professionals to find an adequate service for their child. Some felt that they never did succeed in this last point until latterly (all were positive about the service referred to here).

Siblings offered more detail from another angle. There were some happy memories, but also some less than happy memories. Reactions of visiting friends, birthday parties attended and holidays limited by the siblings' requirements were all mentioned.

Details of life after services became involved was noticeably less detailed, especially if this service was a residential one. Records were not available. Staff had generally moved on or retired. Within the current service, changes were made to records to raise the visibility of the person – to develop less of a record of banal happening (or more commonly, non-events, such as 'had a good night'), and more of a learning log of things learned by the person, or about the person that might inform the person-centred plan.

When it came to gifts, strengths, best days and worst days, things important for and things important to, all were able to contribute in an informed manner.

The histories and other information that informed the plans were created and stored in a number of formats. Photographs were used, as they were felt to be more likely to be easier to understand than signs or symbols (often the symbols available from commercially produced banks of symbols are as vague and difficult to understand as words). Written word was used for those (such as staff and family) who could read – these items were written in the first person, from the individual's point of view. The written items were also stored electronically, so that updating would be easy and not involve totally rewriting the whole.

Of course, limitations have to be acknowledged here. Virtually the whole project consisted of gathering second- or even third-hand information. It is possible that the people involved gave their best opinion but got it wrong. As adults, we are surely well aware of numerous examples of our own parents not knowing us as well as they thought they did, including, perhaps, ill-informed Christmas presents, out-moded career guidance and a general failure to see things from our point of view! It really does emphasise the early point about this approach being one of continual listening and learning – oral history and narratives continue to be written – they are never complete.

A further problem encountered was a parent who refused to take part, making it clear that she thought that the drive for a person-centred approach was merely a service-led drive to tick a box on an inspector's checklist. They refused to take part and influenced other family members so that they did not take part either. Staff contributed their knowledge and a very sketchy history was developed. It was not until the other people in receipt of the service had had their histories written for some time that she decided to volunteer information.

Reader activity 8.6

Referring to the example in the text of the parent who refused to offer information – what would you do if faced with a parent who had information that you wanted to access, but they decided to withhold it as they thought that you were only (or mainly) motivated by a desire to please an inspector?

Bear in mind the following:

- You will probably have a long-term relationship with this parent.
- The person with the learning disability is your client.
- To what extent do you have a right to information from the parent?

Evaluations of attending a small-scale oral history group meeting

The learning disability nursing course at the University of Cumbria incorporates an oral history group comprising people with a learning disability who once lived at the Royal Albert, a local long-stay institution (see Useful addresses). This oral history group is linked to this website. Module evaluations and anecdotal feedback suggested rich learning and so more detailed feedback was sought which may be viewed on this website. A brief summary is useful here.

The experience of the oral history group was reported as having significant impact. One student reported that:

> it was clearly the most memorable learning session I had experienced during the whole 3 years of my nurse training and one that I believe will remain with me throughout my future career.

Another wrote about the way that the experience had already 'stuck':

> myself and my fellow students still discuss these experiences, something which we rarely do about any other sessions we had so long ago (12 months) shows just how effective the experience was, as a teaching method.

The personal nature of the account and the students' emotional response were reported as a significant part of the learning experience. It is clear that the learning is qualitatively different from other learning. Also noteworthy is the clear linkage that students are able to make between the information on the website and their own practice.

One factor with interesting implications for practice is that the experience of attending the oral history group offered the opportunity for students to see people with a learning disability in more positive roles.

In the examples in this section, students perceived people with a learning disability occupying more 'valued' roles than might be typical. The abridged list below compares the roles occupied by members of the oral history group (on the left) to arguably more typical roles occupied by people with a learning disability (on the right):

- *Teller* rather than *listener*.
- *Performer* rather than *audience*.
- *Teacher* rather than *learner*.

All of the roles thus ascribed to people in the oral history group are more powerful and positive than those which might be seen as more typical (Mee 2010).

It can be argued that seeing 'devalued' people in such valued roles should lead to those people having more positive experiences (Wolfensberger 1983). The implications here are that if students carry these more positive cognitive structures into their future practice then the experience for the person with a learning disability is more likely to be positive.

Conclusion

Grant et al (2005:xviii) make the point that "professional" knowledge counts, but so does professional humility. We consider this to be very pertinent to this chapter. A professional who believes that they have all the answers will not be attracted by narratives, oral histories or life story work. It is professionals who have the humility to realise that while they know certain things, the person they are working with is the expert on themselves and the knowledge of their history.

Whether you believe that professional humility is an innate quality, or a skill which can be instilled and developed, it is hoped that the reader possesses it. Further it is hoped that this chapter has given you a feel for this type of work and motivated you to try it. You will be aware by now that there is no one correct way of going about such work. You will also be aware of some of the commoner ethical dilemmas you will probably face, but that awareness is necessary and positive.

At the very least, we hope that after reading this chapter you will try to ensure that the evidence contained in narratives, oral histories and life stories will be incorporated into the body of knowledge and evidence which underpins your practice.

References

Allen, P., 2009. Mental deficiency institutions: have the obituaries been fair and balanced? In: Jukes, M. (Ed.), Learning disability nursing practice. Quay Books, London, pp. 1–38.

Atkinson, D., 2004. Research and empowerment: involving people with learning difficulties in oral and life history work. Disability and Society 19 (7), 691–702.

Atkinson, D., 2005. Narratives and people with learning disabilities. In: Grant, G., Goward, P., Richardson, M., Ramcharan, P. (Eds.), Learning disability: a life cycle approach to valuing people. Open University Press, Maidenhead, pp. 7–27.

Atkinson, D., Walmsley, J., 2000. Oral history and the history of learning disability. In: Bornat, J., Perks, R., Thompson, P., Walmsley, J. (Eds.), Oral history, health and welfare. Routledge, London, pp. 181–204.

Atkinson, D., Williams, F. (Eds.), 1990. 'Know me as I am': an anthology of prose, poetry and art by people with learning difficulties. Hodder and Stoughton in association with the Open University and MENCAP, Kent.

Beauchamp, T.L., Childress, J.F., 2001. The principles of biomedical ethics, fifth ed. Oxford University Press, Oxford.

Birren, J., Deutchman, D., 1991. Guiding autobiography groups for older adults. John Hopkins University Press, London.

Booth, T., Booth, W., 1994. Parenting under pressure: mothers and fathers with learning difficulties. Open University Press, Buckingham.

Braginsky, D., Braginsky, B., 1971. Hansels and Gretels: studies of children in institutions for the mentally retarded. Holt, Reinhart and Winston, New York.

Coleman, P., 1986. Aging and reminiscence processes: social and clinical implications. John Wiley, Chichester.

Cooper, M., 1997. Mabel Cooper's life story. In: Atkinson, D., Jackson, M., Walmsley, J. (Eds.), Forgotten lives: exploring the history of learning disability. British Institute of Learning Disabilities, Kidderminster, pp. 21–34.

Deacon, J., 1974. Tongue tied. Mencap, London.

Edgerton, R.B., 1967. The cloak of competence: stigma in the lives of the mentally retarded. University of California Press, London.

Ellem, K., Wilson, J., Chui, W., Knox, M., 2008. Ethical challenges of life-story research with ex-prisoners with intellectual disability. Disability and Society 23, 497–509.

Fido, R., Potts, M., 1989. It's not true what was written!' Experiences of life in a mental handicap institution. Oral History Autumn, 31–35.

Gilbert, T., 2009. From the workhouse to citizenship: four ages of learning disability. In: Jukes, M. (Ed.), Learning disability nursing practice. Quay Books, London, pp. 101–154.

Gillman, M., Swain, J., Heyman, B., 1997. Life history' or 'case history': the objectification of people with learning difficulties through the tyranny of professional discourse. Disability and Society 12 (5), 675–693.

Goffman, E., 1961. Asylums: essays on the social situation of mental patients and other inmates. C Nichols, Great Britain.

Goodley, D., 1996. Tales of hidden lives: a critical examination of life history research with people who have learning difficulties. Disability and Society 11 (3), 333–348.

Grant, G., Goward, P., Richardson, M., Ramcharan, P. (Eds.), 2005. Learning disability: a life cycle approach to valuing people. Open University Press, Maidenhead.

Hamilton, C., Atkinson, D., 2009. A story to tell: learning from the life-stories of older people with intellectual disabilities in Ireland. British Journal of Learning Disabilities 37, 316–322.

Hunt, N., 1967. The world of Nigel Hunt. Darwen Finlayson, Beaconsfield.

Hussain, F., Raczka, R., 1997. Life story work for people with learning disabilities. British Journal of Learning Disabilities 25 (2), 73–76.

Johnson, K., 1998. Deinstitutionalising women: an ethnographic study of institutional closure. Cambridge University Press, Cambridge.

Jukes, M., 2009. Striving towards ordinariness within a regulatory system. In: Jukes, M. (Ed.), Learning disability nursing practice. Quay Books, London, pp. 39–74.

Kwiatek, E., 2009. Life story work. In: Gates, B., Barr, O. (Eds.), Oxford handbook of learning and intellectual disability nursing. Oxford University Press, Oxford, pp. 74–75.

Mee, S., 2010. You're not to dance with the girls: oral history, changing perception and practice. J. Intellect. Disabil. 14 (1), 33–42.

Meininger, H.P., 2006. Narrating, writing, reading: life story work as an aid to (self) advocacy. British Journal of Learning Disabilities 34, 181–188.

Moses, J.W., Knutsen, T.L., 2007. Ways of knowing. Palgrave Macmillan, Basingstoke.

Ryan, J., Thomas, F., 1981. The politics of mental handicap. Penguin, Harmondsworth.

Sanderson, H., 2007. Person centred planning. In: Gates, B. (Ed.), Learning disabilities: toward inclusion. fifth ed. Churchill Livingstone, London, pp. 301–323.

Thompson, P., 1988. The voice of the past: oral history, second ed. Oxford University Press, Oxford.

Thompson, J., Westwood, L., 2008. Person centred approaches to educating the learning disability workforce. In: Thompson, J., Kilbane, J., Sanderson, H. (Eds.), Person centred practice for professionals. McGraw-Hill, Maidenhead, pp. 95–115.

Traustadottir, R., Johnson, K., 2000. Women with intellectual disabilities: finding a place in the world. Jessica Kingsley, London.

Vernon, A., 1999. The dialectic of multiple identities and the disabled peoples' movement. Disability and Society 14 (3), 385–398.

Wolfensberger, W., 1983. Social role valorisation: a proposed new term for the principle of normalisation. Ment. Retard. 21 (6), 234–239.

Further reading

Atkinson, D., 2010. Narratives and people with learning disabilities. In: Grant, G., Ramcharan, P., Flynn, M., Richardson, M. (Eds.), Learning disability: a life cycle approach. second ed. Open University, Maidenhead, pp. 7–27.

English, S., 2010. Alison's story. Learning Disability Practice 13 (1), 26–27.

Lambie, G.W., Milsom, A., 2010. A narrative approach to supporting students diagnosed with learning disabilities. J. Couns. Dev. 88 (2), 196–203.

Lesseliers, J., Van Hove, G., Vandevelde, S., 2009. Regranting identity to the outgraced – narratives of persons with learning disabilities: methodological considerations. Disability and Society Jun 4, 411–423.

Reid, K.D., Button, J.L., 1995. Anna's story: narratives of personal experience about being labeled learning disabled. J. Learn. Disabil. 28 (10), 602.

Schelly, D., 2008. Problems associated with choice and quality of life for an individual with intellectual disability: a personal assistant's reflexive ethnography. Disability and Society 23 (7), 719–732.

Shaw, S., 2009. The value of analysing learning disability nurses' stories. Learning Disability Practice 12 (7), 32–37.

Yacoub, E., Hall, I., 2009. The sexual lives of men with mild learning disability: a qualitative study. British Journal of Learning Disabilities 37 (1), 5–11.

Useful addresses

The items below are publicly accessible digital archives, or other web-based items which contain narrative, oral history and life story material by people including those with a learning disability.

Ancestry, http://www.ancestry.co.uk.

A Story to Tell: National Institute for Intellectual Disability (NIID), Trinity College Dublin, http://www.tcd.ie/niid/life-stories/.

BBC WW2 People's War, An archive of World War 2 memories – written by the public, gathered by the BBC. http://www.bbc.co.uk/ww2peopleswar/.

Lennox Castle Hospital, Scotland, http://www.secretscotland.org.uk/index.php/Secrets/LennoxCastleHospital#vid.

Museum of disABILITY History, http://www.museumofdisability.org.

Open University Social History of Learning Disability Research Group, http://www.open.ac.uk/hsc/ldsite.

Unlocking the Past: a Royal Albert Hospital Project, http://www.unlockingthepast.org.uk/index/archives/archives_section_list/1/Uni%20Cumbria/.

Person-centred strategies for planning

9

Jo Lay Liane Kirk

CHAPTER CONTENTS

KEY ISSUES

- All people who have a learning disability have the right to a person-centred plan
- Person-centred tools for planning are useful to anyone, not just people who have a learning disability
- Person-centred approaches to planning require people to challenge their previous assumptions and values base
- There are a variety of person-centred tools that support the planning process including PATH, MAPS and Essential Lifestyle Planning
- Facilitators of person-centred plans require training and support to use these tools effectively

Introduction

This chapter will build on the sound exploration of person-centred approaches provided in previous editions of this text. It seeks to develop the reader's knowledge and understanding by harnessing the lived experience of those whose lives have been affected by such approaches. It aims to benefit students, professionals, carers and people who have a learning disability in understanding how the values and principles of person-centred approaches can inform and positively impact on such experiences. The chapter will particularly focus on use of person-centred planning in empowering people with learning disabilities to exercise choice, control and autonomy in their lives. In all of the case illustrations used, names and places have been changed to protect confidentiality.

A person-centred approach to planning has been defined as meaning:

> planning [that] should start with the individual (not with services), and take account of their wishes and aspirations. Person-centred planning is a mechanism for reflecting the needs and preferences of a person with a learning disability and covers such issues as housing, education, employment and leisure.
>
> (Department of Health (DH) 2001a:49)

Although there is some evidence of good practice with regards to facilitating this form of planning, it has been recognised that not all people with learning disabilities have the opportunity to develop plans that place them at the centre (Kinsella 2000a, Robertson et al 2005). The literature proffers a number of reasons for this failure (Mansell & Beadle Brown 2005) such as a lack of time necessary for supporting individuals, the lack of availability of trained facilitators or issues around basic understanding. Indeed, when asked to define a 'person-centred approach', the understanding of individuals beyond recognising the centrality of the person in the process is vague. This chapter attempts to share possibilities for overcoming such barriers to implementing person-centred approaches through developing plans and sharing positive practice in a realistic way. It is essential that we continue to revisit the key features of this person-centred approach if we are to embrace the real values behind person-centredness.

Person-centred values

A person-centred approach or philosophy is one that recognises the values base that underpins concepts of human rights and empowerment. These are the values for learning disability services that have evolved through the development of community support and are based upon principles of inclusion. O'Brien (2004:1) stated that "If person-centred planning did not exist, *Valuing People* would require its invention." The philosophy of person-centredness originates in the work of Carl Rogers, a psychotherapist. Rogers (1961) challenged existing psychotherapy methods based upon Freudian principles. Freud developed the science of psychoanalysis which is based upon the principle that people are unaware of what unconscious factors impact on their behaviour and emotions. It would be the psychoanalyst's role to determine these. Rogers developed the ideal of person-centred counselling (Fadhley 2009). Person-centred counselling recognises that the individual has the ability to self-actualise. Self-actualisation is a term associated with the 'hierarchy of needs' theory developed by Abraham Maslow (1970) that was in turn grounded in the theory of human motivation. Maslow theorised that individuals develop through a process of achieving physical, safety, social and esteem needs before they can achieve self-actualisation. This is clearly illustrated in the now familiar pyramidal design (see Fig. 9.1). The apex represents self-actualisation, the highest need, and one that corresponds with an acceptance and understanding of our potential and development of our competence.

In the context of person-centred counselling, Rogers (1961) believed that the counsellor should support the individual to self-actualise by recognising and developing their understanding of self.

The need for self-actualisation
Experience purpose, meaning and realising all inner potentials.
Esteem need
The need to be a unique individual with self-respect and to enjoy general esteem from others.
Love and belonging needs
The need for belonging, to receive and give love, appreciation, friendship.
Security need
The basic need for social security in a family and a society that protects against hunger and violence.
The physiological needs
The need for food, water, shelter and clothing.

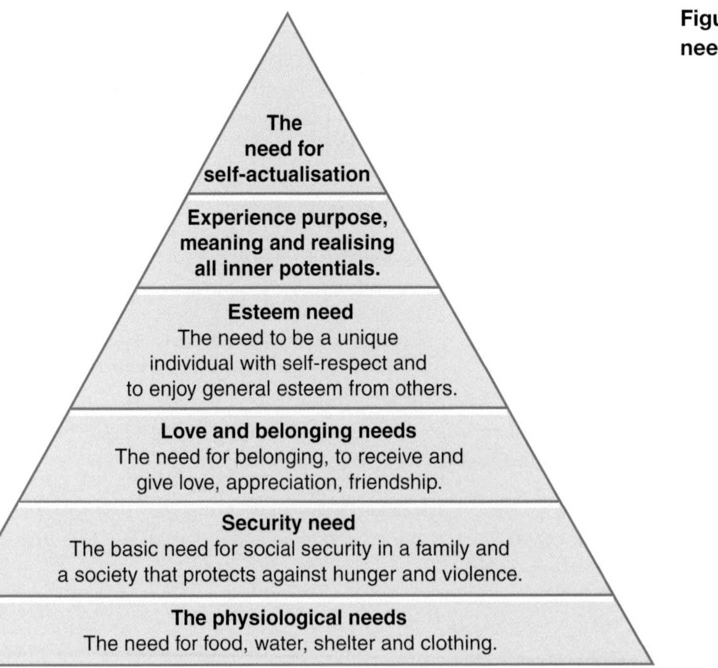

Figure 9.1 • Maslow's hierarchy of needs

He asserted that this could only be achieved if the client–counsellor relationship was genuine and based upon the attributes of warmth, empathy, respect and positive regard. These attributes are also identified by Rungapadiachy (1999) as the skills of an effective communicator and have come to represent the key values that underpin all person-centred approaches including person-centred planning. Such values became explicit within learning disability services following the publication of policy including Scotland's *The Same as You* (Scottish Government 2000) and England's White Paper *Valuing People* in 2001 (DH 2001a). Reader activity 9.1 encourages readers to consider how they might apply these values and principles in practice.

Reader activity 9.1

This exercise requires you to use your imagination and consider what your preferences would be if you were reliant upon a carer. Imagine that due to changed circumstances in your life you are now in need of support with personal care. You are at home awaiting your first visit from a carer. They have been sent by your local authority and although you have been advised to check their identity you do not have a name for the person or know any other details, for example gender, age, etc. You have the verbal communication skills to articulate your views and opinions.

- How are you feeling?
- What information might you have liked to know about them before they made their first visit?
- What would you like to happen at the first visit?
- Can you identify any barriers that might stop this occurring?
- Are you aware of your rights in respect to choice of a carer and control over this process?

You might have considered how you would like the carer to address you. This may be formally using your correct title or informally using your first name. You may have identified that you wish to build a relationship with someone before allowing them to support you with intimate care. You may wish to know more about the carer in addition to their knowledge of you, for example what experience do they have? Where have they worked before? What is their motivation for undertaking this work?

As carers it can be easy to forget what it is like for the recipient of care. Through considering situations from another perspective, we can adapt our behaviour and work practices to become more understanding and reactive to service user needs.

Person-centred planning

When *Valuing People* (DH 2001a) was published, there was a high demand for person-centred planning facilitator training. Many people were trained throughout the UK. The training taught individuals the skills required to develop person-centred plans with an emphasis on values and inclusion as a core of any person-centred work. Person-centred planning has three levels (Simmons, unpublished). The first level is the foundation of any work undertaken in any service which provides support to people. This can be described as the 'person-centredness' of the organisation – the values, attitudes and culture. If this level is not solid enough then any further work undertaken in the name of person-centred planning may not be able to flourish and grow. The second level is the 'practice' level. This is where values are put into practice through person-centred approaches in action. The third level is the plan. This needs to be supported by solid foundations. A core element of facilitator training is recognising the fundamental differences between person-centred planning and traditional ways of planning with people. The person-centred plan doesn't simply include the focus person; it empowers them to take control and own their plan. This is supported by the people they choose to be involved as opposed to a group of professionals who feel they should be involved. Any meetings should be at a place, time and pace that suits the focus person. This may be anywhere from a meeting room, sitting room to a pub. The important point is that the facilitator is clear it is based upon the focus person's choice.

The key features in Box 9.1 challenge us to leave our past experiences and ways of working with people

Box 9.1

Key features of a person-centred plan

1. The person is at the centre.
2. Family and friends are full partners.
3. It reflects the person's capacities, what is important to them and the support they need to make a valued contribution within their community.
4. It incorporates a shared vision and commitment to action that upholds the rights of the focus person.
5. It leads to continuous listening, learning and action that supports the focus person to live the life they choose.

(Adapted from DH 2002)

to focus on their plans and potential as opposed to what we and others might believe is best for them. This involves supporting people to develop their communication skills, opportunities, life experiences and relationships regardless of the impact of their learning disability. The challenge is ours to develop communication strategies that empower people to identify their wishes. Within services today there is discussion around how we make judgements on an individual's capacity or ability to make decisions for themselves. Person-centred values require a belief that everyone has the ability to communicate choices in some way; significant people in the lives of those concerned need to work out what that way is. For people with more complex and multiple disabilities, this highlights the importance of involving family and carers in supporting the person to identify needs (see Case illustration 9.1).

Person-centred planning tools are not tools solely for working with people who have a learning disability but can be tools for our own lives and planning with anyone. An important ground rule of being a person-centred facilitator is never planning with someone if you are not, or have not been, involved in the process in your own life. We all have plans. Some of us are organised in our approach to planning; making lists, seeking advice from those we trust or see as experts. Some people have a more disorganised approach but we all plan. These plans range from what to wear, what to eat and what television channel to watch, to more complex decisions such as where to live, who to live with or what career to choose. These plans are not always straightforward or easy to achieve. We all face barriers such as lack of time, money, resources or necessary support. Sometimes we overcome these barriers, other times we change our plans or change our minds about a course of action. Sometimes we make mistakes and use these as a learning process to change our direction. Unless we recognise all of this in ourselves, we are not fully prepared to support another individual to plan. Through recognising these processes, we strengthen our understanding to support another person to take the same journey. One example of this is by considering whose advice you might seek in making key decisions or plans in your life.

See Reader activity 9.2 on the Evolve website.

Your circle of friends and relationships is probably made up of a range of people with diverse skills and interests. If you were planning to redecorate your sitting room with no previous skills, you would most likely consult with someone who has known skills in this area; likewise if you were developing cooking skills, you might consult a friend who is a culinary wizard and so on. In addition, many of us have a core group of 'intimates' who we continuously share plans and dreams with. The term 'intimate' recognises that this group of individuals have a relationship with us that goes beyond friendship. They are people who know our quirks and behaviours. They will usually be people we love and share a close bond with through family or shared experiences. When supporting an individual with a learning disability to plan in a person-centred context, it is necessary to include and value the people they choose to plan with. The Foundation for People with Learning Disabilities (2009) has produced a booklet called *We can Dream!* This highlights ways of developing person-centred plans with young people who have autistic spectrum conditions through sharing four life stories. The nature of this condition makes the concept of change and developing relationships particularly difficult (see Ch. 10). The booklet provides some practical

Case illustration 9.1

Mandy

Mandy is 45. She has significant communication problems, a profound learning disability and has in the past had a label of 'challenging behaviour'. Her facilitator spent considerable time building her trust to find out what made her unique. All meetings they had resulted in photographs being taken of what they had done and seen (Mandy liked to have her meetings outside). The facilitator would post the photographs to Mandy following their meetings and staff said they were the only things that she did not rip up.

Staff were encouraged to use a communication chart to capture thoughts about why Mandy behaved the way she did. What was it that she was telling staff? It became clear that Mandy was fascinated by babies and that her behaviour would alter if a baby was in her company. She was very calm and relaxed – eventually telling the facilitator that she wanted a baby. This dream was not likely due to Mandy's biological age but the facilitator did not quash this dream. As part of Mandy's plan she was helped to 'sponsor' a baby from the developing world through an agency. She regularly sends letters and birthday and Christmas presents of pencils and pens and in return receives letters about the child's progress. Mandy is always happy when she has received a letter and never destroys it. This has given her a focus. It has also provided staff who support Mandy with a positive example of how they can continue to support her developing communication strategies and tools.

advice on overcoming obstacles and barriers in the planning process including how to develop relationships.

Facilitating the person-centred planning process

This section will consider the key elements that facilitators need to consider. This includes:

- building relationships and working with families
- developing Circles of Support
- knowledge of different planning tools.

Developing relationships and partnerships

This section could be described as 'when not to include your parents'! This does not imply anything negative about parental relationships but gives emphasis to the importance we place on who we plan with. For many of us, the people we choose to plan with will alter depending on a number of criteria such as our age, life experience, confidence levels and knowledge about the reactions and support we believe are likely to come from specific people. People who have a learning disability have the right to the same considerations. This in no way suggests that families should not be included in planning; rather that adults have the right of privacy too. Coles & Short (2008) rightly challenge assumptions that all family involvement can be stifling, protective and controlling by identifying the strength that family support and involvement can bring. This belief is given equal importance in *Valuing People* guidance (DH 2001b). Indeed, many people with a learning disability are more likely to have a person-centred plan if they have involvement with their family (Robertson et al 2005). The importance of this involvement is advocated by the Foundation for People with Learning Disabilities (2003:48) which concludes:

> Family members are usually the only people who will have a continuous relationship with the person with a learning disability. Their contribution needs to be recognised, valued, listened to and acted upon.

Despite this, much of the training and development initiatives for person-centred planning have been given to professionals and organisations who deliver services as opposed to families and carers (Coles & Short 2008). This needs to change for person-centred plans to become a reality for more people. Professionals need to work with families and support them to lead the planning when this is what the individual wants. Box 9.2 outlines important factors in developing this partnership.

Barr (2007) discusses the collaboration that this relationship requires and identifies essential components including recognition of the joint venture where all stakeholders are equally valued within a spirit of cooperation, willing participation with shared planning and decision making, and recognition of expertise based upon knowledge rather than role or title. It is essential that any perceptions of an imbalance of power in planning and decision making are barriers that are broken down. To be able to decide who to plan with depends on having the relationships and support networks to choose from. Person-centred facilitators need to help the individual to engage with family and friends but also build and develop new relationships where necessary.

Many people with a learning disability, particularly older adults, have little or no family contact. A large proportion of people with high support needs have little contact with people other than those paid to support them and will also experience social exclusion. Social exclusion implies a lack or restriction on the resources and services available generally within a community. O'Brien & Lyle O'Brien (1995) believe that involvement and participation with the community are essential in creating person-centred plans. For people with high support needs who are socially excluded, it is necessary to build communities. O'Brien & Lyle O'Brien (1995:1) define this as:

> the intentional creation of relationships and social structures that extend the possibility for shared identity and common action among people, outside usual patterns of economic and administrative action.

Box 9.2

Working in partnership with families

Partnerships between families and professionals require:

1. Openness and honesty – acknowledging barriers and role limitations which exist.
2. Realistic expectations – this may involve recognising barriers or limitations but also challenging these through a problem-solving approach.
3. Mutual respect and trust – a shared values base.
4. Power sharing – keeping the person at the centre.

Morris (2001) identifies five dimensions in which it is most important for people to operate to avoid or combat social exclusion. These are:

1. to have a reasonable standard of living
2. to have reasonable security
3. to participate in activities that have social value
4. to be able to make decisions
5. to utilise support networks including friends, family and community.

To develop this notion of community, we need to support people to find friendships and relationships. Circles of Support have developed as a way to develop relationships and encourage the individual to take strength from the support they provide.

Circles of Support

Circles of Support began to develop in the United Kingdom in the late 1980s after becoming widely established across the UK and Canada (De Marasse 2008). Circles pull groups of people together to support an individual in combating social exclusion through planning. Circles of Support can consist of paid and unpaid workers, but in order to support the philosophy of building therapeutic friendships, they should not consist solely of paid workers. The Circles Network in Warwickshire is an example of a voluntary organisation committed to creating Circles of Support with individuals who are socially excluded. Through their mission statement they encourage people to be the 'architects of their own lives' by:

1. engaging in all aspects of community life
2. increasing confidence, respect and value
3. fostering a variety of interdependent relationships
4. encouraging informed choice and individual control
5. improving personal wellbeing, safety and happiness
6. developing gifts and competencies towards productive, fulfilling aims.

(Circles Network 2008:2)

Circles of Support or friendship were developed from the work of person-centred facilitators Jack Pearpoint, Marsha Forest and Judith Snow (Inclusive Solutions 2009) and are a commonly used tool in the process of person-centred planning. The tool is made up of four concentric circles. The individual who is the focus of the person-centred plan is in the centre of the diagram with people they regard as 'intimates' or close family and friends. Working outwards, the next circle consists of friendship, the third is the circle of participation and the fourth is concerned with exchange (see Fig. 9.2).

The participation circle includes people that we have regular communication with, for example members of the same sports team or class members. These are people who we might not view as friends but rather regular acquaintances. The exchange circle consists of the people paid to be in our lives. This might include paid carers but also service providers such as shop assistants and hairdressers. The relationship circle is a fluid diagram in that people move in and out of the circles at different points in our lives. People in the participation circle may cross into the friendship circle. People in the friendship circle may move out of the circles altogether as life circumstances change and contact is lost.

While this chapter does not explain individual planning tools in detail, Table 9.1 provides a brief overview of specific tools. Some of the different tools are described within the case illustrations provided. Links to further information are provided in the Useful addresses section.

Circles of Support highlight the importance of developing an individual's ability to make choices but need to be within a framework of interdependence. Independence has emerged as a key principle in policy (DH 2001a, Scottish Government 2000)

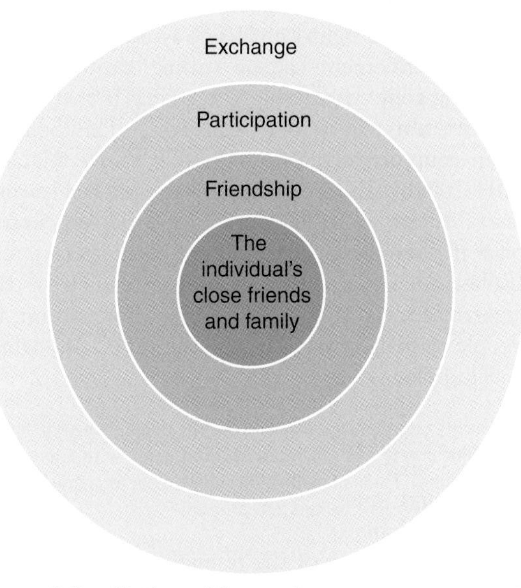

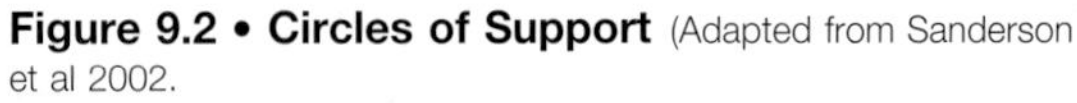
Figure 9.2 • Circles of Support (Adapted from Sanderson et al 2002.

Table 9.1 Person-centred tools for planning

Name of tool	Purpose
Essential Lifestyle Planning (ELP)	• Developed to support people leaving institutions. • A useful tool to support people who have difficulties with communication. • To help develop a support plan.
PATH (Planning Alternative Tomorrows with Hope)	• Focuses on group involvement to raise expectations and make plans for change. • A useful tool for teams and groups.
MAP	• A useful tool to support life transition. • Effective for people who already have a dream in focusing on the action plan and support necessary to implement it.
Personal Futures Planning	• To identify interests, make choices and determine capacity. • To widen and strengthen community networks.
Individual Service Design	• Promotes empathy and understanding through sharing the person's history. • This information is used to develop a life plan based on what is important to the person.

but there is philosophical and sociological debate to be had on the meaning we apply to independence. It can be argued that none of us is ever fully independent (see also Ch. 4).

Circles of Support are key features of many person-centred plans when tools such as Essential Lifestyle Planning are used (see Case illustration 9.2). We rely on the support of family and friends to help achieve our goals and often to help do the things that we find difficult or sometimes do not want to do. This interdependence is important as a means to recognise our own competence as it implies and expects reciprocity. We have to acknowledge where we rely on others in our lives as opposed to being completely independent. This could be practical support such as changing a light bulb, reading or writing a letter. It can also include emotional support in the form of companionship or friendship. This emphasises the value of each individual within the support network. KeyRing is an organisation that exemplifies the positive nature of interdependence in supporting people to live within a supportive interconnected community (see Useful addresses).

Often people ask for a template for a person-centred plan. It is difficult for people to understand that there should be no such templates as the process should remain different for each person. The focus that *Valuing People* (DH 2001a) and subsequent reports and strategy documents have given to person-centred planning provides a good direction as people with a learning disability will have the opportunity to be in control of their lives. We need to be wary that making planning mandatory could result in person-centred planning templates being formulated and plans being generated that look fantastic but may not reflect the person at all. They may just reflect the efficiency of a piece of software or gadget. Person-centred planning only becomes reality when the people who support and guide resources understand their responsibilities. Smull (2000) highlights the issues of making person-centred planning mandatory and argues that unless planning and self-actualisation go together, the plan will remain a plan and not develop into a reality. Barriers to planning have been attributed to several things, including time. It takes time to develop a full person-centred plan that is based on mutual respect. Cultural change has also played a part in the delay of people being able to take control of their lives. If a service was developed with a 'staff know best' culture, the person-centred planning facilitator would have had an uphill battle to help the person have their dreams and aspirations heard. Another barrier that facilitators have had has been the inflexibility of contracting and commissioning within large organisations. When people want something that is not traditionally commissioned, not sitting on the shelf of services, then it has historically been difficult to be able to create a flexible solution for the person. Barriers to person-centred planning have decreased since *Valuing People* (Robertson et al 2005). In individualised budget pilot sites, giving people the opportunity to develop their own support plan with the knowledge of how much money they had to spend has made a significant difference to the planning agenda (HM Government 2007).

facilitator, but in modern society, those people who support people with a learning disability have a duty and responsibility to work and act in a person-centred way at all times. Case illustration 9.5 provides an example of how the facilitator must focus on the key values of person-centred planning to meet the needs of the focus person.

Across the UK there have been a variety of approaches to person-centred planning facilitation. Some areas, such as East Riding of Yorkshire, have invested in stand-alone person-centred planning facilitators whose job it is solely to develop plans for people who want change in their lives. The positive for this model is that plans are generally independent and solely from the person's perspective. One problem with this approach is that all staff need to recognise that you do not always need a person-centred planning facilitator to help someone make meaningful change in their life. Some areas have invested in families and self-advocates to develop their own plans and then to pass on their learning to other family and self-advocates. This approach has many positives as it is led by people who truly know, understand and believe in the individual. The negative may be that families who are already pressured have more pressure put on them. Some areas have commissioned voluntary agencies to deliver their person-centred planning so that the facilitators would be truly independent of any service. However, if the facilitator is viewed as an 'outsider' to statutory services, their influence may be minimal. Some areas have not invested in person-centred planning but are now using person-centred thinking tools 'in house' to direct the personalisation agenda.

Case illustration 9.5

Phillip

Phillip has a learning disability and had in the past been the recipient of both health and social care services. Something happened and Phillip was withdrawn from all services and stayed at home with his parents for several years.

A facilitator was introduced to Phillip when his parents asked if he could have a person-centred plan to help him have a social life. It was clear that Phillip did not want to have anything to do with traditional services for people with a learning disability and it was also clear that he had many gifts, skills and talents around helping others. The facilitator concentrated on the theme of community and what this meant to Phillip. Any work that is person-centred focuses on the positives of people's skills and personality. Phillip has many skills, one of which is having a great memory for facts and information and another skill is Phillip's communication. He likes to talk a lot.

Phillip wanted to be with people and to help people. He tried working voluntarily at a local charity aid station. He became a great hit with the regular volunteers and his confidence grew. He then decided that his dream would be to be a tour guide in a historical house. He frequently visited his local museum and had a planning meeting there. When the staff found out this was a dream of Phillip's, they offered him a voluntary position as a seasonal tour guide. He now shows people around a specific section of the museum and is a valued member of the tour staff. His gift for retaining knowledge and information is invaluable in this job.

Phillip also volunteers at an older people's residential home. The residents enjoy listening to Phillip telling them the day's news and any gossip that he may have. Phillip is an excellent role model and is highly thought of by all people who come into contact with him. He has recently spent time talking to other people about person-centred planning – a role that he will excel at.

Person-centred thinking

As people have started to engage more in the use of person-centred approaches to plan, there has been a growth in the use and understanding of the fundamental elements and questions that arise from the planning tools. Person-centred thinking has evolved as a way of quickly gathering information about the person and translating this into action. An example of this is a one-page profile (Neill et al 2008). This is a snapshot of the individual written in a way that is meaningful to the individual about a certain circumstance. It can show what is important to them and how best to support the person in that situation. A person-centred thinking tool can stand alone, be further developed to inform a support plan or be used to simply ask the added question of what is working and not working in the person's life, leading to real change happening for the person and to the development of a person-centred plan. Essentially a 'thinking tool' can be any strategy used to support the development of a person-centred plan. Sanderson & Goodwin (2006) provide further guidance and examples in their book *Person-centred Thinking*.

Training to use person-centred thinking tools is faster and easier than full facilitation training. To be used successfully, you still need to understand the inner core of being person-centred, but as the tools are fairly self-explanatory, they can be used with great success by the majority of people. The tools can be used on a day-to-day basis helping to direct support and even direct organisational and cultural change. It is clear that no one approach can be the perfect answer. Perhaps the answer in itself, like person-centred planning, is that there needs to be the flexibility and skill to develop a mix and match approach that is tailored to the specific area and its specific issues (see Case illustration 9.6).

Person-centred planning coordination

The following is Liane Kirk's account of developing her role as person-centred planning coordinator for East Riding of Yorkshire in England. This highlights the developing role of planning facilitators and person-centred thinking.

When *Valuing People: a New Strategy for Learning Disability for the 21st Century* (DH 2001a) was published, it placed a real emphasis on person-centred planning as a way of enabling people with a learning disability to take control of their lives. I have worked as a person-centred planning coordinator since then. Large numbers of staff working in health and social care at the time were trained in the tools of person-centred planning facilitation in order to develop plans with people who wanted change in their lives. PATH, MAPS and Essential Lifestyle Planning were identified as key tools and staff became adept at using these.

A small permanent staff team was established that planned independently of any services that an individual attended. Seeing the difference that person-centred planning makes to people's lives is a significant reward to facilitators and to the people who were in the individual's person-centred plans. Changes could be someone moving into their own home; getting a job; getting married, or it could be someone taking control of the way in which they were supported to get up in the morning. It soon became clear that although person-centred planning was making a significant difference in some people's lives, in others there were barriers to the planning process. The main barriers were staff culture (power and control) and elements of the commissioning process not enabling flexibility.

Over the years, time has been spent enabling all staff to understand their roles and responsibilities in working in a person-centred way. Using person-centred thinking tools has helped clarify and consolidate staff approaches and also the significant influence of the development of individual budgets has enabled a change to the commissioning process.

Today facilitators continue to plan with people who want change in their lives; develop person-centred plans into support plans; and also train self advocates, families and health and social care staff

Case illustration 9.6

Charlotte-Ann

Charlotte-Ann was taken into care when she was 2 years old. She has a learning disability and significant emotional damage following her upbringing in a number of different foster homes. Her past has meant she has a really keen sense of justice and will never be afraid of speaking or 'shouting' up on behalf of people that she feels have been treated unfairly. Because of this, Charlotte-Ann has a reputation within services of being a trouble causer and has a label of challenging behaviour.

Charlotte-Ann started her plan while she was living temporarily in a respite unit. She was waiting to move in to her new home with three other people. We worked together on an Essential Lifestyle Plan which gave Charlotte-Ann the opportunity to take control of all aspects of her daily routine. Her plan was prepared and ready for the opening of her new home. Charlotte-Ann wanted to share her plan with the staff to enable her to have a fresh start. She explained in her planning why she acted the way that she did in certain situations and how she wanted staff support to help her. Charlotte-Ann lived in this house for several years. However, her reputation continued to follow her as, because she lived with other people, she always could see injustices in her own and others' support. Charlotte-Ann, at times, needed the support of many professionals and medication to help her relax. We regularly updated her plan and formed a circle of support to help Charlotte-Ann safeguard her plan and future wishes. Her dream was to live in her own place, to have a boyfriend and to have a job that paid.

Charlotte-Ann was offered a council house last year. We worked together to update her plan and translate it into a support plan which enabled Charlotte-Ann to take control over interviewing and employing her own support staff. Staff were given a copy of her support plan which became in effect their contract of employment. Since moving to her own home, she has fewer support hours as she is happy in her own home doing the things that she wants to do. Charlotte-Ann's circle of support remains the guardian of her person-centred support plan but currently she no longer needs other professional input or medication. She is seeking employment and currently waiting for the right man to come along – painting her bedroom 'sexy pink' in preparation!

in the tools of person-centred planning. Working in a person-centred way is everyone's responsibility, no longer confined to learning disability services but embedded in all health and social provision. This in itself brings new challenges, but by being creative and having the knowledge that if person-centred thinking is at the heart of any service then people's lives will change – for the better.

Conclusion

Person-centred planning strategies have sought to challenge the core beliefs and philosophy in which we support people with learning disabilities and diminish the stereotypes and labels that have impacted so negatively on their lives. Promoting equality through empowerment enables people with a learning disability to take control of their lives through decision making. Duffy & Sanderson (2005) talk about 'self-determination' and cite that it is human services' lack of support for this that has limited the use and potential of person-centred working in this sector. This chapter has sought to highlight through the case illustrations that promoting empowerment is possible and achievable. Services must strive to continue to develop the voices of people with learning disabilities and person-centred thinking provides strategies and tools for doing this.

References

Atkinson, D., Walmsley, J., 1999. Using autobiographical approaches with people with learning difficulties. Disability and Society 14 (2), 203–216.

Barr, O., 2007. Working effectively with families of people with learning disabilities. In: Gates, B. (Ed.), 2008 Learning disabilities: toward inclusion. fifth ed. Churchill Livingstone, London.

Circles Network, 2008. Circles Network impact report. Available at:http://www.circlesnetwork.org.uk/Impact%20Report/circles-network-impact-report.pdf (accessed on 27.02.10.).

Coles, B., Short, A., 2008. Families leading person-centred planning. In: Thompson, J., Kilbane, J., Sanderson, H. (Eds.), Person-centred practice for professionals. Open University Press, Maidenhead.

De Marasse, R., 2008. Circles of Support. Circles Network, Warwickshire. Available at: http://www.circlesnetwork.org.uk/circles_of_support.htm (accessed 27.02.10.).

Department of Health, 2001a. Valuing people: a new strategy for learning disability for the 21st century. HMSO, London.

Department of Health, 2001b. Family matters: counting families. HMSO, London.

Department of Health, 2002. Valuing people: a new strategy for learning disability for the 21st century: planning with people towards person-centred approaches. Guidance for implementation groups. HMSO, London.

Duffy, S., Sanderson, S., 2005. Relationships between care management and person-centred planning. In: Cambridge, P., Carnaby, S. (Eds.), Person-centred planning and care management with people with learning disabilities. Jessica Kingsley, London.

Fadhley, C., 2009. On becoming a person by Carl R Rodgers. Review of Carl Rodgers' book on person-centred philosophy. Available at: http://philosophybooks.suite101.com/article.cfm/on_becoming_a_person_by_carl_r_rogers (accessed 7.02.10.).

Foundation for People with Learning Disabilities, 2003. Learning with families: a training resource. Available at: http://www.learningdisabilities.org.uk/publications/?EntryId5=15153 (accessed 26.02.10.).

Foundation for People with Learning Disabilities, 2009. We can dream! Ways of planning for the future for young people with autistic spectrum disorders. Available at: http://www.learningdisabilities.org.uk/publications/?entryid5=32524 (accessed 25.02.10.).

HM Government, (ministerial concordat), 2007. Putting people first: a shared vision and commitment to the transformation of adult social care. HMSO, London.

Inclusive Solutions, 2009. What is a circle of friends?. Available at: http://www.inclusive-solutions.com/whatisacircle.asp (accessed 28.02.10.).

Kinsella, P., 2000a. What are the barriers in relation to person-centred planning?. Joseph Rowntree Foundation, York. Available at: http://www.paradigm-uk.org/Resources/5/o/z/Joseph%20Rowntree%20Foundation%20PCP%20Article.pdf (accessed 25.02.10.).

Kinsella, P., 2000b. Person-centred risk assessment. Paradigm, Birkenhead.

Mansell, J., Beadle Brown, J., 2005. Person-centred planning and person-centred action. In: Cambridge, P., Carnaby, S. (Eds.), Person-centred planning and care management with people with learning disabilities. Jessica Kingsley, London.

Maslow, A.H., 1970. Motivation and personality, second ed. Harper & Row, New York.

Morris, J., 2001. That kind of life? Social exclusion and young disabled people with high level support needs. Manuscript copy of report published by SCOPE in 2001. Available at: http://www.leeds.ac.uk/disability-studies/archiveuk/morris/Social%20Exclusion%20and%20young%20disabled%20people%20with%20high%20levels%20of%20support%20needs.pdf (accessed 26.02.10.).

Neill, M., Sanderson, H., Bailey, G., 2008. One page profile to person-centred plan or support plan.

Available at: http://www.helensandersonassociates.co.uk/media/13258/one%20page%20profile%20to%20person%20centred%20or%20support%20plan.pdf (accessed 16.02.10.).

Nind, M., Hewett, D., 2001. A practical guide to intensive interaction. BILD, Kidderminster.

O'Brien, J., 2004. If person-centred planning did not exist, Valuing People would require its invention. J. Appl. Res. Intellect. Disabil. 17, 11–15.

O'Brien, J., Lyle O'Brien, C., 1995. Unfolding capacity: people with disabilities and their allies building better communities together. Available at: http://thechp.syr.edu/unfoldin.htm (accessed 26.02.10.).

Pearpoint, J., O'Brien, J., Forest, M., 2001. PATH – a workbook for planning positive possible futures. Planning Alternative Tomorrows with Hope for schools, organisations, businesses, families. Inclusion Press, Toronto.

Robertson, J., Emerson, E., Hatton, C., et al., 2005. The impact of person-centred planning. Institute for Health Research, Lancaster University, Lancaster.

Rogers, C.R., 1961. On becoming a person: a therapist's view of psychotherapy. Houghton-Mifflin, Boston.

Rungapadiachy, D., 1999. Interpersonal communication and psychology for healthcare professionals: theory and practice. Butterworth Heinemann, London.

Sanderson, H., Goodwin, G., 2006. Person-centred thinking. The Learning Community for Person-centred Practice, Stockport.

Sanderson, H., Kennedy, J., Ritchie, P., Goodwin, G., 2002. People, plans and possibilities: exploring person-centred planning. Scottish Human Services, Edinburgh.

Scottish Government, 2000. The same as you? A review of services for people with a learning disability. HMSO, Edinburgh.

Smull, M., 2000. A plan is not an outcome. In: Smull, M. (Ed.), Selected writings by Michael W Smull on Essential Lifestyle Planning, self determination and organizational change, Available at: http://learningcommunity.us/documents/listenlearnact.pdf (accessed 21.09.10.).

Snow, J., 1997. On dreaming. Available at: http://www.ecac-parentcenter.org/packets/friends/dreaming.shtml (accessed 10.03.10.).

Titterton, M., 2005. Risk and risk taking in health and social welfare. Jessica Kingsley, London.

Further reading

Falvey, M., Forrest, M., Pearpoint, J., Rosenberg, R., 1997. All my life's a circle. Using the tools: circles, MAPS and PATH. Inclusion Press, Toronto.

O'Brien, J., Lyle O'Brien, C., 1998. A little book about person-centred planning. Inclusion Press, Toronto.

Pitts, J., 2009. BILD guide: an introduction to personalisation. British Institute of Learning Disabilities, Kidderminster.

Poll, C., Kennedy, J., Sanderson, H., 2009. In community: practical lessons in supporting isolated people to be part of community. HSA Press, Stockport, in association with In Control Publications.

Thompson, J., Kilbane, J., Sanderson, H., 2008. Person-centred practice for professionals. Open University Press, Maidenhead.

Useful addresses

British Institute of Learning Disabilities:, http://www.bild.org.uk.

The Circles Network:, http://www.circlesnetwork.org.uk.

Helen Sanderson Associates:, http://www.helensandersonassociates.co.uk.

Inclusive Solutions:, http://www.inclusive-solutions.com.

In Control:, http://www.in-control.org.uk.

KeyRing:, http://www.keyring.org.

Michael Smull – The Learning Community (Essential Lifestyle Planning):, http://www.learningcommunity.us.

Publications by John O'Brien and Connie Lyle O'Brien:, http://thechp.syr.edu.

Say it Works:, http://www.sayitworks.co.uk.

Social Care Institute for Excellence:, http://www.scie.org.uk.

Valuing People Now:, http://www.valuingpeople.gov.uk.

Inclusive research: people with learning disabilities can be the "artists of their lives"

10

Anna Marriott Val Williams

CHAPTER CONTENTS

KEY ISSUES

- Inclusive research covers a wide variety of models and methods by which people with learning disabilities get involved in the process of doing research. This can range from research which is initiated and controlled by people with learning disabilities to active participation in specific stages of the research process
- For people with learning disabilities to be in control of research, they need to be involved from the outset, and to take part in choosing research questions and designing the research
- One of the most important aspects of inclusive research is to ensure that it is set up with good support
- A whole range of data collection methods is represented in the inclusive research literature, and people with learning disabilities have participated as interviewers, focus group facilitators, life story researchers and as observers through video recording of natural interactions
- The involvement of people with learning disabilities in the dissemination of research can help to make the messages more powerful
- It is important to ensure that the needs and voices of *all* people with learning disabilities are included in research. There are creative ways of working with people with higher support needs to make sure that they can be involved

Introduction

> *Some people may think that people with learning difficulties cannot be researchers, but we know that we can do it. In a lot of research, we are the exhibits. But now we are not just part of the picture – we are the artists of our lives.*
>
> (Gramlich et al 2002:120)

Taking a meaningful part in research may appear to be a difficult achievement for people who, by definition, have some measure of cognitive impairment. Some readers of this book may feel that they themselves would find research daunting. Yet inclusive researchers have developed a range of models in which people with learning disabilities can and do take active roles, beyond simply being research participants or subjects of research.

Research can and does take place in many different contexts. In this chapter there are examples of small, local projects that are relevant to the immediate concerns of groups of individuals. There are also examples of national, fully funded projects that aim to influence the worlds of policy and practice. We hope to show that becoming a researcher and supporting inclusion are both compatible and achievable for a vast range of people. The words 'inclusive research' were adopted by Walmsley (2001), because of the ongoing debate about whether people with learning disabilities really can initiate their own research independently. Research involving people with learning disabilities is often referred to as 'participatory': in other words, they are participating in someone else's research. However, in order to avoid making assumptions about the status of the research, the term 'inclusive' research was adopted by Walmsley (2001), to cover a wide variety of models and methods by which people with learning disabilities get involved in the process of doing research. This can range from research which is initiated and controlled by people with learning disabilities (Williams 1999) to active participation in specific stages of the research process (Walmsley & Johnson 2003, Ward & Simons 1998). This chapter aims to give an overview of some of the issues, but also to offer positive examples of practice in inclusive research.

In the opening quotation to this chapter, Stacey Gramlich captures perfectly the sense of power, ownership and achievement in becoming the 'artist' rather than the exhibit. His comment was made at the end of a 2-year period of direct experience in a paid job on a national research project about direct payments (Gramlich et al 2002, Williams et al 2005). Yet despite such testimonies, there are still concerns and tensions about the whole endeavour of inclusive research. This chapter will start by exploring some of these tensions, with a brief overview of the development of inclusive research since the 1990s. We will then move on to practice-based suggestions, based on real life examples of inclusive projects, focusing in turn on the various stages involved in a research cycle:

- Deciding what research should be carried out.
- Planning the context and control of research.
- Supporting inclusive research.
- Learning research skills.
- Collecting data.
- Owning the research: saying what it all means.
- Dissemination.

This chapter does not provide a cookbook approach; each research project is different and the way in which people with learning disabilities can get involved is bound to vary. For instance, people with learning disabilities who take part in research are often among the more able people with mild learning disabilities. We agree with Barton (2005) that the challenge for inclusive research is to include the concerns and voices of those whose voices are less often heard, people with higher support needs. This chapter is largely based on experience within the Norah Fry Research Centre but we also draw on the growing body of published literature and accounts. Reviewing this range of literature serves also to underpin the diversity of the field. We hope above all that this chapter will encourage readers to have a go, to share and develop skills with people with learning disabilities, and to enable them also to be the 'artists of their lives'.

Nature of emancipatory research

Until comparatively recently, research about disabled people was generally commissioned and led by academics who were not themselves disabled. The roots of criticism about this situation can be traced back to the 1960s. It is since the 1990s, in particular, that disabled people have articulated their exclusion from research as oppression; in order to fight back, and to have a voice in their own concerns as disabled people, research is construed as a powerful weapon (Campbell & Oliver 1996). Disabled activists in the UK developed their own model of research that would assist in their struggle, rather than be part of their oppression (Oliver 1992, Zarb 1992). They suggested a clear way forward, which they termed 'emancipatory research'. Recognising that all social research is influenced by the perceptions and world view of the researcher, they argued that they should create their own knowledge, based on the social model of disability (Oliver 1990). In what is now a landmark special journal issue about emancipatory research, Oliver (1992) advocated for research which would be 'on the side' of disabled people, by adopting the ideas in the social model of disability. Instead of focusing on the individual problems of disability, emancipatory research would focus on the barriers faced by disabled people in society and create a momentum for positive change. Issues of power are central to this new paradigm, in which the roles of 'researcher' and 'researched' are essentially flipped over.

How does this new paradigm of emancipatory research apply to people with learning disabilities? Until the 1990s, people with learning disabilities were often not even considered to be suitable research *respondents*.

> The field had been dominated by eugenics, psychology, educational studies and medical investigations, in which people with learning difficulties were tested, counted, observed, analysed, described and frequently pathologised, but never asked for their views.
>
> (Walmsley 2001:188)

'User views' were more frequently collected from parents, carers or professionals rather than from people with learning disabilities themselves (Goodley 2001). This was not just about exclusion from the *process* of research, but also from the *products*. More than any other group of individuals, people with learning disabilities were almost universally excluded from the vast body of learned knowledge about them. At the Norah Fry Research Centre, the *Plain Facts* series has for several years delivered easy-read information about research studies directly to people with learning disabilities (Townsley & Gyde 1997). While this has had a leading role in bringing research 'into the open', nevertheless making this information accessible to people with learning disabilities produces its own tensions about how decisions are made about accessible summaries. It is true that abstract research information can be hard to translate into 'easy read', and quite clearly "some information is by its nature more complex and harder to understand" (Rodgers & Namaganda 2005:53). Accessible information is one of the keys, however, to successful research inclusion, and is a major theme in this chapter.

Research makes a difference, but on whose terms?

In the face of these difficulties, why should people with learning disabilities in fact want to get involved in actually doing research? At the collective level, the answer is that research matters to their lives. Indeed, it is considered so important to make sure that research has an effect on both policy and practice that governmental bodies such as the Social Care Institute for Excellence (SCIE) in the UK have been created precisely to ensure that research knowledge is disseminated and used (see, for instance, Walter et al 2004). The concept of 'using research evidence' can also be problematic however. Research can do a range of different things, including raising awareness, changing attitudes, policy or practice, and should, as Oliver (1992) observed, produce "changes ... in outcomes for service users' (Walter et al 2004:9). The notion of changing outcomes for service users is important. However, the big questions are: On whose terms are these changes made? Who gets to define both the questions and answers?

The move towards inclusion in research concerns itself with those questions, and is closely bound up with the whole shift towards 'service users' having a voice in the policies and practices underpinning their own support (Beresford 2001). Instead of seeing disabled people as passive recipients of services, the goal of English public policy (Department of Health (DH) 2006a, 2009) is now to engage with disabled people as citizens.

This shift towards active citizenship and having a voice is also reflected in the growth of the self-advocacy movement, in which people with learning disabilities represent their own affairs and support each other to develop a collective voice (Goodley 2000, Sutcliffe & Simons 1994). Self-advocacy groups give people with learning disabilities a chance to discuss their *own* issues, on their own terms (see Ch. 7). People bring their individual, real life experiences, and, based on these experiences, they articulate a collective voice, as is illustrated in Williams (in press). Inclusive research is closely bound up with self-advocacy, campaigning for change and collective action (Chapman & McNulty 2004, Townson et al 2004). Therefore, even when inclusive research is situated in universities, or indeed within services, it is defined by a certain campaigning spirit. In other words, if it did not have that edge to it, perhaps we would not call it truly inclusive. This is the difference between doing academic research and research which informs the collective consciousness of a movement.

Deciding what research should be carried out

For research to be truly emancipatory (Oliver 1992), it must not only be controlled by disabled people but it should stem from their own agenda. However, although people with learning disabilities are increasingly being more involved in research projects (Walmsley & Johnson 2003), their participation in larger, academic projects is often only considered once a project has been designed and funding obtained.

The Learning Disabilities Research Initiative (LDRI) was a series of 13 research studies commissioned by the Department of Health in England to inform the implementation of *Valuing People* (DH 2001). All the projects commissioned as part of this initiative had to include people with learning disabilities in some way in the project design. One of these projects was specifically designed to explore the various roles and experiences of people with learning disabilities within the other 12 projects (DH 2006b). The researchers in this project concluded that none of the 12 projects they were studying had involved people with learning disabilities at the initial stages, despite the fact that the research group of people with learning disabilities had been involved in commissioning the research projects. They nevertheless felt that they had not been consulted in relation to constructing a research question nor had they been able to give any input into the study designs. It was clear from the interviews with people with learning disabilities that they *did* think they needed to be involved from the very beginning.

At a local level, service users of a provider organisation may well have a clear idea about what they want to find out. For instance, people with learning disabilities at a specialist residential college took part in designing research with one of their tutors, who was an MSc student at Norah Fry Research Centre. They decided that they wanted to find out more about funding and running their own activities within the houses where they lived. One of the advantages of people with learning disabilities choosing the research question is that it should ensure this is meaningful to the people it concerns. Moreover, research can be a slow and frustrating process at times and at these points a genuine desire to find the answer to the research question can be a powerful motivator. For instance, the Burton Street Group chose to explore the views of people with learning disabilities about day centres and the fact that this was a subject close to their hearts helped the researchers to maintain focus.

> We believe that researchers need to pick research areas that they are really interested in as research is a long haul.
>
> (Abell et al 2007:123)

Bridging the gap between the world of academia and the real lives of people with learning disabilities was one of the major challenges in a scoping study that aimed to include people with learning disabilities in establishing the research priorities in the field of learning disability (see Box 10.1). The methodology adopted here led to a research conversation taking

Box 10.1

People with learning disabilities involved in setting the research agenda

Shaping Our Future (2007–2008)

This UK-wide project was a scoping study commissioned by the National Institute for Health and the overall aim of the study was to work with relevant stakeholders to reach a consensus on the research gaps in the field of learning disability that need to be addressed. The academic research team worked with a group of representatives of local People First organisations, known as the 'Ideas Group'. The main stages of the research were:

First round of consultation workshops

At this point the focus was on individuals telling their own stories and voicing their concerns rather than on possible research questions. Although it was important that other stakeholder groups were able to have a voice, the structure of the workshops was designed to foreground the views and issues raised by people with learning disabilities themselves. In order to facilitate this, there was a morning session solely for people with learning disabilities. Their views then provided a backdrop for the afternoon discussions when family members and professionals joined the workshops.

Literature review

A systematic literature review was conducted on the six priority areas identified in the workshops.

Second round of consultation workshops

Accessible summaries of the research reviews were presented and participants shared their own detailed stories and recent experiences that related to the themes. This method enabled the research team to capture individual narratives and it also helped participants to refer back to their lived experiences and to consider how research could have a purpose in these real life events.

Researchers' focus group

Researchers were asked to respond to the research gaps identified through the consultation workshops

Validation exercise

A questionnaire was sent out to national development and policy organisations in order to explore how they viewed the identified research gaps and how they perceived them to fit with their own agenda.

For full details of this study, please see Williams et al (2008).

Reader activity 10.1

What is the most important topic for our research? People with learning disabilities may need some support to think about what matters to them. If working with a small group of people, the most important thing is that they have a say about the topic.

- Find some pictures relating to different aspects of people's lives (e.g. leisure activities; work; family; housing) and ask some people with learning disabilities to come and talk about the pictures.
- Have a large flipchart, or board, so that the group can be asked to decide which picture represents the most important issue to them.
- They can put that picture up on the board, and you can record the main points about their discussion.
- Ask them what they want to find out about that topic and write those points around the picture.

place, between the primary stakeholders (people with learning disabilities themselves) and also family members and professionals. Most importantly, that conversation took place within the framework of a literature review, so that at least some of the existing body of research could inform the views and opinions of people with learning disabilities.

Planning the context and control of the research

Another important consideration in the initial stages of a research project, alongside deciding 'what to research', is the question of *who* will do what. In inclusive research, there is often a team of people involved, and this type of research has been called 'participatory' and is sometimes seen as a pre-stage to people being actually in control of the research (Zarb 1992). However, ideas can be shared in a team, and a team approach generates creativity. When the issues for people with higher support needs are considered, there is almost bound to be a team approach, perhaps with others involved who are close to the individual and can advocate for them. This type of approach, which may involve family members and friends as researchers, simply follows the principles of person-centred practice, as Sheehy & Nind (2005:37) point out:

> We cannot ask people with profound and multiple learning disabilities directly, but by asking those who do know them well, we do the next best thing ... within this collaborative framework the features of enabling and disabling environments and interactions ... can be shared

Even if only one person with learning disabilities is involved, there is generally a supporter or facilitator as well, and so the big question is about what roles these people will take up, and how these relate to each other. Roles are related to context, and so this section will also consider the question of location and management of the research.

The terms used to describe people with learning disabilities in research projects are many and various; if they form a research group, they are often referred to simply as group members (Abell et al 2007, Williams 1999). The term 'co-researcher' has also featured and Williams et al. (2009a) referred to 'self-advocate researchers'. In fact, when people doing research are asked about their title, unsurprisingly, they mostly say 'researchers'. It might be thought that terminology does not matter. However, the choice of term can express many underlying issues. For example, if the non-disabled researcher has a different title from that given to the people with learning disabilities, then it surely implies a different role. On the whole, the way in which roles are set up is central to ensuring that the research project includes people with learning disabilities successfully, on their own terms.

Starting first with research situated in universities or other academic contexts, one of Oliver's (1992) central dissatisfactions with the status quo was that most research simply benefits the careers of academic researchers, rather than the people it is focused on. Therefore, one of the important messages is that research should be recognised as a paid job, and that people with learning disabilities should have research posts, as academic researchers may do. The role of people with learning disabilities needs to be carefully planned as it is likely to be resource intensive, both in terms of time and money (DH 2006b).

There are many decisions to make in relation to the various roles people with learning disabilities may have within a study and how these work in practice. In academic research, the most 'basic' level of involvement is generally considered to be membership of an advisory group (Tarleton et al 2004, Ward & Simons 1998). The majority of the studies in the LDRI (DH 2006b) did succeed in including people with learning disabilities in their advisory groups. Some of these had a traditional format, with representation from a range of professionals and one to three people with learning disabilities attending. There was some evidence that this approach could lead to the people with learning disabilities comprising a small minority of the advisory group and not always being included effectively. In some research studies at Norah Fry Research Centre, the group of people with learning disabilities offering advice has expressly requested to be consulted directly as a discrete group, rather than participating in a large, multidisciplinary advisory meeting (Davies & Evans 2010). This reflects their previous experiences of attending meetings where the discussion is not accessible to them and they do not feel properly included. The disadvantage of this approach is that people with learning disabilities cannot influence the discussions of the professionals. Such issues need to be weighed up and, more importantly, there needs to be open discussion about the exact way in which people with learning disabilities do wish to participate.

Academic research is not always situated within universities. At Norah Fry Research Centre, and elsewhere, much of the research is carried out in partnership, and in some cases this can mean that people with learning disabilities are in control of their own research group. For instance, in some inclusive research studies, people with learning disabilities have been given a choice about how they wished to participate. This enables people to gain a variety of experience and to start to explore where their individual strengths lie. The Burton Street Research Group (Abell et al 2007) made a conscious decision that they would have a different chairperson each week to ensure that everybody had a chance to undertake this role. It is probably true to say that the further research is removed from the constraints of funders and academia, the more freedom there is for people with learning disabilities to exert control. For instance, Palmer et al (1999) was a small group of four people with learning disabilities who got together to find out 'whether other people with learning disabilities were hitting their head against a brick wall like we are'. They had voluntary support from a university researcher (Williams 1999), but their methods and research questions were entirely in their own hands.

People First groups have played major international roles in promoting inclusive research. Central England People First was pivotal in setting up a special interest research group in the International Association for the Scientific Study of Intellectual Disability in 1996, and this still exists in 2010. The self-advocacy movement provides a context for the collective voice of people with intellectual disabilities at a global level, and so it is natural that this context should provide the basis for inclusive research. At international level, Reinforce, a self-advocacy organisation in Australia, has generated a number of different research projects, including research about plain English, and about self-advocacy itself and deinstitutionalisation (Walmsley & Johnson 2003:129). In England, Dorset People First (see Useful addresses) have led research about hate crime and safety issues for people with learning disabilities, and the Carlisle Research Group opted for an approach in which members selected the roles they wished to have, as well as the way in which they wanted to work. Some chose to undertake interviews totally independently, while others wanted support, with the technical equipment for example (Chapman & McNulty 2004). It is often possible for a self-advocacy group to provide the base and management for a project, so the research can be controlled by the collective body of people with learning disabilities. This is illustrated below in the following section, as well as in Box 10.2, which outlines the questions that may need to be considered about context and control in setting up inclusive research.

Supporting inclusive research

One of the important roles in an inclusive research project is that of supporter. The relationship between the 'supporter' and the researchers with learning disabilities is pivotal to the success of the project, although the nature of this role can be contentious.

> If people with learning difficulties require support in order to conduct research, the roles which non-disabled people will play are likely to have significant implications for the way in which the research is undertaken.
>
> (Chappell 2000:41)

Support is contingent on the setting, and it is perhaps easier to adopt a facilitative role when working within the traditions of self-advocacy. Williams et al (2005) were involved in a research project which was essentially set up as a partnership between an academic institution and a self-advocacy organisation. Williams took up the role of 'research supporter', with Simons as principal researcher. It was the research supporter who had regular, weekly contact with the whole team and worked very much to enable the self-advocate researchers to occupy strong positions, so that their

Box 10.2

Context and control in inclusive research

Skills for Support

Set up as a partnership project, this was a 2-year, national study funded by the UK Big Lottery from 2005–2007. The central goal was to explore what direct payments users with learning disabilities want from their personal assistants. The work was based in an organisation of disabled people (a centre for inclusive living called 'WECIL') and the academic partner was Norah Fry Research Centre at the University of Bristol. The lead researcher was Val Williams, but two people with learning disabilities (self-advocate researchers) were employed by WECIL to be the central disabled researchers. The project budget also included money for a research supporter, also employed by WECIL; additionally one of the two self-advocate researchers had a personal assistant, who effectively became part of the support available to the team. There were many issues that were raised by this large team approach, which are set out below:

How are personnel selected?

In this project, we felt it was very important for the two self-advocate researchers to be in post first, so that they could have a say in selecting their own supporter, as well as the PA. However, they did not select the lead researcher.

How did the research remain answerable to disabled people?

It was extremely important for this project to be sited within an organisation of disabled people; that gave it both direction and a wider perspective. Additionally, an advisory group met regularly which consisted of disabled people and representatives of national organisations.

Whose job is it to make sure that the research gets done?

Although this task belonged to everyone, it was always emphasised that the lead researcher was responsible for making sure the project did what it said it would.

How do the self-advocate researchers get support?

In this case, both the self-advocate researchers had separate, private supervision sessions with the project manager from WECIL, who was a disabled person with a visual impairment.

How do the self-advocate researchers remain central to the process of research?

It would be very easy for the views of the self-advocates to be lost in a large team approach. The key to ensuring they remain central is to give them ways to make decisions, and in this project it was done on a day-to-day basis by enabling them to decide what tasks they were going to do. One of the two researchers also chaired every meeting; and most importantly, they made decisions about the findings from the research.

What happened when things went wrong?

There were several points at which the whole team felt the need to revisit their roles, to rethink how they worked together. Time spent in those discussions was never wasted, because they were a way for everyone to have a fair say about *how* we worked.

(Ponting et al 2010, Williams et al 2009a, 2009b)

views and insights led the research. Williams et al (2005) discussed the need for research supporters to divest themselves of power and step back to let people with learning disabilities take control of the research process.

Roles within a research project are not always static. Chapman & McNulty (2004) describe the process of research within a People First (self-advocacy) organisation. Initially Chapman's own role was as a self-advocacy supporter, however the research group chose to shift over to becoming a 'cooperative' instead of a self-advocacy group, so that it could be recognised that research supporters have a distinct role from that of self-advocacy supporters. In effect, as Chapman & McNulty acknowledge, the research supporter has to advise, actively teach skills and enlarge the horizons of the research, in a way that would be beyond the brief of a self-advocacy supporter. In this case the people with learning disabilities expressly wanted the supporters to be equally involved and not to just stay in the background. The group acknowledged the crucial role of their research supporter and wanted to be honest about how the relationship had worked and the contributions made by all the different team members to the project. The group was aware that other self-advocacy groups might be critical of this stance but felt they were able to maintain control of the project, while recognising their reliance on their research supporter in particular areas. Moreover they knew how inaccessible academic writing and techniques are. They felt that any self-advocacy group would need some fairly proactive support, in order to tackle research. They were adamant that:

> It is also essential to discuss the role of the supporter, whether a researcher or advocacy supporter, because unless the process is clearly out in the open it cannot be challenged by others or improved upon.
>
> (Chapman & McNulty 2004:78)

Another group was concerned that a supporter was dominating their group and they videoed their own interactions and used this as a method to observe how often she interrupted (Abell et al 2007). They reflected on this as a group and discussed who else might be able to fulfil some of the roles she had taken on. In this way they were able to bring a better balance to their work. Williams et al (2009a and b) also found that it was necessary to devote time and energy to reflections on people's roles within the team (see Box 10.2).

As with any teamwork, it is vital to pay attention to individuals' interests and abilities. For example, often a research supporter is needed to act as a translator in order to ensure that people with learning disabilities can access, and understand the implications of, existing published research (see Rodgers et al 2004 and Ch. 6 in this book for guidelines about accessible information).

Ultimately people with learning disabilities are the experts on their own lives. As one research supporter said:

> in some areas I can only have opinions and . . . in general these opinions are not important compared with people in this group who have actually lived through what they are talking about.
>
> (Chapman & McNulty, 2004:81)

See Reader activity 10.2 on the Evolve website.

The central goal of providing good support is to ensure the people with learning disabilities in any research team really do have a powerful voice, and this can come about through the structures set up by the whole team. Research within a service provider organisation, for instance, may include service users of that organisation, and so it is important to ensure they have independent support which will enable them to speak up. The most vital thing here is to ensure that the role descriptions for the whole team are very clear, and that the people appointed for those roles have the right skills and aptitudes which include listening and stepping back at the right moments. These were the views of the two self-advocate researchers, when asked about the team approach at the end of the 'Skills for Support' project:

> There are ups and downs to team work. One of the up sides was that we both [Lisa and Kerrie] got to know each other. We were friends at school. But it's also tough at times. Working in a team is sometimes hard, and we'd have liked to be more independent at times. That's where a PA comes in – it's good if people can get Access to Work money to pay for a PA to help them be independent.
>
> The research supporter's job was to help us do the research. She translates what we wanted, and she helped

Box 10.3

Supporting a local action research project

Working in the garden

One of the tasks of a supporter is to help people with learning disabilities see that they can be researchers. A group of people with learning disabilities in Ennis, County Clare were discussing possible areas of concern in their lives. In the discussion, the garden attached to the local sheltered workshop was discussed. People in the group were really concerned that as the workshop was closing, the garden was at risk. Most of them had worked there for long periods of time. They decided to tell its story and met up with Kelley Johnson who helped them to think about their work as a local research project.

A supporter is not always necessary. Often she or he has to step back, so that people with learning disabilities themselves can decide what to do in a project. It is important that researchers with learning disabilities are in control of the day-to-day decisions and planning.

During the research, the group of people in Ireland:

- found old photographs of the land before the garden was developed and some articles about the work that was done
- learned to use a digital camera and recorder
- visited the places in the garden that were important to them, took photographs and recorded their stories
- interviewed other people with learning disabilities and managers about the garden and what it meant to them.

Another key task for the supporter is to act as translator. Kelley helped the research by providing some plain English guides to interviews; she was also there as a facilitator for their learning, and helped them to use the camera and record their stories. Once all the stories were collected, one member of the research team with some support put them together with the photographs, to make a book, *The Garden Story* (Minogue et al 2007) which was published by the service. Having support to do their own research meant that the people with learning disabilities had their own voices heard, and that managers of their service realised how much the garden meant to them. In this way, a research supporter is very much like an ally or an advocate; she is someone who is on the side of the researchers with learning disabilities.

> us out as well as the team. The research advisor [lead researcher] researches, and also helps us with the project. It's very good to have a research advisor we think, because she can advise us on what to do and what not to do, and help us make our decisions. It's good to have a laugh with your research advisor, and to have someone who can make you feel relaxed and cool. This team's been really brilliant, it has. Without the team, we'd be lost wouldn't we?
>
> (Lisa Ponting and Kerrie Ford in conversation: August 2007)

Learning research skills

People with learning disabilities, like any new researchers, will need to learn research skills. However, this opens up some more contentious issues. Being cast in the role of student is not necessarily a powerful position; studying research skills can mean that people with learning disabilities simply take on yet another set of learning hurdles, which are necessary for them to 'prove' themselves (Williams et al 2005). However, our experience at Norah Fry Research Centre has been that research skills training need not necessarily become 'technical'; in fact, both supporters and people with learning disabilities can probably best learn together. It is important to establish exactly what researchers with learning disabilities will need to learn (see Box 10.4) and also to think of innovative teaching methods that will help them to gain the essential skills.

Bjornsdottir & Trausdottir (2010) worked with a small group of young people with learning disabilities in Iceland, using a life history approach. One of the key needs for learning in that study, as in many across the globe, is that the researchers with learning disabilities needed to find out more about the life conditions that had affected others with learning disabilities. In this case, the history of institutionalisation in Iceland was not necessarily known to all those in the group, but they could learn and relate to those issues, and this helped them to see their own lives in perspective.

Another commonly identified training need by researchers with learning disabilities relates to research terminology. People need to learn some research jargon in order to feel properly included in meetings and conferences, for example. Williams et al (2005) described how the team they worked with attached a sense of power to the technical research terms and therefore wanted to learn them. This can be part of the process of helping people to feel confident and knowledgeable. Some research teams have chosen to draw up a training programme and to decide together what this needs to include. The Burton Street Group took this approach and devised an 11-week programme to cover all the topics identified by group members (Abell et al

Box 10.4

Learning research skills

'Journey to Independence' (Gramlich et al 2002) was a national research project about direct payments for people with learning disabilities. The research team consisted of three people with learning disabilities, employed by a People First (self-advocacy) organisation, and they had support from the Norah Fry Research Centre.

During the course of this project, some attempts were made to set up training both for the self-advocate researchers as well as the supporters in the organisation. What we found was that research training was better carried out during the course of actually doing the research, and so a set of leaflets was developed which aimed to help each individual identify their own learning goals.

General skills

Some of the skills identified by the team were actually generic, transferable skills which would be useful for many jobs. We listed these as:

- office skills, including computer skills
- team work – being able to work with other people
- punctuality and persistence in the job
- planning your own work.

Self-advocacy skills

Many of the things that researchers with learning disabilities need to learn are actually the same things that self-advocates generally learn about. Inclusive research depends on having a strong voice, and so self-advocacy skills include:

- speaking up for yourself
- listening to other people in the group
- taking part in meetings

Finally, we listed some of the specific skills that were actually related to doing research. We divided these into:

- planning research
- understanding research question and topics
- interviewing other people
- finding out information in different ways (including by using the Internet)
- working out what research findings mean
- disseminating research.

(Research skills leaflets produced by this group are available at the Norah Fry Research Centre, Bristol University; see Useful addresses)

2007). In contrast, the Carlisle Group did not undertake formal training; they opted to use an approach where they discussed what was important in individuals' lives and the research supporter tried to identify where it was relevant to introduce 'research points' into these discussions (Chapman & McNulty 2004).

Some examples of activities to include in research skills training are given at the end of this chapter. For instance, video and role play can be useful ways of teaching people with learning disabilities about interviewing techniques. Some people find it very helpful to watch themselves on video, and participating in role plays can also assist with exploring how it feels to be the person being interviewed. This can help the person that will be conducting the interviews develop a sense of empathy with the research participant, which may improve their interview skills. There is also a need for training about analysis, as this is a stage of research at which people with learning disabilities are often excluded. There is a lot of scope for creative thinking in how to make analysis accessible. One group described how they learnt about thematic analysis by reading film reviews and looking for common aspects (Abell et al 2007). In Williams et al (2009a), the team took some transcripts of conversations between support staff and people with learning disabilities from a book by Rapley (2004) and role played them, to see how they would improve the support for themselves.

Training needs to be done at appropriate stages; some people with learning disabilities will have difficulty in retaining new ideas and therefore it may not be helpful to undertake training about analysis methods prior to the start of data collection. This was the approach taken by the research team on *Let Me In* (DH 2006b). However, despite the training the research team received, they still encountered unanticipated difficulties once they had begun interviewing people for their study. Sometimes the interviews were distressing and the researchers then needed some emotional support. They were able to reflect on this and felt that they needed to set limits on what could be talked about. This suggests that in order to protect both participants and researchers, there may be a need for learning about setting boundaries and perhaps assertiveness training.

Finally, it is important to remember that all researchers need appropriate training, not just the members of the team who have learning disabilities. *Let Me In* found no evidence that professionals within mixed advisory groups had received training on how to work alongside people with learning disabilities. Consequently, these advisory groups did not set ground rules and establish appropriate ways for all members to work together.

Reader activity 10.3

Learning to do interviews (or 'not just sticking to the questions')

A good way to start a training session for a group of people with learning disabilities is to ask them to get into pairs and find out something about each other. They report it back, and you can then point out that 'everyone has found something out. They are all researchers!'

- In groups, people can decide on two or three key questions for interviews.
- People can practise doing interviews on video. When you watch back the video, ask people to listen carefully to what the other person said in their response to the questions.
- If possible, find points at which the researchers could have followed up with another question.

Collecting data

The collection of data is often the most memorable part of a research project for the researchers with learning disabilities who are involved. When asked some years afterwards about their project relating to day services, for instance, members of a group called 'Connect in the North' talked first about the problems and achievement of travelling to their research interviews (Goodwin & Williams 2004). This is the point at which the plans and preparation come to fruition, and the research starts to feel as if it is really happening.

In social research, there are different ways of collecting data, according to the type of analytic methodology adopted. Quantitative research generally uses tools such as surveys, checklists or measures which will produce a large amount of data, in order to establish widespread or generalisable findings. It is more common for inclusive research projects to use qualitative methods, perhaps because of the difficulties posed by abstract data which need a measure of skill to interpret successfully. Survey methods should not, however, be overlooked. Like all aspects of inclusive research, it is possible to make survey data accessible, through pictorial graphs or charts; indeed, some projects (Williams et al 2009a) have found that researchers with learning disabilities particularly enjoyed coding survey returns.

This whole range of data collection methods is represented in the inclusive research literature, and people with learning disabilities have participated as interviewers (Heslop et al 2005); focus group facilitators (Palmer & Turner 1998); life story researchers (Johnson 2009); and as observers through video recording of natural interactions (Williams et al 2009a).

Whatever the data collection method, one of the central benefits of people with learning disabilities taking up roles as researchers is intended to be that they can identify better with the people they are researching. This should lead to people being more relaxed, and possibly giving more honest answers to questions. However, in some inclusive projects, we have found that peer identification is not necessarily a 'given', and may have to be worked at. This happens even when people with learning disabilities are supposedly interviewing others with the same impairment. For instance, in Palmer et al (1999), the research team took pains to compose their own research questions with great sensitivity. They themselves had an interest in the issues of labelling, and they wanted to ask a question about being labelled as having a learning disability, without being rude to the people they were interviewing. They therefore came up with the following wording:

> What do you think about people being labelled?

However, as Williams (in press) explores, the very first time they asked this question in a focus group, they were met with some confusion. The people they were interviewing did not know whether the labelling applied to them, nor whether the interviewers identified themselves as 'people with learning difficulties'. It took some subtle work on the part of all participants to sort out this issue.

It is easy to misjudge or doubt what people with learning disabilities can achieve as researchers. In relation to interviewing, Williams (1999) felt worried at one point that the research team members would not be able to ask questions and listen respectfully to what research participants said. It seemed that their own opinions were so strong, that they would much prefer simply to answer their own questions and to speak up about their own views. However, she was proved wrong: in fact, what transpired from analysis of this research project (Williams in press) was that inclusive research tended to be characterised by a certain openness. The members of the research team were quite prepared to discuss their own opinions, at the same time as listening to the participants' views. In the end, this made for a much richer and more natural research conversation, and one in which all participants could take part in working out their points of view together.

When approaching methods of data collection it is useful to think laterally about creative and new ways that inclusive research projects can operate. For instance, Johnson (2009) has worked with people with learning disabilities on life story research, where the individual researcher focuses on his or her own past history. This is possible at an individual level, or within a group, and some researchers (Andrews 2009) have used pictorial methods very successfully, where people with learning disabilities have been given cameras to take photos of significant people and events in their lives. This is very similar to the production of a photographic record (e.g. for a person-centred plan), but can be used within research for people to discuss the significance of events in their lives.

In Ponting et al. (2010) (same project as Williams et al 2009a), data collection was partly carried out by making videos of people with learning disabilities working with their personal assistants. Video has many advantages, whatever analytic method is planned, since it is a naturally accessible format. People with learning disabilities can return to video data easily, while paper records of interviews, or even audio data, are much more dense and difficult. Some projects have included researchers with higher support needs by using pictorial and video methods, alongside drama and role play. Interactive role play is becoming increasingly recognised as a means of data collection, since it enables participants to directly explore their own issues and questions in an open fashion. As such, it is ideally suited as a data collection method for people whose focus is on the present here-and-now, rather than on abstract meanings. An example is given in Box 10.5.

Owning the research: saying what it all means

The reason people with learning disabilities are involved in research at all is that the research is about their own lives, and/or the lives of people with whom they identify. The whole idea of inclusive research would be rather meaningless if people left their own life experience at the doorstep of the research

Box 10.5

Data collection methods used by Rooots

'Rooots' was the name (correctly spelt!) for a group of people with learning disabilities from black and minority ethnic groups who met in Leeds. They carried out research relating to their own identity as black people with learning disabilities, and used primarily active and creative methods to involve all members of the group. Information about their project was included in Goodwin & Williams (2004) and is available as video footage on the CD-ROM from that project.

Rooots included several members who had higher support needs. Some people did not use words to communicate; others had very short concentration spans, and difficulty in understanding. There were also people with multiple impairments (i.e. physical impairments and learning disability), and thus the group had quite a mixed profile. It was not useful for them to sit down and discuss research in the abstract; they aimed to get out and about to do research in a more concrete way.

Among the methods Rooots members used to collect their research data were:

- the use of dance and drama, to express their individual feelings and views about themselves
- creating their own video about their own experiences, within the group and outside the group
- making individual picture books to express their opinions, and talking about these within the group
- going out into the neighbouring area, to discover the community resources that existed for black and minority ethnic people. This was a direct way of involving people with learning disabilities within their own community
- creating role plays which illustrated key themes about being black and having a learning disability.

project. That was why Goodwin & Williams (2004) called their exploration of involvement in research *Our Lives, Our Research*. The two terms go together, and both are about ownership and power.

In order to ensure the research truly represents the perspective and life of the researchers with learning disabilities, the way in which analysis is carried out becomes crucial. Their views, and their lives, have to be central to that analysis. This stage is often viewed as particularly problematic (Richardson 2002); the research team in *Let Me In* reflected on their experience of the analysis stage:

> We found analysis difficult because you have to deal with a lot of information at the same time and work on it until patterns become clear. This is hard work and takes quite a long time.
>
> (DH 2006b:34)

However, using the training they had received, they looked at the interview data and thought about the differences and similarities between the sites. This helped them to find patterns in the data and they also looked for examples of particularly good or poor practice.

It is important to explore ways in which researchers with learning disabilities can be kept central to the analysis stage, as the inclusion of their perspective in the research findings is the whole point of their inclusion. They often have a different way of seeing things, which academic researchers can learn a lot from. Indeed, one of the central tasks of support in inclusive projects is to encourage people with learning disabilities to understand the importance of their own perspective. Their learning disability can actually be their advantage. One of the members of the team who worked on Journey To Independence commented:

> Other research is clouded by the fact it's done by professionals, it's from their point of view and they're effectively only guessing how we feel.
>
> (Tarleton et al 2004:79–80)

Analysis is often thought about both as a technical activity, and also as something which should be independent of the views and subjectivity of the researcher (Bryman 2008). However, many qualitative methods in particular acknowledge and take into account the perspective of the researcher. Creative, but systematic, methods of analysis are needed, so that the findings of inclusive research can be trusted as robust and reliable. What is important in inclusive research is that the perspectives which prevail are those of the researchers with learning disabilities. In fact, one of the keys to getting this right is to think in terms of ownership, rather than the technical skills involved in analysis. If people with learning disabilities really are in the driving seat of a research project throughout, then methods for analysis often fall into place. Some examples are given in Box 10.6.

When researchers with learning disabilities discuss the meaning of research that they themselves have set up and initiated, the stage of analysis is not always a discrete activity.

In traditional qualitative research projects, the analysis comes after the data collection, and follows transcription and coding of data. However, inclusive research often benefits from several chances to reflect and to respond to data; it can be valuable to have a quick and immediate chance to discuss what has been learnt, so that those views can be

Box 10.6

Ways to include people with learning disabilities in the analysis of research

- **Visual methods** are often useful. In Gramlich et al (2002), for instance, the team took photographs on all their research visits to different sites where they were finding out how people with learning disabilities managed their direct payments. They spoke with managers, direct payments organisers, people with learning disabilities and families – sometimes as many as ten interviews in each site, resulting in a mass of data! What they did was to construct a visual map for each area they had visited, by making a 'story' of that area. A fictional person with learning disabilities was created, who approached that area to get direct payments, and the photos helped the team recall and discuss what they felt about the things they had learnt from each person. This method required plenty of wall space for the picture maps, but was successful in giving the team an idea of the 'big picture'.
- **Repeated discussions** are used in nearly all inclusive projects. Richardson (2002), for instance, supported people with learning disabilities to write stories about their experience of living in hospital. His own analysis of the stories, and selection of words for those stories, were taken back to the group several times, until each person was happy with the meaning assigned to the story.
- **Interpreting your own photos** can be useful if the research topic is about the lives of the people with learning disabilities; they can be involved in taking their own significant photos (Andrews 2009). People with learning disabilities were given cameras in this study in order to take pictures of significant people or moments in their own life. Their analysis therefore depended on how they saw the photo, and in explaining why they took the photo in the first place.
- **Checking out findings with different groups** can be done by taking the analysis from one group of people to another group, for their opinion and discussion. Iterative processes like this can give greater depth and validity to the analysis. In Williams (in press), the interpretation of 'self-advocacy' emerged from the initial research by a small group of people with learning disabilities (Palmer & Turner 1998) but was then discussed with a wider group of self-advocates; it was their views that helped to shape the subsequent analysis (Williams in press).
- **Video is invaluable for analysis.** If it is available, it can be edited and the research team can return to it several times. In Ponting et al (2010), the researchers with learning disabilities can be seen discussing their interpretation of video clips they had helped to film, showing personal assistants working with people with learning disabilities. Their involvement in analysis is discussed in greater detail in Williams et al (2009a and b). They were able to select the extracts from videos which they felt were interesting, so that these formed the basis for a conversation analysis approach.

returned to and broadened later. A tip for any inclusive project is to have an audio recorder or notebook available for the stop at the service station on the way back after an interview! With sensitive listening, a supporter or academic researcher can build the larger analysis or report around the insights of the researchers with learning disabilities, making for a richer and more meaningful final result.

Dissemination

Finally, we will consider some examples of how people with learning disabilities have disseminated research successfully. Their voice and their direct messages about the research are important in making sure that research has an impact at many different levels. It is vital to remember people with learning disabilities themselves are one of the audiences for the research findings. This means it is necessary to think about how the findings of the research can be made meaningful to people with learning disabilities and how they will hear about them. This can involve the production of easy-read project summaries, which follow existing recommendations in relation to fonts, layout and use of pictures. One of the LDRI studies in England explored the best ways of making materials accessible for people with learning disabilities; the findings are presented in *Information For All,* a pack of 13 booklets, and are also available in a CD format (Rodgers et al 2004). Increasingly researchers must think about ways to produce information in a range of formats and also how to use the wide range of media outlets for dissemination. There is a traditional reliance on the production of written information and yet clearly this may not be the most appropriate format for people with learning disabilities. There is evidence that they prefer to learn via websites and DVDs (Marriott & Tarleton 2009).

It can be very powerful when people with learning disabilities present their own research at conferences. The Burton Street Group said this was "a chance to be there and get your message across"

(Abell et al 2007:123) and highlighted it as one of the most positive aspects of the research process. Williams et al (2005) also identified this as being empowering for people with learning disabilities:

> I think my power started up when talking in conferences and to people, and that's what has given me more confidence and strength.
>
> (Gramlich in Williams et al 2005:11)

It can be difficult to stand up alone and present at conferences; one method of providing support to a person with learning disabilities without dominating is the 'interview technique'. The supporter can ask pre-arranged questions which act as prompts for the person with learning disabilities. It can help them keep to time and yet, as they are responding, they are still in control of the presentation. Chapman & McNulty (2004) described how this method worked well in helping a member of the team to build up confidence. Subsequently he was able to move onto using symbols and pictures to represent the questions and ultimately was able to present at a large international conference independently.

The academic requirement is that research should be published in peer-reviewed journals, as this is both a test of quality and also will enable it to permeate the academic world and be available on an ongoing basis to other researchers. The Carlisle Group described the process of writing an academic article collaboratively (Chapman & McNulty 2004). The group would not have been able to undertake this task without support, as the invitation to submit to the journal was not in an accessible format and they only had limited access to a computer. Therefore the supporter typed up the article but every word was agreed upon by the group. They decided they wanted to include pictures; their preference was for digital photos but time limitations prevented this and so they pictorialised their article using a mixture of photos, clip art and CHANGE picture bank images. At times they found it difficult to reach a consensus on the wording; they wanted to keep the article free from jargon and yet it needed to be academic enough to be suitable for the journal.

The impact made by inclusive research, like that of all social research, is hard to measure. However, on the whole it seems more likely that inclusive research will turn towards practical types of impact, and generate outputs that can have a direct influence on others in the field. Many of the research projects at Norah Fry Research Centre do produce some practical outputs, as well as the academic articles and conference dissemination necessary in the academic world. For instance, a training pack based on the research can have a direct effect on practice (Mallett et al 2003 (Bridging the Divide pack), Ponting et al 2010 (Skills for Support), Townsley et al 1997 (Training Staff handbook)). People with learning disabilities have also taken part in training based on sexuality research in Australia, as outlined in Box 10.7. Training based on research can also make a very tangible difference (Jefferson et al 2005, Williams & Heslop 2006), and those who are involved in producing such dissemination materials may not necessarily be the people actually participating in the original research, as is also outlined in Box 10.7 (Heslop & Macaulay 2009).

Box 10.7

Disseminating inclusive research

Hidden Pain? was a 3-year research project that explored the views of people with learning disabilities about their self-injury and the study provided considerable insights into their individual experiences (Heslop & Macaulay 2009). This work generated a set of resources to be used by people with learning disabilities who self-injure, as well as their family members and the professionals who are working with them. One of the resources was a DVD which was made in conjunction with a local theatre group of people with learning disabilities. The actors tell stories based on the experiences of the people who took part in the project. This format means that it is accessible to people with learning disabilities themselves but also it has had a powerful impact when clips have been shown at conferences (Davies & Evans 2010).

Living Safer Sexual Lives was an Australian research project, in which adults with intellectual disabilities (learning disabilities) told their own stories about their experiences, in a life story approach. There was also a reference group for the project, which took on a more and more important role as the research continued. One way in which they became central was at the dissemination stage, when they were involved in listening to the stories and editing them. Two members of the reference group were employed to read the stories on video, and these were subsequently used in sexuality workshops for service providers, along with plain English booklets which the reference group had helped to edit.

Kelley Johnson, who led this project, describes and critiques the processes of involvement in Walmsley & Johnson (2003:109–125).

Conclusion

We hope that this chapter has served to encourage people to think about an inclusive approach to research. As we have described, there are various levels at which this can happen. We want people to remember that just because they may not be able to reach the 'gold standard' of emancipatory research, it does not mean that their research will not be strengthened by the inclusion of people with learning disabilities in whatever ways are possible. Inclusive research can draw on existing research methodologies, such as life stories or action research. It can also lead to new, creative methodologies. Inclusive research is an interesting process that sits on the edge of research, self-advocacy and community development – which is what makes it so exciting. Those who wish to involve people with learning disabilities in research will learn much for themselves, and will find that they can also contribute to this growing field.

For the future, it is important that everyone continues to ensure that people with learning disabilities are central to matters that concern them. This may well be done together with people with other impairments, as people with learning disabilities increasingly identify their issues with those of the disabled people's movement more generally. In that case, however, it will be vital that the issues about accessibility, communication and support of inclusive research are not overlooked. If it is simply assumed that people with learning disabilities can participate in generic disability forums, then their needs and voices can easily be ignored, and so specific efforts will need to be made in order to ensure that people with learning disabilities can exert their own power. The answers to these issues lie within good self-advocacy practice, and so a conversation between disabled people's organisations and self-advocacy groups can be very productive.

Finally, as Barton (2005) points out, there is a continuing need to ensure that the needs and voices of *all* people with learning disabilities are included in research. People with higher support needs may not have the cognitive or communication skills to take part in any kind of 'conventional' research process in their own right. However, this chapter has indicated some of the more creative ways in which they can be involved. This will include the person-centred practices of listening to and involving those who are closest to the individual, but it is going to be important that this is done in such a way that people with learning disabilities really are at the centre of their own lives, and of their own research.

References

Abell, S., Ashmore, J., Beart, S., et al., 2007. Including everyone in research: the Burton Street Research Group. British Journal of Learning Disabilities 35 (2), 121–124.

Andrews, V., 2009. Exploring what is important to people with Down syndrome living in a residential service in Ireland: a preliminary participatory research study. MSc Thesis, Trinity College, Dublin.

Barton, L., 2005. Emancipatory research and disabled people: some observations and questions. Educational Review 57 (3), 317–327.

Beresford, P., 2001. Service users, social policy and the future of welfare. Critical Social Policy 21 (4), 494–512.

Bjornsdottir, K., Traustadottir, R., 2010. Stuck in the land of disability? The intersection of learning difficulties, class, gender and religion. Disability and Society 25 (1), 49–62.

Bryman, A., 2008. Social research methods. Oxford University Press, Oxford.

Campbell, J., Oliver, M., 1996. Disability politics: understanding our past, changing our future. Routledge, London.

Chapman, R., McNulty, N., 2004. Building bridges? The role of research support in self-advocacy. British Journal of Learning Disabilities 32, 77–85.

Chappell, A., 2000. Emergence of participatory methodology in learning difficulty research: understanding the context. British Journal of Learning Disabilities 28, 38–43.

Davies, R., Evans, D., 2010. Public involvement in research: how can organisations collaborate to improve involvement? Report of the University of the West of England. Available at: http://hls.uwe.ac.uk/suci/Default.aspx?pageid=9.

Department of Health, 2001. Valuing people: a new strategy for learning disability in the 21st century: a White Paper. Department of Health, London.

Department of Health, 2006a. Our health, our care, our say. Department of Health, London.

Department of Health, 2006b. Let me in, I'm a researcher. Department of Health, London.

Department of Health, 2009. Valuing people now: from progress to transformation. Department of Health, London.

Goodley, D., 2000. Self-advocacy in the lives of people with learning difficulties. Buckingham Open University Press, Buckingham.

Goodley, D., 2001. Learning difficulties', the social model of disability and impairment: challenging epistemologies. Disability and Society 16 (2), 207–231.

Goodwin, J., Williams, V., 2004. Our lives, our research: CD ROM produced as part of Plain Facts. Norah Fry Research Centre, University of Bristol.

Gramlich, S., McBride, G., Snelham, N., et al., 2002. Journey to independence: what self advocates tell us about direct payments. British Institute for Learning Disabilities, Kidderminster.

Heslop, P., Macaulay, F., 2009. Hidden pain? Self-injury and people with learning disabilities. Final report. Bristol Crisis Service for Women, Bristol.

Heslop, P., Folkes, L., Rodgers, J., 2005. The knowledge people with learning disabilities and their carers have about psychotropic medication. Learning Disability Review 10, 10–18.

Jefferson, E., Irish, M., Jones, C., et al., 2005. We are the strongest link: a pack to help people with learning disabilities support each other. Available at: http://www.learningdisabilities.org.uk (follow links to publications).

Johnson, K., 2009. No longer researching about us without us: a researcher's reflections on rights and inclusive research in Ireland. British Journal of Learning Disabilities 37, 250–256.

Mallett, R., Power, M., Helsop, P., 2003. All change: transition into adult life – a resource for young people with learning difficulties, family carers and professionals. Pavilion, Brighton.

Marriott, A., Tarleton, B., 2009. Finding the right help. NSPCC, London.

Minogue, G., Rynne, J., Johnson, K., et al., 2007. The garden story. The University of Dublin, Dublin.

Oliver, M., 1990. The politics of disablement. Macmillan, Basingstoke.

Oliver, M., 1992. Changing the social relations of research production? Disability and Society 7 (2), 101–114.

Palmer, N., Turner, F., 1998. Self advocacy: doing our own research. Royal College of Speech and Language Therapy Bulletin August, 12–13.

Palmer, N., Peacock, C., Turner, F., et al., 1999. Telling people what we think. In: Swain, J., French, S. (Eds.), Therapy and learning difficulties. Butterworth Heinemann, Oxford, pp. 33–46.

Ponting, L., Ford, K., 2007. (in conversation). Transcript available from val.williams@bristol.ac.uk.

Ponting, L., Ford, K., Williams, V., et al., 2010. Training personal assistants. Pavilion, Brighton.

Rapley, M., 2004. The social construction of intellectual disability. Cambridge University Press, Cambridge.

Richardson, M., 2002. Involving people in the analysis: listening, reflecting, discounting nothing. J. Learn. Disabil. 6 (1), 47–60.

Rodgers, J., Namaganda, S., 2005. Making information easier for people with learning disabilities. British Journal of Learning Disabilities 33, 52–58.

Rodgers, J., Townsley, R., Tarleton, B., et al., 2004. Information for all: guidance. Available at: http://www.easyinfo.org.uk (accessed 21.04.10.).

Sheehy, K., Nind, M., 2005. Emotional well-being for all: mental health and people with profound and multiple learning disabilities. British Journal of Learning Disabilities 33, 34–38.

Sutcliffe, J., Simons, K., 1994. Self advocacy and adults with learning difficulties. National Institute of Adult Continuing Education, Leicester.

Tarleton, B., Williams, V., Palmer, N., et al., 2004. An equal relationship? People with learning difficulties getting involved in research. In: Smyth, M., Williamson, E. (Eds.), Researchers and their 'subjects': ethics, power, knowledge and consent. Policy Press, Bristol, pp. 73–90.

Townsley, R., Gyde, G., 1997. Plain facts. Information about research for people with learning difficulties. Norah Fry Research Centre, Bristol.

Townsley, R., Howarth, J., LeGrys, P., et al., 1997. Getting involved in choosing staff. Pavilion, Brighton.

Townson, L., Macaulay, S., Harkness, E., et al., 2004. We are all in the same boat: 'doing people-led research'. British Journal of Learning Disabilities 32, 72–76.

Walmsley, J., 2001. Normalisation, emancipatory research and inclusive research in learning disability. Disability and Society 16 (2), 187–205.

Walmsley, J., Johnson, K., 2003. Inclusive research with people with learning disabilities: past, present and futures. Jessica Kingsley, London.

Walter, I., Nutley, S., Percy-Smith, J., et al., 2004. Improving the use of research in social care practice. In: Knowledge Review, vol. 7. Social Care Institute for Excellence, London, Available at: http://www.scie.org.uk/publications/knowledgereviews/kr07.pdf.

Ward, L., Simons, K., 1998. Practising partnership: involving people with learning difficulties in research. British Journal of Learning Disabilities 26, 128–131.

Williams, V., 1999. Researching together. British Journal of Learning Disabilities 27, 48–51.

Williams, V., 2005. Disability and discourse: analysing inclusive conversations with people with intellectual disabilities. Wiley-Blackwell, Oxford.

Williams, V., Heslop, P., 2006. Filling the emotional gap at transition: young people with learning difficulties and friendship. Tizard Learning Disability Review 11 (4), 28–37.

Williams, V., Simons, K., Swindon People First Research Team, 2005. More researching together. British Journal of Learning Disabilities 32, 1–9.

Williams, V., Marriott, A., Townsley, R., 2008. Shaping our future: a scoping and consultation exercise to establish research priorities in learning disabilities for the next ten years. Report for the National Co-ordinating Centre for NIHR Service Delivery and Organisation. Available at: http://www.sdo.nihr.ac.uk/files/adhoc/152-research-summary.pdf.

Williams, V., Ponting, L., Ford, K., et al., 2009a. Skills for Support: personal assistants and people with learning disabilities. British Journal of Learning Disabilities 38, 59–67.

Williams, V., Ponting, L., Ford, K., et al., 2009b. I do like the subtle touch: interactions between people with learning disabilities and their personal assistants. Disability and Society 24 (7), 815–828.

Zarb, G., 1992. On the road to Damascus: first steps towards changing the relations of research production. Disability, Handicap and Society 7 (2), 125–138.

Further reading

Barnes, C., Mercer, G., 1997. Doing disability research. The Disability Press, Leeds.

Clough, P., Barton, L. (Eds.), 1998. Articulating with difficulty: research voices in inclusive education. Paul Chapman, London.

Faulkner, A., 2004. An exploration of guidelines for ethical conduct of research carried out by mental health service users and survivors. Policy Press, Bristol.

Lowes, L., Hulatt, I., 2005. Involving service users in health and social care research. Routledge, London.

Smyth, M., Williamson, E. (Eds.), 2004. Researchers and their 'subjects': ethics, power, knowledge and consent. Policy Press, Bristol.

Walmsley, J., Johnson, K., 2003. Inclusive research with people with learning disabilities: past, present and futures. Jessica Kingsley, London.

Useful addresses

Research based in self-advocacy organisations

Follow the links to People First organisations in the UK, for example.

Central England People First, http://www.peoplefirst.org.uk/.

Dorset People First, http://www.dorsetpeoplefirst.co.uk/.

Cumbria People First, http://www.peoplefirstcumbria.co.uk/.

Practical support and networking about service user involvement in research

'Involve' organisation, http://www.invo.org.uk/.

Folk.us, http://www.folkus.org.uk/.

Norah Fry Research Centre

General information, http://www.bristol.ac.uk/norahfry.

Inclusive Theory and Practice (MSc), http://www.bristol.ac.uk/norahfry/teaching-learning/masters.

Producing easy-read information

Easyinfo: http://www.easyinfo.org.uk.

CHANGE, http://www.changepeople.co.uk/uploaded/ CHANGE_How_to_Make_Info_Accessible_guide.pdf.

Inspired Services: http://www.inspiredservices.org.uk/.

Positive risk taking

11

Andy Alaszewski Helen Alaszewski

CHAPTER CONTENTS

Key issues

- Risk assessment and management continue to be major preoccupations in the 21st century. However there are tensions between ensuring individual and collective safety and facilitating positive risk taking especially in an increasingly blame-oriented environment
- People with learning disabilities, their relatives, carers and professionals often define risk in different ways. Risk is often associated with dangerousness and harm and therefore to be avoided. However there is also awareness that risk is part of everyday life and that successful risk taking has positive benefits
- It is important that people with learning disabilities are given the opportunity to take risks; risk taking is part of normal everyday life, can be seen as a human right and provides opportunities for personal learning and development
- Agencies which provide support for people with learning disabilities and their families need to have policies and structures that enable individuals to take positive risks. Such policies and structures should have a clear and balanced definition of risk, that emphasises the importance

of empowerment of people with learning disabilities, procedures intended to facilitate decision making that enable positive risk taking and methods for following through on decisions
- An important way of facilitating risk taking is through relationships where another person, a relative, friend or professional, acts with and for a person. Such relationships can be effective when the agent understands the interests and preferences of the person on whose behalf they are acting and has the skills and capacity to make decisions that support these interests and choices
- Positive risk taking requires trust and effective communication between all the key stakeholders

Introduction

In this chapter we explore the importance of positive risk taking for people with learning disabilities and the challenges of ensuring they have the resources and support that enables them to take reasonable risks. It examines the increasing importance of risk in contemporary society, the benefits of successful risk taking and some of the difficulties of risk taking and the ways in which they can be overcome.

The nature of positive risk taking

Risk assessment and management have become a major preoccupation and an important ideology in the 21st century. As with many ideologies (see Alaszewski & Brown 2011), risk is intrinsically complex and used in different ways for different purposes. On the one hand politicians claim the aim of government is to create a safer, less risky society providing all citizens with cradle to grave protection from harm, yet on the other hand there is criticism of individuals who are unwilling to take risks, for example parents who overprotect their children (Furedi 2002). This means that practitioners who are supporting people with learning disabilities are simultaneously expected to ensure they are safe, and if they do not are blamed, but at the same time provide them with opportunities to take risks.

Defining risk

Society's ambiguity towards risk is evident in the way it is discussed and defined. In the late 1990s, the authors of this chapter participated in a number of studies that explored the ways in which health and social care agencies support vulnerable people and manage risk (see Alaszewski et al 1998, 1999, 2000). As part of these projects, we interviewed service providers, people with learning disabilities and their relatives. While practitioners acknowledged risk was an important part of practice, they often found it difficult to define risk. Some practitioners described risk in terms of dangers, often citing specific incidents when things had gone wrong. For example, a student on a learning disability branch of a nursing degree course provided the following negative image:

> Somewhere I used to work – I took a client to a supermarket and he completely smashed the place up and there were children hanging around. It could have been a risk.

However, other practitioners viewed risk very differently. One qualified learning disability nurse stressed risk could be considered as an opportunity and that it depended on the perceptions of both the practitioner and the person with learning disabilities:

> In the learning disabilities field we talk a lot about risk because . . . clients have not taken risks or not been allowed to take risks . . . And it can be anything from something very small like putting the kettle on, which was often regarded as high risk for several people . . . it's entirely down to the individual as to what you would class a risk as being; something that's a risk to you or I may not be a risk to someone else . . . [It] depends on your own abilities, your own perceptions and also the person with learning disabilities – their perceptions of what a risk would be.

A number of practitioners did try to reconcile these two contrasting approaches to risk, arguing that risk involved balancing the danger of things going wrong against the benefits of risk taking. A learning disability lecturer discussed risk in the following way:

> Well, risk is a very important area in learning disability and anybody working in that area needs to be concerned with it. It is enabling the people you work with to do something, but taking into account the risk that may be involved . . . for example, you might have somebody who is suffering from epilepsy and you may want them to take part in a certain activity – you need to make a judgement about what the risk to that person is and that's got to be balanced with the experience that they get by taking part, so it's taking account of the risk involved without devaluing the person by not letting them take part.

We also asked people with a learning disability and their relatives to discuss risk. While some relatives claimed they were not particularly worried about risk as it was part of everyday life: "Well I think living life is a risk, so it doesn't really enter my mind"; for most, risk was seen in terms of a threat or hazard. They related risk to their everyday life and to challenges of providing care for a vulnerable person and in particular to the danger that existed outside the relatively protected environment of the home. One mother discussed the risk her daughter was exposed to outside the home:

> Well my daughter is at risk if she tries to walk and people expect her to walk because she looks quite normal; but if they expect her to walk then she's likely to fall, so she's at risk whenever she's out of my sight really.

Indeed, some parents noted that their strategies to protect their children might actually create new risks:

> She's at risk all the time so I've taken the key out of the door. This could be a real problem if we need to get her out quickly.

The people with learning disabilities also tended to see risk as a threat. For example, two service users stressed the dangers of living in the community:

> Anthony: I used to live in an old house and there was a risk of fire because of electrical faults.
>
> Brenda: When it gets dark ... there is the risk of being abused. If you go out at night – people on skate boards – you get abused if you don't get out of the way.

Some service users felt that risk had been used to deprive them of opportunities:

> Jean: If I say something they take no notice. At college I wanted to put my name down for a Christmas dinner and they made it so I couldn't. They shouldn't have done that. That's the risk of college – being ignored ...
>
> Simon: Our group organised a disco. Most people live in the city – it was in the city – but people wouldn't go because it was in the city on a Friday night and they said it wouldn't be safe.
>
> Tom: And my holiday. I was going to Spain but the staff said they were having difficulties getting some people able to go. The travel firm was seeing people in wheelchairs as a risk.
>
> Jean: We're not taken seriously.

However those participants who had successfully taken risks felt it was a positive experience:

> I went to [major seaside landmark] – there was a sand dune – it was hard to get up – we went up. We took pictures. It was risky but worth it. Someone was with us.

These individuals were aware of the risks of everyday life and the ways in which they impacted on them. However, they were also keen to stress that they were responsible and capable of learning about and managing risks. Indeed, one participant stressed the way in which she helped a less able colleague deal with hazards:

> I go with Joseph to [a large supermarket] because he doesn't understand roads and can't understand money. He throws his money away. If he had a £10 note he would just give it away.

Risk: managing uncertainty and allocating blame

The ambiguities about risk that are evident in these accounts are intrinsic to the concept of risk which can be used in different and contradictory ways. It can be used to describe the ways in which we seek to manage and control an uncertain future. In this sense, it refers to the choices individuals and groups make both about their desired future and the best way of achieving that. Rational risk taking involves a structured approach to uncertainty, that is using knowledge from past experience to consider what might happen in the future and possible consequences of different outcomes (Zinn 2008). Risk involves imagining the future and identifying those aspects that individuals would like to change (Heyman et al 2010). For example, screening programmes focus on particular health hazards such as breast cancer and the actions that can be taken to minimise the harm from this hazard. Dowie (1999) provided a conceptual framework for such risk taking that involves identifying the possible outcomes of courses of action, an assessment of the probability or likelihood of such outcomes and an evaluation of the desirability or value of different outcomes. For example, if a young person is offered drugs at a party and then refuses the offer, they can be certain that they will neither get high nor be harmed. However, if they accept the drugs, they are likely to get high. They may experience no side effects but they may experience serious side effects and be permanently disabled or even die. Dowie argued that the actual decision which an individual makes depends on their preferences, for example being safe versus getting high, and their knowledge of the likely outcomes. For example, the case of Leah Betts who died after taking Ecstasy paradoxically resulted in an increase in the consumption of Ecstasy:

> The detailed publicity and information which came out about Ecstasy as a result of her death communicated to a wider public two separate things ... First, that the probability of dying was very low, if various precautions were taken ... Second, that the outcome in terms of the enjoyment and activity made possible from consumption were high ...
>
> (Dowie 1999:50)

However, there is also a forensic use of risk. Douglas (1990) has argued the concept of risk is increasingly used in the same way as sin was in religious societies – to identify (moral) failing and to allocate blame. This underpins the development of a 'blame culture', in which all harmful events are seen as a product of human agency, every misfortune is someone's fault and "under the banner of risk reduction, a new blaming system" has developed (Douglas 1992:16). Thus when a major misfortune occurs, for example a vulnerable person is killed, this private misfortune then becomes a public disaster and the mass media, especially the tabloid press, identifies the agencies which failed to identify and prevent the risk. They then call for the punishment of the 'guilty' party. In such circumstances, an inquiry or investigation takes place which, in using the benefit of hindsight, identifies those who failed to effectively identify and manage the risk (Alaszewski & Brown 2011).

There have been a number of well publicised incidents where people with learning disabilities have suffered when risk taking has gone wrong. Some of these incidents relate to leisure activities. In 1998, four adults with learning disabilities died during a canal holiday. The Director of Social Services for Cumbria justified the risk taking in the following way:

> Canal holidays are a common activity at this centre and this group has been on holiday together before. Of the four who died, some had attended the day centre for the best part of 20 years. They had been active members of the local community, taking part in many ordinary community events and involved in education, health and employment schemes in Barrow.
>
> (Mike Siegel quoted in The Guardian 1998:10).

The spokesperson for the local authority responsible for the safety of the lock where the accident occurred said:

> It has got all the hallmarks of a tragic accident and there will be a full and thorough investigation.
>
> (Gillian Taylor quoted in BBC News 1998).

More recently the failures of risk taking in relation to people with learning disabilities have been associated with the hazards of living in the community. In 2006 and 2007, three men with learning disabilities were murdered in separate disability hate crimes (VOICE UK, Respond and the Ann Craft Trust 2007). The case of Steven Hoskin exemplifies the high price of failed risk taking. He was in his late 30s when rehoused in a bed-sit in the Cornish market town of St Austell and was excited about having a home of his own, a dog and having new friends. Despite visits from care workers, these new friends abused him for over a year before forcing him to jump to his death from a 70 foot viaduct (Morris 2007).

There is naturally a desire to learn from such incidents and to take action to prevent people with learning disabilities from suffering. Most agencies providing support for people with learning disabilities have an adult abuse policy. Poole Social Services (undated) adult abuse policy states that: "Together we can safeguard and protect vulnerable adults, and prevent and stop abuse from happening". However, Carson & Bain (2008:38) have argued that:

> Risk-taking involves potential harms as well as benefits and uncertainty. There should be a constant drive to reduce the degrees of uncertainty involved in risk-taking and to increase the potential for successful risk management. That can be achieved by using risk-taking as an opportunity to learn and develop more information to assist in the future. Risk-taking should be associated primarily with learning, not with blame or liability.

Of course, in a perfect world, risk takers would be protected from blame and liability. The reality is that official bodies responsible for regulating services see

Reader activity 11.1

Over a period of 7 days, read one quality and one tabloid newspaper. Identify any articles that refer to either risk to, or the care and support of, vulnerable adults and children. Consider and reflect on the ways in which risk is used in these articles and particularly if it is used synonymously with danger or is used in a more balanced way.

You can use printed version of newspapers. These are usually available in public or college libraries, or most newspapers have websites such as:

- http://www.guardian.co.uk/
- http://www.mirror.co.uk/
- http://www.thesun.co.uk/sol/homepage/
- http://www.thetimes.co.uk/tto/news/

risk in terms of safety. The Nursing and Midwifery Council (NMC) defines its role in terms of safety: "We exist to safeguard the health and wellbeing of the public" (NMC undated) and, in its code of practice, makes it clear that nurses are responsible for minimising risk, for example "You must act without delay if you believe that you, a colleague or anyone else may be putting someone at risk" (NMC 2010). Similarly the Care Quality Commission (CQC 2010), the agency responsible for monitoring the quality of health and social care, has a 'Managing Risk' section on its website. This section makes no reference to positive risk taking but does include a discussion of safeguarding which it defines in the following way:

> Safeguarding means enabling people to live their lives free from harm, abuse and neglect, and to have their health, wellbeing and human rights protected.
>
> (CQC 2010)

Despite the apparent risk aversion of various regulatory agencies, Carson (undated) argues that "acting professionally requires risk-taking where, by definition, harm can – and sometimes will – occur however well the decisions were taken". Therefore the issue is not whether to take risks, but rather to balance the potential benefits of exciting and challenging activities against the harm and threat of blame if things go wrong. Positive risk taking involves managing uncertainty – identifying a desired future and choosing the best way of creating this future while acknowledging and taking action to prevent undesired and harmful outcomes.

The importance of positive risk taking

There are two major reasons for ensuring that people with learning disability have the opportunity to take risks; one relates to the human rights of people with a learning disability and the other to the practical benefits that come from successful risk taking.

Human rights and risk taking

The human rights approach was initially grounded in a critique of the traditional institutions that deprived individuals of their human right to participate in everyday life and experience and manage its risks. The report of the Inquiry into Normansfield Hospital (National Health Service (NHS) 1978) spelt out the limitations of the culture of protection and control that stemmed from the in-charge consultant's concern about being held responsible for any untoward incident. This 'safety first' culture provoked a strike in the hospital during which 200 patients with learning disabilities were exposed to serious danger. In the USA, the human rights movement underpinned the development of the normalisation philosophy that stressed the importance of risk taking:

> Many who work with the handicapped, impaired, disadvantaged, and aged tend to be overzealous in their attempts to 'protect', 'comfort', 'keep safe', 'take care', and 'watch' . . . they will overprotect and emotionally smother the intended beneficiary. In fact, such overprotection endangers the client's human dignity, and tends to keep him from experiencing the risk-taking of ordinary life which is necessary for human growth and development.
>
> (Perske 1972:195).

In the UK, the Jay Committee (1979) was heavily influenced by the normalisation philosophy which in the UK was being promoted by the Campaign for Mentally Handicapped People and by voluntary organisations such as Barnardo's (see Alaszewski & Ong 1980). The Jay Committee stressed the centrality of reasonable risk taking:

> The question of risk, which at this stage [childhood] involves such things as climbing and running, and later in life hazards of other kinds, is one of extreme delicacy for those who care. Staff are likely to receive harsh criticism when accidents or injury occurs, yet if we entirely cushion people against these dangers we immediately restrict their lives and their chances of development. This restriction can be cloaked in respectability and defended on the grounds of protecting mentally handicapped people and keeping them safe, but it can also endanger human dignity. Each of us lives in a world which is not always safe, secure and predictable; mentally handicapped people too need to assume a fair and prudent share of risk.
>
> (Jay Committee 1979: para. 121)

As services shifted from health-oriented institutional services to educational and social care community support so the importance of reasonable risk taking was endorsed by the relevant regulatory agencies. The Social Services Inspectorate accepted that people with learning disabilities had the right to normal life experiences but that agencies should use effective methods of assessing risk to ensure that these rights were exercised safely. An Inspectorate report stressed that agencies supporting adults with learning disabilities should address "issues of autonomy and of risk in policy and practice for seeking life-styles and activities for users to bring them into the mainstream of society" (Fruin 1998: para 6.5). The report included examples of such everyday activities as "getting the bus, not a taxi, to the day centre, working in potentially hazardous environments, having a boyfriend or girlfriend, [or] raising children".

The *Valuing People* strategy for developing services in England did not explicitly discuss positive risk taking but did emphasise that people with learning disabilities should be able "to lead full and purposeful lives in their communities" (Department of Health 2001:7). The strategy implicitly addressed positive risk taking in terms of choice:

> **Choice:** Like other people, people with learning disabilities want a real say in where they live, what work they should do and who looks after them. But for too many people with learning disabilities, these are currently unattainable goals. We believe that everyone should be able to make choices. This includes people with severe and profound disabilities who, with the right help and support, can make important choices and express preferences about their day to day lives.
>
> (Department of Health 2001:24)

The practical benefits of successful risk taking

As Carson & Bain (2008) have noted, risk taking is a part of everyday life. Both mundane activities such as crossing a road or cooking a meal or more fateful decisions such as seeking medical care or developing an intimate relationship can have unpredicted and harmful outcomes. In theory, this should generate a continual sense of fear and anxiety but in reality, most adults disregard or bracket out the possibility that things may go wrong. They have successfully learnt to accomplish activities such as crossing the road or cooking a meal and are confident in their ability to successfully safely perform them. Indeed, they do it as a matter of habit relying on risk management strategies that do not require the time and intellectual energy of rational decision making but are more effective than passively relying on faith or hope. Such in-between strategies (Zinn 2008) include intuition, trust or emotion and underpin routine and habitual decision making such as deciding what and where to eat. Therefore the nature, importance and benefit of risk taking are often most clear in relatively atypical situations.

See Reader activity 11.2 on the Evolve website.

Taking high risks

In contemporary societies, some individuals voluntarily undertake high-risk activities. In some cases, these activities are part of occupations such as motor or horse racing, but more often it is a leisure activity such as mountain climbing or parachute jumping. It is difficult to understand why individuals should expose themselves to serious injury and death. However those that take part see it as a personal challenge. While they are doing it, they often experience fear as well as the thrill of danger. When they have successfully achieved this, they feel a sense of achievement and self-worth. Thus Damon Hill, a Grand Prix motor racing driver, when asked to comment on the death of his team mate Aryton Senna in a racing accident, said:

> I think every driver thought of that . . . It's not something I really want to dwell on, but it made every driver consider whether they really wanted to do this. But you think to yourself, well, that's what I planned to do with my life, and it's what I love doing . . . I love to do something exciting. If there's no risk, there's no life.
>
> (Williams 1994:3)

Parker & Stanworth (2005) noted that in taking high risks such as charity parachute jumping, the 'going for it' creates self-worth that can play an important part in the development of personal identity and social standing within a group. They noted that those who participate in charity parachute jumping take a 'cultivated risk'; they demonstrate a key facet of their personality, their courageousness, but do so responsibly for the collective good.

> By taking the risks [stet] of death (and injury) and of being able to go through with the jump, they had *made themselves* courageous, and in a context where there are very clear criteria of success . . . Moreover, crucially, this courage was exercised in a good cause. The charity element of the jumping further contributed to the jumper's virtue. They were able to present themselves as not only showing courage but also putting themselves on the line for others, not just for themselves.
>
> (Parker & Stanworth 2005:329, italics in the original)

See Reader activity 11.3 on the Evolve website.

Adolescents and risk taking: learning and developing an identity

Adolescence tends to be a period of experimentation in which young people move from dependency in which others take decisions and risks on their behalf to one in which they are competent adults taking risks and being responsible for the outcome of such risk taking. The development of autonomous risk taking involves a transfer of responsibility and power, and while such transfer may take place smoothly with mutual agreement, more often there is tension especially over the dangerousness of activities such as meeting friends in town centres or consuming alcohol. Jenkins (2006), in a study which included interviews with 15 parents and young people (11–15-year-olds) who had been treated in accident and emergency department for injuries sustained outside the home, found that the relationships between parents and their children were complex. Parents were clearly anxious about their children's safety but also wanted to let them experiment and learn: "You can't wrap them in cotton wool". The young people wanted to demonstrate they were responsible and could safely take risks:

> In relation to injury prevention, while parents were concerned about the risk of injury this was often seen as being offset by the advantages participation in outdoor recreation brings ... In short, these are 'good' parents not because they 'abandon' their anxieties but because they find practical solutions to competing cultural viewpoints. While parents framed the need for their child to access the outside world in terms of their future social development, young people tended to present themselves as being socially competent already and, as such, capable of managing physical risk.
>
> (Jenkins 2006:391)

Thus the development of risk taking involved negotiation between parents and their children and, as in all negotiations, they were influenced by the power and resources of the parties. Jenkins draws attention to some of the strategies used by parents such as surveillance by stealth and the young persons' awareness of and ability to resist such strategies. The following extract is a mother and her daughter's retelling of the story of the young person's first unsupervised trip to the cinema:

> Mother: Oh yes, I dropped them off in town and went scatty because there was supposed to be four of them and only one of them was there by that time. So you sort of go round and round the block, unbeknown to them. Go round and round the block watching everybody else turn up until there were four of them, until there were five of them, now there's six of them, now I can leave.
>
> Young Person: Didn't you see me wave like, the ninth time you went round?
>
> Interviewer: Right, and did you know? You were saying about driving round to check how many people had arrived, did you know that at the time?
>
> Young Person: What that she went past like twenty times? Oh yeah. You see the white car and you thought, 'I know that car.' And it goes past again and your mum's looking at you like this through the window you know? Ah, I'll play with her now. So we pushed some of them round the corner to hide them. She just kept going round and round and round [laughs].

For young people, risk taking can be an important source of learning and a way of building social relations and a personal identity. Some adolescents will miscalculate, and get it wrong and accidentally harm themselves or others, but most will get it right and become competent adults. Parents of young people including those with learning disabilities are likely to feel anxious about such risk taking but often choose to manage their anxiety, recognising the benefits of risk taking.

These two examples, although atypical, highlight the core challenge of enabling people with learning disabilities to take risks. Mountain climbers and parachute jumpers are often seriously injured or die through their participation in a leisure activity. Although this may be considered tragic and a waste of a life, we take the collective view that they have the right to take the risk and do what they wanted to with their body and life. However, when Steven Hoskin died because he wanted to join and be part of an urban gang, there was collective shock and a sense that services had failed to protect a vulnerable man (VOICE UK, Respond and the Ann Craft Trust 2007). We noted above that for many young people adolescence is a period of experimentation, risk taking and rebellion. While parents may not approve of and be concerned that the risk taking is dangerous, their capacity to control such activities is often limited. Adolescents often have the resources to resist control, for example the legitimisation of dangerous activities by their peer group and access to 'concealed' spaces in which they can participate in such activities. Stanley (2005) described the ways in which adolescents who live in rural areas used local seaside towns to escape adult surveillance. In contrast, young people with learning disabilities are generally subject to higher levels of supervision and the resources they can draw on are more restricted. They can seek greater autonomy and control over risk taking and some more able individuals described their 'adolescent' rebelliousness:

> Why am I rebellious? I don't know, to tell you the truth. It was probably because at school I used to be a goodie, goodie, so I wanted to change my role a bit, and I knew damn well I would get a clipped ear from my Mum and Dad. But because Mum and Dad weren't around I knew I could do what I wanted.
>
> (Eve in Peterborough Voices 1997:7)

Although the capacity of most people with learning disabilities to take and learn from risks is more restricted, some parents have enabled their son or daughter to move into supported living. In our study of risk in community practice (Alaszewski et al 2000), we talked to parents of young adults with learning disability. One parent reflected on "when is it the right time to let your child go? It's scary because you don't want to hold them back". However, a small but vocal group of parents indicated that their children did not have the mental capacity to be engaged in risk taking and move beyond childhood:

> Sarah: And at the end of the day, as I always say they're just children in adults' bodies ... well they are, most of them ... four year olds in 20-plus bodies.
>
> Bill: They'll never grow up, I mean, he loves his mum and he loves Christmas, but it's as a child. Mark expects to see a big pile of toys on the chair when he comes down and he always picks the biggest out first to open and that sort of thing.

These parents recognised that their assessment of risk differed from that of service providers, but as one mother whose daughter attended a day centre put it:

> Professionals will encourage you to let them move on. But you've brought them up and you've cared for them ... You know their capabilities more than anybody else.

Impediments to positive risk taking and ways of overcoming them

It is possible to help people with a learning disability take reasonable risks but this requires overcoming organisational and individual barriers.

Overcoming organisational barriers to positive risk taking

In the mid-1990s, we conducted an Economic and Social Research Council project that examined the ways in which health and social care agencies were developing risk management policies (Alaszewski et al 1998). At the time, less than a half of the agencies we contacted had such policies and there was little evidence that the staff they employed were aware of or used the policies. This situation changed post-1997 with the development of policies such as clinical governance. All health and social care agencies were expected to put in place risk management policies to ensure the safety of those using their services and to maintain public confidence in these services (Alaszewski 2002, 2003a).

In 1999, we (Alaszewski et al 1999) published the findings of a study funded by the Mental Health Foundation on the development of risk policies by agencies supporting people with learning disabilities and their families. Most of the agencies did have clear and explicit policies for managing risk but there were separate risk-management and risk-taking policies. The risk-management policy usually formed part of the agency's health and safety management that often formed part of the central directorate or management team. The specified aim of such policies was to keep staff and those using the agency safe. However, agencies were also aware of reputational risk, that is if they failed to prevent accidents and injuries then their reputation could be damaged, and in the case this was linked to the development of an increasing hostile environment, that is a tabloid press looking for scandal and relatives willing to complain, use the media or sue the agency:

> I think the litigation mentality [is] growing everywhere. We're certainly becoming very, very mindful of the business that we're in and the associated problems with it and also the potential now for people suing you or your organisation.

In our study of agencies supporting adults with learning disabilities, all respondents accepted that ensuring safety was a prime objective for their agencies. Those working in the public sector saw this as part of national guidelines while those in the independent sector saw it as a requirement to win contracts, gain registration and pass inspections. One independent sector manager described the pressure to develop a risk management policy in the following way:

> We are in the independent sector and our contracts are with the statutory sector. So, yes, the people in the statutory sector ... are [commissioning services] from us ... increasingly do address issues of risk. Essentially, it seems to me, the way they are doing that is through obliging the providers they purchase from to have in situ policies that address risk and all sorts of related issues, i.e. abuse, harassment.

The risk management policies were framed in terms of health and safety. They were based on the assumption that risks or hazards could be objectively identified through a process of risk assessment and that such assessments informed a process of rational decision making that would minimise harm and maximise safety. One NHS trust supporting individuals with learning disabilities had a health and safety policy which included general guidance for identifying hazards plus a check-list of over 50 risk factors with the advice to staff that they should:

> Look out for the hazards you could reasonably accept to result in significant harm in your work place . . . Particular attention may need to be paid to specific hazards when undertaking an assessment of risk around individuals. Things that may not normally present a hazard like a particular work process or lifestyle could be a major source of risk.

One private sector manager indicated that the agency subcontracted risk management to another company that:

> does all of our risk assessments for health and safety, and brings in our guidelines and policies, and advises the staff and the manager directly, and provides training as well.

While risk management and safety policies tended to be organisation wide, there were also mechanisms for assessing risks for individual users, and these formed part of individuals' life or care plans. The broader framework of organisational policies on risk including specific policies on abuse, personal care, sexual relations or the management of complex needs informed these care plans. One manager in an NHS service described planning in the following way:

> I think it's down to the individual assessment and the services that we set up around individuals, yes, so very much a sort of personal development plan.

Alongside their risk management policies with emphasis on health and safety and risk assessment, some agencies had policies and practices encouraging user empowerment and positive risk taking. Such policies involved three interlinked elements:

1. *Aims and definitions* which emphasised the importance of empowerment of people with learning disabilities.
2. *Procedures* intended to facilitate decision making that enabled positive risk taking.
3. *Methods of following through on the decision.*

In each of these areas it is possible to identify key components of good practice. In Box 11.1 we give examples of good practice in specifying aims for positive risk taking and in providing working definitions of risk.

A risk-taking policy should address the key processes involved in assessing and managing risk, especially planning, decision making, recording and communicating decisions. The planning aspect should involve the ways in which hazards and opportunities should be identified and balanced and should start from the service user's wishes and needs (see Box 11.2 for an example of the ways in which a non-profit agency placed the user at the centre of the planning process).

Such a process helps identify the key information which then needs to be used in a decision-making process. Generally it is assumed that decision making is unproblematic as it is based on the 'facts' generated by risk assessment. However it is important to recognise and put in place mechanisms for dealing with disagreement about objectives and the hazards involved in achieving them. Good practice in managing tensions over risk is shown in Box 11.3.

In this bureaucratic approach to risk taking, it is important that all decisions and the reasons for them are recorded so that if things do not work out as anticipated there is a paper trail enabling any investigators to understand how and why the risk was taken and assuring them that those involved in the decision acted responsibly and rationally.

While the existence of positive risk-taking policies is important, their impact is limited in a number of ways and include the subordination of risk taking to the maintenance of safety, bureaucratic formalism and intrinsic paternalism. For care staff, this means that facilitating is a complex balancing act which Robertson & Collinson (in press) describe in the following way:

> Many staff are keenly aware of the various pressures on them to achieve the best overall outcomes. Not only do they seek satisfied and safe service users, but also the avoidance of harm to anyone else. Service integrity has to be maintained, but staff also have to protect their own integrity in terms of their personal safety and confidence. In endeavouring to promote autonomy and improving lives for service users staff seek to get the balance of control over risk taking right. In so doing, they wrestle with a different form of self-control that is concerned with managing anxiety that they are dealing with the least known about, least organisationally supported, yet most significant aspects of the service user's life. The choice is whether to take calculated positive risks for the best outcome or to retreat into conservative interventions with the potential for collateral damage that they bring.

Box 11.1

Good practice: aims and definitions

Key issue

The agency policies should acknowledge the benefits of risk taking and provide a link to and balance between issues of safety and those of empowerment. The risk-taking policy should have an explicit definition of risk that recognises the benefits of risk taking. While the potential dangers of risk taking are recognised, these should be set alongside the benefits.

Aims example 1

(NHS trust) "The trust recognises that users of services for learning disabilities, as part of their right to ordinary living opportunities, will be exposed to hazards of daily life. The Directorate acknowledges that if service users are to continue their process of acquiring skills for independence and integration into the local community, they must be allowed to take calculated risks".

Aims example 2

(For-profit agency) "It is our belief that people with a learning disability are entitled to participate in activities and exploit opportunities available to anyone else. We also recognise that our service users are vulnerable to harm and exploitation and need protection. We will strive to achieve an accountable balance between these apparently opposing positions . . . It is our intention to fulfil our duty of care to service users and staffing protecting them from harm, which arises from negligent action, but that is balanced by enabling service users to enjoy freedom, to participate in activities, which involve an element of planned and responsibly managed risk."

Risk definition example 1

(Not-for-profit agency) "A risk situation where benefits can be gained but harms are also possible".

Risk definition example 2

(Local authority Social Services Department) "Risk does not necessarily mean that people are placed in dangerous situations, but that something can go wrong. It may in some situations involve an element of danger".

Risk definition example 3

(NHS trust) "When considering risks, staff are asked to consider the probable outcomes of any activity and whether these outcomes will be beneficial or harmful. Staff will also need to consider the likelihood that these outcomes will occur . . . Risk can be said to occur when two or more outcomes of an activity are possible but not certain".

Box 11.2

Good practice: placing individual's wishes and needs at the centre of the planning process

Key issue

It is important that individuals do not get lost in the planning process. Therefore it is important that the individual's wishes are considered before possible risks are considered.

Example 1: Giving priority to an individual's needs and wishes

Before risks can be assessed, an individual's needs and objectives have to be identified. This can be done in a number of ways:

- Through goal planning.
- Observations from staff, family, friends and other agencies.
- Giving people information about resources and opportunities available to enable them to make informed choices.
- Different forums for people to express themselves, e.g. quality action groups, residents' meetings, community forums.
- Building on and developing individual skills.

Example 2: Developing risk assessment from individual preferences

Questions from preliminary risk assessment forms:

- What is this person's objective?
- What things have led to this objective being chosen?
- How will achieving this improve the person's life?

Subordination of risk taking to the maintenance of safety

While risk taking policies focus on the needs and rights of people with learning disabilities to take reasonable risk, the risk management policies also consider staff and others and there may be circumstances in which a positive risk taken by a person with a learning disability is a threat to a member of staff or some other person to whom the agency has a duty of care. In such circumstances, the risk management policy is likely to override the positive risk-taking policy.

Box 11.3

Good practice: managing tensions over risk

Key issue

Participants in planning and decision making may differ in their assessment of the potential benefits and possible hazards of activities which a person with a learning disability would like to undertake. In such circumstances it is important that a process exists for identifying, discussing and resolving these differences.

Example 1: Identifying disagreement

When an individual has identified something they wish to do which involves an element of risk, a full discussion should take place between that individual and a staff member. This discussion should look specifically at what the person wishes to do and what it is likely to entail. It is important to highlight the risks and consequences involved to the individual before continuing. During this meeting a preliminary risk assessment form should be completed with as much information as possible.

Example 2: Assessing the acceptability of risk

The meeting should aim to make a decision on the acceptability of risk that is summarised on a risk-assessment form in the following way:

- Can a decision be taken at this point as to whether this is an acceptable or unacceptable risk?
- If acceptable, please give the reasons why and also the ways in which the person will be enabled to take the risk.
- If unacceptable, please give the reasons why.

Example 3: Planning risk taking

If the risk is considered potentially acceptable then a further meeting may be needed for more detailed planning. This meeting should include the introduction of information contained in the preliminary risk assessment form including the objective, the risks and the other areas highlighted. If individuals are able and wish to do so, they should present this information themselves; if not, it should be presented by somebody of their choice. There should follow a general discussion of the information presented, adding any new points and considerations. The aim should be to reach a joint decision either to go ahead with the risk because it is acceptable or because it is not too great. If all those present are not able to agree then further discussion may need to take place or a majority decision be adhered to.

Bureaucratic formalism

The procedures described above are highly formal, often involving meetings of all interested parties during which negotiations take place at the end of which an agreement should be reached, recorded and communicated to all stakeholders. While such formal contracts may be necessary, they are likely to be intimidating and agreements are likely to be relatively general and perhaps can address important and fateful issues in a person's life but cannot deal with the details of everyday life.

Avoiding paternalism

It is clear that while people with learning disabilities may have an input into the process, the final decisions about which risks they take are often made for them. However as the *Valuing People* strategy noted:

> People with learning disabilities often feel excluded and unheard. They want to be fully part of our society, not marginalised or forgotten. They told us advocacy and direct payments were key to helping them gain greater independence and control.
>
> (DH 2001:11)

In the case of children and adults who experience serious problems with communication, it is inevitably difficult to find out how they like to experience life. For these individuals, it is important efforts are made to ascertain their preferences, especially the type of activities they appear to enjoy and the ways such activities can be facilitated. In the case of individuals with less severe disabilities who can, for example, use language to make their preferences clear, it is important that ways are found for engaging them in decision making and not creating complex time-consuming systems that they find alien and frustrating. In both cases, good communication and relationships can play an important part in facilitating reasonable risk taking.

Methods of facilitating spontaneity and informality in risk taking: advocacy, trust and communication

Bureaucratic systems provide one way of making decisions that are rational and grounded in a review of the key issues and protect the reputation of the agency if things go wrong. However, such decision making takes time and effort and is not suited to the quick day-to-day decision making that forms the basis of everyday life, for example what to eat or wear or when to go to sleep. Within institutions, such decision making was embedded within the routines of the institution, and no one had to think about it (Alaszewski 1986). Now that care and support are provided at home and in the community, these decisions have to be made and thought about each day. It is important that such decisions express individual preferences of people with learning disabilities and this can be facilitated through advocacy, trust and communication.

Developing effective advocacy

Contemporary society is based on the assumption that individuals have the knowledge and capacity to make everyday decisions for themselves. However, where individuals find it difficult to access or use appropriate information then this assumption is called into question. Collectively society can intervene to control some of the uncertainty through some form of regulation and the bureaucratic management of risk taking such as the example of regulation described above. However, as we noted, this process is cumbersome and inflexible. One way of overcoming such inflexibility is through the use of advocates, that is individuals who are willing to act for and on behalf of a person. Such relationships depend on the advocate being able to understand the interests and preferences of the person on whose behalf they are acting and having the skills to make decisions that support these interests and choices. If the advocate is effective then they can manage "the potentially high costs associated with the actual process of decision making and those associated with making the wrong decision (i.e. anxiety costs)" (McGuire et al 1988:186). Most people with learning disabilities have ready-made advocates – their relatives, especially parents – and this relationship often works well. For example, Christine, who attended a day centre, described the ways in which she made the day-to-day decisions and her mother's role in facilitating this by looking after her money for her:

> What makes me really happy is playing my music centre – playing my Abba tapes and the Eastenders record I've got. I like to lie on my bed to listen to my music. Sometimes I watch the telly. I bought it myself. I don't know how much money I've got. Mum does it for me.
>
> (Atkinson & Williams 1990:30).

However, in some circumstances there are difficulties. As we noted above in our discussion of adolescents, parents and their children do not always have the same interests and perceptions, but when they disagree, adolescents often have the resources to resist. In contrast, many people with learning disabilities find it difficult to resist well-meaning paternalism. Professionals and support workers often see parents as over-protective and motivated to keep their charges in a state of pseudo-childhood (Heyman & Huckle 1993:1562). Parents can put their own interests above those they should be acting for:

> The notion of parental 'overprotection' . . . incorporates a covert value judgement that parents ought to encourage people with learning difficulties to take more risks. The concept of 'letting go' . . . implies that parents avoid risk for adults with learning difficulties for selfish reasons, because they do not want to give up the parental role.
>
> (Heyman et al 1998:211)

If agreement cannot be reached over acceptable risk taking, then it may be necessary to identify an individual who is able and willing to act on their behalf and that person should not have a vested interest, that is should be independent of all the main stakeholders. Mencap provides such support, for example through their Children's Rights Officers and Advocates (CROAs), a membership organisation that provides a variety of advocacy services to support children and promote their rights (Mencap undated).

If independent advocates are to facilitate risk taking then they need the trust of all the key participants and the ability to communicate effectively.

Building trust and communicating effectively

Risk involves dealing with the uncertainties of everyday life. One important resource for managing such uncertainties is trust, which should form the basis of advocacy. A person with learning disability should be able to trust, that is have confidence, that their agent has the ability to act in and represent their interests (Alaszewski 2003b). However, where an independent advocate becomes involved, this often indicates that there is some tension between stakeholders, that is the person with learning disabilities, their parents or relatives and employed carers and professionals. The relationship between the person with learning disabilities and their parents or professional carers may have broken down and become one of distrust. Some agencies recognise the possibility of tension with relatives albeit not professional carers. One social service department included the following statement in their specification of who should be involved in decision making:

> There may be some occasions when the person who has a learning disability may express a wish not to involve close relatives in planning and making decisions about their lives. Where this is the case, consideration needs to be given to the importance of their relatives accepting and co-operating with the plans or decisions. Where exclusion from decision making process of relatives may lead to conflict, this needs to be explained and discussed with the person with a learning disability.
>
> (Alaszewski et al 1999:40)

There is scope for the relationship between parents and professional carers to break down, especially over risk taking. Parents are aware of, and concerned about, the vulnerability of the person with learning disabilities. Parents often have horror stories where their child had been exposed to unacceptable risks (Heyman & Huckle 1993:1560). In our own study (Alaszewski et al 2000), we were also told horror stories such as:

> We went to two or three places with Amy ... One of the places was the queerest place I've ever been in my life. We took Amy through the door and the first thing we got was two blokes fighting ... there was one of them on the floor and the other one was kicking the crap out of him ... I didn't want to leave her there ... The other place; well while Amy was there she lost three-quarters of her finger. We don't know how she lost it ... She lost about an inch and half of her finger and they said she must have bitten it off ... it's a great person that could have bitten off like that, never mind a handicapped person ... We think she lost it in a door or something like that.

However, the participants in our study were not opposed to risk taking per se. Indeed they recognised that day care and residential facilities could provide opportunities that they could not provide themselves:

> When my sister came here they wanted her to go sailing, now she can't even swim ... she doesn't like water. So I wouldn't have let her go, to be honest, but they were happy to do that.

They wanted to be able to trust that the individuals supporting their relative would take reasonable risks. One parent stressed the importance of trust in the following way:

> With most of children not able to speak, you have to have trust, because they couldn't really tell us if there was something wrong; anyway ... we have to believe that what we are told happens to them does happen.

This trust comes from effective communication both with the staff providing the support and also with the service user. Relatives recognised that sometimes things might not work out as planned but they wanted staff to be open and honest when things went wrong:

> I mean that they have a very good policy of communication with us so if there are any problems they do ring, they don't just sweep anything under the carpet ... you're not thinking, 'Oh, what's going on behind my back?' all the time or anything.

Communication with the person with learning disabilities is more limited but crucial. Relatives want evidence that things are well. We conclude with two extracts in which parents indicated how communication helped them build trust in a service:

> When John was being moved around, trying to find a residential spot for him, we tried three residential homes, and, although he can't talk, he can't tell us, he walked out of one and he just wouldn't entertain it and the social worker said, 'Well he's voted with his feet, hasn't he!'

Reader activity 11.4

1. Identify two or three people you trust and write down two or more reasons for your trust in them and at least one occasion in which your trust has been well placed.
2. Identify one or more person with learning disabilities who you know and consider whether they can trust you and why this should be.

This exercise requires reflection on your own circumstances and those of a person with learning disability that you know and to examine the nature of trust, which is a complex concept involving rational (previous knowledge and experience) and non-rational elements (it is essentially an act of faith). You can revisit some of the reading outlined in Reader activity 11.3, in particular Zinn's article in the special issue on 'Living with Risk and Uncertainty' (Zinn J O 2008 Heading into the unknown: everyday strategies for managing risk and uncertainty. Health, Risk and Society 10(5). Available at: http://www.informaworld.com/smpp/title~db=all~content=g904609569). A keyword search of the Health, Risk and Society website should identify a range of articles that explore trust issues in health and social care, such as Alaszewski A 2003 Risk, trust and health. Health, Risk and Society 5(3):235–239.

> Now when we came here, he didn't know this place from another and the first thing he did was settle himself down on the settee and looked as if he was at home. The atmosphere had obviously got to him.

> Eric is happy here, I think they must be doing the right things or he wouldn't be happy. I don't feel that I really need to know more than that and I know Eric doesn't. He doesn't care about policies, he doesn't understand that sort of thing . . . He just knows that his friends are here and he likes it, he has fun.

Conclusion

Risk has become a major preoccupation of the early 21st century. Governments aim to provide citizens with a safe, secure environment and protection from cradle to grave. However, there are also concerns that society is becoming more risk averse, for example with parents depriving their children of the opportunity to experience and learn from risk taking.

However risk is a complex, ambiguous concept. It can be used to describe the ways in which individuals seek to manage and control an uncertain future. In this sense it refers to the choices individuals and groups make both about their desired future and the best way of achieving this imagined future. However, risk is increasingly used in the same way as sin was in religious societies – to identify failings and to allocate blame in the context of disasters. This underpins the development of a 'blame culture', in which all harmful events are seen as a product of human agency and every misfortune is someone's fault. Such ambiguities are evident in the accounts which people with learning disabilities, their relatives and professional carers give of risk. They do acknowledge the potential benefits of risk and that risk-taking is part of everyday life but they are concerned that things can easily go wrong and people can be harmed if risk is not effectively assessed and managed.

Risk taking is a part of everyday life. Since people with learning disabilities should have the right to normal life experiences, they should also have the right to take positive risks. Agencies which support people with learning disabilities should use effective methods of assessing risk to ensure that such rights are exercised as safely as possible. Successful positive risk taking provides opportunities for learning and for developing a sense of self that can counteract stigmatisation. It can also enable individuals to establish themselves within social groups.

Agencies providing support for people with learning disabilities should have positive risk-taking policies. Such policies should include: a clear statement of values that acknowledges the benefits of risk taking and provides a link and balance between issues of safety and those of empowerment; an explicit definition of risk that recognises the benefits of risk taking; and should address the key processes involved in assessing and managing risk, especially planning, decision making, recording and communicating decisions.

Bureaucratic systems provide one way of making decisions that are rational and grounded in a review of the key issues and protect the reputation of the agency if things go wrong. However, such decision making takes time and effort and is not suited to the quick day-to-day decision making that forms the basis of everyday life. They need to be complemented by more informal mechanisms. Agency relations grounded in trust and good communication provide a way of articulating and meeting the needs of people with learning disabilities and enabling them to take positive risks.

References

Alaszewski, A., 1986. Institutional care and the mentally handicapped: the mental handicap hospital. Croom Helm, London.

Alaszewski, A., 2002. The impact of the Bristol Royal Infirmary disaster and inquiry on public services in the UK. J. Interprof. Care 16 (4), 371–378.

Alaszewski, A., 2003a. Risk, clinical governance and best value: restoring confidence in health and social care. In: Pickering, S., Thompson, J. (Eds.), Clinical governance and best value: meeting the modernisation agenda. Churchill Livingstone, Edinburgh, pp. 171–182.

Alaszewski, A., 2003b. Risk, trust and health. Health, Risk and Society 5 (3), 235–239.

Alaszewski, A., Brown, P., 2011. The challenges of making health policy: an introductory text. Polity Press, Cambridge.

Alaszewski, A., Ong, B.N., 1980. Normalisation in practice. Routledge, London.

Alaszewski, A., Harrison, L., Manthorpe, J., 1998. Risk, health and welfare: policies, strategies and practice. Open University Press, Buckingham.

Alaszewski, H., Parker, A., Alaszewski, A., 1999. Empowerment and protection: the development of policies and practices in risk assessment and risk management in services for adults with learning disabilities. The Mental Health Foundation, London.

Alaszewski, A., Alaszewski, H., Ayer, S., Manthorpe, J., 2000. Managing risk in community practice: nursing, risk and decision making. Baillière Tindall, Edinburgh.

Atkinson, D., Williams, F., 1990. 'Know me as I am': an anthology of prose, poetry and art by people with learning difficulties. Hodder and Stoughton, London.

BBC News, 1998. Four die in canal accident. BBC News. Available at: http://news.bbc.co.uk/1/hi/uk/154436.stm (accessed 10.06.10.).

Borough of Poole, (undated). Adult abuse. Available at: http://www.boroughofpoole.com/adult_social_services_commissioning/services/ref:S464832144DAD0/aka:Adult+Abuse/ (accessed 10 June 2010).

Care Quality Commission, 2010. Safeguarding. Available at: http://www.cqc.org.uk/guidanceforallhealthcarestaff/managingrisk/safeguarding.cfm (accessed 10.06.10.).

Carson, D., (undated). Positve professional risk-taking. Available at: http://sites.google.com/site/dcccarson/our-company/positive-professional-risk-taking (accessed 10.06.10.).

Carson, D., Bain, A., 2008. Professional risk and working with people: decision-making in health, social care and criminal justice. Jessica Kingsley, London and Philadephia.

Department of Health, 2001. Valuing people: a new strategy for learning disability for the 21st century. Cm 5086. The Stationery Office, London.

Douglas, M., 1990. Risk as a forensic resource. Dædalus, Journal of the American Academcy of Arts and Science 119, 1–16.

Douglas, M., 1992. Risk and blame: essays in cultural theory. Routledge, London.

Dowie, J., 1999. Communication for better decisions: not about 'risk. Health, Risk and Society 1 (1), 41–53.

Fruin, D., 1998. Moving into the mainstream: the report of a national inspection of services for adults with learning disabilities. Department of Health, Social Care Group, SSI, London.

Furedi, F., 2002. Paranoid parenting: why ignoring the experts may be best for your child. Chicago Review Press, Chicago.

Heyman, B., Huckle, S., 1993. Not worth the risk? Attitudes of adults with learning difficulties and their informal carers to the hazards of everyday life. Soc. Sci. Med. 37, 1557–1564.

Heyman, B., Huckle, S., Handyside, E. C., 1998. Freedom of the locality for people with learning difficulties. In: Heyman, B. (Ed.), Risk, health and health care: a qualitative approach. Arnold, London.

Heyman, B., Shaw, M., Alaszewski, A., Titterton, M., 2010. Risk, safety and clinical practice: health care through the lens of risk. Oxford University Press, Oxford.

Jay Committee, 1979. Report of the Committee of Enquiry into Mental Handicap Nursing and Care, Chairman Peggy Jay, vol, 1. Cmnd-1. HMSO, London.

Jenkins, N.E., 2006. You can't wrap them up in cotton wool!' Constructing risk in young people's access to outdoor play. Health, Risk and Society 8, 379–393.

McGuire, A., Henderson, J., Mooney, G., 1988. The economics of health care: an introductory text. Routledge, London.

Mencap, (undated). Children Rights Officers and Advocates - CROA. Available at: http://www.mencap.org.uk/organisations.asp?id=1372 (accessed 12.06.10.).

Morris, S., 2007. Tortured, drugged and killed, a month after care visits stopped. The Guardian. 4 August 2007 Available at: http://www.guardian.co.uk/society/2007/aug/04/socialcare.crime (accessed 10.06.10.).

National Health Service, 1978. Report of the Committee of Inquiry into Normansfield Hospital. Cmnd 7357. HMSO, London.

Nursing and Midwifery Council, (undated). General public. Available at: http://www.nmc-uk.org/General-public/ (accessed 10.06.10.).

Nursing and Midwifery Council, 2010. The code in full. Available at: http://www.nmc-uk.org/Nurses-and-midwives/The-code/The-code-in-full/ (accessed 10.06.10.).

Parker, J., Stanworth, H., 2005. Go for it!' Towards a critical realist approach to voluntary risk-taking. Health, Risk and Society 7 (4), 319–336.

Perske, R., 1972. The dignity of risk. In: Wolfensberger, W. (Ed.), The principles of normalization in human services. National Institute on Mental Retardation, Toronto.

Peterborough Voices, 1997. Peterborough Voices: extraordinary people, extraordinary lives. Peterborough Council for Voluntary Services, Peterborough.

Robertson, J., Collinson, C., in press. Positive risk taking: whose risk is it? An exploration in community outreach teams in adult mental health and learning disability services. Health, Risk and Society 11.

Stanley, N., 2005. Thrills and spills: young people's sexual behaviour and attitudes in seaside and rural areas. Health, Risk and Society 7 (4), 337–348.

The Guardian, 1998. Four die as canal boat sinks – disabled trippers trapped after narrow boat is snagged in lock. The Guardian, 20 August 1998 p. 5.

VOICE UK, Respond and the Ann Craft Trust, 2007. Disability hate crime against adults with learning disabilities: supplemental evidence to the Joint Committee on Human Rights Inquiry into Human Rights of Adults with Learning Disabilities. Available at: http://www.voiceuk.org.uk/pdfs/SupplementalEvidence HumanRights_Disability_Hate_Crime.pdf (accessed 10.06.10.).

Williams, R., 1994. Hill drives back the shadows. The Independent on Sunday 25 September p, 3.

Zinn, J.O., 2008. Heading into the unknown: everyday strategies for managing risk and uncertainty. Health, Risk and Society 10 (5), 439–450.

Further reading

There is a substantial and growing literature on risk. This literature can be accessed through specialised journals, through the practitioner-oriented publications and through more theoretical analyses.

Journals

There are several specialist journals that include articles on risk and health including Risk Analysis (http://www.wiley.com/bw/journal.asp?ref=0272-4332), Journal of Risk Research (http://www.tandf.co.uk/journals/titles/13669877.asp) and Health, Risk and Society (http://www.tandf.co.uk/journals/chrs) which has a strong social science orientation and includes qualitative articles that explore the nature of risk in health and social care.

Practitioner-oriented publications

There is a range of practitioner-oriented publications which all provide helpful advice and guidance and are informed by risk research. The book by Heyman and his colleagues takes a more theoretical approach and is recommended for further reading.

Alaszewski, H., Parker, A., Alaszewski, A., 1999. Empowerment and protection: the development of policies and practices in risk assessment and risk management in services for adults with learning disabilities. The Mental Health Foundation, London. Update available from: http://www.learningdisabilities.org.uk/publications/?esctl544701_entryid5=22293&q=0%c2%acempowerment+and+protection%c2%ac.

Alaszewski, A., Alaszewski, H., Ayer, S., Manthorpe, J., 2000. Managing risk in community practice: nursing, risk and decision making. Baillière Tindall, Edinburgh.

Carson, D., Bain, A., 2008. Professional risk and working with people: decision-making in health, social care and criminal justice. Jessica Kingsley, London and Philadelphia.

Heyman, B. (Ed.), 1998. Risk, health and health care: a qualitative approach. Arnold, London.

Heyman, B., Shaw, M., Alaszewski, A., Titterton, M., 2010. Risk, safety and clinical practice: health care through the lens of risk. Oxford University Press, Oxford.

Pritchard, J., Kemshall, H., 1995. Good practice in risk assessment and management 1. Jessica Kingsley, London and Philadelphia.

Pritchard, J., Kemshall, H., 1997. Good practice in risk assessment and risk management 2. Jessica Kingsley, London and Philadelphia.

Sellars, C., 2002. Risk Assessment in people with learning disabilities. BPS Blackwell, Oxford.

Titterton, M., 2004. Risk and risk taking in health and social welfare. Jessica Kingsley, London and Philadelphia.

Theoretical analyses

There are a lot of theoretical texts on risk, some of them fairly complicated. Adam's and Lupton's books on risk are readable introductions, and Douglas' essays on risk and blame provide a good introduction to the ways in which risk is used in contemporatry societies.

Adams, J., 1995. Risk. UCL Press, London.

Beck, U., 1992. Risk society: towards a new modernity. Sage, London.

Breakwell, G.M., 2007. The psychology of risk. Cambridge University Press, Cambridge.

Douglas, M., 1992. Risk and blame: essays in cultural theory. Routledge, London.

Franklin, J. (Ed.), 1998. The politics of the risk society. Polity Press, Cambridge.

Hood, C., Rothstein, H., Baldwin, R., 2004. The government of risk: understanding risk regulation regimes. Oxford University Press, Oxford.

Luhmann, N., 1993. Risk: a sociological theory. Aldine Transaction, New Brunswick.

Lupton, D., 1999. Risk. Routledge, London.

Power, M., 2007. Organized uncertainty: designing a world of risk management. Oxford University Press, Oxford.

Taylor-Gooby, P., Zinn, J., 2006. Risk in social science. Oxford University Press, Oxford.

Tulloch, J., Lupton, D., 2003. Risk and everyday life. Sage, London.

Zinn, J.O. (Ed.), 2008. Social theories of risk and uncertainty. Blackwell, Oxford.

Useful addresses

David Carson, Reader in Law and Behavioural Sciences at the Institute of Criminal Justice Studies, University of Portsmouth, provides workshops without the university on 'Positive approaches to professional risk-taking in human services', 'Developing expert witness skills' and 'Investigations: from fact-finding to proof', Further information can be accessed via his website: http://sites.google.com/site/dcccarson/.

The Foundation for People with Learning Disabilities "works to promote the rights, quality of life and opportunities of people with learning disabilities and their families." The Foundation provides a consultancy service which works "with local authorities, the voluntary and private sector, the National Health Service, parent groups and self-advocates to improve services and promote tailor-made solutions", Further information can be accessed via its website: http://www.learningdisabilities.org.uk/welcome/.

The King's Fund is a major health and social care resource and 'think tank'. It has in the past conducted major studies of services for people with learning disabilities and a key word search of its library database using 'learning disabilities' and 'risk' indicates that it can provide access to 44 key texts, Further information can be accessed via its website: http://www.kingsfund.org.uk/.

The King's Centre for Risk Management supports a wide range of projects and academic fellowships, helping to translate its risk research into practical, policy-relevant solutions and is a centre for advanced postgraduate studies in risk. Further information can be accessed via its website: http://www.kcl.ac.uk/projects/kcrm/.

The Learning Disability Coalition includes 15 organisations that campaign to improve services and support for people with learning disabilities. Its policy and statitics webpage provides access to a useful range of evidence, Further information can be accessed via its website: http://www.learningdisabilitycoalition.org.uk/policyandstatistics.asp.

Mencap is a national charity that "works with people with a learning disability to change laws and services, challenge prejudice and directly support thousands of people to live their lives as they choose". Further information can be accessed via its website: http://www.mencap.org.uk/.

Safeguarding against abuse and harm

12

Caroline White

CHAPTER CONTENTS

KEY ISSUES

- People with learning disabilities are at risk of abuse, neglect and harm in a variety of settings and circumstances
- While individuals may demonstrate resilience and coping strategies, the emotional impact of abuse for people with learning disabilities and their families may be significant
- Practitioners should have an understanding of abuse and take steps to prevent the onset of abuse; respond to abuse which occurs; and provide support to those who have been abused
- People with learning disabilities have the potential to play an active role in their own protection; this should be recognised, while ensuring that individuals are not isolated from the support of practitioners

Introduction

Recent UK policy has been underpinned by significant principles which highlight the importance of rights, inclusion, choice and independence in the lives of people with learning disabilities (Department of Health (DH) 2001). However, in contrast to these important policy aims, inquiries, investigations and research have indicated that people with learning disabilities face risks of abuse, neglect and harm. Such abuse and harm may have a profound impact on individuals' lives, and may prevent them from accessing and enjoying the opportunities presented within current service and policy agendas. Those who support people with learning disabilities need an awareness of the risks they face and their rights to live lives in which they are safe from abuse and mistreatment. At the same time, there is a need to strive to ensure that awareness of risk does not detract from individuals' rights to make informed choices, to choose to take risks, to develop friendships and relationships and to strive towards independence (see also Chs 11 and 28). As Fyson (2009:23–24) has questioned;

> what value does freedom from abuse have if it comes at the cost of losing all independence? ... What value does independence have if it comes at the cost of being abused?

This chapter will give examples of how people with learning disabilities have been abused in a range of settings and circumstances, and will outline some of the current policy and legislation developed to reduce risks of abuse and to support people who have been abused. It outlines contemporary definitions of abuse and explores the different kinds of abuse currently recognised within UK policy and practice. Some of the underlying reasons why people with learning disabilities appear to be at risk of abuse will be explored, as well as some of the potential consequences of abuse. Practice responses to prevent the onset of abuse and to support people with learning disabilities who have been abused will be outlined. Finally, the importance of seeking to move towards enabling people with learning disabilities to play active roles in their own protection will be highlighted.

It is important to note that much of our knowledge of the abuse of people with learning disabilities is based on research regarding sexual abuse. Therefore, inevitably, discussion of this form of abuse will dominate within this chapter. However, it should not be forgotten that there are other serious and significant forms of abuse which may cause harm and distress to people with learning disabilities.

Background and historical overview

An early scandal concerning the abuse of people with learning disabilities was reported by the Ely Hospital Inquiry in 1968/1969, which concerned the treatment of people with learning disabilities in a long-stay hospital, typical of service provision for people with learning disabilities at that time. The abuses reported included examples of cruel and threatening treatment (such as beatings, hosing patients down with cold water), theft of items belonging to the hospital and the patients, and a lack of care and indifference by senior staff to complaints (Butler & Drakeford 2005). Further examples of abuses within learning disability services were revealed by inquiries during the 1960s and 1970s (Martin 1984) leading to some recognition of the failings within institutional care at that time. However, any ideas or assumptions that such abuses were due to outmoded practice and service delivery have been challenged by more recent examples of abuse within contemporary services. For example, in 2006, an inquiry into services for people with learning disabilities in Cornwall found examples of abuse and ill treatment of people with learning disabilities. These included hitting, mocking, withholding food, giving cold showers, inappropriate use of residents' money and violence between residents. It was reported that "one person spent 16 hours a day tied to their bed or wheelchair, for what staff wrongly believed was for that person's own protection" (Commission for Social Care Inspection/Healthcare Commission 2006:5). Such abuses have highlighted the risks faced by people with learning disabilities in settings designed to offer support and care, and to promote the safety and wellbeing of individuals.

Much attention has been focused on the abuse of people with learning disabilities in institutions and service settings. However, people with learning disabilities have been abused in other settings and situations, although accounts of such abuses are less prevalent within the literature.

A significant case of abuse within the family setting concerned Beverley Lewis, a young deafblind woman with learning disabilities. She "had a warm personality and a lot to offer. At the age of 23 she died, wrapped in newspapers and weighing less than 5 stone" (Powerhouse 1996:139). Beverley's mother had deteriorating mental health difficulties and had refused to accept help. Although family members tried to draw attention to the situation of Beverley and her mother, professionals had been unable to gain access to Beverley. Following Beverley's death, the responses of the professionals concerned were criticised as poorly coordinated, with a lack of clear responsibilities (Sense 2000).

Examples of abuse affecting people with learning disabilities within the wider community have also been highlighted. In 2006, Steven Hoskin, a young man with learning disabilities, was killed by his 'friends'. On the night of his death he was subjected to violent behaviours, verbal abuse and humiliation and was given a lethal dose of painkillers. He was then taken to a local viaduct, where he was forced over the safety rail and kicked until he let go (Flynn 2007). Such abuse may also be labelled as 'disability hate crime': this refers to crimes which are perceived to be motivated by an individual's disabilities (Better Days/Coast2Coast/Inclusion North 2008).

The above cases highlight the risks faced by people with learning disabilities of abuse, neglect and hate crime. It is also useful to be aware that people with learning disabilities report bullying as a significant issue (Mencap 1999). Reports of bullying, while serious in their own right, should be considered carefully, and not dismissed as relatively minor problems, since the term 'bullying' may be used by some people with learning disabilities to describe abusive and criminal experiences (Quarmby 2008).

The risks faced by people with learning disabilities are apparent in a variety of settings and contexts, including formal care services, the family home and when living independently in the community; therefore it should not be assumed that changing the setting in which individuals live or the style of services offered will automatically make people safer. The above cases illustrate the need for practitioners to recognise signs of abuse and to act appropriately and effectively to prevent and respond to abuse and harm.

Policy and legislation

In response to the risks faced by people with learning disabilities and other vulnerable groups (such as older people and people with mental health needs), policy and legislation have been developed.

In 2000, the Department of Health published *No Secrets*, which aimed to ensure a 'consistent and effective response' where there are concerns or evidence of abuse (DH 2000:6). This guidance covers England and Northern Ireland; similar guidance *In Safe Hands* (National Assembly for Wales 2000) was published in Wales. These documents define abuse and highlight the need for policies and guidance to safeguard adults against abuse and harm. While giving the lead responsibility for adult safeguarding to social services departments, these policies stress the importance of multi-agency working, indicating a wide-reaching, cross-agency responsibility for adult safeguarding and protection, emphasising that 'safeguarding is everyone's business' (DH 2008:5). The work of *No Secrets* was further developed within *Safeguarding Adults* (Association of Directors of Social Services (ADSS) 2005) which extended the focus of concern to include "all work which enables an adult *'who is or may be eligible for community care services'* to retain independence, wellbeing and choice *and* to access their human right to live a life that is free from abuse and neglect" (ADSS 2005:5). It replaced the previously widely used term 'adult protection' with that of adult safeguarding.

No Secrets and *In Safe Hands* have arguably played a significant role in influencing policy and practice; they provide guidance to agencies, but fall short of providing adult safeguarding legislation. A somewhat different situation exists in Scotland where the introduction of the Adult Support and Protection (Scotland) Act 2007 (implemented in 2008) provides specific legislative powers with regard to adult safeguarding which include:

- a duty to make inquiries about people at risk of harm
- powers to examine records (such as agency files, financial records)
- powers for the local authority to apply for court orders, which enable them to:
  - remove the adult at risk to another place to carry out an assessment
  - remove the adult to a place of safety to prevent harm, for up to 7 days
  - ban specific people from contact with the adult to prevent harm.

(Armstrong 2008, Mackay 2008)

Although potentially giving local authorities significant powers to intervene in the lives of those at risk of abuse, the principles of the Act state that any interventions taken must:

- benefit the adult
- be the least restrictive intervention possible
- consider the wishes of the adult, past and present, as well as the views of the people who are important to them
- involve the participation of the adult as much as possible.

(Armstrong 2008, Mackay 2008)

Although there is no specific adult safeguarding legislation in England, Northern Ireland and Wales, there are other pieces of legislation which do addre the abuse of vulnerable adults. For example Mental Capacity Act 2005 (and similarly the with Incapacity (Scotland) Act 2000), offers guidance with regard to decision making where individuals lack capacity and introduces a new offence of *'the ill-treatment or wilful neglect of a person lacking capacity'* (Brammer 2010). Additionally, the Sexual Offenses Act (2003) emphasises the importance of consent and introduces offences against 'persons with a mental disorder' who are unable to consent to sexual activity or who are vulnerable to being coerced through bribes or threats (Brammer 2010). Also of significance is the Disability Discrimination Act 2005 which requires public authorities to "have due regard to the need to eliminate harassment of and unlawful discrimination against disabled persons" (Brammer 2010:156).

At the time of writing, both *No Secrets* and *In Safe Hands* are under review. The review processes aim to strengthen adult safeguarding work, to ensure such work reflects developing policy and government vision, identify areas where improvements can be made and consider whether adult safeguarding legislation should be introduced (DH 2008, Magill et al 2010).

Definitions and categories of abuse

Definitions of abuse have been much debated. However *No Secrets* (DH 2000:9) offers a clear definition of abuse which is currently widely used. This definition states that:

> Abuse is a violation of an individual's human and civil rights by any other person or persons.

It also acknowledged that such abuse may "result in significant harm and exploitation" (DH 2000:9). *No Secrets* identified a range of underlying reasons for abusive behaviour, which include "deliberate intent, negligence or ignorance" (DH 2000:10).

Reader activity 12.1

Adult safeguarding legislation has been introduced in Scotland, but not at the time of writing in the rest of the UK.

s about whether legislation should
ughout the UK?
tial advantages of such legislation?
ny risks or disadvantages of
egislation?

No Secrets identified six categories of abuse: sexual; physical; psychological; financial/material; neglect and acts of omission; discriminatory abuse. These abuses may occur in isolation, or as multiple abuses (for example, within a single incident, an individual may be physically assaulted, sexually and psychologically abused.) Each of these categories of abuse will be discussed below.

Sexual abuse

Sexual abuse occurs when an individual is subjected to sexual acts in the absence of meaningful consent (Brown & Turk 1992, Brown et al 1995). The category of sexual abuse includes acts labelled as contact and non-contact abuse (Brown & Turk 1992). Contact abuse includes acts such as rape, penetration, masturbation and sexual touch. Non-contact abuse includes acts which do not involve touch, such as harassment, indecent exposure, involvement in pornography, which can also be distressing and harmful.

A key issue to consider with regard to sexual abuse is that of consent. Brown & Turk (1992) define sexual abuse as occurring when:

- the person withholds consent (in such cases, people with learning disabilities are protected by the laws against rape and sexual assault which protect all members of society)
- the person is unable to give consent, for example because they lack the capacity to understand sexual acts. Individuals may be unable to consent to sexual acts if they do not understand the potential risks or consequences (e.g. pregnancy), or if they do not appreciate that certain behaviours or relationships (such as incestuous relationships) are inappropriate, illegal or not socially sanctioned
- there are barriers which prevent the individual from exercising free choice and expressing consent or dissent. Such barriers include the use of force, threats or bribes, an imbalance of power between the person with a learning disability and their abusers. The balance of power within some relationships, for example where the abuser is a family member, a staff member or someone in a high status or authority role, may make it very difficult for an individual with learning disabilities to say no, or withhold consent.

Recognition of the risks of exploitation by those in positions of trust and authority underpins recent legislation. The Sexual Offences Act 2003 sets clear boundaries around the relationships between workers (such as care workers, doctors and therapists) whose roles include face-to-face contact with people who lack capacity.

Under the terms of the Act, such workers who engage in sexual activity with the people they support commit an offence (Brammer 2010).

Working to establish whether consent has been given or withheld can be complex, especially perhaps when both individuals have a learning disability. However, it is an issue which requires clear and careful consideration. In the absence of such consideration there are risks either that safe, consenting and mutually satisfying relationships are prohibited, or that relationships in which one individual is frightened, hurt and exploited are supported. People are placed at risk both when their rights to a consenting sexual life are ignored, and when a desire to support choice and adult lifestyles mean that indicators of fear, distress and a lack of meaningful consent are ignored.

Physical abuse

Although concerns about sexual abuse have dominated the literature, physical abuse probably occurs more frequently (Brown 1999, 2003, Brown & Stein 1998). This category of abuse includes acts of physical assault such as hitting, slapping, kicking and pushing, as well as insensitive personal care, the misuse or overuse of medication and of restraint (Brown 1999, DH 2000).

Psychological abuse

This type of abuse is also sometimes referred to as emotional abuse. Behaviours such as making threats, controlling, blaming, harassment, verbal abuse (such as shouting and swearing), 'cold shouldering' and isolating people from their support networks are all forms of psychological abuse (DH 2000, Gaylard 2008).

Financial and material abuse

This category of abuse includes theft of money (both small amounts of cash as well as large sums of money) and an individual's possessions, fraud and placing people under pressure to change the terms of their wills (DH 2000). Careful consideration is required by services to enable people with learning disabilities to manage their own money and make financial choices, while at the same time protecting them from abuse and exploitation (Livingstone 2006).

Neglect and acts of omission

The types of abuse defined above involve acting or doing something *to* another person. In contrast, neglect involves a failure or omission to do something for another. This includes failing to meet basic physical, social and health care needs, for example failing to provide adequate nutrition, heating, medication, access to medical and dental care, social care or educational services (Brown 1999, DH 2000).

Discriminatory abuse

This is abuse which is grounded in discrimination based on an individual's race, gender, disability, sexual orientation or religion. A refusal to respect an individual's religious or cultural needs, for example by failing to provide an appropriate diet (Brown 2003), or belittling an individual on the grounds of their disability would constitute discriminatory abuse.

No Secrets also highlights the issue of institutional abuse. This is not clearly and consistently defined within the literature. *No Secrets* suggests that:

> Repeated instances of poor care may be an indication of more serious problems and this is sometimes referred to as institutional abuse.
>
> (DH 2000:10)

Brown (2007) has noted that institutional abuse is not a 'type' of abuse, but instead consists of a range of factors which interact together to promote poor or abusive practice. These factors include:

- poor quality environments
- rigid and oppressive routines
- neglecting the needs and wishes of residents
- practice which does not reflect accepted professional behaviours (for example inappropriate responses to challenging behaviours)
- acts of cruelty from individuals or staff groups
- negligent practice and exposing residents to risks.

Settings of abuse

With regard to sexual abuse, Brown et al (1995) and McCormack et al (2005) have explored the settings in which abuse occurs. They found that individuals were most frequently abused at home (this included abuse within the family home and residential services). Additionally abuse was found to occur in day services, in the perpetrator's home, in public places and leisure facilities. These studies highlight the risks to individuals within settings where there would be an expectation of safety, such as the home or service settings (Brown et al 1995), as well as risks within the community and public places.

Perpetrators of abuse

Brown et al (1995) and McCormack et al (2005) also identified a range of perpetrators of sexual abuse. These included:

- other people with learning disabilities
- family members
- staff members
- volunteers
- other known adults
- strangers.

Although there is a public and media perception that strangers pose considerable risk (Peckham 2007), both studies found that this group accounted for a very small proportion of the abuse identified (1–5%). While the risks from strangers should not be ignored, both studies indicate that abuse is more significantly perpetrated by known individuals, often those within the support networks of people with learning disabilities, with whom there would be an expectation of a safe and trusting relationship.

Both studies indicated that a significant proportion of abuse (over 50% in each study) was perpetrated by peers with a learning disability, who may share a service setting with those they abuse. The issue of abuse between service users, while prevalent, is often overlooked. The label of 'challenging behaviour' is often used within services (see Ch. 18). This may reduce the stigma attached to such behaviours, but can also distort and soften perceptions of the behaviours, so that the impact upon others may not be recognised and abusive behaviours remain unreported and unchallenged (Brown 1999, 2003, Joyce 2003). In such circumstances:

> many people with learning disabilities are encouraged by staff to tolerate behaviours from their peers that few other people would want to put up with from their friends, flatmates or colleagues.
>
> (McCarthy & Thompson 1996:213–214).

Where people with learning disabilities present with challenging behaviours, there is a need to consider clearly the impact of these behaviours on other service users, and to respond effectively and in ways which recognise and respect their feelings and needs for safety and security. A clear acknowledgement of abuse between service users helps ensure both that those at risk of being abused are protected, and that those at risk of abusing receive appropriate support to manage their behaviour.

The impact of abuse

Understanding, recognising and responding to the abuse of people with learning disabilities is a vital area of work, because of the potential costs and consequences to those who are abused. McCarthy (1999), who carried out research into the sexual experiences of women with learning disabilities, found high levels of sexual abuse among the women that she interviewed. Her work highlighted the resilience of the women and she observed that, although some experienced difficulties:

> generally speaking . . . the personal strength and resilience shown by the women in coming to terms with what had happened to them and in some cases was continuing to happen, was to their great credit.
>
> (McCarthy 1999:217)

McCarthy's work offers an important reminder that people with learning disabilities who have experienced abuse should not be perceived simply as 'victims', but as survivors with personal coping skills and resources.

However, there is also evidence that the experience of abuse can, for some individuals, be traumatic, distressing and have a profound impact upon their lives. Our understanding of the impact of abuse comes largely from research with individuals who have been sexually abused; less is known about the effects of other kinds of abuse.

Two key studies (O'Callaghan et al 2003, Sequeira et al 2003) explored the impact of abuse on people with learning disabilities, the majority of whom had been sexually abused. O'Callaghan et al (2003) identified that the experience of abuse had had a devastating, profound and long-lasting impact upon survivors. Both studies identified symptoms of post-traumatic stress disorder and a range of behavioural and mental health problems among the survivors. O'Callaghan et al presented case studies in which the following effects of abuse were evidenced:

1. Behavioural changes including:
   - self-harming
   - challenging behaviours
   - stopping communicating
   - avoiding places associated with the abuse
   - re-enacting the abuse, including demonstrating sexualised behaviours.
2. Emotional changes including:
   - appearing depressed
   - showing signs of fear

- becoming tearful and withdrawn
- experiencing flashbacks and nightmares

3. Physical changes, including weight loss.

They also found that abuse could lead to other consequences for survivors. For example, the majority (89%) experienced changes to their services, either moving to different residential placements or stopping using respite services, following the abuse. While these changes may have been intended to protect individuals from repeated abuse and further harm, these findings suggest that survivors of abuse are at risk of experiencing change, discontinuity and disruption, at a time when they are especially vulnerable (O'Callaghan et al 2003). In contrast, the Association for Residential Care (ARC)/ National Association for the Protection from Sexual Abuse of Adults and Children with Learning Disabilities (NAPSAC) (1996) have recommended that moving the person who has been abused should only be considered as a last resort.

O'Callaghan et al's study also highlighted the profound consequences for the families of those who had been abused. These included feelings of distrust of other people and services, feelings of guilt and anger, developing mental health problems (such as depression) and personal problems (such as alcohol abuse, problems in their relationship with their partner). While the provision of therapeutic support to survivors of abuse was identified as 'patchy', they found that, although family members were experiencing trauma, they were offered little support.

The profound consequences of abuse reported in the above studies may not be shared by all survivors of abuse. O'Callaghan et al note, for example, that the survivors in their study had experienced very severe forms of multiple abuse, and may therefore not be typical of all survivors. However, these studies do highlight the potentially significant consequences of abuse, stressing the importance of acting to prevent abuse and indicating a need to provide sensitive support to those who have been abused, and their families.

Why are people with learning disabilities abused?

This chapter has identified that people with learning disabilities are a population at risk of abuse and neglect. This section explores some of the underlying reasons for these risks.

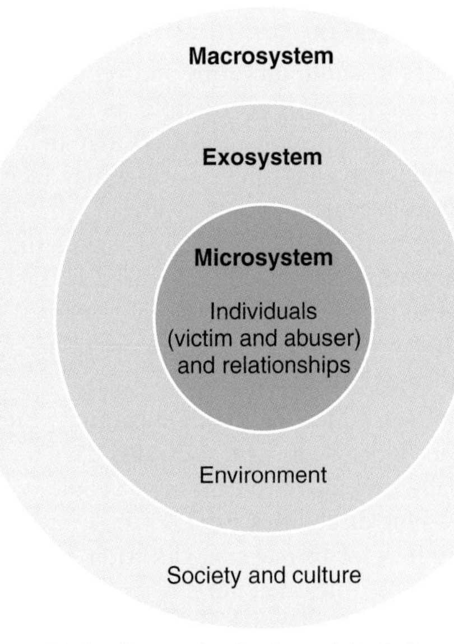

Figure 12.1 • An ecological model of abuse (Adapted from Sobsey 1994 and Hollomotz 2009)

A key message with regard to the causes of abuse is that there are no easy or simple explanations. Instead there are a wide range of factors which place people with learning disabilities at risk (Joyce 2003, Wishart 2003). Sobsey (1994) and Hollomotz (2009) have both proposed 'ecological models' of abuse. These models are helpful in highlighting the range of risk factors for abuse and the interactions between them. These risk factors are grouped within three systems (Fig. 12.1):

1. The microsystem – which is concerned with individuals, i.e. those who are abused, those who carry out abuse, and the relationships between them.
2. The exosystem – which is concerned with the environments in which people with learning disabilities live.
3. The macrosystem – which is concerned with wider cultural and societal factors.

Each of these will be considered in greater detail.

The microsystem

This section will consider the characteristics and behaviours of individuals.

People who are abused

A number of risk factors associated with people with learning disabilities themselves have been identified. These include the following:

- An inability to recognise risky or abusive situations (Hollomotz 2009).
- Difficulties in communicating and reporting abusive experiences. For example, individuals whose communication is impaired may be vulnerable to ongoing abuse as they may face difficulties in making others aware of what is happening to them. Sobsey (1994) notes that communication may also be impaired by factors external to individuals, for example, where individuals are isolated from support or are not listened to or believed.
- A lack of sex education. Sex education, while important in its own right, may also have a potentially protective role. Where people with learning disabilities have not had opportunities for formal sex education, their only opportunities to learn about sex and sexual relationships may come through personal experience, including experiences of abuse (McCarthy 1999, Sobsey 1994). Sex education can provide individuals with opportunities to learn about consent and their right to say no, an opportunity to recognise the importance of sex as an act which should be enjoyed (not endured) by both partners, and to learn a vocabulary which can assist the reporting of sexual abuse (ARC/NAPSAC 1996, McCarthy 1999, Wishart 2003).
- Cultures of compliance. Services delivered to people with learning disabilities have been characterised as cultures in which service users are expected to do as they are told. In such settings, individuals may learn to comply with requests or demands made by abusers (Sobsey 1994, Wishart 2003). A need for opportunities to develop assertiveness skills to counter such service expectations has been advocated (Brown 2003, Sobsey 1994, Wishart 2003).

A focus on individuals can be useful in highlighting areas in which change and development are required; for example the provision of sex education and assertiveness training, steps to reduce individual isolation. However, this is also a focus which has been criticised. Considering the risks associated with individuals may lead to 'victim blaming' in which the reasons for the abuse are perceived to be the fault of the individual (Brown 2003, Sobsey 1994, Wishart 2003). However, the ecological model highlights the importance of exploring factors beyond the individual, such as wider environmental and cultural factors. Sobsey (1994:103) has observed that "society's response to disability may be more important than the disability itself".

Individual abusers

When we think of the characteristics of those who abuse, we are apt to depict abusers as individuals who abuse deliberately and maliciously, for their own gratification. Martin (1984) has termed this the 'bad apple' model. While this model accounts for some of the underlying reasons for abuse, especially with regard to sexual abuse (Brown 2007), there is a strong consensus that individuals' behaviours are also shaped or influenced by external factors (for example Brown 2007, Manthorpe & Stanley 1999, Martin 1984), the significance of which will be explored below.

The exosystem

The environments in which people with learning disabilities live can expose them to significant risk. This has been most clearly documented with regard to residential services. Research and inquiries have indicated that "in certain circumstances, it is possible for a culture of abuse and exploitation to become established and flourish in services" (Cambridge 1999:303). Key elements of service environments and cultures which promote abuse include the following:

- *The quality of management.* Research and inquiries into abusive services have highlighted the significance of management. Where leadership in services or organisations is weak and supervision of staff is infrequent, managers will lack opportunities to challenge poor or abusive practice and to set positive standards for the provision of care (Cambridge 1999, Marsland et al 2006, 2007).
- *Staff skills and competence.* A staff group which is skilled, knowledgeable and well trained will be aware of accepted practice and able to recognise poor or abusive practice (White et al 2003). Where staff lack such skills and awareness, people with learning disabilities may be vulnerable to abuse, which may be perpetrated unintentionally, and this abuse may remain unrecognised and unchallenged. For example, where staff lack training and support in working with people with learning disabilities who have aggressive or challenging behaviours, there is a risk that they may respond

inappropriately or aggressively to episodes of violent behaviour through a lack of awareness of the most appropriate, safe and dignified responses.

- *Staff attitudes and behaviours*. How staff perceive the people with learning disabilities they support is important and can influence the ways they treat individuals. Wardhaugh & Wilding (1993) introduced the term 'neutralisation of normal moral concerns' to describe the process by which people receiving care may become dehumanised or perceived as 'other'. Where people with learning disabilities are perceived as of lesser value than staff or other members of society, there is a risk that poor or abusive treatment, which would normally be viewed as unacceptable, can be justified.
- *The staff culture*. The culture among the staff group can influence the attitudes which are held in the service and the ways in which residents are treated. Strong staff cliques or the presence of friendship/family groups working together can make it hard for other staff to challenge poor practice or encourage other ways of doing things (White et al 2003). Staff groups may become intimidating, suppressing the reporting of concerns (Cambridge 1999). In such teams, staff who disagree with the prevailing way of doing things may be bullied, ostracised or isolated.
- *Isolation*. Although residential homes are now typically placed within the community (in contrast with historically segregated services), services for people with learning disabilities can still be isolated from the support and vigilance of external professionals, family and friends. This isolation can "help the unacceptable become the norm" (Cotshill Hospital Report in Martin 1984:58). Isolation may allow abuse to occur (because ideas about good practice are not being brought into the service) and enables abuse to remain concealed (because there are few external people to observe and report poor practice) (Sobsey 1994 in White et al 2003).

This exploration of the exosystem, or the environments in which support is provided, helps to illustrate how, while individual attributes and characteristics are important (and individual responsibility for behaviour should not be ignored), the services, settings and cultures in which people with learning disabilities live are also significant. For example, where services are poorly managed, isolated from external support and staff are given little training, abusive practice may develop and become entrenched. Such settings may provide a safe haven for those whose individual characteristics predispose them to abuse others, as well as creating the conditions in which well-intentioned staff commit acts of abuse, or fail to challenge the abuses of others (Marsland et al 2007).

The macrosystem

Wider cultural and societal factors may contribute towards the vulnerability of people with learning disabilities. Cultural beliefs about the lack of value of the lives of people with learning disabilities may influence and be used to justify individual behaviours, as has been indicated above. Other cultural views and attitudes may also be significant. For example, Flynn & Brown (1997:40) highlighted the significance of sexism and stereotypical views of male and female behaviour. They identified a service in which the sexual abuse of a woman with learning disabilities was accepted and not taken seriously due to the prevailing attitude that 'men will sow their wild oats' and that women are to blame for 'encouraging' the abuse. Such attitudes fail to acknowledge the significance of abusive actions and to recognise the hurt and harm that such behaviours may cause for women.

Responding to abuse and harm

The findings with regard to the impact of abuse demonstrate the importance of taking steps to prevent people with learning disabilities from being abused, and of responding wisely and appropriately when abuse does take place.

Brown (2003) and May-Chahal et al (2006) have offered useful models for considering the prevention of abuse, which will be used within this section. These models define three levels of prevention:

1. Primary prevention, which includes strategies to reduce risk and prevent the onset of abuse.
2. Secondary prevention, which is concerned with ensuring the prompt identification of abuse, and responding effectively to prevent the reoccurrence of abuse.
3. Tertiary prevention, which focuses on the need to support individuals who have been abused, seeking to reduce the impact of the harm and trauma that may follow on from abusive experiences.

Primary prevention

As has already been seen, the experience of abuse can lead to hurt, harm and distress. Therefore, a critical element of adult safeguarding work concerns actions to prevent abuse from happening at all. *No Secrets* (DH 2000:6) recognised the importance of primary prevention stating that "agencies' primary aim should be to prevent abuse where possible". However, it has been argued that 'we are better able to respond to abuse which has already occurred than to protect people before they are abused' (White et al 2003:2). This section will consider two forms of primary prevention:

- Actions to identify unsuitable or inappropriate workers.
- The recognition of 'early indicators' of abuse.

Actions to identify unsuitable or inappropriate workers

There is a particular irony that people with learning disabilities, as other adults at risk and children, may be abused by those who are paid to offer support, care and protection. Thus providers of residential, day and domiciliary services are expected to take steps to ensure a safe and competent workforce. These steps include the adoption of positive recruitment practice, which may act as a barrier to the employment of unsuitable workers. Current recruitment practice is underpinned by The Safeguarding Vulnerable Groups Act 2006 which was passed in response to the Bichard Inquiry into the Soham murders (Brammer 2010). This Act creates a Vetting and Barring Scheme, overseen by the Independent Safeguarding Authority (ISA), which will act to reduce the likelihood of unsuitable individuals gaining paid employment or volunteering to work with vulnerable adults or children. The new Act creates the following (Brammer 2010, ISA 2010, Mandelstam 2009):

- A barring list. Individuals included on the list cannot work, or seek to work, with vulnerable adults if carrying out 'regulated activity'. Regulated activity is carried out frequently and by the same person and includes such roles as providing care, assistance, training and teaching, treatment and therapy for vulnerable adults.
- A requirement for individuals who wish to work with vulnerable adults to register with the ISA. Registration is only permitted where individuals are judged not to pose a risk to vulnerable adults.
- A requirement for employers to check the register. Employers who permit individuals who are on the barred list to engage in regulated activity commit an offence.
- A requirement for employers to inform the ISA about individuals who have caused harm or pose a risk of harm. This reduces the risk of those who have been dismissed for poor conduct, or who have resigned prior to dismissal, from gaining employment elsewhere.

At the time of writing the UK coalition government has announced its intention to review the system for registration and barring (ISA 2010).

The proposed Vetting and Barring Scheme may contribute to primary prevention by excluding some unsuitable individuals from the workforce. However, such individuals can only be listed where harmful behaviour has been recognised, taken seriously and reported to the ISA, meaning there is potential for some unsuitable individuals to 'slip through the net'. Therefore, reference to the barring lists and registration status of potential employees should be seen as part of a wider approach to positive recruitment practices (Brammer 2010). An important element of positive and inclusive employment practice is to involve people with learning disabilities in the recruitment and selection process. Such a strategy is an important sign that services are committed to the rights of people with learning disabilities to make choices and be in control of their lives (Townsley et al 1997). Townsley et al also recognise the expert experience that people with learning disabilities have in working alongside and receiving help from staff, an expertise which may mean they are well placed to identify applicants with whom they do not feel comfortable, safe or secure. Therefore, including people with learning disabilities in the selection process may help contribute to the identification of unsuitable staff.

While efforts to screen out unsuitable individuals can play an important role in preventing abuse, this approach has been criticised as focusing energy and resources on individuals who are perceived as causing risk, with less emphasis placed on other factors which promote abuse (Manthorpe & Stanley 1999).

The recognition of 'early indicators' of abuse

Marsland et al (2006, 2007) carried out research regarding the abuse of people with learning disabilities in residential settings, which aimed to contribute to the prevention of abuse. This research identified 'early indicators' of abuse in such settings. Early indicators are signs or warnings that service conditions are such that residents are being placed at significant risk of abuse and neglect in the places they live (these indicators are distinct from the indicators of abuse detailed in Box 12.2, which are signs that abuse may already have taken place). Recognising and responding to the presence of early indicators in a service can enable practitioners to take steps at an early stage to protect residents and prevent the onset of abuse. This research builds on explanations of abuse which recognise the importance of service environments and cultures in promoting the conditions in which abuse of residents can occur. It also recognises the inherent abilities and skills of practitioners, such as community nurses, social workers and psychologists, who visit services as part of their professional role, to recognise and respond to signs that 'something is wrong'.

The early indicators identified were grouped under six key headings. Examples of the early indicators identified are presented in Box 12.1.

Secondary prevention: responding effectively

The previous section highlighted the importance of acting to prevent abuse from happening at all. However, it is unfortunate but inevitable that some abuse will occur. Therefore it is vital that such abuse is recognised and that effective and appropriate actions are taken to:

- investigate the suspected abuse
- support the person(s) who has been abused
- prevent the person from being abused again
- prevent others from being abused

(Brown 2003, McCormack et al 2005)

This section will consider the following key issues:

- Recognising abuse.
- Responding to abuse.
- Taking action.

Box 12.1

Early indicators of abuse in residential services

1. The decisions, attitudes and actions of managers

- The managers can't or don't want to make decisions or take responsibility for things.
- The managers don't make sure staff meetings and supervision take place.
- The manager has relatively little experience of working with people with learning disabilities and/or little understanding of the care needs of people with learning disabilities.

2. The behaviours and attitudes of staff

- Members of staff do not manage behaviours in a safe, professional or dignified way.
- Restraint is used frequently and as a first option before other approaches are tried.
- The members of staff do not appear to value people with learning disabilities and treat them as different from themselves and other people.
- There is denial or a lack of concern where the possibility of abuse is raised.

3. The behaviours of people with learning disabilities

- Residents are expressing emotional changes – for example becoming withdrawn, weepy or anxious.
- There are residents who control, bully or harm other residents.

4. Isolation

- There is little input from outsiders and external professionals.
- Members of staff try to manage very complex situations (such as aggression, severe distress) without or against the advice of external professionals.
- Important meetings are arranged at very short notice.

5. Service design, placement planning and commissioning

- Agreed programmes or plans are not being carried out.
- The residents are incompatible.
- Residents with a history of abusing are placed alongside other vulnerable people.

6. Fundamental care and the quality of the environment

- There is poor or inadequate support for residents with health problems who become ill or have special needs (e.g. sensory impairments).
- Residents are not given support to change inappropriate or harmful behaviours.
- There are no or few activities for residents

(Marsland et al 2007)

Reader activity 12.2

Read the following case study and consider whether there are any circumstances which give you cause for concern.

You are the community nurse for Leo, a young man with learning disabilities. Leo has lived at Rowan Hall residential home for the past year. He settled in well and began to make friends with the other four residents. Two months ago, Ellie, the oldest resident, moved to a nursing home and a new resident, Harry, moved in.

On your recent visits you have noticed a change in Leo. He seems unsettled, jumpy and weepy. You discuss his behaviour with staff members who agree 'he's been a bit demanding and all over the place lately', but seem unconcerned. You ask them to keep a daily diary of Leo's activities and emotions. However, when you visit 3 weeks later, there are only a couple of entries in the diary.

You telephone the manager, Kevin, to request that a review meeting is held for Leo. He tells you one is happening later in the week. He apologises for not letting you know, saying he hadn't realised that you might want to come. You ask who else will be attending. Kevin says he's not sure if they have managed to speak with Leo's social worker yet. His dad will not be coming because 'Thursdays are always difficult for him'.

You attend Leo's review. At the review, you raise your concerns about the changes you have seen in Leo. Kevin says that they are having 'teething troubles' with the new resident group and that things haven't quite settled down yet. One staff member says she thinks Leo might be scared of Harry who is often distressed, agitated and shouts and threatens people. Kevin disagrees as he says that Harry only shouts and gets angry with the two women service users 'so it would make no sense for Leo to be getting so upset about that'. You suggest it might be a good idea to arrange some training for the staff in supporting Harry and managing his behaviours. Kevin says he doesn't think that will be needed. A previous manager bought a guide to supporting challenging behaviour – he will find it and make sure the staff refer to that if they think it is necessary. Meanwhile he just wants to let Harry settle in without a fuss, saying 'the last thing we want is for his placement to break down like the last one'.

Recognising abuse

Effective responses to abuse depend upon first recognising that abuse has taken place. The recognition of abuse depends upon closely listening to people with learning disabilities. This includes listening carefully to the things they say, as well as attending to the non-verbal ways in which individuals communicate fear and distress.

Abuse may come to light through disclosure, in which one individual informs another that they have been abused, witnessed abuse or have abused someone else. Disclosures may offer detailed and clear information about what has happened, or a partial disclosure may be made in which the person with learning disabilities indicates that they are being abused, for example mentioning secrets, repeating threats others have made (ARC/NAPSAC 1996). Good practice in responding to disclosures has been identified (ARC/NAPSAC 1996); this includes:

- **Listening** to the person, and believing them. However, you should not ask for details about what happened – this will happen in any later investigation
- **Explaining** what you will do and that you cannot keep what they have told you a secret
- **Recording** what they say, using their own words
- **Taking action**. Follow agency policies regarding safeguarding. Report immediately to a manager. Do not discuss what you have been told with the alleged abuser. (ARC/NAPSAC 1996)

Making a disclosure may be a stressful experience (Joyce 2003) and people with learning disabilities may need encouragement to express and discuss negative feelings and experiences, and to trust that others are willing to listen if they raise difficult and painful issues. Bruder & Stenfert Kroese (2005) highlight the importance of regularly making the time to ask people with learning disabilities how they are and whether anything or anyone has upset them. Taking such steps can help create a culture in which people with learning disabilities feel able and permitted to disclose difficult, abusive or hurtful experiences.

Research has indicated that most abuse comes to light as a result of self-disclosure by people with learning disabilities (Brown et al 1995, McCormack et al 2005). While this is an important means of bringing abuse into the open, people with learning disabilities may be unable to report abusive experiences, due to communication impairments, fear or intimidation. As Brown & Stein (1998:386–387) have noted:

> The dynamics of abuse militate *against* disclosure or discovery, victims are often ashamed or bullied, threats are used to maintain secrecy and the person's credibility called into question if they do try to put what is happening to them into words or to use formal complaints systems.

Given these barriers to disclosure, it is vital that people in the support networks of people with learning disabilities (such as families, friends, staff and professionals) are vigilant to and able to recognise signs that abuse may have occurred. Indicators of abuse have been identified; examples are given in Box 12.2.

Working with indicators of abuse may be complex and problematic. Many of the indicators have multiple potential causes so are not clear and unambiguous. For example, depression is associated with abuse, however, it may also be a response to bereavement, change or other factors. Despite these limitations, the signs listed below highlight that something is very wrong for individuals, and the possibility that abuse is occurring should be considered as one of a range of possible causes.

Box 12.2

Examples of indicators of abuse

Behavioural changes

- Depression.
- Sudden withdrawal from activities.
- Loss of skills.
- Self-injury.
- Disturbed sleep patterns.

Physical signs and medical symptoms

- Bruising.
- Finger marks, slap marks or kick marks.
- Fractures.
- Weight loss.
- Genital infections and sexually transmitted diseases.
- Difficulty sitting or walking.

Circumstantial signs

- Torn underwear.
- Stained underwear.

Financial indicators

- Sudden or unexplained inability to pay bills.
- Sudden or unexplained withdrawal of money from bank accounts.
- Disparity between income/savings and living conditions.

The behaviours of others

- A practitioner or staff member's behaviour towards an individual changing.
- A practitioner/staff member who is secretive and defensive when discussing the person with learning disabilities with colleagues.

(ARC/NAPSAC 1996, Dakin 2007, Nursing and Midwtifery Council 2002)

Reader activity 12.3

You are the care coordinator for Rachel, a young woman with learning disabilities. Rachel lives at home with her mum Barbara, and goes to respite once a month which she enjoys.

Barbara phones to talk to you about Rachel. She tells you that in the last few weeks Rachel has 'not been herself at all'. She has taken to spending a lot of time shut in her room and is reluctant to leave the house. She is eating very little and often says she feels sick. Rachel seems in 'very low spirits' but will not speak to Barbara about what is upsetting her. Rachel is due to go to the respite unit next weekend, but cried and said she didn't want to go when Barbara reminded her.

- What are possible explanations for Rachel's behaviour and distress?
- What initial steps might you take to understand better what is happening for Rachel?

Responding to abuse

The recognition of abuse, or the possibility of abuse, is an important step. Once abuse has been disclosed, witnessed or suspected, it is essential that this is reported, so that actions can be taken to support the person who has been abused and ensure their future safety.

Ignoring abuse, or concerns about abuse, is not an option. *The Code: Standards of Conduct for Nurses and Midwives* (Nursing and Midwifery Council (NMC) 2008) is clear about the professional duty to report concerns, for example stating:

> you must disclose information if you believe that someone may be at risk of harm, in line with the law of the country in which you are practising.
>
> (NMC 2008:2)

and:

> you must act without delay if you believe that you, a colleague or anyone else may be putting someone at risk.
>
> (NMC 2008:3)

This need to report concerns about abuse and risks to service users is also reflected in guidance for social care workers and nurses and midwives working in settings beyond the UK (An Bord Altranais 2000, General Social Care Council 2002).

Following from *No Secrets* (DH 2000) and *In Safe Hands* (National Assembly for Wales 2000) local authorities have developed multi-agency policies to ensure effective responses to actual or suspected abuse. Concerns or evidence of abuse should therefore

Reader activity 12.4

An important element of adult safeguarding is for practitioners to be sure that they know what to do when they have concerns or evidence of abuse. Look up the adult protection/adult safeguarding policy for your local area. You may find this on the website for your local authority area.

be reported in line with local policies. It is essential to be familiar with these policies and your responsibilities, and to know where you should report concerns about abuse and neglect.

Although there is a professional duty to report concerns, this is not always easy. In some situations or settings, people may lack faith that their concerns will be taken seriously and fear the possible consequences of reporting, such as intimidation or harassment by colleagues; in such circumstances, reporting can be a courageous act (Calcraft 2005). Where managers are involved in abusive or poor practice, or fail to respond to reports of abuse, workers may take their concerns outside the usual management structures and report to external agencies; such action is referred to as 'whistleblowing' (Calcraft 2005, Gaylard 2008). The Public Interest Disclosure Act 1998 was developed to offer support and protection to whistleblowers. Under the terms of the Act, individuals who report concerns in good faith should not be discriminated against, lose their job or experience victimisation (Calcraft 2005, Gaylard 2008).

See Reader activity 12.5 on the Evolve website.

Once abuse has been reported, an investigation may take place, the purpose of which includes:

- establishing the facts
- assessing the needs of the person who has been abused
- deciding what further actions are required (DH 2000).

Taking action

A range of actions may be taken where abuse has occurred (ARC/NAPSAC 1996, Brown 2003, Brown & Stein 1998, DH 2000, Martin 2003). These include:

- disciplining staff members
- providing training to staff members to improve practice
- planning how to protect the individual from abuse by another person with learning disabilities
- providing additional services or support, or amending existing services (for example providing same gender care or services if required)
- an individual moving to a new service. Ideally the person who has been abused should not have to move.

Additionally legal action should be considered where a crime has been committed, and the involvement of the police sought. Historically, people with learning disabilities have not been considered reliable witnesses (Corbett et al 1996). The Youth and Criminal Evidence Act 1999 recognises that giving evidence in court can be a stressful and intimidating process. It therefore identified 'special measures' to support vulnerable witnesses. These include the following (Brammer 2010):

- Giving evidence behind screens or via video link.
- The use of videotaped evidence.
- The removal of wigs and gowns in court.
- Examination by an intermediary who is skilled in communication and can explain the question asked, and the witness' responses to the court.

The use of special measures may enable people with learning disabilities who have experienced crime to take legal action against an abuser.

Where a vulnerable adult is being interviewed as a suspect or charged with an offence, they are entitled, under the Police and Criminal Evidence Act 1984, to the support of an appropriate adult. The role of the appropriate adult includes (Brammer 2010):

- advising the suspect
- observing whether the interview is carried out properly and fairly
- facilitating communication.

Tertiary prevention: emotional support and aftercare

As has already been seen, the experience of abuse can be traumatic and distressing. Therefore, in addition to taking practical action to ensure the safety of individuals and reduce the risk of future abuse, it is also important to consider the emotional needs of those who have been abused.

Approaches to respond to the trauma of abuse have been described. Workers such as Sinason (1992) and Corbett et al (1996) have written accounts of providing therapy to people with learning disabilities who have been abused. Such therapy can provide an important space in which the voice of the person who has been abused can be heard, believed and respected, and in which support and empathy can be offered (Corbett et al 1996). Perhaps contrary to expectations, Sinason (1992) states that levels of intelligence or verbal abilities are not prerequisites for benefitting from therapy, and Corbett (2003) presents an account of providing therapeutic support to a person with learning disabilities who used little verbal communication.

Group work may also offer an important source of support for people with learning disabilities who have been abused, in which participants may gain support from group workers as well as other group members. Peckham et al (2007) described the work of a support group for women survivors of sexual abuse. They concluded that the participants appeared to develop increased sexual knowledge, and that symptoms of depression and trauma decreased. They also identified an initial increase in challenging behaviour, which later improved, illustrating the emotional demands which such work asks of participants.

Some common themes emerge from the accounts of providing individual or group support to people with learning disabilities. First, such work is complex and may require significant time (and therefore resources). Second, the provision of such support is a skilled role, requiring training, support and supervision. (However, while the provision of therapeutic support may be a specialist role, this is not to suggest that other practitioners should not be willing to hear and acknowledge painful experiences and to take a supportive and empathetic approach.) Third, it is apparent that accessing appropriate emotional support for people with learning disabilities who have been abused can be difficult, and therefore support needs may remain unmet.

The apparent paucity of specialist provision offers a reminder that the ability of generic services to support people with learning disabilities should be explored. Howlett & Danby (2007) carried out a pilot project to make the support of a mainstream rape counselling service available to women with learning disabilities. They concluded that the service:

> provided a respectful, empowering environment in which women with learning disabilities have been able to explore their experiences of sexual abuse. It offered them the opportunity ... to resolve feelings about what had happened to them in the past, thereby promoting self-esteem and control of their lives, enabling them to move towards a stronger future.
>
> (Howlett & Danby 2007:9)

This section suggests that finding appropriate and skilled sources of emotional support to reduce the impact of abuse may be difficult. However, where the experience of abuse appears to have been traumatic, steps should be taken to attempt to identify – or develop – appropriate and compassionate sources of support.

Safeguarding – towards inclusion

Work to safeguard people with learning disabilities, which has often used the language of 'vulnerability' and 'protection', is open to charges of paternalism; as Collins & Walford (2008:7) have observed, historically such work was "for vulnerable adults, but not with them". In a book that considers the journey of people with learning disabilities 'towards inclusion', it is important to reflect upon how the focus of safeguarding work could move towards greater partnership working with people with learning disabilities.

Projects which have attempted such partnership work have identified a lack of information and awareness of abuse as a potential barrier to people with learning disabilities acting to protect themselves and report abuse, and have recognised their fundamental right to be able to access such information. Without information, knowledge and awareness about abuse and safeguarding, there is a risk that people with learning disabilities may become:

- disempowered, not recognising their treatment and experiences as abusive and harmful
- silenced, not knowing how to report their experiences
- isolated from sources of support.

(Miklasz & White 2008:4)

People with learning disabilities themselves have also identified this need for information, stating:

> Abuse can happen anywhere ... You can't be kept totally safe from abuse. But I need to know what to do or who can help.
>
> (DH 2009:15)

Different approaches have been adopted to raise awareness and provide accessible information about abuse to people with learning disabilities. Bearder & Ball (1997) and Miklasz & White (2008) have provided accounts of projects which used drama to raise awareness. In Wales, college-based 'Keeping Safe' courses have been developed (Collins & Walford 2008). The aims of these projects have included enabling people with learning disabilities to identify abusive situations and to recognise that abuse is always wrong, to develop personal safety plans, and to consider who they could tell if they have been abused or frightened.

The projects described above represent important attempts to ensure that people with learning disabilities have opportunities to consider how to avoid risky situations and to identify appropriate sources of support to whom they can disclose abuse if necessary. However, this work should never be perceived as a substitute for good support and detection of abuse by practitioners. Accessing information, while important, may not be sufficient to enable people to report abusive or harmful experiences, for example where they are afraid or intimidated. McCarthy & Thompson (1996) have cautioned that an emphasis on education risks 'victim blaming' when people with learning disabilities 'fail' to avoid abuse, offering a reminder that steps to empower people with learning disabilities must take place alongside attempts to change the behaviours of others, as well as the environmental and societal factors that place individuals at risk (Hollomotz 2009). However, despite the importance of ensuring that the full weight of responsibility is not placed upon people with learning disabilities, it remains important to identify ways of ensuring that they have opportunities to become active participants in their own protection.

Conclusion

This chapter has highlighted the risks faced by people with learning disabilities in their lives. Such abuse can be distressing and traumatic, although the resilience and coping skills of this group should not be overlooked. The risks of abuse for people with learning disabilities means that practitioners have a professional duty to take steps to prevent the onset of abuse, to recognise and respond to the abuse of individuals, as well as to work alongside them, ensuring they have the necessary skills and knowledge to enable them to address their own protection.

References

An Bord Altranais, 2000. The code of professional conduct for each nurse and midwife. Available at: http://www.nursingboard.ie/en/policies-guidelines.aspx?page2 (accessed 19.04.10.).

Armstrong, J., 2008. The Scottish legislation: the way forward? In: Mantell, A., Scragg, T. (Eds.), Safeguarding adults in social work. Learning Matters, Exeter, pp. 60–71.

Association of Directors of Social Services, 2005. Safeguarding adults. A national framework of standards for good practice and outcomes in adult protection work. Association of Directors of Social Services, London.

Association for Residential Care/ National Association for the Protection from Sexual Abuse of Adults and Children with Learning Disabilities (ARC/NAPSAC), 1996. It could never happen here! The prevention and treatment of sexual abuse of people with learning disabilities in residential settings. In: Churchill, J., Craft, A., Holding, A., Horrocks, C. (Eds.), ARC/NAPSAC, Chesterfield/Nottingham.

Bearder, C., Ball, L., 1997. Towards educating adults with learning disabilities on issues of abuse: a report of an innovative use of dance, drama and mime. Journal of Learning Disabilities for Nursing, Health and Social Care 1, 120–130.

Better Days/Coast2Coast/Inclusion North, 2008. Learning disability hate crime. Good practice guidance for crime and disorder reduction partnerships and learning disability partnership boards. Available at: http://www.inclusionnorth.org/documents/Hate%20Crime%20Good%20Practice%20Guide.pdf (accessed 21.04.10.).

Brammer, A., 2010. Social work law, third ed. Pearson Education, Harlow.

Brown, H., 1999. Abuse of people with learning disabilities – layers of concern and analysis. In: Stanley, N., Manthorpe, J., Penhale, B. (Eds.), Institutional abuse: perspectives across the lifecourse. Routledge, London, pp. 89–109.

Brown, H., 2003. Safeguarding adults and children with disabilities against abuse. Council of Europe Publishing, Strasbourg.

Brown, H., 2007. Editorial. The Journal of Adult Protection 9, 2–5.

Brown, H., Stein, J., 1998. Implementing adult abuse policies in Kent and East Sussex. J. Soc. Policy 27, 371–396.

Brown, H., Turk, V., 1992. Defining sexual abuse as it affects adults with learning disabilities. Mental Handicap 20, 44–55.

Brown, H., Stein, J., Turk, V., 1995. The sexual abuse of adults with learning disabilities: report of a second two-year incidence survey. Mental Handicap Research 8, 3–24.

Bruder, C., Stenfert Kroese, B., 2005. The efficacy of interventions designed to prevent and protect people with intellectual disabilities from sexual abuse: a review of the literature. The Journal of Adult Protection 7, 13–27.

Butler, I., Drakeford, M., 2005. Scandal, social policy and social welfare, second ed. ASW/Policy Press, Bristol.

Calcraft, R., 2005. Blowing the whistle on the abuse of adults with learning disabilities. Ann Craft Trust, Nottingham.

Cambridge, P., 1999. The first hit: a case study of the physical abuse of people with learning disabilities and challenging behaviours in a residential service. Disability and Society 14, 285–308.

Collins, M., Walford, M., 2008. Helping vulnerable adults keep safe. The Journal of Adult Protection 10, 7–12.

Commission for Social Care Inspection/ Healthcare Commission, 2006. Joint investigation into the provision of services for people with learning disabilities at Cornwall Partnership NHS Trust. Commission for Healthcare, Audit and Inspection, London.

Corbett, A., 2003. The psychotherapeutic needs of people with learning disabilities who have been sexually abused. The Journal of Adult Protection 5, 28–33.

Corbett, A., Cottis, T., Morris, S., 1996. Witnessing, nurturing, protesting. Therapeutic responses to sexual abuse of people with learning disabilities. David Fulton, London.

Dakin, M., 2007. Whose secret? Protecting vulnerable adults from abuse. Pavilion, Brighton.

Department of Health, 2000. No secrets. Guidance on developing and implementing multi-agency policies and procedures to protect vulnerable adults from abuse. Department of Health, London.

Department of Health, 2001. Valuing people: a new strategy for learning disability for the 21st Century. Department of Health, London.

Department of Health, 2008. Safeguarding Adults. A consultation on the review of the 'No secrets' guidance. Department of Health, London.

Department of Health, 2009. Safeguarding adults. Report on the consultation on the review of 'No secrets'. Department of Health, London.

Flynn, M., 2007. The murder of Steven Hoskin. A serious case review executive summary. Cornwall Adult Protection Committee. Available at: http://www.nwtdt.com/Cornwall/Steven%20Hoskins%20executive%20summary.pdf (accessed 12.01.10.).

Flynn, M., Brown, H., 1997. The responsibilities of commissioners, purchasers and providers: lessons from the recent National Development Team-led inquiries. In: Churchill, J., Brown, H., Craft, A., Horrocks, C. (Eds.), There are no easy answers: the provision of continuing care and treatment to adults with learning disabilities who sexually abuse others. ARC/NAPSAC, Chesterfield/ Nottingham.

Fyson, R., 2009. Independence and learning disabilities: why we must also recognise vulnerability. The Journal of Adult Protection 11, 18–25.

Gaylard, D., 2008. Policy and practice. In: Mantell, A., Scragg, T. (Eds.), Safeguarding adults in social work. Learning Matters, Exeter, pp. 9–30.

General Social Care Council, 2002. Codes of practice for social care workers. General Social Care Council, London.

Hollomotz, A., 2009. Beyond 'vulnerability': an ecological model approach to conceptualizing risk of sexual violence against people with learning difficulties. British Journal of Social Work 39, 99–112.

Howlett, S., Danby, J., 2007. Learning disability and sexual abuse: use of a women-only counselling service by women with a learning disability: a pilot study. Learning Disability Review 12, 4–15.

Independent Safeguarding Authority, 2010. Available at: http://www.isa-gov.org.uk (accessed 4.02.10 and 21/11/10.).

Joyce, T., 2003. An audit of investigations into allegations of abuse involving adults with intellectual disability. J. Intellect. Disabil. Res. 47, 606–616.

Livingstone, J., 2006. My money matters. Guidance on the best practice in handling the money of people with learning disabilities. ARC, Chesterfield.

McCarthy, M., 1999. Sexuality and women with learning disabilities. Jessica Kingsley, London.

McCarthy, M., Thompson, D., 1996. Sexual abuse by design: an examination of the issues in learning disability services. Disability and Society 11, 205–218.

McCormack, B., Kavanagh, D., Caffrey, S., Power, A., 2005. Investigating sexual abuse: findings of a 15 year longitudinal study. J. Appl. Res. Intellect. Disabil. 18, 217–227.

Mackay, K., 2008. The Scottish adult support and protection framework. The Journal of Adult Protection 10, 25–35.

Magill, J., Yeates, V., Longley, M., 2010. Review of In Safe Hands. A review of the Welsh Assembly Government's guidance on the protection of vulnerable adults in Wales. Welsh Institute for Health and Social Care. University of Glamorgan, Pontypridd.

Mandelstam, M., 2009. Safeguarding vulnerable adults and the law. Jessica Kingsley, London.

Manthorpe, J., Stanley, N., 1999. Conclusion. Shifting the focus from 'bad apples' to users' rights. In: Stanley, N., Manthorpe, J., Penhale, B. (Eds.), Institutional abuse: perspectives across the lifecourse. Routledge, London, pp. 223–240.

Marsland, D., Oakes, P., Tweddell, I., White, C., 2006. Abuse in care? A practical guide to protecting people with learning disabilities from abuse in residential services. University of Hull, Hull.

Marsland, D., Oakes, P., White, C., 2007. Abuse in care? The identification of early indicators of the abuse of people with learning disabilities in residential settings. The Journal of Adult Protection 9, 6–20.

Martin, J., 1984. Hospitals in trouble. Basil Blackwell, Oxford.

Martin, J., 2003. Safeguarding adults. Russell House, Lyme Regis.

May-Chahal, C., Bertotti, T., Blasio, P., Di, Cerezo, M.A., Gerard, M., Grevot, A., Lamers, F., McGrath, K., Thorpe, D.H., Thyen, U., Al-Hamad, A., 2006. Child maltreatment in the family: a European perspective. European Journal of Social Work 9, 3–20.

Mencap, 1999. Living in fear. The need to combat bullying of people with a learning disability. Mencap, London.

Miklasz, H., White, C., 2008. Acting to protect. Using drama to inform people with learning disabilities about abuse. Ann Craft Trust Bulletin 63, 4–9.

National Assembly for Wales, 2000. In safe hands. Implementing adult protection in Wales. National Assembly for Wales, Cardiff.

Nursing and Midwifery Council, 2002. Practitioner–client relationships and the prevention of abuse. Available at: http://www.nmc-uk.org/aDisplayDocument.aspx?documentID=520 (accessed 18.02.10.).

Nursing and Midwifery Council, 2008. The code. Standards of conduct, performance and ethics for nurses and midwives. Available at: http://www.nmc-uk.org/Documents/Standards/nmcTheCodeStandardsofConductPerformanceAndEthicsForNursesAndMidwives_TextVersion.pdf (accessed 18.02.10.).

O'Callaghan, A.C., Murphy, G., Clare, I. C.H., 2003. Symptoms of abuse in adults with severe learning disabilities. Final report to the Department of Health. Tizard Centre. University of Kent, Canterbury.

Peckham, N.G., 2007. The vulnerability and sexual abuse of people with learning disabilities. British Journal of Learning Disabilities 35, 131–137.

Peckham, N.G., Corbett, A., Howlett, S., et al., 2007. The delivery of a survivors group for learning disabled women who have been abused. British Journal of Learning Disabilities 35, 236–244.

Powerhouse, 1996. Power in the house. Women with learning difficulties organising against abuse. In: Morris, J. (Ed.), Encounters with strangers; feminism and disability. The Women's Press, London.

Quarmby, K., 2008. Getting away with murder. Disabled people's experiences of hate crime in the UK. Scope, London.

Sense, 2000. Would 'No secrets' have saved Beverley? Talking Sense 46 (3) Available at: http://www.sense.org.uk/publicationslibrary/allpubs/talking-sense/tsarticles/2000/nosecret.htm.

Sequeira, H., Howlin, P., Hollins, S., 2003. Psychological symptoms associated with sexual abuse in people with learning disabilities: case control study. Br. J. Psychiatry 183, 451–456.

Sinason, V., 1992. Mental handicap and the human condition. New approaches from the Tavistock. Free Association Press, London.

Sobsey, D., 1994. Sexual abuse of individuals with intellectual disability. In: Craft, A. (Ed.), Practice issues in sexuality and learning disabilities. Routledge, London.

Townsley, R., Howarth, J., Le Grys, P., Macadam, M., 1997. Getting involved in choosing staff. A resource pack for supporters, trainers and staff working with people with learning disabilities. Pavilion, Brighton.

Wardhaugh, J., Wilding, P., 1993. Towards an explanation of the corruption of care. Critical Social Policy 37, 4–31.

White, C., Holland, E., Marsland, D., Oakes, P., 2003. The identification of environments and cultures that promote the abuse of people with intellectual disabilities: a review of the literature. J. Appl. Res. Intellect. Disabil. 16, 1–9.

Wishart, G., 2003. The sexual abuse of people with learning difficulties: do we need a social model approach to vulnerability? The Journal of Adult Protection 5, 14–27.

Further reading

Brammer, A., 2010. Adult protection in social work law, third ed. Pearson Education, Harlow.

Brown, H., 1999. Abuse of people with learning disabilities – layers of concern and analysis. In: Stanley, N., Manthorpe, J., Penhale, B. (Eds.), Institutional abuse: perspectives across the lifecourse. Routledge, London, pp. 89–109.

O'Callaghan, A.C., Murphy, G., Clare, C.H.C., 2003. The impact of abuse on men and women with severe learning disabilities and their families. British Journal of Learning Disabilities 31, 175–180.

White, C., Holland, E., Marsland, D., Oakes, P., 2003. The identification of environments and cultures that promote the abuse of people with intellectual disabilities: a review of the literature. J. Appl. Res. Intellect. Disabil. 16, 1–9.

Useful addresses

The following organisations can provide information, resources and advice where there are concerns about the abuse of people with learning disabilities.

The Ann Craft Trust,
Centre for Social Work,
University of Nottingham,
University Park,
Nottingham NG7 2RD,
Tel: 0115 951 5400:
http://www.anncrafttrust.org.

Respond,
3rd Floor,
24–32 Stephenson Way,
London NW1 2HD,
Tel: 020 7383 0700
Helpline 080 8808 0700:
http://www.respond.org.uk.

Voice UK,
Rooms 100–106,
Kelvin House,
RTC Business Centre,
London Road,
Derby DE24 8UP,
Tel: 01332 291 042,
Helpline: 080 8802 8686:
http://www.voiceuk.org.uk.

Section 3

Overcoming challenges to good health

13 Enabling good health

Kim Scarborough Matthew Godsell

CHAPTER CONTENTS

KEY ISSUES

- Social and organisational factors have contributed to the inequalities separating the health of people with learning disabilities from the health of the rest of the population
- To develop effective strategies for promoting health and wellbeing, practitioners need to combine their knowledge of individual patients or clients and their families with a sound understanding of their communities
- Advocacy, enablement and mediation are key actions in promoting good health
- A range of person-centred strategies exist to encourage positive health behaviours among people with learning disabilities
- Ensuring accessibility to such interventions is a key role of health and social care providers with effective communication a core component of this process
- Continual monitoring and evaluation of how health inequalities are being tackled is important at a strategic, local and personal level

Introduction

This chapter will examine the social and political context in which health and social care is delivered. It also identifies some of the ways in which services and professionals will be expected to perform to reduce health inequalities. *Enablement, Mediation and Advocacy* introduces a model that combines these activities with practitioners' knowledge of their local community so that they are encouraged to think strategically about promoting health. Social determinants of health will be considered and how a combination of 'top-down' and 'bottom-up' strategies can change the dynamic that connects social institutions, practitioners and people with learning disabilities. Detail focusing on the nature of interventions that improve health will be provided. Material includes health action plans (and alternatives to them), behavioural change, motivational interviewing, providing support to keep people healthy and managing illness.

Finally, the focus returns to larger scale initiatives and developments, addressing monitoring and evaluating health care, teaching and training health care workers and new roles for learning disabilities practitioners.

Health and difference: discrimination and prejudice

Since the production of the World Health Organization's (WHO) definition of health in 1946, the definitions and models that represent the essential components of health and wellbeing have gone through a succession of revisions and changes. These revisions and changes have responded to and precipitated changes in the practice and delivery of health and social care, policy and the production of evidence that supports practice. The definition that was produced in 1946 was regarded as an improvement on the concepts that preceded it because it represented health and wellbeing as something more sophisticated than a smooth running machine that performed most efficiently and effectively when it was not impeded by disease or infirmity. The WHO (1946) definition has three core components:

> Health is a state of complete physical, mental and social wellbeing.

A complete state might mean balancing physical, mental and social elements. It might also refer to an optimum state which cannot be improved. The interpretation and application of these components warrant further exploration because they can be used to illustrate how some conceptions of health and wellbeing might become divisive and exclusive. Although the original definition is embedded in a larger body of work that sought to improve health across the globe, the links that connect physical and mental health and social wellbeing might be seen by a contemporary practitioner as contentious.

When a state of 'completeness' is associated with an optimum level of performance or an enduring balanced state, the definition will best serve those populations where the aim of an intervention is to restore an individual so that they might perform at an optimum level or to restore equilibrium. People with long-term conditions, for example people with learning disabilities, people with a mental illness and people with physical impairments, have been set apart from those people that might be restored to a peak level of performance or have their equilibrium restored. They are perceived by some groups within society as possessing less value or merit than people without those conditions in the same way that a jigsaw puzzle with a piece missing might be described as incomplete or broken when it is contrasted with a complete, finished puzzle. In a social system where economic conditions dictate that the resources that have been dedicated to health care are under constant scrutiny, there is likely to be much debate around the funding that is allocated to a minority group like people with learning disabilities. Funding may be contested on the grounds that the interests of a small group are being promoted before the interests of the majority; a movement that will be viewed by some people as running counter to the utilitarian values embedded in an organisation like the National Health Service (NHS).

While any discussion about utilitarian values and merit may appear abstract in a chapter on enabling health and wellbeing, the inequitable distribution of resources within the health and social care systems has consequences which are observable and measurable at the point of delivery. At a macro level, decisions about the resources that have been allocated to a specific group of clients, patients or service users will determine how many practitioners with specialised knowledge are available to deliver a dedicated service. Similar decisions will also determine how much preparation (teaching, supervision and training) is available to support generic practitioners who have acquired more responsibility for extending their services to a broader population. At a micro level, beliefs about the rights and status of people with learning disabilities and their entitlement to health services are going to shape the ways in which people respond to them at reception desks, in waiting areas, surgeries and treatment rooms.

Equity is recognised as a principle that informs the delivery of health and social care services in the United Kingdom. Many of the professions that contribute to health and social care have a code of conduct or ethos which embraces diversity. A belief that health services should be available to everyone, irrespective of their ability to pay for them, was a cornerstone in the foundation of the NHS. The *Standards of Conduct, Performance and Ethics for Nurses and Midwives* produced by the Nursing and Midwifery Council (NMC 2008) states that nurses and midwives "must not discriminate in any way against those in your care" and that they must "demonstrate a personal and professional commitment to equality and diversity". Despite the widespread recognition that this principle has received from nursing and other professional groups, there is a considerable body of evidence which shows that recognition has not been translated into actions that promote and maintain the health of people with learning disabilities. The Disability Rights Commission (2006) has gathered data about the health inequalities experienced by people with learning disabilities and/or mental health problems, and Mencap (2004, 2007) has gathered evidence about the inadequate treatment that people with learning disabilities have received in primary and secondary care. The Parliamentary and Health Service Ombudsman and Local Government Ombudsman (2009) have also reported on the deaths of six people while in the care of the NHS. The evidence reveals that people with learning disabilities have not received the same benefits from health services as the rest of the population. Some of the material goes a stage further; showing that health care practitioners have been instrumental in perpetuating inequalities and excluding people from the services and treatment that they need.

Guidance on improving the delivery of services has addressed two different groups; practitioners that have intermittent contact and specialists. The report produced by Sir Jonathan Michael (Michael 2008:36) has made recommendations for improving the understanding of practitioners with limited personal experience of people with learning disabilities. The recommendation suggests that the curricula for undergraduate and postgraduate clinical training must address learning disabilities. It also states that people with learning disabilities and carers should be involved in delivering training. Another recommendation is better record keeping and data collection so that people with learning disabilities can be identified by the health service and their pathways of care tracked (Michael 2008:37). *Valuing People* (Department of Health (DH) 2001a:60) identified a historical problem that has led to an imbalance in the delivery of health services from specialist and mainstream providers. It stated that mainstream services had been slow in acquiring the capacity and skills to meet the needs of people with learning disabilities whereas NHS specialists had been slow to devolve some aspects of their service to other providers. It may have been the case that specialised services and practitioners were compelled to acquire exclusive responsibility because precedent suggested that without them many people with learning disabilities would be excluded from health care. It may also be argued that the problem was created because specialised practitioners protected their interests by defending their professional 'territory'. It may be a 'chicken and egg' style debate, nevertheless the document contained an explicit acknowledgement that the imbalance between mainstream and specialist services was "the most important issue" the NHS needed to address.

The White Paper (DH 2001a, p.69) described four complementary tasks that should be undertaken by specialists working in learning disabilities services. The aim of these tasks was to establish a better balance between the input from mainstream and specialist services. Specialists were encouraged to develop:

- a health promotion role; working closely with the local health promotion team
- a health facilitation role; working with primary care teams, community health professionals and staff involved in delivering secondary health care
- a teaching role; to enable a wide range of staff, including those who work in social services and the independent sector, to become more familiar with how to support people with learning disabilities to have their health needs met
- a service development role; contributing their knowledge of health issues to planning processes.

Shaping the Future (Northway et al 2006) referred to similar skills in a vision for learning disabilities nursing. Contributors stated that the "breadth, depth and combination of skills and knowledge" (p. 9) acquired by learning disabilities nurses gave them a unique opportunity to enhance the delivery of care for people with learning disabilities. This document placed particular emphasis on leadership and directed learning disabilities nurses to improve standards of care by providing the sort of leadership that inspired and influenced others. Contributors made specific reference to the range of personal, cognitive and social qualities described in the *NHS Leadership Qualities Framework* (NHS Modernisation Agency Leadership Centre 2003) that contribute to effective leadership. The clusters that they identified are:

- personal qualities – self-belief, self-awareness, self-management, drive for improvement and personal integrity
- setting direction – broad scanning, intellectual flexibility, seizing the future, political astuteness and drive for results
- delivering the service – leading change through people, holding to account, empowering others, effective and strategic thinking and collaborative working.

Enablement, mediation and advocacy

The Ottawa Charter (WHO 1986:1) added to the original WHO (1946) definition by declaring that health is:

> ... a resource for everyday life, not the objective of living. Health is a positive concept emphasizing social and personal resources as well as physical capacities.

This definition locates health in a dynamic relationship that draws on social resources in addition to personal resources. A similar understanding has been used to establish the philosophical and ideological foundation that supports the policy expressed in *Valuing People* (DH 2001a) and *Valuing People Now* (HM Government 2009). Health is part of a network of services that extends into housing, work, education, transport, leisure, social activities and the judicial system. The links that connect health with a wide range of resources and services are a helpful way of encouraging practitioners to appraise the relationship between people's health and their environment. When this understanding is applied to the lives of people with learning disabilities, it reveals a heterogeneous population that has complex relationships with a diverse range of professionals and services. People occupy social networks that reflect significant differences related to income, accommodation, social class, gender, age and family structure as well as communities that have different ethnic identities and sexual preferences. The resources that determine the quality of 'everyday life' might be distributed unevenly between these groups. People with severe cognitive and physical impairments and/or enduring mental health issues are likely to have to dedicate a significant amount of their resources towards the maintenance of their health. This might mean that the amount of time and money at their disposal for social and leisure activities is restricted. Conversely some people with milder impairments and good health may be in a position that enables them to make more choices from a greater range of options that determine their lifestyle. The fact that some people have fewer choices suggests that the pursuit of health may not feel like a resource that is accessible on an everyday basis and those people may be more inclined to feel that the attainment of stable or better health has become the 'objective' of living.

To develop effective strategies for promoting health and wellbeing, practitioners need to combine their knowledge of individual patients or clients and their families with a sound understanding of their communities. This type of knowledge might include information about the characteristics which make some sectors within a population more vulnerable or susceptible to a wider range of risks than other sectors. The Centre for Disability Research (Emerson & Hatton 2008:14) produced information which looks at the characteristics that distinguish different sections of the population with learning disabilities. One in five people (19%) with learning disabilities smoked cigarettes. This rate was highest in people with mild to moderate disabilities (30%), 11% of people with severe disabilities smoked and 4% of people with profound and multiple disabilities. Rates of smoking were higher in people living in private households (rather than supported accommodation). One in five people with learning disabilities (20%) reported that they exercised three or more times per week. This was highest among people with mild to moderate learning disabilities (23%), 11% of people with severe learning disabilities exercised (three or more times per week) and 9% of people with profound and multiple disabilities. The rates of exercising were higher in people living in private households (26% of people with mild to moderate learning disabilities living in private households exercised three or more times per week whereas the figure for people with mild to moderate disabilities living in supported accommodation was 16%). The report also stated that the uptake of all health services was higher for people living in supported accommodation than it was for people living in private households. People living in private households were more likely to live in areas characterised by higher levels of hardship and deprivation (Emerson & Hatton 2008:9). The finding reinforces a statement made by the Healthcare Commission (2005:4) which asserted that people with learning disabilities "are among the most deprived and excluded populations in the UK".

The emblem for the First International Conference on Health Promotion (see Fig. 13.1) held in Ottawa (WHO 1986) identified activities that required practitioners to utilise their knowledge of local communities.

The three wings represent the activities (reorienting health services, creating supportive environments, developing personal skills and strengthening community action) that will extend health promotion into different communities. The three activities

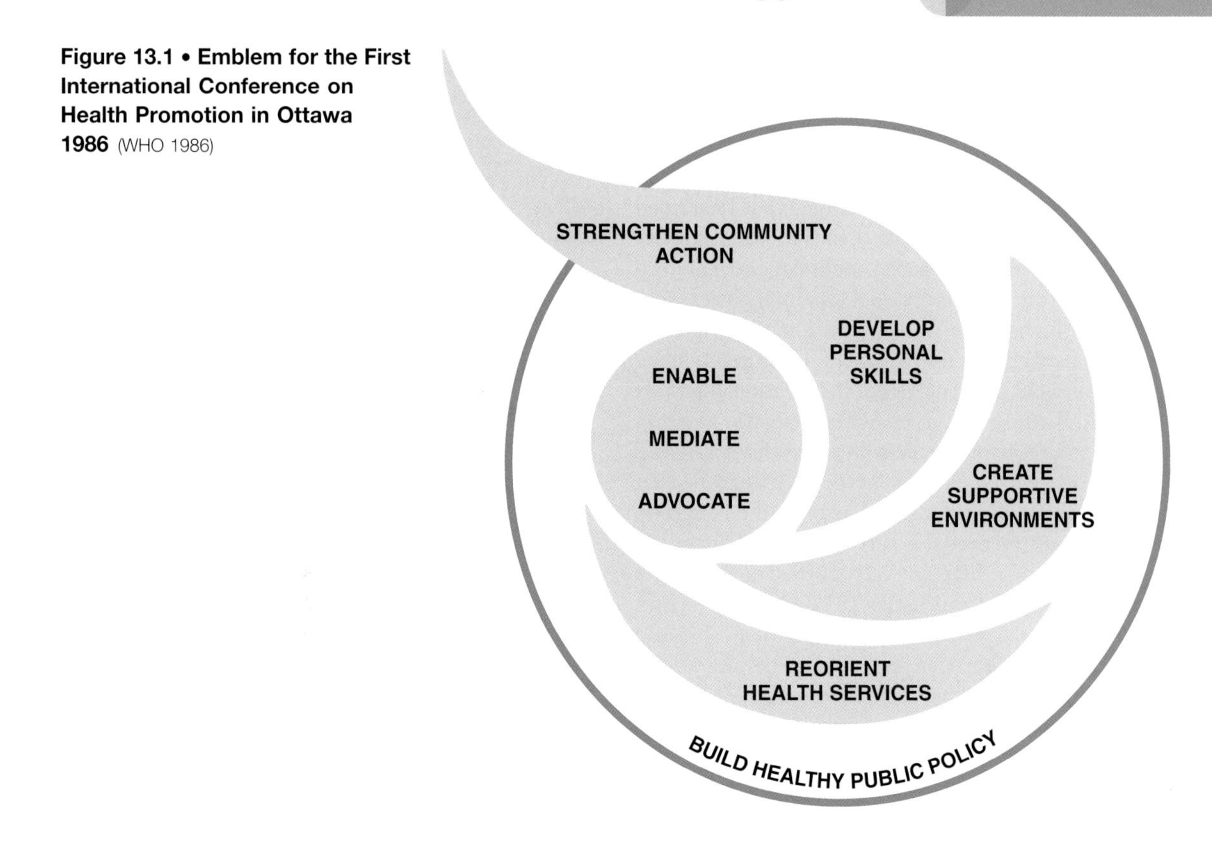

Figure 13.1 • Emblem for the First International Conference on Health Promotion in Ottawa 1986 (WHO 1986)

in the circle towards the middle of the emblem represent the actions that practitioners might take to promote change. Advocacy requires practitioners to work towards creating an environment where the political, social, economic, cultural, environmental, behavioural and biological factors leading to good health are most likely to flourish. Enablement requires practitioners to develop resources that people can use to improve their health and provide the encouragement and support that they need to use them. Mediation means that practitioners should act to facilitate networks and connections that bring different services and services providers (for example statutory, private and voluntary providers) together to improve health.

The NMC Code (2008) stipulates that all nurses and midwives must advocate for people in their care by helping them to access relevant health and social services, information and support. Although The Code does not make explicit references to activities that have been defined as enablement and mediation, there are other standards that describe similar activities. Nurses must collaborate with people in their care by supporting them so that they can improve and maintain their own health. Nurses must also share information and work effectively in teams by consulting and taking advice from colleagues. A service that is moving towards equity, one that is capable of reducing health inequalities for people with learning disabilities, will use advocacy in different ways. Practitioners inexperienced in working with people with learning disabilities will have to recognise that they are entitled to the same level of service as the rest of the population – even when this entitlement leads to them receiving more time or attention if this is what it takes to provide them with access to a service. Specialised practitioners will have to take on an enhanced and expanded role so that they might work and liaise with other services in order to educate, train and support colleagues with dissimilar backgrounds. They will also have to embrace the principle that investing time in developing collaborative relationships with other health workers is likely to be an investment that is as important as the relationships that they have developed with people with learning disabilities and carers.

The social determinants of health

The model developed by Dahlgren & Whitehead (1991) provided a series of headings that described the social determinants of health. Social determinants are a range of social, political and environmental factors and individual characteristics that influence the health of a person or a population. This model is particularly useful when practitioners need to develop a detailed analysis of the relationships that link an individual or a group with a specific environment. At the core of the model are the characteristics linked to age, sex and/or hereditary factors that define an individual or group. The individual or group at the core of the model is surrounded by concentric arcs representing different factors that may interact with the core characteristics to determine health. The distance that separates the individual or group from different arcs can be used to evaluate the impact of a range of factors that combine to shape the health of a citizen or a community. These main determinants of health are shown at Figure 13.2.

The idea of 'choice' (explored in detail in Ch. 21) will be used to show how multiple factors operating at different levels can have a bearing on health. People might not be able to make choices about their age or their genetic make up but they may be able to make choices about the lifestyles they lead. The decisions that they make might influence their diet, the amount of exercise they take, the extent to which they socialise with other people or their level of sexual activity. Similarly people might make decisions about how they engage with their community. In its broadest sense, this means a group of people that share common interests or features as well as people that live close to each other. Consequently, choices might involve the people an individual likes to associate with as well as where they live. The model can also encourage practitioners to focus on areas where choices are constrained. Some people with learning disabilities may not be able to convey their choices, others do not have the resources they need to move away from their families, to relocate themselves in a new neighbourhood or to quit their job and look for a better one.

Change is a dynamic process that can originate in the external layers as well as the core so socioeconomic, cultural and environmental conditions can have an impact on the individual as well as individuals or groups making an impact on those conditions. Individuals may combine and use their influence to instigate change in their communities, or at national level, by forming pressure groups and leading campaigns. The activity of the groups involved in *Nothing About Us Without Us* (DH 2001b) gave people with learning disabilities a chance to represent their views on health and health services so that they were included in the development of the policies that were articulated in *Valuing People* (DH 2001a). The emergence of learning disability partnership boards has also created opportunities for people with learning disabilities and carers to communicate their views on the suitability of local services and to suggest areas where improvements can be made. These developments can be seen as changes that have enabled the users of services to influence the providers of services. This sort of communication is 'bottom-upwards' but there is also 'top-downwards' communication where a powerful body

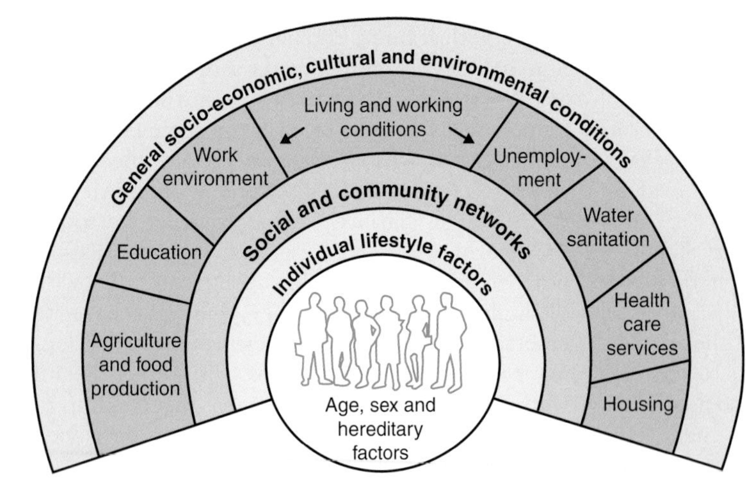

Figure 13.2 • Dahlgren & Whitehead's determinants of health model (Dahlgren & Whitehead 1991: http://www.pharmacymeetspublichealth.org.uk/publichealthbackground_determinants.html)

or agency, for example central government or the Department of Health, instigate large-scale change by implementing legislation or issuing guidance. In this instance, legislation or policy may regulate the behaviour of individuals or organisations (for example services providing employment, health or education). The Disability Discrimination Act (Her Majesty's Stationery Office (HMSO) 1995, 2005a) and the Mental Capacity Act (HMSO 2005b) are pieces of legislation that have a bearing on the treatment that people with learning disabilities receive in the NHS. The Disability Discrimination Act made it unlawful to discriminate against people with disabilities and a legal requirement for service providers to make 'reasonable adjustments' to accommodate them.

Giraud-Saunders (2009) has produced a single equality scheme for improving access for people with learning disabilities. *Equal Access* provides practical examples and best practice as well as the top tips shown in Box 13.1 (Giraud-Saunders 2009:32) for making improvements.

The Mental Capacity Act (HMSO 2005b) established the principle that everything must be done in the best interests of the patient. This means that a person is assumed to have the capacity to make decisions about care or treatment unless there is evidence to the contrary. The Act was implemented to protect people that are especially vulnerable by giving practitioners a framework that told them who should make decisions and the situations in which those decisions might be made. The Act also gave authority to the role of independent mental capacity advocate (IMCA) (see Ch. 7). NHS bodies and local authorities have a duty to consult IMCAs when certain decisions must be made about people that lack capacity but have no family, friends or others to advocate for them. Like the Disability Discrimination Act, the Mental Capacity Act and the Adults with Incapacity (Scotland) Act 2000 state that practical steps should be taken to present information to individuals with learning disabilities so that they can make sense of it. This type of legislation has been implemented to change the behaviour of practitioners and other people providing services that have an immediate impact on living and working conditions. At an interpersonal level it has been designed to change the ways in which practitioners and organisations communicate with people with learning disabilities. At a societal level it has added legal sanctions to the principle that people with learning disabilities have the same rights and entitlements as everyone else.

Interventions that improve health

Health action planning

Health action planning is a key strategy for health improvement and reducing health inequalities experienced by people with learning disabilities

Box 13.1

Top tips

- Communicate – check how the person communicates, use easy English, provide easy-read information, show and tell.
- Speak to the person – ask questions in different ways to check whether they have understood.
- Check whether family carers or other supporters have something to add – they may have important information.
- Use simple words to explain what will happen, what the health problem is, what equipment is for. Let the person see and touch equipment.
- See the person, not the disability – don't allow assumptions about capacity or what is 'normal' for that person to colour your judgement about investigations or treatment.
- Be flexible – be prepared to change the way you usually do things; be creative in offering reasonable adjustments that go beyond physical access.
- Involve local people with learning disabilities in carrying out equality impact assessments and service audits, and then planning reasonable adjustments.
- Offer your staff training so they are confident in supporting people with learning disabilities – involve people with learning disabilities and family carers as trainers.
- Be aware that getting it right for people with learning disabilities will also help people with dementia and people who find written and spoken English difficult.
- Capture and use data about people with learning disabilities to improve your services – use clinical coding and 'flags' to track their usage and experiences.
- Get to know your local learning disability service and find out what support they can offer you to improve your services.

(DH 2001a). *Valuing People* (DH 2001a) aimed for all people with a learning disability to have a health action plan (HAP) by July 2005, which would be led by an identified health facilitator in partnership with the individual and primary care providers. With communication processes between primary, secondary and tertiary care cited as contributing to poor health outcomes, health action planning is now seen as a way of improving health knowledge for the individual, their family and paid carers and is a useful way to promote communication between health professionals (DH 2007a, National Patient Safety Agency 2004). *Valuing People* (DH 2001a:64) suggested a HAP should contain information about:

- health interventions
- oral/dental care
- fitness and mobility
- continence
- sensory impairments
- nutrition needs
- emotional needs
- medications including side effects
- screening test details.

It also identified key times when HAPs were required with the importance of HAPs for teenagers in transition restated in *Valuing People Now* (HM Government 2009):

- transitions (child–adult services)
- leaving and moving home
- changes in health status
- retirement
- transition for those living with older family carers.

(DH 2001a:64)

The Department of Health (2002) stated that HAPs should be individualised, reflect person-centred planning philosophies with no set format. However, standardised formats for HAPs have been developed, often with accessible words and graphics in the form of booklets and health passports. Examples can be accessed via the web resources at the end of this chapter. Although the consultation (DH 2007d) that preceded *Valuing People Now* stated that the objectives for implementing health action planning have not been achieved, there have been a range of activities to develop, implement and evaluate health action planning. Evaluations by Joseph & Wood (2008) and Buckinghamshire County Council (BCC) with the Ridgeway Partnership (RP) NHS Trust (2008) indicated general satisfaction with HAP documents but also identified issues of how relevant these set formats are for people with severe and profound disabilities or for people who are literate, further recognising that if standardised formats are used, they need to accommodate people's cognitive abilities. Northamptonshire's evaluation (Joseph & Wood 2008) identified that plans should be developed with people close to the person with learning disabilities to ensure they were realistic and could be updated when health changes occurred. This could be support workers and family carers as opposed to being health practitioner led. They also identified that parents and people with learning disabilities could be reluctant to ask health care staff to fill in the HAP, meaning it quickly becomes out of date. Identifying who is responsible for ensuring HAPs are recorded and kept up to date can be an issue that practitioners need to consider. HAPs do provide a focus for keeping health information together, improve communication and are generally liked by people with learning disabilities (BCC with the RP NHS Trust 2008, Joseph & Wood 2008).

Alternatives to a health action plan

People may be offered personalised care plans, especially where they have a long-term health condition (DH 2007a). These plans are written with the involvement of health care staff and, like a HAP, cover both physical and mental health needs and consider the educational and social needs that impact on health. As with HAPs, they aim to reduce health inequalities and support self-care and independence.

Keeping a health diary can promote more self and carer awareness of health status and can improve communication with health professionals. Lennox et al (2008) used a health diary to promote health advocacy. This diary contained sections called *All About Me, Health Communication Tips, For the Doctor* and *Medical Records* (p. 485). Although their research did not show that communication improved as a result of keeping the diary, there were sufficient indications of this to lead to further research.

Health passports have been used in Buckinghamshire for a number of years and have proved to be a useful tool in supporting access to health services (BCC and RP NHS Trust 2008). They are a tool that reflects 'reasonable adjustment' providing people with learning disabilities an aide memoire and health professionals with relevant personal information about ways to communicate with the individual and what other health input the person is receiving. Health passports are a patient-held record which the person with learning disabilities takes to health appointments. It contains information for health professionals and easily understood information for the individual who owns it. Health diary pages help people remember outcomes of health appointments and are often written by health professionals using accessible language or graphics (Talkback 2009). They may contain details of medication, treatments and records of health symptoms that are being monitored, therefore contributing to on-going monitoring and evaluation of health interventions. Mencap believes all people with learning disabilities should have a health passport, and in 2009 commenced a campaign for hospitals and primary care trusts (PCTs) to use them to improve access to health services (Mencap 2009).

Health promotion

Health promotion aims to encourage positive changes in the health of communities and individuals through people taking more control of their environment and lifestyle. There are four main approaches to health promotion. These are radical, educational, preventative and self-empowering (Bright 1997). Bright discusses that radical health promotion is a systems approach usually taken by government who seek to make social and economic changes to improve health. Educational is about providing information to enable informed health choices. Preventative is about changing behaviours to prevent illness and disease and self-empowerment concerns individual growth. Health promotion can therefore entail health screening programmes, health education aimed at communities and individuals and behavioural change approaches through support groups and individual coaching.

Health education

All health professionals have a role in seeking opportunities to improve people's health through health educational activities (DH 2006). Although research indicates lower rates of smoking, alcohol consumption and drug taking in people with learning disabilities than the general population, as they become more a part of their local communities it is envisaged they will be increasingly exposed to such health risks. Taggart (2007) identified that people with learning disabilities may use alcohol and drugs to feel included in communities. Alcohol consumption was identified within 35% of respondents in a study by Walsh et al (2008) with 10% of people with learning disabilities in the study drinking alcohol every week. They also found that 9.9% of their respondents smoked while Gale et al (2009) identified that people with learning disabilities had higher rates of asthma (12%) than the local population (6%) and people with learning disabilities, especially men, who had asthma were also smokers. With increased access to tobacco, alcohol and drugs, people need access to health education about these topics and equal access to smoking cessation, drug and alcohol management programmes. Gale et al (2009) recognised that smoking cessation programmes should be a health priority for people with learning disabilities.

Health education is often supported with written and audio-visual materials. This can include campaigns such as *Change4Life* (NHS 2010) which promotes active lifestyles through television commercials, advertisements, leaflets and planned activities. Health education can also be promoted through face-to-face meetings or giving resources such as leaflets or tapes. Health care staff can provide sessions about specific health education topics such as smoking cessation. All contact provides an opportunity for health education.

Accessible health resources

Face-to-face contact

The language of health and illness is varied, sometimes colloquial and jargon filled. People with mild learning disabilities may appear to understand the language you use, however even easily managed health problems such as constipation can go undetected when individuals do not admit their lack of understanding or feel embarrassed (Coleman & Spurling 2010). Accessible information starts with the use of appropriate vocabulary and consideration of people's cognitive abilities. Having longer health appointments is essential so that levels of understanding can be assessed. Mencap (2000, 2008) recommends using objects and images to augment the spoken word and promote understanding while the inclusion of a health advocate, family member or support staff may also be appropriate. Working with individuals to build their health language and understanding may also highlight areas of misunderstanding and provide opportunities for more specific health education.

Case illustration 13.1

When working with a group of six people with learning disabilities to improve their knowledge of healthy eating, the learning disabilities nurse suggested an activity to plan a healthy day's food and drink. The group produced posters about meals, drinks and snacks. When talking about their poster it became apparent that four people felt it was *essential* to drink probiotic drinks every day, with one person believing this prevented cancer; one person understood the *5-a-day* (see Useful addresses) campaign encouraging people to eat five portions of fruit and vegetables each day, and two people felt you should never have any fat, cheese or milk in your diet as they caused obesity. No one understood about food groups. Doing this activity provided an opportunity to explore the language of health each person used and identify misunderstandings and learning needs for future sessions.

Written information

Accessible information includes the information given to people to support and extend what has been discussed during a health consultation. This aids memory, understanding and supports decision making and compliance with treatment plans. A key action for implementing *Valuing People Now* is the provision of accessible resources to parents who have learning disabilities and accessible materials about making complaints (DH 2009a). Even when people with learning disabilities can read, such information is often confusing and badly structured (Glaysher 2005). The use of symbols to support text is widely used in the belief it improves understanding, however Poncelas & Murphy (2007) found little evidence to support this. They identified that the use of easy words alone had the same impact as easy words and Makaton symbols together although there was some indication that symbols aided memory if the document was read with people.

Reader activity 13.1

Use the internet to identify at least four pieces of accessible health information for people with learning disabilities. Review this material using the information in the text and in Chapter 6.

- Of the resources you reviewed, which do you consider are accessible?
- How might you improve those you feel are not accessible?

Behaviour change

Behaviour change can be supported by the process outlined in Figure 13.3 (DH 2008). When a person is supported to work through these stages, the individual can develop self-efficiency through developing confidence in their own ability to successfully make changes in their life (see Bandura 1995 for more about self-efficacy). To maximise opportunities for success, SMART goals can be developed:

- S Specific
- M Measurable
- A Achievable
- R Realistic
- T Time limited

In Case illustration 13.2, Julie was attending a healthy eating group. In addition, Julie had one-to-one coaching to help her consider her own health and agree an area to improve. Julie's coach helped her develop SMART goals and worked with her to make an accessible diary so she could monitor progress. Julie coped with Saturday's setback because she had developed strategies. The group celebrated successes, and rewards were built in. Recognition and rewards are considered to be an essential aspect of human motivation and success and need to be part of the behaviour change plan (Bandura 1995). Frey et al (2005) identified that awards and recognising achievement helped sustain motivation in people with learning disabilities. As Julie developed belief in her ability to succeed, the goals became harder. Working in this way can help motivate people to succeed and overcome setbacks which helps develop self-efficacy (Bandura 1995).

The Department of Health in 2004 proposed the development of health trainers. Health trainers are recruited from local communities where people are at higher risk of poor health. They motivate individuals to improve their health through practical support and health education as described in the practice example (DH 2009a). In Bristol, people with learning disabilities have been trained as health trainers, supporting other people with learning disabilities to improve their health (Scarborough et al 2009). Their work has included supporting people at health appointments including health screening, health education activities and helping individuals develop health action plans and health goals. This type of individual work can keep people focused on achieving health goals and provides support when motivation is low. Health trainers need to understand their own values, attitudes and beliefs

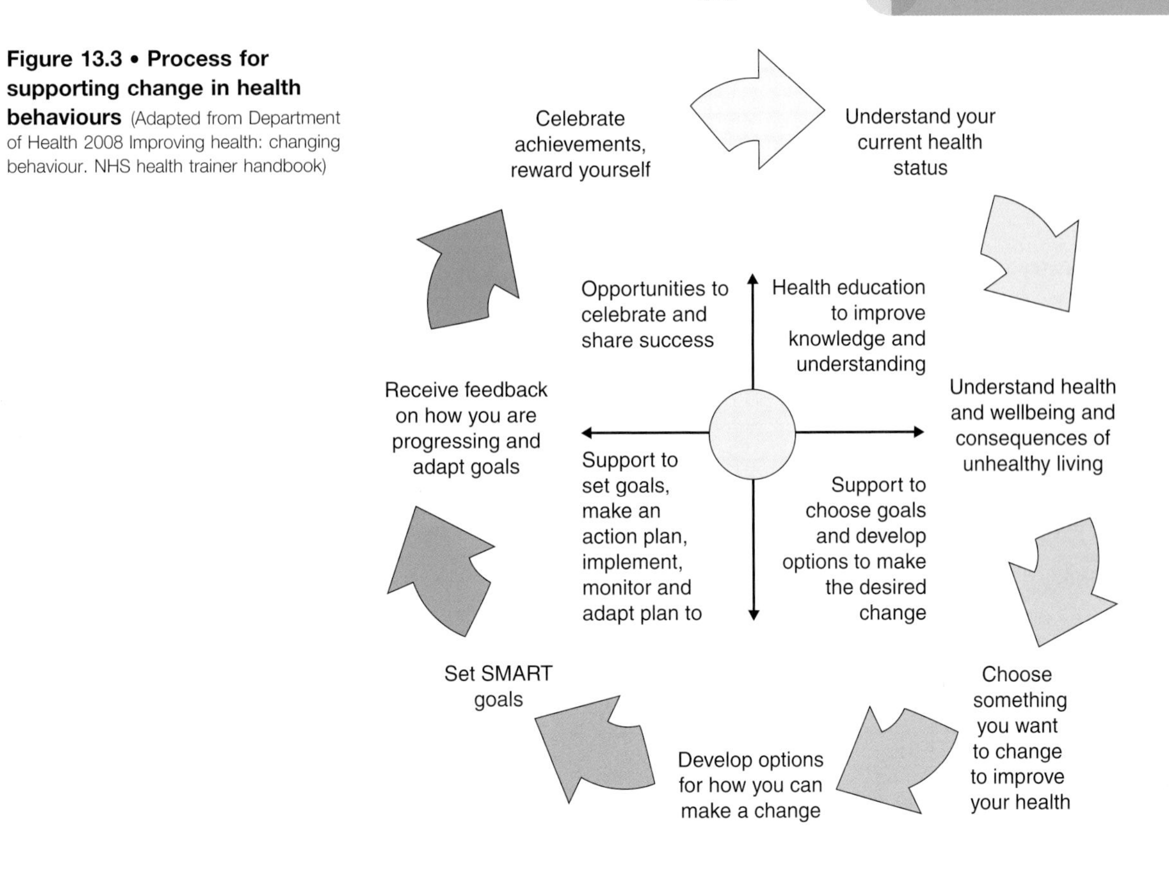

Figure 13.3 • Process for supporting change in health behaviours (Adapted from Department of Health 2008 Improving health: changing behaviour. NHS health trainer handbook)

Case illustration 13.2

Julie does not meet the *5-a-day* (see Useful addresses) target, limits herself to a selection of fruit and vegetables and is unsure of how to prepare and cook new things. Having discussed healthy eating and Julie's current health, she would like to improve her diet. Julie has set herself SMART goals and has discussed what to do on more difficult days when she needs to eat more fruit and vegetables. Julie will be honest in her food diary and start again the next day even if she did not eat as well as hoped the previous day. Julie can telephone the coach between 10 am and 3 pm if she needs support achieving her goals.

Week 1

1. Julie will eat two portions of vegetables and one piece of fruit for 4 out of 7 days.
2. Julie will choose a type of fruit she has not eaten before at the healthy eating session, she will prepare it and then will eat it during the session.

Week 2

1. Julie will eat two portions of vegetable and two pieces of fruit for 4 out of 7 days.
2. Julie will choose a salad vegetable she has not eaten before at the healthy eating session, she will prepare it and will eat it during the session.

Week 3

1. Julie will eat two portions of vegetable and two pieces of fruit for 5 out of 7 days
2. Julie will choose a vegetable she has not eaten before at the healthy eating session, she will learn how to cook it and will eat it during the session.

It is helpful to have an accessible recording system and Julie will complete a pictorial food diary so she can monitor how she is progressing with her goals (see Fig. 13.4).

Julie succeeded in her goal with support and was rewarded verbally, with recognition of her success by other group members and, in week 4, with a visit to a hotel where the group were shown how to make a vegetable curry.

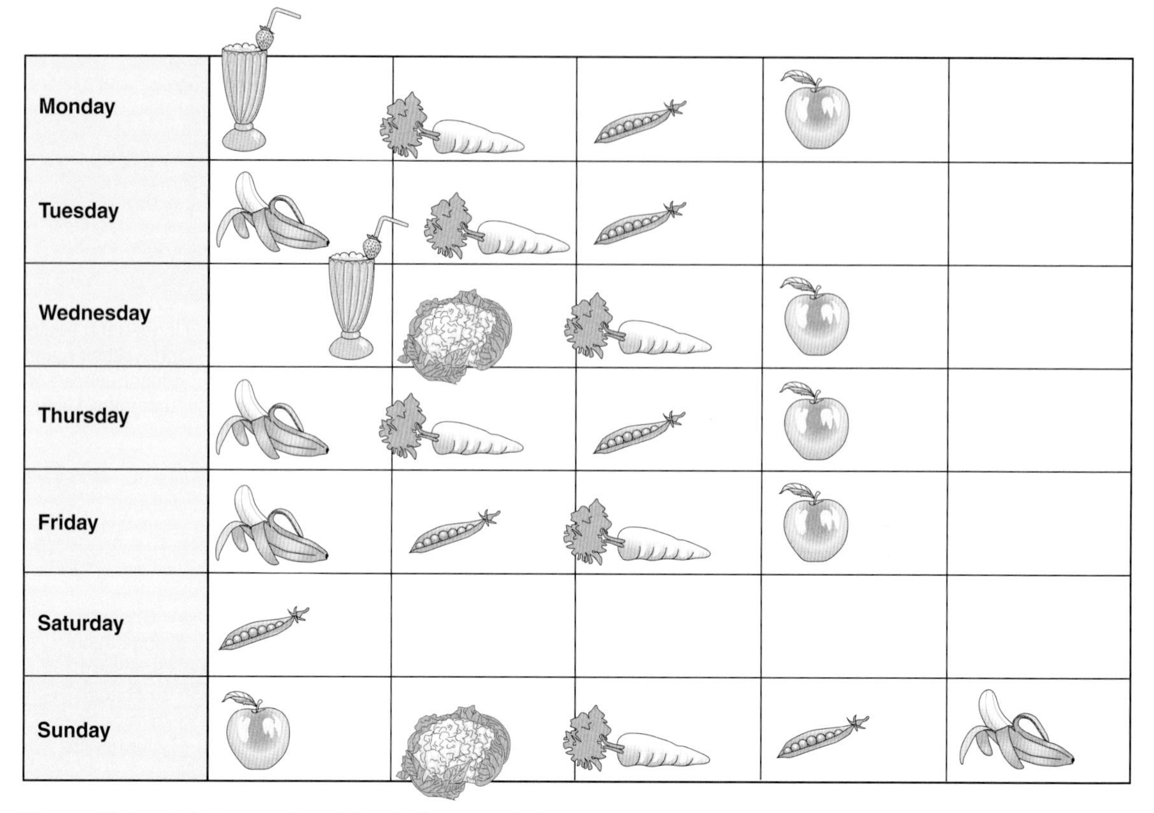

Figure 13.4 • Julie's completed food diary, week 3

about healthy living so they can ensure they are not forcing their own health agenda on the individuals they are supporting as it is important that people choose their own health goals to maximise success (DH 2008). Helping people make their own healthy lifestyle choices means providing information about general health topics, and others more specific to the individual, in a way that the individual can understand including helping them recognise the impact of unhealthy choices (DH 2004). For staff supporting individuals with learning disabilities, it can be difficult to find appropriate meaningful health education materials (Russ 2006), meaning materials may need to be developed to meet the individual's health needs.

Accessible recording systems contribute to action plans and are useful in evaluation. Food diaries can improve an individual's understanding of food consumption, however keeping such diaries can be difficult for people with learning disabilities. Work on 'food on film' by Humphries et al (2008) involved a group of nine people with learning disabilities photographing their food intake as an aide memoire for interviews about eating. People were able to take photographs which helped them to remember what they had eaten and improved communication between the interviewer and the person with a learning disability. While a photograph cannot indicate food qualities or additives, it did raise awareness of food preferences, portion size and nutritional balance such as food groups.

With obesity and inactivity linked to higher risks of coronary heart disease, there have been studies exploring how to increase activity and decrease obesity in people with learning disabilities. Programmes which have provided opportunities for planned activities providing support and goal setting have been successful in increasing activity levels also resulting in weight loss (see Moss 2009).

Motivational interviewing

Another approach to helping people change health behaviours is motivational interviewing which has been recommended in a variety of government initiatives including its use by health trainers (DH 2004) and the *Let's Get Moving* initiative (DH 2010) in general practice. Rollnick et al (2008) refer to motivational interviewing as conversations that are based on collaboration and support for individual autonomy. Rollnick et al (2008:7–10) use four principles represented by RULE:

R Resist the righting reflex – you can't and should not try to put things right
U Understand your patient's motivations
L Listen to the person
E Empower the person

Motivational interviewing is not about judging people or telling them what to do or developing a relationship where they argue or feel a need to justify their position. It is about active listening, understanding the individual and helping them identify their motivations and guiding them to make choices. The use of motivational interviewing has been shown to produce positive outcomes in relation to weight management, diet and activity levels and alcohol consumption in the general population (Burke et al 2003, Rubak et al 2005). Although there is limited published research as to the effectiveness of motivational interviewing specifically with people with learning disabilities, there are indications of its usefulness with people with mild learning disabilities (Mendel & Hipkins 2002, Rose & Walker 2000).

Motivational interviewing is carried out either on a one-to-one basis or in groups with an aim to support people to change their behaviour. It usually requires repeated sessions where a therapeutic relationship is developed. Mendel & Hipkin (2002:155) used a FRAMES model to decide structure and content of sessions:

F Feedback personal to the individual
R Responsibility of the individual for changing their own behaviour
A Advice given non-confrontationally about health risks
M Menu of possible goals and ways to achieve
E Empathy raising self-esteem
S Self-efficacy in developing self-belief

The need to support individuals to develop a belief in their own abilities and effect change in their health behaviours requires skill not only in communication but also in careful goal setting that enables successes and develops coping strategies for setbacks.

Supporting people to keep healthy

Annual health checks

Annual health checks for people with learning disabilities are a reliable way of identifying new health problems, monitoring changes in a person's health status and improving health outcomes (Felce et al 2008, Lennox et al 2007). Checks are offered to people with learning disabilities usually through GP surgeries (DH 2007a). These checks include:

- family history and risk factors
- immunisation record
- health screening and health promotion
- vision and hearing
- chronic illnesses including epilepsy
- physical examination including fitness, mobility and posture
- review of mental health and emotional needs
- syndrome-specific check
- medication review
- oral health.

(DH 2007a:18–19)

Checklists have been developed to standardise annual health checks. The *Cardiff Health Check* (Kerr 2001) includes all the above plus behavioural disturbances and communication needs. The *Comprehensive Health Assessment Programme* (CHAP) developed by Lennox et al (2007) entailed a carer-completed medical history section and a GP-led health assessment leading to a HAP. Because people with learning disabilities may experience difficulties in remembering and communicating their health history, the involvement of a health advocate (often a family member or support worker) who is well informed about the person's past and current health status is important. This role should be undertaken by someone who knows the person with learning disabilities and who can offer support to improve how the GP and individual communicate. The GP requires reliable information to complete the health check and make appropriate suggestions for health interventions; therefore forward planning for an annual health check is good practice. Lennox et al (2007) also identified how high staff turnover can have a negative impact on knowledge of an individual's health history meaning that having this information recorded is essential.

Consent for health checks requires accessible information and time to discuss both the process and reasons for the check and the possibility of other health interventions if problems are identified. The Department of Health have published *Seeking Consent: Working with People with Learning Disabilities* (DH 2001b) which outlines good practice in this area. Health care professionals need to be conversant with consent and capacity guidance including the Mental Capacity Act (HMSO 2005b). Behavioural consent is discussed in *Equal Access to Breast and Cervical Screening for Disabled Women* (NHS Cancer Screening 2006). This means that when a woman with learning disabilities participates in screening, responding to simple requests and is not overly anxious, screening can continue. The role of staff includes supporting the woman with learning disabilities to access information in a way she can best understand. Staff also need to inform screening services of the person's access, information and familiarisation requirements. It is important to ensure the individual's needs are addressed to increase the likelihood of them cooperating with screening processes. Screening units should provide familiarisation visits if needed to reduce anxiety. Where access needs can be planned for, gentle empathic support during screening can be provided to help the individual participate. If a woman is considered to be unsuitable for undertaking breast screening due to problems associated with comprehension, cooperation in testing or physical ability to be tested, the *Equal Access* document (NHS Cancer Screening 2006) states that staff should support the person in breast awareness. However, this is problematic in itself as staff may be unsure how to support women with learning disabilities with breast self-examination or what to look for when providing personal care. These issues need to be discussed within the support team, including the woman and significant others where appropriate, and an individual plan developed with health education and staff education provided as appropriate. Difficulties accessing screening, health tests or interventions may need to be discussed with a health professional experienced in working with people with learning disabilities.

Health facilitators

The role of health facilitators was developed as a result of the *Valuing People* White Paper (DH 2001a) with a remit for supporting individuals to access health care. Originally linked to community learning disabilities teams, health facilitators were tasked with ensuring people with learning disabilities were registered with GPs by 2004 and had a HAP by 2005. By 2003, people with a learning disability should have had access to a health facilitator. The new guidance on health facilitation (DH 2009c) states that health facilitators can be family members, advocates and health and social care staff. With the implementation of annual health checks, where GPs and practice nurses take a lead role in health assessment, the development of individual HAPs is now moving into primary care (DH 2007a). Where people have complex needs in relation to their health and/or communication, the Department of Health (2007a) recommends partnership working between GP staff and specialist learning disabilities services to ensure equity of health outcomes for individuals, and health facilitators may be involved in partnership working.

But, as discussed in *Health Action Planning and Health Facilitation for People with Learning Disabilities* (DH 2009c), health facilitation does not stop at working with individuals. It includes health professionals and managers working at a strategic level to audit health initiatives and influence commissioning of health services for people with learning disabilities. Working at a strategic level entails close collaboration with stakeholders including people with learning disabilities, family carers, learning disabilities partnership boards, health and social care providers and commissioners (DH 2009c).

The expert patient programme

People with learning disabilities may have associated long-term conditions which need to be managed (DH 2001a). The expert patient programme is designed to help people understand their own long-term health condition and develop confidence in managing their health and improving their quality of life (DH 2007c). It has been run successfully for people with learning disabilities in Bristol and Staffordshire and raised the issue of a lack of accessible health materials for people with learning disabilities (Russ 2006). Wilson et al (2008) developed the expert patient programme further by running and evaluating an expert patient programme for four groups of people with learning disabilities. They were able to use accessible materials that people generally understood but found sessions were too intense. The individuals reported changes in how they self-managed their health behaviour, for example requesting medication reviews, exercising more and cooking healthy meals with friends.

Managing illness

Part of maintaining health is receiving the most appropriate health care when experiencing mental distress, physical illness and dental problems. Most acute illnesses are managed in primary care. There have been developments in the role of learning disabilities nurses in partnership working between specialist learning disabilities teams and primary care staff. Also the role of the GP liaison nurse has been developed (Foundation for People with Learning Disabilities (FPLD) 2006). People with learning disabilities also access secondary health care. Walsh et al (2008) identified that 15% of respondents with learning disabilities had accessed accident and emergency in the last year and 17% of respondents required at least one overnight stay as an in-patient during a 12-month period. This may be a difficult experience for people with learning disabilities and, in response, the role of hospital liaison nurse has evolved. Backer et al (2009) reviewed the literature concerning accessing secondary health care and consolidated recommendations for improvements. Although wary of generalising their findings across the health services, they did identify common themes such as providing staff education, improving communication skills and systems, having accessible information, using tools such as health and communication passports and HAPs and working closely with significant others, especially family carers. The use of integrated care pathways and protocols with good admission and discharge planning were areas that had a positive impact on care in the limited research they critiqued, as did the use of specialist assessment tools. They found hospital liaison posts were being developed with positive outcomes being reported. Such roles are not new; NHS Lothian established its liaison nurse service in 1999 and has completed a service evaluation (MacArthur & Brown 2009). The evaluation of four of their liaison services identified how the liaison nurses raised the profile of people with learning disabilities, improved health outcomes as well as having an impact at strategic level, on practice development and on staff education. The role of the liaison nurse is complex (see Fig. 13.5), encompassing the need for a visible presence within the health care setting, working with individuals and local staff while also working in partnership to develop care pathways, policies and procedures. The significance of their role as advocates was strongly promoted by people with learning disabilities and family carers who commented on how it facilitated choice and autonomy.

Garvey's (2008) work in establishing a hospital liaison service mirrored many of the roles described in the Lothian services including working with individuals in admission and discharge planning, protocol developments, educational activities and linking with specialist learning disabilities teams.

Monitoring and evaluating care at national and local levels

National and local monitoring

Monitoring how health inequalities are being tackled is important at a strategic, local and personal level, however reliable data from PCTs, specifically about people with learning disabilities' health, satisfaction of services and uptake of health care services, has been poor (Giraud-Saunders et al 2003). At a national level, Learning Disability Metrics (NHS and Healthcare Commission 2007) have been developed (Box 13.2).

A project was established with the Foundation of People with Learning Disabilities (FPLD) and 10 PCTs to use the Learning Disability Metrics to provide a focus for improvements in services (FPLD 2006). The project identified that a number of factors improved the chances of being successful. Key was the commitment by senior managers to the project with partnership working between GP services, acute services, information technology (IT) services and specialist learning disabilities services. Important roles in successful projects were GP practice managers, practice nurses and learning disabilities nurses (especially health facilitators), self-advocates and IT managers. Problems arose when senior management and GP services had a low commitment to change. Inhibiting factors included a perception that expertise in caring for people with learning disabilities was lacking and that meeting people's needs would be too difficult (FPLD 2006). Such perceptions need to be challenged, with learning disabilities practitioners helping other health care professionals see how they can support people through education, partnership working and role modelling. The project led to improvements in partnership working, developing learning disability registers, raising awareness of the health inequalities experienced by people with learning disabilities and the need for people with learning disabilities to be included in public participation groups.

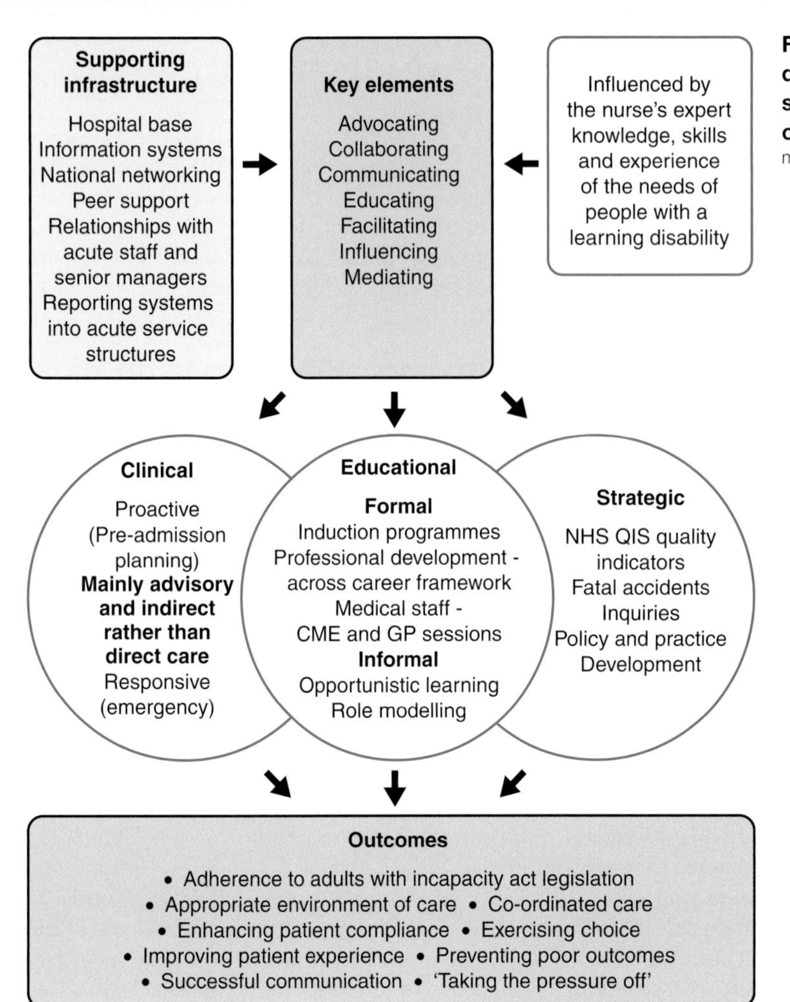

Figure 13.5 • Model of learning disability liaison services – role, supportive infrastructure and outcomes (Permission granted by juliet.macarthur@ed.ac.uk)

Box 13.2

Learning Disabilities Better Metrics topics

('People' refers to patients with learning disabilities.)

- GPs identify and record patients with learning disabilities.
- GPs record numbers of people who have/are offered annual health checks and health action plans.
- PCTs identify health facilitators.
- PCTs annually review people in NHS-funded hospital beds and record percentage of people exceeding a 12-month stay.
- PCTs record number of people with challenging behaviour, mental health or forensic needs in out-of-area placements.
- PCTs ensure that people with dual diagnosis access mental health services.
- PCTs record how many people have been screened for dysphagia (National Patient Safety Agency 2007) in the last 3 years and have a regularly reviewed dysphagia plan.
- PCTs survey people and their family carers about how understandable information provided about their health and treatment was.
- PCTs record number of people on patient forums.
- PCTs record number of people who are in-patients including long-stay and campus provision with independent health advocates.
- Acute hospitals identify patients with learning disabilities and provide appropriate support.
- PCTs ensure quarterly monitoring of access and take-up rates for people with learning disabilities to check and promote equal access to benefits in mainstream services, national service frameworks and plans.

(NHS and Healthcare Commission 2007)

Individual and local level

The use of HAPs provides a system for monitoring and evaluating health care at an individual level. They should also feed into a data collection system whereby service deficits can be identified and recommendations for service change can be considered (DH 2002, 2009c).

The involvement of people with learning disabilities and family carers is embedded in the patient and public involvement agenda and is seen as an essential aspect of need assessment, service design, service delivery and service evaluation (DH 2009d). It is about active partnerships in the transformation of health care including involvement in decision-making processes and commissioning of services but also in the ongoing monitoring of services at individual, local, regional and national levels. Local involvement networks (LINKs) were established in 2008 (HMSO 2007) to facilitate everyone in the local community having a voice in the planning and delivery of NHS services. How to ensure the voice of people with learning disabilities is included can be an aspect of the hospital liaison nurse (Garvey 2008), or it might be the voluntary organisations such as People First (see Useful addresses) who take this role. The most empowering change in health care may be the implementation of personalised health budgets; from November 2009, PCTs in England that are in the pilot scheme will be able to give direct payments (HMSO 2009) enabling individuals to have control over their health spending.

Teaching and training health care workers

It is now considered to be good practice to involve people with learning disabilities and family carers in the education of health staff (DH 2009d, Michael 2008). Registered nurses for people with learning disabilities (RNLD) are often required to teach health and social care professionals (DH 2007d). RNLDs must be competent communicators able to present the realities of health inequalities within a context of positive lives, human rights, choices and inclusion. The ability to co-train with people with learning disabilities and family carers is becoming an additional required skill for RNLDs with roles in liaison nursing, community nursing and lecturing. Successful co-training is about listening to each other, sharing power, respecting what each other brings to the learning experience, planning and reviewing (British Institute of Learning Disabilities 2007).

New roles for learning disabilities practitioners

Many new roles have already been discussed including liaison nurses in primary and secondary care, health facilitators, health trainers and staff trainers. Other roles include continuing health care nurses who access and review health needs and develop complex care plans for people with learning disabilities establishing their eligibility for continuing health care funding. These assessments include health conditions, treatments, complexity in interacting health needs and the difficulties in managing them, level and timing of intervention required and stability of health needs (DH 2009e). RNLDs are also specialising in forensic services, prison health, brain injury, specialist outreach teams and children's health. There are also RNLD and allied health professional (AHP) consultants in learning disabilities. The common link between these roles is the need to work in partnership with a range of health and social care services, people with learning disabilities and their carers.

Conclusion

At the start of this chapter, improving the health and wellbeing of people with learning disabilities was located in a broader context that identified the need to make services more inclusive. Much of the evidence related to health has been focused on the inequalities that separate people with learning disabilities from the rest of the population, however this chapter has also described some of the strategies that might help to close that gap. These strategies are not the prerogative of learning disabilities specialists. They will be utilised by practitioners that work with people with learning disabilties most of the time but they might also be adopted by practitioners that work with them less frequently. The key points to bear in mind from this chapter are as follow:

- Equitable treatment and anti-discriminatory practice are professional and legal requirements.
- Practitioners need to understand the communities they work with as well as the individuals that they provide care for.
- Communication with clients with learning disabilities and carers needs to address the specific needs of discrete groups and/or individuals because people with learning disabilities are not a homogeneous group.
- Be SMART, remember RULE, and do not forget FRAMES.

References

Backer, C., Chapman, M., Mitchell, D., 2009. Access to secondary healthcare for people with intellectual disabilities: a review of the literature. J. Appl. Res. Intellect. Disabil. 22, 514–525.

Bandura, A., 1995. Self-efficacy in changing societies. Cambridge University Press, Cambridge.

Bright, J., 1997. Health promotion in clinical practice. Baillière Tindall, London.

British Institute of Learning Disabilities (BILD), 2007. Partnerships in training. BILD, Kidderminster.

Buckinghamshire County Council, Ridgeway Partnership NHS Trust, 2008. Health passports: a survey improving healthcare access for people with a learning disability. Available at:http://valuingpeople.gov.uk/dynamic/valuingpeople118.jsp (accessed 14.02.10.).

Burke, B., Arkowitz, H., Menchola, M., 2003. The efficacy of motivational interviewing: a meta-analysis of controlled clinical trials. J. Consult. Clin. Psychol. 71 (5), 843–861.

Coleman, J., Spurling, G., 2010. Easily missed? Constipation in people with learning disability. Br. Med. J. 340, c222. Available at:http://www.bmj.com/cgi/content/full/340/jan26_1/c222 (accessed 16.02.10.).

Dahlgren, G., Whitehead, M., 1991. Policies and strategies to promote social equity in health. Institute for Futures Studies, Stockholm.

Department of Health, 2001a. Valuing people: a new strategy for learning disability for the 21st century. Available at:http://www.archive.official-documents.co.uk/document/cm50/5086/5086.pdf (accessed 01.03.10.).

Department of Health, 2001b. Nothing about us without us. DH, London.

Department of Health, 2002. Action for health health action plans and health facilitation. Detailed good practice guidance on implementation for learning disability partnership boards. Available at:http://www.dh.gov.uk/prod_consum_dh/groups/dh_digitalassets/@dh/@en/documents/digitalasset/dh_4079650.pdf (accessed 20.02.10.).

Department of Health, 2004. Choosing health: making healthy choices easier. Available at:http://www.dh.gov.uk/en/Publicationsandstatistics/Publications/PublicationsPolicyAndGuidance/DH_4094550 (accessed 14.02.10.).

Department of Health, 2006. Our health, our care, our say. Available at: http://www.dh.gov.uk/en/Publicationsandstatistics/Publications/PublicationsPolicyAndGuidance/Browsable/DH_4127552 (accessed 14.02.10.).

Department of Health, 2007a. Primary care service framework: management of health for people with learning disabilities in primary care. Available at:http://www.pcc.nhs.uk/uploads/primary_care_service_frameworks/primary_care_service_framework__ld_v3_final.pdf (accessed 15.02.10.).

Department of Health, 2007c. The expert patients programme. Available at:http://webarchive.nationalarchives.gov.uk/+/ www.dh.gov.uk/en/Aboutus/MinistersandDepartmentLeaders/ChiefMedicalOfficer/ProgressOnPolicy/ProgressBrowsableDocument/DH_4102757 (accessed 14.02.10.).

Department of Health, 2007d. Good practice in learning disability nursing. NHS, London.

Department of Health, 2008. Improving health: changing behaviour. NHS health trainer handbook. Available at: http://www.dh.gov.uk/prod_consum_dh/groups/dh_digitalassets/@dh/@en/documents/digitalasset/dh_085778.pdf (accessed 20.02.10.).

Department of Health, 2009a. Key actions for making Valuing People Now happen locally and regionally – primary care trusts (and strategic health authorities) (2009–2012). Department of Health, London.

Department of Health, 2009c. Health action planning and health facilitation for people with learning disabilities: good practice guidance. Department of Health, London.

Department of Health, 2009d. World class commissioning for the health and wellbeing of people with learning disabilities: improving the health and wellbeing of people with learning disabilities. Available at: http://www.dh.gov.uk/en/Publicationsandstatistics/Publications/PublicationsPolicyAndGuidance/DH_109088 (accessed 20.02.10.).

Department of Health, 2009e. NHS-funded nursing care practice guide (revised). Available at:http://www.dh.gov.uk/prod_consum_dh/groups/dh_digitalassets/documents/digitalasset/dh_106225.pdf (accessed 20.02.10.).

Department of Health, 2010. Let's get moving introducing a new physical activity care pathway. Available at: http://www.dh.gov.uk/en/Publichealth/Healthimprovement/PhysicalActivity/DH_099438 (accessed 20.02.10.).

Disability Rights Commission, 2006. Equal treatment: closing the gap. A formal investigation into physical health inequalities experienced by people with learning disabilities and/or mental health problems. Available at:http://83.137.212.42/sitearchive/DRC/library/health_investigation.html#Finalreportsandsummaries (accessed 02.03.10.).

Emerson, E., Hatton, C., 2008. People with learning disabilities in England. Centre for Disability Research, University of Lancaster. Available at: http://www.mencap.org.uk/document.asp?id=3160 (accessed 15.03.10.).

Felce, D., Baxter, H., Lowe, K., et al., 2008. The impact of repeated health checks for adults with intellectual disabilities. J. Appl. Res. Intellect. Disabil. 21, 585–596.

Foundation for People with Learning Disabilities (FPLD), 2006. Better health, better metrics. A project to use clinically relevant measures of performance to improve local service quality. Available at:http://www.learningdisabilities.org.uk/our-work/improving-service/better-health/ (accessed 14.02.10.).

Frey, G., Buchanan, A., Rosser Sandt, D., 2005. I'd rather watch TV': An examination of physical activity in adults with mental retardation. Ment. Retard. 43 (4), 241–254.

Gale, L., Naqvi, H., Russ, L., 2009. Asthma, smoking and BMI in adults with intellectual disabilities: a community-based survey. J. Intellect. Disabil. Res. 53 (9), 787–796.

Garvey, F., 2008. Setting up a learning disabilities acute liaison team. NursingTimes.net. Available at: http://www.nursingtimes.net/nursing-practice-clinical-research/setting-up-a-learning-disability-acute-liaison-team/1732222.article (accessed 20.02.10.).

Giraud-Saunders, A., 2009. Equal access? A practical guide for the NHS: creating a single equality scheme that includes improving access for people with learning disabilities. Department of Health. Available at:http://www.dh.gov.uk/dr_consum_dh/groups/dh_digitalassets/documents/digitalasset/dh_109751.pdf (accessed 23.03.10.).

Giraud-Saunders, A., Gregory, M., Poxton, R., et al., 2003. Valuing health for all: PCTs and the health of people with learning disabilities. Journal of Integrated Care 11 (3), 26–33.

Glaysher, K., 2005. Making hospitals friendlier and easier to use for people with learning disabilities: a project looking at service-users' perspectives. In: Shaw, T., Sanders, K. (Eds.), Foundation of Nursing Studies Dissemination Series, vol. 3. 1–4 1.

Healthcare Commission, 2005. Draft three year strategy for assessing and encouraging improvement in the health and healthcare of adults with learning disabilities 2006–2009. Healthcare Commission, London.

Her Majesty's Stationery Office, 1995. Disability Discrimination Act. The Stationery Office, London.

Her Majesty's Stationery Office, 2005a. Disability Discrimination Act. The Stationery Office, London.

Her Majesty's Stationery Office, 2005b. Mental Capacity Act. The Stationery Office, London.

Her Majesty's Stationery Office, 2007. Local Government and Public Involvement in Health Act. The Stationery Office, London.

Her Majesty's Stationery Office, 2009. Health Act. Available at: http://www.dh.gov.uk/en/Publicationsandstatistics/Legislation/Actsandbills/DH_093280#_1 (accessed 03.03.10.).

HM Government, 2009. Valuing people now: a new three-year strategy for people with learning disabilities. Making it happen for everyone. Available at:http://www.dh.gov.uk/en/Publicationsandstatistics/Publications/PublicationsPolicyAndGuidance/DH_093377 (accessed 01.03.10.).

Humphries, K., Traci, M.A., Seekins, T., 2008. Food on film: pilot test of an innovative method for recording food intake of adults with intellectual disabilities living in the community. J. Appl. Res. Intellect. Disabil. 21, 168–173.

Joseph, K., Wood, S., 2008. An evaluation of health action planning in Northamptonshire. Northamptonshire Healthcare NHS Trust and Northamptonshire Primary Care Trust, Northampton.

Kerr, M., 2001. Cardiff health check. Welsh Centre for Learning Disabilities, Cardiff University, Cardiff.

Lennox, N., Bain, C., Rey-Conde, T., et al., 2007. Effect of a comprehensive health assessment programme for Australian adults with intellectual disability: a cluster randomised trial. Int. J. Epidemiol. 36, 139–146.

Lennox, N., Rey-Conde, T., Faint, S., 2008. A pilot of intervention to improve health care in adolescents with intellectual disabilities. J. Appl. Res. Intellect. Disabil. 21, 484–489.

MacArthur, J., Brown, M., 2009. Learning disability liaison nursing services in South East Scotland: a mixed methods impact and outcome research study. Lothian Learning Disability Research Group. Available at:http://www.debramooreassociates.com/Resources/LD_Liaison_Nursing_Briefing_Paper_Dec%2009.pdf (accessed 20.02.10.).

Mencap, 2000. Am I making myself clear?. Available at:http://november5th.net/resources/Mencap/Making-Myself-Clear.pdf (accessed 07.05.10.).

Mencap, 2004. Treat me right! Better health for people with learning disabilities. Mencap National Centre, London.

Mencap, 2007. Death by indifference. Mencap National Centre, London Following up the Treat Me Right report.

Mencap, 2008. Make it clear. Mencap, London.

Mencap, 2009. Health passports. Available at:http://www.mencap.org.uk/document.asp?id=11985 (accessed 15.02.10.).

Mendel, E., Hipkins, J., 2002. Motivating learning disabled offenders with alcohol-related problems: a pilot study. British Journal of Learning Disabilities 30, 153–158.

Michael, J., 2008. Healthcare for all: report of the independent inquiry into access to healthcare for people with learning disabilities. Available at:http://www.dh.gov.uk/en/Publicationsandstatistics/Publications/PublicationsPolicyAndGuidance/DH_099255 (accessed 1.02.10.).

Moss, S., 2009. Changes in coronary heart disease risk profile of adults with intellectual disabilities following a physical activity intervention. J. Intellect. Disabil. Res. 53 (8), 735–744.

National Health Service Cancer Screening Programmes, 2006. Equal access to breast and cervical screening for disabled women. NHS Cancer Screening Programmes, Sheffield.

National Health Service and Healthcare Commission, 2007. The Better Metrics project. List of metrics. Available at:http://www.cqc.org.uk/_db/_documents/List_of_metrics-The_Better_Metrics_project_v8-Nov07.pdf (accessed 14.02.10.).

National Patient Safety Agency, 2004. Understanding the patient safety issues for people with learning disabilities. NPSA, London.

National Patient Safety Agency, 2007. Problems swallowing? Ensuring safer practice for adults with learning disabilities who have dysphagia. Available at:http://www.npsa.nhs.uk/resources/dysphagia (accessed 20.02.10.).

NHS, 2010. Change4Life. Available at: http://www.nhs.uk/change4life/Pages/change-for-life.aspx (accessed 31.07.10.).

NHS Modernisation Agency Leadership Centre, 2003. NHS leadership qualities framework. NHS Executive, London.

Northway, R., Hutchinson, C., Kingdon, A., 2006. Shaping the future: a vision for learning disability nursing. United Kingdom Learning Disability Consultant Nurse Network, UK.

Nursing and Midwifery Council, 2008. The code: standards of conduct, performance and ethics for nurses and midwives. Available at:http://www.nmc-uk.org/aArticle.aspx?ArticleID=3056 (accessed 27.02.10.).

Parliamentary and Health Service Ombudsman and Local Government Ombudsman, 2009. Six lives: the provision of public services for people with learning disabilities. Available at:http://www.ombudsman.org.uk/improving-public-service/reports-and-consultations/reports/health/six-lives-the-provision-of-public-services-to-people-with-learning-disabilities (accessed 15.03.10.).

Poncelas, A., Murphy, G., 2007. Accessible information for people with intellectual disabilities: do symbols really help? J. Appl. Res. Intellect. Disabil. 20, 466–474.

Rollnick, S., Miller, W., Butler, C., 2008. Motivational interviewing in health care: helping patients change behaviour. The Guildford Press, Guildford.

Rose, J., Walker, S., 2000. Working with a man who has Prader–Willi syndrome and his support staff using motivational principles. Behavioral and Cognitive Psychotherapy 28, 293–302.

Rubak, S., Sandboek, A., Lauritzen, T., Christensen, B., 2005. Motivational interviewing: a systematic review and meta-analysis. Br. J. Gen. Pract. 55, 305–312.

Russ, L., 2006. Managing long-term health conditions: the expert patient programme and people with learning difficulties. Bristol Primary Care Trust, Bristol.

Scarborough, K., Kerswell, S., Godsell, M., 2009. Health trainers, educators and communities: changing the dynamic in service provision for people with learning disabilities. New Types of Worker in Health and Social Care Conference. Heathrow Airport, London.

Taggart, L., 2007. Listening to people with intellectual disabilities who misuse alcohol and drugs. Health and Social Care in the Community 15 (4), 360–368.

Talkback, 2009. Health passports. Available at:http://www.healthpassport.co.uk (accessed 15.02.10.).

Walsh, P., Hall, L., Ryan, D., 2008. Health indicators for people with intellectual disability: using an indicator set. Available at:http://ec.europa.eu/health/ph_projects/2004/action1/docs/action1_2004_frep_14_en.pdf (accessed 20.02.10.).

Wilson, P., Goodman, C., Shaw, H., 2008. Evaluation of a modified chronic disease self-management programme for people with learning difficulties. Valuing People Support Team with CSIP and University of Hertfordshire, Hertford.

World Health Organization, 1946. Preamble to the Constitution of the World Health Organization as adopted by the International Health Conference, New York. WHO, Geneva 19–22 June, 1946; signed on 22 July 1946 by the representatives of 61 states (official records of the World Health Organization, No. 2, p. 100 and entered into force on 7 April 1948).

World Health Organization, 1986. Ottawa charter for health promotion. WHO, Geneva. Available at:http://www.who.int/healthpromotion/conferences/previous/ottawa/en/ (accessed 01.02.10.).

Further reading

Bhaumik, S., Watson, J., Thorp, C., et al., 2007. Body mass index in adults with intellectual disability: distribution, associations and service implications: a population-based prevalence study. J. Intellect. Disabil. Res. 52 (4), 287–298.

DiMascio, F., Hamilton, K., Smith, L., 2003. Professional consensus statement: the nutritional care of adults with a learning disability in care settings. Available at:http://www.bda.uk.com/publications/statements/AdultsLearningDisabilityStatement0804.pdf (accessed 14.02.10.).

Fairclough, J., Burton, S., Craven, J., et al., 2008. Home enteral tube feeding for adults with a learning disability. British Dietetic Association. Available at:http://www.bda.uk.com/publications/statements/index.html (accessed 14.02.10.).

Hamilton, S., Hankey, C.R., Miller, S., Boyle, S., 2007. A review of weight loss interventions for adults with intellectual disabilities. Obes. Rev. 8, 339–345.

Melville, C., Cooper, S., Morrison, J., et al., 2007. The prevalence and determinants of obesity in adults with intellectual disabilities. J. Appl. Res. Intellect. Disabil. 21, 425–437.

Useful addresses

Healthy eating

5-a-day: http://www.nhs.uk/livewell/5aday/pages/5adayhome.aspx/.

British Dietetic Association: http://www.bda.uk.com/.

Food Standards Agency: http://www.eatwell.gov.uk/healthydiet/eatwellplate/.

General information about healthy eating and drinking and specific information about healthy eating and drinking and people with learning disabilities.

National Patient Safety Agency: http://www.nrls.npsa.nhs.uk/resources/?entryid45=59823.

Reviews formats for care plans, meal plans and assessments, safe swallowing documents.

NHS Evidence – National Library for Public Health: http://www.library.nhs.uk/PUBLICHEALTH/ViewResource.aspx?resID=311255.

Evidence about healthy lifestyles and people with learning disabilities.

People First – A voice for people with learning difficulties: http://www.peoplefirstltd.com/.

Skills for Health (SfH): https://tools.skillsforhealth.org.uk/suite/show/id/49.

Competency framework for dysphagia, undertaking a comprehensive dysphagia assessment.

Health action plans

There are many examples of health action plans available and a selection are shown below. These links do not indicate our endorsement. These are currently available or best resources. You should consider first and foremost how any format is suitable for the individual you are supporting. The links are given so you may consider a variety of sources.

My health action plan. Bedfordshire Health Local Implementation Team: http://www.bedfordshire.gov.uk/Resources/PDF/L/LearningDisabilities/Health%20action%20plan%20for%20women.pdf.

Health Passport Talkback UK: http://www.healthpassport.co.uk.

My Health Action Plan. Mencap: http://www.pmldnetwork.org/resources/mencap_hap.pdf.

Health Action Plan Haringey Council: http://www.haringey.gov.uk/index/social_care_and_health/learningdisabilities/be_healthy.htm.

Health action planning. Bristol Community Learning Disability Teams, also resources for making a hospital information book: http://www.bristollearningdifficulties.nhs.uk/HAP.htm.

Accessible health information

There are ranges of accessible books on health topics to purchase. These are excellent resources to use with people with learning disabilities to provide a teaching resource and aide memoire leading to improved understanding. Understanding health issues that impact on you enables people to make decisions about their health and promotes good practice in consent.

The Books Beyond Words *series is available from http://www.rcpsych.ac.uk/bbw:.*

Bob Tells All (About abuse)
Feeling Blue
Getting on with Epilepsy
Going to the Doctor
I Can Get Through It (About abuse)
Jenny Speaks Out (About abuse)
Keeping Healthy 'Down Below'
Looking After My Breasts

Your Good Health Books *are available from http://www.bild.org.uk:.*

Alcohol and Smoking
Breathe Easy
Coping with Stress
Epilepsy
Getting Older – Feeling Good
If you are Ill . . .
Looking after your Teeth
Pregnancy and Childbirth
Seeing and Hearing
Using medicine safely

Accessible health information and videos about health care: http://www.lookupinfo.org/:.

Alcohol
Asthma
Back
Blood pressure
Breast examination
Calling an ambulance
Colds and flu
Coming for a drink
CT scan
Diabetes
Epilepsy
Healthy eating

Making accessible resources

Guide for people with sensory loss, communication needs and people from ethnic minorities: http://easyinfo.org.uk/dynamic/easyinfo46.jsp

Physical health

14

Caroline Dalton O'Connor Maria Caples Lynne Marsh

CHAPTER CONTENTS

KEY ISSUES

- People with learning disabilities can experience coexisting physical disabilities
- These physical disabilities can significantly impact on the quality of life of such individuals
- Such physical disabilities include disorders of movement, eating, swallowing and nutrition difficulties as well as bladder and bowel difficulties
- Appropriate assessment and management of these conditions can significantly increase the quality of life of people with learning disabilities
- It is imperative that people with learning disabilities and their families are central to the care planning process

Introduction

The purpose of this chapter is to develop the reader's awareness of the impact on quality of life of a range of physical health conditions that may arise as the result of the manifestation of a physical disability in individuals with learning disabilities across the life-span. Best practice in optimising the health status of affected individuals will be discussed utilising contemporary evidence to support a range of possible interventions. Such interventions recognise the necessity of working in a person-centred way and hence build on the approaches to health outlined in the previous chapter. The complexity of such physical health conditions among people with learning disabilities often necessitates a multi-disciplinary approach, therefore the range of professionals that could be involved in the provision of support is discussed. While 'physical disability' is an umbrella term encompassing a wide range of conditions, this chapter will specifically focus on disorders of movement, eating, swallowing and nutrition and bladder and bowel difficulties.

Physical disabilities: an overview

There are many causes of physical disabilities which impact on individuals with learning disabilities to a lesser or greater degree. Genetic causes can be linked to specific syndromes or conditions such as Down syndrome, Prader–Willi and Fragile X (some of which are discussed in Ch. 2), though this is not an exhaustive list. Aside from genetics, it must be noted that environmental factors also play a role in causing and exacerbating physical disabilities such as those experienced by people who have cerebral palsy. Such factors can include complications of prematurity, birth trauma, adverse domestic and social circumstances as well as accidental injury and infection. While understanding the cause of an individual's physical disability is important, understanding the manner in which it impacts on the individual's capacity to live a happy and productive life requires full consideration.

Physical disabilities, in addition to a learning disability, have a marked impact on the individual's capacity to exercise control over their lives and it is implicit that appropriate supports are available to individuals cognisant of their rights to respect, dignity, choice, self-determination and independence. Thus the individual with a learning disability must be central to the development of all aspects of supports. These supports must be fit for purpose and meet the needs of individuals who require them.

Person-centred assessment and interventions

When undertaking an assessment of the needs of people with learning disabilities who present with physical disabilities, the basic principles of person-centredness should be adhered to (see Table 14.1).

Table 14.1 Principles of person-centred assessment

Principles	Indicators
Person is at the centre of the assessment process.	• The person is involved in the assessment. • Communication used to include appropriate language and the use of augmentative communication strategies. • Consultation with the individual regarding who is involved and where and when the assessment takes place.
Assessment should be important to the person reflecting the supports they require.	• Assessment should identify and document the person's needs and requirements. • Professional assessments should be incorporated into the overall plan as required. • Actions should reflect the persons needs and not what is available. • Consultation should identify areas of concern.
Inclusion of family members and significant others.	• Discuss with the individual who should be included in the assessment. • Encourage and support those involved in the assessment process.
Long-term goals.	• Care provision reflects the outcome of the assessment. • Assessment is an ongoing process. • Assessment should evolve over time reflecting changing needs of the individual. • Assessment should reflect the individuals past, present and future goals.

(Aldridge 2009)

The process should fully involve the individual and, where appropriate and necessary, their families should be communicated with and integrated into the decision-making process leading to the development of appropriate and responsive interventions. When developing therapeutic interventions, the individual and their families should be made aware of the range of options and services available to them. It is important that this information is communicated in an accessible format (see Ch. 6). Additionally short-and long-term goals should be clearly identified to ensure that any interventions implemented are fit for purpose.

Disorders of movement

There are two systems in the body concerned with movement: the skeletal system and the muscular system, often referred together as 'the musculoskeletal system'. The musculoskeletal system is comprised of bones, muscles, joints, cartilage, tendons, ligaments and connective tissue. The bones provide structure and support to the body and protect vital organs such as the heart and brain. Bone is continually regenerating throughout the lifespan; as an individual ages, the 'building up' process slows down. After the age of 30, it is easier to lose bone than to build it up. Between the ages of 40 and 50, more bone mass is lost than is produced.

Normal movement occurs only if there is an intact musculoskeletal system, nervous system and undamaged inner ear structures (Berman et al 2008). Moreover, movement and positioning of the body are possible through the joints and associated voluntary skeletal muscles which are under the conscious control of the person. The impact of musculoskeletal problems experienced by an individual with learning disabilities varies from slight problems with balance that might necessitate the use of walking aids, to partial or total dependence on a wheelchair.

When musculoskeletal disorders are evident, the risk of skin breakdown, aspiration and constipation is significantly increased. These factors can be further exacerbated by poor positioning, inadequate/inappropriate seating or equipment. Additionally the individual is at a higher risk of developing serious respiratory problems, fractures, osteoporosis, hip and spinal problems including spinal curvatures, all of which ultimately impact on overall functional ability. These immobility-related conditions can further exacerbate the physical health of the individual leading to muscle atrophy (wasting), a reduction in muscle mass and potentially hip and spinal problems (Hong 2005). Significantly, those with cerebral palsy and profound and multiple disabilities commonly experience spasticity and joint contractures due to their neuromuscular difficulties.

It is important to recognise that disorders of the musculoskeletal system have far reaching implications not only for the physical health of the individual but also on their psychological and social wellbeing, affecting their overall quality of life.

Spasticity

Spasticity is where there is increased muscle tone due to a loss of control of spinal reflexes and exaggerated reflexes resulting in joint contractures (Batshaw 2002). For many, spasticity leads to the shortening of muscles which can decrease the range of movement within the limbs over time. The condition can be divided into five subcategories depending on muscles and areas of the body affected: monoplegia (one limb affected), hemiplegia (one side of body affected), diplegia (spasticity predominately in both legs), triplegia (spasticity in three limbs) and quadriplegia (spasticity in all four limbs) (see Fig. 14.1).

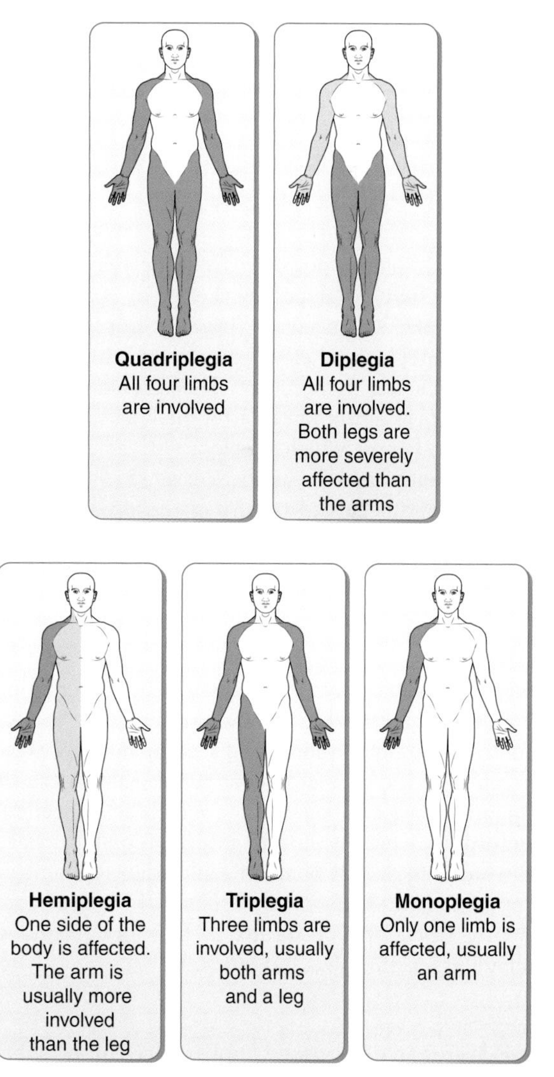

Figure 14.1 • Categories of spasticity (http://www.ofcp.on.ca/guide.html)

The consequences of this condition are overall muscle weakness, decreased range of functional ability and impaired coordination. Without appropriate interventions to manage this condition, the physical health of the individual will continue to deteriorate.

There is a broad spectrum of possible interventions available to individuals who experience spasticity ranging from passive movement exercises, correct positioning, physiotherapy, medication such as muscle relaxants, orthotics and ultimately surgical interventions. The management of this condition requires the input of a range of professionals dependent on individual needs, and may include nurses, physiotherapists, occupational therapists, GP and medical/surgical consultants. Ultimately the cause of and extent to which spasticity is present will dictate the professional involvement and forms of treatment required.

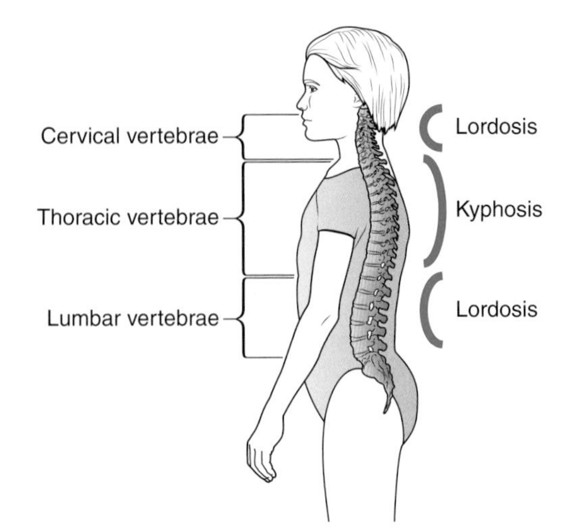

Figure 14.2 • Different curvatures of the spine (http://www.eorthopod.com/sites/default/files/images/)

Curvatures of the spine: kyphosis, lordosis and scoliosis

The spinal column normally has four spinal curves which are fully developed by the age of 10. At birth there is one slight curve (primary curve) which appears late in fetal development which becomes the thoracic and sacral curve. The secondary curves do not appear until months after birth and consist of the cervical curve which develops with achievement of head control and the lumbar curve which develops when a child begins to stand. For those who do not achieve these milestones, abnormal curvatures of the spine including kyphosis, lordosis and scoliosis can occur.

Kyphosis

Kyphosis is excessive roundness of the upper spine commonly referred to as a humpback. It is also referred to as kypho-lordosis if accompanied by exaggeration of the normal lumbar curve. Known causes include changes in bones of the vertebrae, congenital deformity, changes in the intervertebral cartilage discs due to loss of bone, or faulty development of supporting muscles of the spine. If muscles are poorly developed, it results in flat foot, rounded shoulders, clumsiness and lethargy.

Lordosis

Lordosis is an exaggerated lumbar curve in the spine where there is an obvious inward unnatural curvature in the lower back. Lordosis is often seen in obesity, pregnancy and in those with weak muscles. The signs of lordosis includes slumped posture, forward-flexing neck, protruding abdomen, pelvis pushed forward, hyperextended knees, low back pain and fatigue (Kozier et al 2008) (see Fig. 14.2).

Scoliosis

Scoliosis is any side to side curve of the spine with one single curve or two or more curves occurring in opposite directions. Identified causes include idiopathic (cause unknown), congenital deformity especially spina bifida, rickets, paralysis of the back or abdominal muscles and faulty posture. The most serious complication of this condition is reduction in the size of the thoracic cavity compromising the capacity of the lungs and heart to function effectively. With this condition, the person is prone to developing pressure ulcers, back pain and gross deformity of the whole trunk. Early indicators of scoliosis are unequal shoulder heights and slanting of the waist (Batshaw et al 2007) (see Fig. 14.3).

Management of curvatures of the spine

The management of spinal curvatures is highly dependent on the cause and the severity of the condition. For developmental causes such as poor posture, interventions addressing general health, posture and exercise will be warranted. Structural and fixed anomalies are more difficult and at times impossible to treat and correct. However, it is imperative that there is no further structural deterioration so the use of a variety of orthotic aids should be

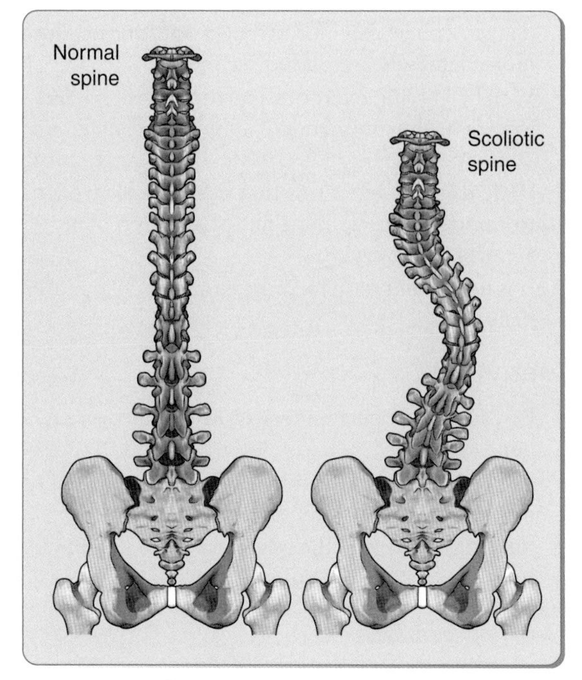

Figure 14.3 • Scoliosis

considered including permanent spinal support braces and moulded or supported seating which may be considered to slow deterioration.

Congenital dislocation of the hips

Congenital dislocation of the hip, now referred to as development dislocation of the hip, is most commonly found in girls and ranges in severity (Batshaw et al 2007). Dislocation of the hip occurs when the head of the femur is partially or completely displaced out from the hip socket. This condition was previously believed to occur exclusively in the womb, however it is now recognised that it may occur gradually after birth. Early diagnosis is essential as non-surgical management such as a Pavlik harness (a harness which ensures hips are kept in normal alignment) are very successful in the first 6 months of life. Corrective surgery may be required in the event that non-surgical interventions are unsuccessful.

Dyspraxia

Dyspraxia is referred to as a developmental coordination disorder (DCD), a complex condition with many signs and symptoms. The Dyspraxia Foundation (2010) defines it as "an impairment or immaturity in the organisation of movement which leads to associated problems with language, perception and thought". It presents primarily with difficulties with gross motor movement, for example jumping, running, climbing and catching. The person may present with poor posture due to low muscle tone. Additionally they may have difficulties with small movements of the fingers including using a pen, knife and fork, tying of shoe laces, buttons or zips. Dyspraxia often affects the ability of the person to process information from the senses and may lead to being over- or undersensitive to input from any of the senses. Oversensitivity includes distress at loud noises and fear response on swings due to a lack of awareness of body position in space and spatial relationships. Undersensitivity includes low response to pain and perhaps not responding to name being called. Those with dyspraxia may also have poor body awareness and may appear to be clumsy and bang into objects.

Early diagnosis and intervention is important if difficulties are evident in these areas. Therefore, a comprehensive assessment needs to be undertaken inclusive of the individual themselves, family members, support staff and the multi-disciplinary team such as the GP, psychologist, occupational therapist, speech and language therapist and the physiotherapist.

Osteoporosis

Osteoporosis is a disease characterised by low bone mass and structural deterioration of bone tissue caused by an imbalance between calcium reabsorption and bone formation. As a result, bones become fragile resulting in a high risk of fractures especially of the hip, spine and wrist although any bone may be affected. Osteoporosis is often called a 'silent disease' as it occurs without symptoms often diagnosed initially as a result of a break in a bone. However, for some, localised pain may present as an early indication of a break. In people with learning disabilities, it is beginning to occur more frequently than previously observed as many are now living longer and presenting with age-related conditions. Significantly, women with learning disabilities occasionally present with late onset of menstruation (menarche) and early onset of menopause, limiting oestrogen production which is a factor known to increase the risk of osteoporosis (Lohiya et al 2004). Other risk factors for osteoporosis are outlined in Table 14.2.

Table 14.2 Risk factors for osteoporosis

Risk	Related to
Lifestyle	• Cigarette smoking. • Excessive alcohol consumption. • Inadequate calcium intake. • Little or no weight-bearing exercise.
Medication/ chronic diseases	• Rheumatoid arthritis. • Endocrine disorders, e.g. underactive thyroid. • Seizure disorders, e.g. epilepsy.
Gender (women)	Lack of oestrogen caused by: • Early menopause (before age of 45). • Early hysterectomy (before age of 45) especially when both ovaries have been removed, i.e. oopherectomy. • Missing periods for 6 months or more, excluding pregnancy, but as result of overexercising/overdieting.
Drugs	• Antacids (neutralises stomach acid). • Gonadotrophin-releasing hormones. • Methotrexate: for cancer treatment. • Cyclosporin A: an immunosuppressive drug. • Heparin (blood thinner).

Early diagnosis is paramount and it is the GP who is often required to carry out a detailed health history of the individual, family history and lifestyle factors as part of the initial assessment. A bone mineral density test is also required for a definitive diagnosis.

Upon diagnosis, an intervention can slow down or arrest the progression of this disease. Numerous interventions are available including advice on weight-bearing exercises such as walking or lifting weights. Indeed, lost bone can be replaced in most people if treated correctly in accordance to that advised by the GP. Such treatments are aimed at strengthening bone, reducing the risk of fractures, managing pain relief, maintaining bone density, stopping or slowing the rate of calcium reabsorption, reducing discomfort, maintaining a satisfactory lifestyle, preserving physical function and promoting healthy eating.

Management of osteoporosis

Exercise

- Family doctor to be consulted prior to commencing any exercise regimes.
- Lack of exercise can contribute to lower bone density (bones become stronger and denser the more demands are placed on them).
- Weight-bearing exercises including walking and jogging are recommended to build and maintain bone mass.
- Weight-lifting exercises that use muscle strength to improve muscle mass and strengthen bone are also encouraged.
- It is best to exercise for approximately 30 minutes daily.

Lifestyle factors

- Be careful of being underweight as this decreases bone density.
- Diet rich in calcium and vitamin D is essential as it helps the absorption of calcium.
- Sunshine promotes the manufacture of vitamin D.
- Reduce smoking, caffeine and alcohol intake.

Diet and nutrition

The following calcium intake is recommended for all people, with or without osteoporosis:

- 800 mg/day for children 1–10 years of age
- 1000 mg/day for men, premenopausal women and postmenopausal women also taking oestrogen
- 1200 mg/day for teenagers and young adults 11–24 years of age
- 1500 mg/day for postmenopausal women not taking oestrogen
- 1200–1500 mg/day for pregnant and nursing mothers

The total daily intake of calcium should not exceed 2000 mg (National Institutes of Health 2000).

Foods rich in calcium include dairy products, some green vegetables, some juices, breakfast cereals, soya milk, fortified bread and bottled water.

Medications

Hormone replacement therapy (HRT) restores levels of oestrogen to premenopausal levels thus slowing bone loss and maintaining bone level. The risks and benefits of HRT need to be assessed individually and carefully discussed due to risks and side effects including breast cancer (Hopkins 2005).

Both men and women with a learning disability are at risk of osteoporosis due to inactivity as a consequence of impaired mobility and long-term use of medications such as antiepileptic drugs, however women are at an increased risk due to the effects of the menopause. Indeed, specific attention must be paid to other medications being taken in addition to calcium as calcium could impact on their absorption (Rubin & Crocker 2006). Additionally, analgesics may need to be prescribed and taken as directed to relieve pain following a break.

Pain assessment and management

Numerous reports such as *Treat me Right!* (Mencap 2004) and *Death by Indifference* (Mencap 2007) have identified that pain experienced by people with a learning disability is poorly recognised by professionals thus impacting on the health and wellbeing of this population. Pain is subjective and multidimensional, impacting differently on each individual. "Pain is whatever the experiencing person says it is existing whenever he says it does" (McCaffery 1968:95 cited in Dougherty & Lister 2008). However, for those with a learning disability, communicating where and how pain is impacting on their daily lives can be a significant barrier to its successful management. Often those with a learning disability may be completely reliant on the observations and actions of others to ensure effective pain management. However, it is evident that underdiagnosis of pain, underutilisation of pain assessments and the misconception that people with a learning disability have higher pain thresholds than the general population limit effective management of pain (Beacroft & Dodd 2009). For those individuals who have the capacity to self-assess and identify their personal level of pain, augmentative and alternative communication devices can be used and include easy-read assessment tools or visual analogue pain scales. For those who are dependent on others to identify the presence or absence of pain, effective management requires the use of appropriate pain assessment tools such as Disability Distress Assessment Tool (DisDat) (Northumberland Tyne & Wear NHS Trust and St Oswald's Hospice 2008), or the Pain and Discomfort Scale (PADS) (Bodfish et al 2001). Additionally, observation of the individual and knowledge of any general health issues are fundamentally important to successful pain management. Information from family and significant others relating to how the individual expresses pain is also vitally important.

Expression of pain is multi-faceted and may include self-injurious behaviour, grimacing, crying, sweating profusely and pallor. In contrast, the person may be withdrawn, reluctant to engage in activities and have a poor appetite. The treatment of pain is unique to the individual and the ultimate aim of treatment is to identify and treat the cause of the pain. In the event that the cause of the pain cannot be treated, the aim then becomes to ensure the effective management of pain ensuring a positive outcome and good quality of life for the individual.

Reader activity 14.1

Hannah is a 48-year-old lady who has a mild learning disability and lives at home with her sister Julie. She has worked all her adult life until recently retiring due to ill health. Hannah has recently broken her wrist and following investigations has been diagnosed with osteoporosis. In addition, her sister has noticed lately that her posture has become more stooped and she also appears to be experiencing pain. Although Hannah is not complaining, she does recognise that osteoporosis is impacting on her quality of life. While Julie is alarmed by the overall deterioration in her sister's health, they have approached you for support around minimising the impact osteoporosis is having on her quality of life.

- How would you work in a person-centred way to:
    - minimise the effects of osteoporosis?
    - ensure adequate calcium intake?
- What other actions might you consider to support Hannah and her sister?
- What factors influenced your decision?

Nutrition and hydration

Nutritional issues impact significantly on the quality of life of people with learning disabilities from both a physical and social perspective. Food plays an essential role in peoples lives; not only does it ensure adequate nutrition but can also be a means of social contact. However, for many people with learning disabilities and their families, mealtimes can be a source of stress and anxiety considering that 30–35% have difficulties with eating and drinking (Telch & Telch 2003) resulting in slow growth, inadequate weight gain, dehydration and malnutrition (Royal College of Physicians and British Society of Gastroenterology 2010). Conversely, obesity can also negatively impact on a person's wellbeing contributing to health issues relating to mobility, gastrointestinal disorders and cardiorespiratory conditions. Individuals with a severe or profound level of learning disability are at an increased risk of being underweight and malnourished (Brown 2009) in comparison to their peers with mild or moderate level of learning disabilities who have a higher risk of being obese (Melville et al 2007). Living arrangements have been identified as significantly impacting on nutrition with individuals living in congregate settings presenting with lower levels of obesity compared to their peers living at home or independently, suggesting that the environment is a crucial influencing factor with respect to weight (Melville et al 2007). Table 14.3 provides key definitions relating to nutrition and hydration.

Obesity

The World Health Organization (2004) has identified obesity as a major health concern on an international level for those with and without learning disabilities. It is generally accepted that people with learning disabilities are at an increased risk of being overweight or becoming obese in comparison to their peers in the general population. The International Association for the Scientific Study of Intellectual Disabilities (Lennox et al 2002) has indicated that managing obesity in this population should be a priority as it can reduce life expectancy and place people at an increased risk of developing serious health conditions such as heart disease, diabetes and cancer (Bradley 2005).

Table 14.3 Definitions of nutrition and hydration

Term	Definition
Underweight or overweight	An individual can be defined as being under- or overweight when they weigh less or more than the recommended weight as identified by body mass index (BMI).
Malnourished	The state of being poorly nourished which may be caused by inadequate food or essential nutrients either from poor absorption, eating and drinking difficulties and metabolic disorders.
Dehydrated	Loss or removal of fluid where fluid intake fails to replace fluid lost from the body due to excessive sweating, polyuria (excessive urination), vomiting, diarrhoea and eating and drinking difficulties.
Obesity	The accumulation and excessive storage of fat on the body. Caused by excessive calorie intake. Level of obesity is calculated using body mass index. Morbid obesity is classified when body weight is 70% more than the ideal weight for specific individuals.

(Freshwater & Maslin-Prothero 2005)

Some determinants of obesity in the learning disability population include gender (women are more at risk), increasing age starting from 34 years of age onwards, level of learning disability (people with a mild or moderate learning disability are at an increased risk), the manifestation of specific syndromes (Down syndrome and Prader–Willi), the side effects of medications (anti-depressants and anti-epileptic drugs) and living arrangements (those living at home or independently are at higher risk) (Melville et al 2007). Thus obesity presents many challenges for individuals with learning disabilities and their carers and a variety of interventions can be employed in the management of this condition. Such interventions may include advice with exercise and diet, participation in health promotion initiatives, access to a dietician and behavioural interventions. Behavioural interventions may be particularly beneficial in the development of life skills around food preparation, food consumption and maintenance of balanced diets and exercise plans (Sharma 2006).

See Reader activity 14.2 on the Evolve website.

Disorders of eating and swallowing

There are three phases of normal swallowing: oral (mouth), pharyngeal (swallowing reflex is triggered) and oesophageal (movement of food along the oesophagus into the stomach) (Dalton 2009). When eating, food is placed in the mouth. Effective lip closure is essential to prevent spillage. Food is then chewed, sucked and mixed with saliva to create a bolus (ball) which is then swallowed. Biting and chewing reduces the size of food to manageable lumps which is pushed by the tongue into the oesophagus and onwards to the stomach for digestion. Food is prevented from entering the airway through the actions of the epiglottis (see Fig. 14.4).

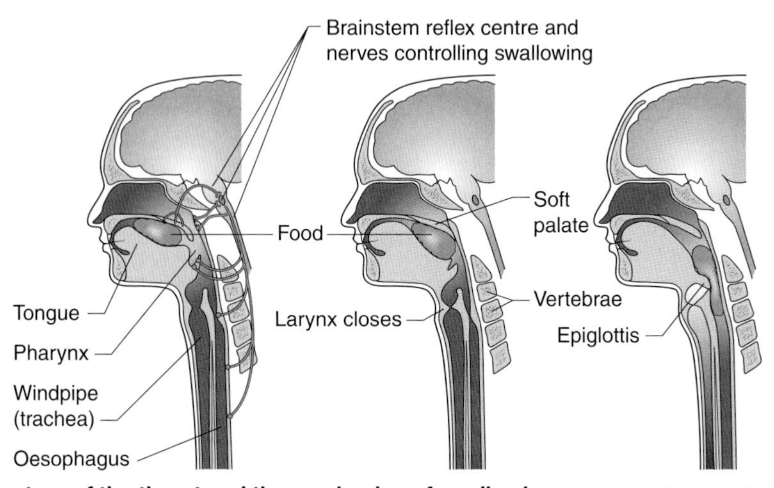

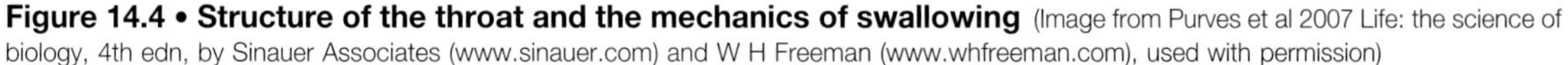
Figure 14.4 • Structure of the throat and the mechanics of swallowing (Image from Purves et al 2007 Life: the science of biology, 4th edn, by Sinauer Associates (www.sinauer.com) and W H Freeman (www.whfreeman.com), used with permission)

While for the majority of people with learning disabilities, eating and drinking are an automatic social activity, for some, disorders of eating and swallowing are more prevalent due to reduced or heightened oral sensation, abnormalities of the mouth such as cleft lip or palate, uncoordinated and involuntary movements as a result of conditions such as cerebral palsy or behaviour problems that interfere with one's ability to participate appropriately at mealtimes, for example hyperactivity. Some common features of these disorders include excessive drooling, difficulty with chewing, difficulty or delay with swallowing, tongue thrust, pocketing of food, coughing, choking and regurgitation.

Gastro-oesophageal reflux disease (GORD)

GORD is a condition which involves the backward flow of stomach contents into the oesophagus (throat) resulting in a burning sensation in the chest (Seeley et al 2010). Signs include chest pain, vomiting, refusal or fear of eating, recurrent wheezing and heartburn. Stomach contents entering the airway may cause coughing and choking, potentially leading to recurrent episodes of aspiration pneumonia (Pawlyn & Carnaby 2009). Consequently, GORD causes irritation and distress making mealtimes an uncomfortable experience.

According to Bohmer et al (2001), GORD can be present in up to 50% of people with learning disabilities and as such is a significant area of concern. Indeed the presence of a learning disability may often lead to underdiagnosis of this condition as some individuals may be unable to express symptoms of discomfort. Additionally, GORD can be exacerbated as a result of coexisting conditions such as cerebral palsy, postural abnormalities (scoliosis) and enteral feeding where correct upright positioning of an individual is not maintained for an adequate amount of time post administration of the enteral feed. Enteral feeding involves the provision of nutrient-rich fluids via small-bore feeding tubes through the nose (nasogastric), the stomach (gastrostomy) or the jejunum (jejunostomy).

Aspiration pneumonia

Aspiration pneumonia occurs when food is aspirated (inhaled) into the lungs (Pawlyn & Carnaby 2009). The signs of this include coughing and choking, gagging, wheezing, lengthy feeding times, recurrent chest infections, high temperature and change of facial colour. The individual may appear flushed, pale or cyanosed (bluish discolouration of the skin as there is not enough oxygen in the blood). It should be noted that 'silent' aspiration may occur where the above signs are absent but the individual experiences recurrent episodes of chest infections or pneumonia and further investigations are warranted. These investigations may include some or all of the following: arterial blood gases (checks for levels of oxygen, carbon dioxide and acidity levels in blood), chest X-rays, sputum collection (phlegm), complete blood counts and swallowing studies (Walsh 2002). At this stage, referral to a physiotherapist, speech and language therapist and dietician would be warranted for assessment of needs.

Dysphagia

Dysphagia is a disorder of swallowing where problems can occur during any phase of swallowing from the point where food is taken into the mouth, the bolus is prepared and is pushed into the stomach via the oesophagus (Rubin & Crocker 2006). Dysphagia is potentially a life-threatening condition that can cause dehydration, malnutrition, asphyxiation, aspiration ultimately causing respiratory tract infections, a leading cause of mortality among people with learning disabilities (Chadwick et al 2006, Mencap 2004). Malnutrition as reported by Mencap (2007) was the cause of the death of Martin, a 43-year-old man with learning disabilities who was left without food for 26 days following a stroke.

Therefore the importance of providing support to those with eating and swallowing difficulties cannot be underestimated and it is essential that the signs and symptoms are recognised and taken seriously. Some of the more common signs of dysphagia include coughing while eating, choking, obvious distress, drooling, spillage of food and saliva, pocketing of food in the cheeks, difficulty with chewing, coughing when not eating, tiring during eating and regurgitation. Changes in speech pattern may also be noted. All people identified as poorly nourished or at risk of malnutrition should have a nutritional assessment completed as a matter of urgency. While there are many nutritional assessment tools available, the Malnutrition Universal Screening Tool (MUST) (British Association for Parenteral and Enteral Nutrition 2003) is often used to identify such individuals.

Management of disorders of eating and swallowing

The management of conditions relating to eating and drinking difficulties requires the input of the multi-disciplinary team, to include the individual themselves, family members, speech and language therapist, nurse, occupational therapist, physiotherapist and support staff. Concerns relating to management of disorders of eating and swallowing should be dealt with promptly and appropriately through appropriate assessment. If any of the aforementioned signs are evident, a referral to a speech and language therapist (SLT) who has expertise in dysphagia is the first line of intervention. Once the SLT carries out the assessment, a planned intervention will be identified and implemented to support the individual.

Any intervention must be planned in conjunction with the individual, significant others and members of the multi-disciplinary team as identified above. Interventions are dependent on the severity of the presenting condition and can vary from simple modifications to diet to enteral feeding. All eating and swallowing interventions should have at their core the potential to minimise the risk of aspiration and facilitate adequate nutrition and hydration. Such interventions may include the use of medication, correct positioning during and after meals, the use of appropriate eating utensils and adaptation of eating utensils as required. In addition, attention should be paid to the presentation of food and to ensure choice to optimise the person's appetite for and enjoyment of food. Of specific importance are strategies that include changes to the texture and consistency of food ranging from pureed, minced, ground, chopped and modified regular foods (see Table 14.4).

Fluids may also need to be thickened and there are many products available on the market for this purpose. Fluid textures range from 'thin' such as water, teas and coffee to naturally 'thick' fluids such as milk. Fluids which are thickened using commercial thickeners can be classified under three distinct categories:

1. Fluid leaves a thin coat on the back of a spoon and can be sucked through a straw or drunk from a cup.
2. Fluid leaves a thick coat on the back of a spoon, cannot be drunk through a straw but can be from a cup.
3. Fluids need to be taken from a spoon.

(British Dietetic Association 2009)

Bearing in mind the specific needs of individuals and the impact of dysphagia, particular food types should be avoided such as stringy foods(runner beans); mixed-consistency foods (muesli with milk); crunchy/crumbly foods (toast, dry biscuits) and hard foods such as boiled sweets.

Prior to any planned intervention, including enteral feeds, the person must be made comfortable in an environment that is conducive to eating and drinking with specific emphasis on the social aspect of eating. This can be achieved through effective communication, gaining trust and consent using a person-centred approach where the needs and requirements of the individual are central to the care planning process. This is particularly important given the findings of the Commission for Healthcare Audit and Inspection (2007) who highlighted issues around mealtime regimes for people with learning disabilities; lack of choice in food available and poor communication between staff and people with learning disabilities in residential services were identified as specific areas of concern (see Table 14.5).

Table 14.4 National descriptors of texture

Texture	Description of food texture	Food examples
A	• A smooth, pouring, uniform consistency. • A food that has been pureed and sieved to remove particles. • A thickener may be added to maintain stability. • Cannot be eaten with a fork.	• Tinned tomato soup. • Thin custard.
B	• A smooth, uniform consistency. • A food that has been pureed and sieved to remove particles. • A thickener may be added to maintain stability. • Cannot be eaten with a fork. • Drops rather than pours from a spoon but cannot be piped and layered. • Thicker than A.	• Soft whipped cream. • Thick custard.
C	• A thick, smooth, uniform consistency. • A food that has been pureed and sieved to remove particles. • A thickener may be added to maintain stability. • Can be eaten with a fork or spoon. • Will hold its own shape on a plate, and can be moulded, layered and piped. • No chewing required.	• Mousse. • Smooth fromage frais.
D	• Food that is moist, with some variation in texture. • Has not been pureed or sieved. • These foods may be served or coated with a thick gravy or sauce. • Foods easily mashed with a fork. • Meat should be prepared as C. • Requires very little chewing.	• Flaked fish in thick sauce. • Stewed apple and thick custard.
E	• Dishes consisting of soft, moist food. • Foods can be broken into pieces with a fork. • Dishes can be made up of solids and thick sauces or gravies. • Avoid foods which cause a choking hazard.	• Tender meat casseroles (approx ×1.5 cm diced pieces). • Sponge and custard.
Normal	Any foods.	Include all foods.

British Dietetic Association (2009). National descriptors for texture modification in adults. Birmingham: British Dietetic Association

Oral health

People with learning disabilities often experience poorer oral health than the general population (Yoshihara et al 2005). Regrettably oral disease has not been prioritised when compared with other complex medical conditions identified in this population despite the severity of its impact on the overall health of the individual. Poor oral health leads to dental caries, periodontal disease (gum disease), pain, poor nutritional intake and poor quality of life. Specific issues also arise in this population including bruxism (grinding of teeth), overgrowth of gingival tissues (gums) as a side effect of long-term use of certain medications and altered saliva production (xerostomia; dry mouth) (Doyle & Dalton 2008). A comprehensive oral assessment should be undertaken and an individualised oral care plan should be developed to meet each individual's needs in consultation with the dentist and dental hygienist.

Bladder and bowel function

Elimination is a private and independent bodily function of the bladder and bowel and is not usually a cause of concern until difficulties arise. The embarrassment often associated with discussing these functions can

Table 14.5 Intervention strategy to support adequate nutritional intake

Before meals	During meals	After meals
• Avoid unpleasant or uncomfortable treatments before offering food or drink. • Offer the toilet or change incontinence wear to promote comfort. • Position individual in comfortable chair in upright position. • Take cognisance of individual's likes and dislikes and offer range and choice of food and drink. • Ensure consistency of food is correct for individual. • Ascertain level of independence and provide appropriate supports to maintain independence. • Be aware of and adhere to any eating and drinking programme in place. • Ensure adequate time for the meal.	• Massage the cheeks to encourage chewing if appropriate. • Present food in an appetising manner. • Heating small amounts of food at a time should be considered particularly if the person needs a lot of time to eat the meal in full. • Use appropriate eating and drinking utensils. • Use appropriate communication to engage with the individual during meal times. • Sit with the person and maintain eye contact and attention (one support/individual). • Observe for signs of coughing, choking, distress, changes in colour of face. • Give adequate time for the person to chew and swallow each mouthful. • Adequate fluids offered according to personal preferences. • Avoid distractions.	• Ensure that the individual is satisfied with the meal. • Check the mouth is clear of food. • Attend to personal hygiene needs. • Ensure the person remains in an upright position for at least 30 minutes following the meal. • Ensure comfort of the individual. • Document food and fluid intake.

Reader activity 14.3

Louise is 5 years old and has cerebral palsy which affects all four of her limbs. She has a severe learning disability which limits her ability to communicate verbally. She is unable to walk and uses a specially adapted wheelchair. She lives at home with her parents and her mother is her full-time carer. Louise and her mother access both mainstream and specialist learning disabilities services for support particularly around Louise's feeding difficulties. Louise has dysphagia which means that she has difficulty chewing and swallowing and experiences episodes of coughing and choking when eating and drinking. In addition, Louise also experiences tongue thrust and jaw weakness which creates difficulties with drinking. She has been hospitalised on one occasion with aspiration pneumonia. Recently there has been a deterioration in her overall physical health with a significant weight loss noted and occasional dehydration. Meal times can be distressful and her mother is seeking support to minimise the risk of aspiration and to facilitate adequate food and fluid intake.

- How would you minimise the effects of dysphagia?
- How would you ensure adequate food and fluid intake?
- What other actions might you consider to support Louise and her mother?
- What factors have influenced your decision?

lead to non-disclosure of problems and their presence can negatively impact on both the person and their family through social isolation. At times, even in the event that problems are recognised, difficulties in accessing appropriate professional supports may often occur (Pawlyn & Carnaby 2009). Bowel and bladder problems are an important general health issue that often go unrecognised as symptoms are frequently masked due to the presence of a learning disability, communication difficulties, physical disabilities and withdrawal (Bohmer et al 2001). The elimination process is very subjective and varies from person to person. People usually urinate up to five times a day and their bowels open from between three times a week to three times a day (Kozier et al 2008) dependent on nutritional intake and coexisting conditions (see Table 14.6). Knowing what is normal for an individual can assist in recognising irregularities.

Urinary incontinence

Urinary incontinence is an inability to store urine in the bladder (Palwyn & Carnaby 2009). Normally an individual is aware of the urge to pass urine, but in the case of polyuria (excessive production of urine), infection, constipation and reduced mobility and manual dexterity, this ability is impaired. Notably people with spina bifida are at a higher risk of developing a neurogenic

Table 14.6 Normal process of elimination	
Urinary elimination	**Bowel elimination**
Urine collects in the bladder (1500 ml per day on average per adult).	Faeces pass along the intestine towards the rectum.
Pressure activates nerve endings stimulating the urge to urinate.	Sensory nerves in the rectum are activated stimulating the urge to defaecate.
Urethral sphincter muscle relaxes.	Anal sphincter muscle relaxes.
Person passes urine.	Person passes faeces.

bladder where the individual does not recognise fullness leading to involuntary urination (Berman et al 2008). The bladder becomes flaccid, distended or spastic with frequent involuntary urination.

For those with learning disabilities who are trying to achieve urinary continence, the issue can be further compounded by reduced mobility and cognitive impairments. In this instance, there can be failure to recognise signals which indicate the bladder needs to be emptied. Urinary incontinence is individual and not all cases can be cured but can successfully be managed. The prerequisites for achieving urinary continence include the ability to store urine, sit properly on the toilet and pass urine voluntarily. However, in order to achieve continence, people with learning disability need support from the multi-disciplinary team specifically in relation to education of healthy bladder and bowel, diet, nutrition and exercise as first line of intervention. It is not advisable to immediately resort to using incontinence pads or aids as these lead to dependence and learned helplessness. It is essential that a comprehensive continence assessment is conducted to ensure that dignity, respect and independence are at the core of all interventions as this condition is still under-reported and undertreated for this population (Stenson & Danaher 2005).

The ability to achieve continence varies from person to person depending on the severity of learning disability and associated conditions. Environmental adaptations such as raised toilets, grab rails, foot supports and hoists can be used to support continence in this situation. Appropriate continence wear may also have to be considered to ensure the dignity and comfort of the individual.

Urinary retention

Urinary retention has been defined as "the accumulation of urine in the bladder due to inability to void" (Freshwater & Maslin-Prothero 2005:639). Contributory factors may include obstruction of the urethra (bladder stone), enlargement of the prostate, nerve damage (spina bifida and multiple sclerosis), embarrassment or fear and weak bladder muscles. Additionally cystocoele (bladder droops into vagina), constipation, narrowing of the urethra and surgery also contribute to this condition. The signs and symptoms are quite varied and may include discomfort, pain, abdominal distension, feeling a need to urinate but unable to do so, leakage of urine between trips to the toilet and feeling of incomplete emptying of the bladder (National Institute of Diabetes and Digestive and Kidney Disease 2007). Management of urinary retention varies from person to person and can include conservative methods such as correct positioning of the individual, promoting relaxation and avoiding delay when the urge to empty their bladder arises. If these approaches fail, the use of cholinergic drugs to stimulate the bladder may be required. Additionally, urinary catheterisation may be necessary and types of catheterisation may range from intermittent self-catheterisation to an indwelling Foley catheter and ultimately long-term suprapubic catheterisation depending on the severity of the condition.

Intermittent self-catheterisation

Intermittent self-catheterisation is carried out by the individual at 3–4-hourly intervals throughout the day to maintain dryness, promote comfort, prevent infection and improve quality of life. This method is the approach of choice for those who can understand the technique and who have the capacity to self-catheterise. Those with spina bifida or impaired bladder function benefit from this intervention. It is important that the person uses the toilet prior to catheterisation as this technique is used to completely empty the residual urine from the bladder, further promoting normal bladder function. As this technique requires the introduction of a catheter (hollow tube used to remove urine from the bladder) to the bladder, it is essential that excellent personal hygiene is maintained. This must include washing of hands with warm water and soap, washing of the perineum (area that lies between the vulva and anus in females and between the scrotum and anus in males, often referred to as the pelvic floor) (Freshwater & Maslin-Prothero 2005) and washing of equipment.

There is a possible risk of tissue damage, pain and urinary tract infection during catheterisation. In this event the person needs to seek medical attention to resolve any of these issues.

Faecal incontinence

Faecal incontinence is a sign or symptom of an underlying condition relating to neuromuscular conditions, physical disabilities, spinal cord trauma, behavioural difficulties, failure to recognise the urge to defaecate and difficulties with dressing or undressing. There is a loss of voluntary ability to control the exit of faeces from the bowel, therefore it is imperative that the cause (or causes) for each individual is diagnosed promptly as many factors are relatively simple to reverse (National Institute for Clinical Excellence (NICE) 2007). Moreover, faecal incontinence has remained a largely hidden problem due primarily to the embarrassment and shame experienced by individuals. Indeed, Cassidy et al (2002) in their research identified that 26% of people with learning disability experience problems with faecal continence. Faecal incontinence is further compounded by the presence of a learning disability and treatment is often not prioritised or even considered as there can be a perception that faecal incontinence is symptomatic of a learning disability as opposed to a skill that can be taught.

Thus the management of this condition needs to be prompt, appropriate and include members of the multi-disciplinary team including the continence advisor to identify appropriate treatment strategies. Strategies may include use of skills training programmes, education, appropriate and accessible toileting facilities, changes to diet and lifestyle and use of appropriate continence aids.

A comprehensive assessment of bowel pattern needs to be undertaken to establish the extent of the problem and, following this, interventions can be planned and implemented accordingly. The process begins with identifying reversible factors such as clothing, diet and exercise, progressing to the use of specialised continence aids with surgery being the last.

Skin integrity

It is a function of the skin to prevent infection, regulate body temperature, maintain fluid and chemical balance and produce vitamin D. In addition, one's ability to respond to pain, temperature and touch is regulated by nerve endings in the skin (Clark 2009). If skin integrity is compromised, infections and decubitus ulcers (pressure sores) may occur. Common risk factors include immobility, friction, pressure due to poor positioning, poor nutritional intake, age and moisture (Ebersole et al 2008). Therefore, personal hygiene and attention to skin integrity are of paramount importance for people who experience urinary and faecal incontinence. As part of a person-centred care approach, an assessment of the skin should be undertaken to determine an individual's level of risk. Given the intimate nature of such an assessment, the personal integrity and dignity of the individual should be of the foremost concern. In addition, the individual's cultural and religious beliefs must be addressed. Discretion in undertaking this form of assessment and discussion of outcomes should be of paramount importance in maintaining the respect and dignity of the individual. When undertaking an assessment of the skin formal assessment tools such as The Waterlow Score (Waterlow 2005) and Braden Scale (Braden & Bergstrom 1989) should be considered. These tools examine features such as skin type, continence, mobility and malnutrition. In the event of an identified risk to skin integrity, care should include a balanced diet, adequate fluid intake, good personal hygiene, use of appropriate skin care products, changes in positioning, correct use of and adaptation of equipment and clothing from natural fibres such as cotton.

Constipation

Many disorders of digestion are evident specifically for people with learning disability. Constipation is one of the most common digestive complaints for this population, occurring in 19% of children with learning disabilities (Wallace 2007) and 69% of adults with learning disabilities (Bohmer et al 2001). Notably, constipation has received insufficient attention in terms of recognition, prevention and management despite the fact that it can be managed and treated quite easily. People with cerebral palsy and Down syndrome are at a high risk of suffering from constipation. However, constipation is not exclusive to these populations and affects many others across the lifespan with learning disabilities. Many factors including immobility, hypotonia (low muscle tone), eating and swallowing difficulties as well as mobility limitations have all been recognised as contributing to this condition.

Indeed constipation can be further exacerbated by environmental, physical and psychological factors though this is not an exhaustive list (see Table 14.7). Arguably sedentary lifestyles, lack of exercise and increased longevity among people with learning disabilities further increases the risk of developing constipation (Marsh et al 2010). Symptoms of constipation include straining, hard stool, halitosis, infrequent defaecation and vomiting. Moreover, if a person has fewer than three bowel movements per week with associated abdominal fullness, pain or bloating with symptoms persisting for at least three months, this would indicate that the person is constipated (Folden et al 2002).

In addition, in cases of chronic constipation, faecal fluid can leak from the bowel and can be misdiagnosed as diarrhoea and often anti-diarrhoeal medications are inappropriately prescribed. If faecal overflow occurs, it is important to continue with the planned intervention as the person is still constipated.

Categories of constipation

Constipation can be primary (unknown cause), secondary (physiological diseases or conditions which affect bowel function) and iatrogenic (side effects of medications) (Kyle 2006). Primary or idiopathic constipation is largely associated with lifestyle changes with no underlying medical cause. In almost 90% of children, constipation is thought to be functional (no organic cause) or idiopathic in nature (Benninga 2004). Secondary constipation may be a consequence of physiological diseases or conditions which affect bowel function (see Table 14.8).

Management of constipation

Given the personal and subjective nature of this condition, the person must be at the centre of any intervention supported by significant others and members of the multi-disciplinary team including the nurse, physiotherapist, the GP and the dietician. In this instance, referral to the dietician is the first port of call as the dietician will carry out an nutritional assessment, identify a planned intervention and consider the appropriate supports required to promote the healthy bowel. Any interventions are dependent on the severity of the condition and can vary from simple modifications to diet and lifestyle to medical interventions. People with learning disability are frequently prescribed many medications and constipation is a notable side effect. It is essential that those supporting this population are aware of this and take appropriate action to combat these side

Table 14.7 Factors influencing constipation

Environmental	• Poor diet. • Lack of exercise. • Change in routine and diet. • Low-fibre diet. • Poor fluid intake. • Toilet training. • Inadequate toileting facilities. • Increased use of a bed pan.
Physical	• Stressful events. • Reduced physical exercise. • Pregnancy. • Irritable bowel syndrome. • Pelvic floor muscle damage.
Psychological	• Social isolation – withdrawal from community activities due to embarrassement. • Loneliness and anxiety leading to depression.

Table 14.8 Categories of constipation

Categories	Associated with
Primary (idiopathic constipation – unknown origin).	• Largely lifestyle changes with no underlying medical cause.
Secondary (physiological diseases or conditions which affect bowel function).	• Parkinson's disease. • Multiple sclerosis. • Spinal cord damage. • Cerebral palsy. • Diabetes mellitus (metabolic disorder affecting blood sugar level). • Hypothyroidism (low thyroid hormone production). • Depression.
Iatrogenic (common side effect of polypharmacy – use of two or more medications).	• Anti-depressants. • Iron supplements. • Calcium channel blockers. • Anti-emetics (controls vomiting). • Anti-epileptics (see Ch. 16).

Table 14.9 Toilet use

Before visiting the toilet	During toileting	After toileting
• Ensure toilet is accessible at all times and free from clutter. • Ascertain level of independence of individual and ability to get to the toilet. • Ensure bathroom is well ventilated, warm and clean. • If unable to access the bathroom, offer a commode or bedpan to promote independence. • Ensure that room is of adequate size to accomodate support staff if needed. • Ensure that the toilet is of appropriate height (see seating position during toileting).	• Ensure privacy at all times. • Ensure that individual can adjust their clothing. • Ensure adequate time is given. • Ensure that the person is seated with knees higher than hips, leaning forward, elbows on knees and sitting upright with feet supported if necessary. • Avoid distractions. • Be supportive and observe the individual for signs of distress, pain or discomfort.	• Ensure comfort of the individual and offer assistance if necessary. • Attend to personal hygiene needs. • Document bowel movement using the Bristol stool form scale (Lewis & Heaton 1997).

effects. This can be achieved through knowledge, and regular review, of medications and awareness of side effects. The aim of all interventions is to minimise discomfort, promote normal bowel function thus ensuring dignity, respect and independence. It is essential to promote comfort when using the toilet and this can be achieved quite easily (see Table 14.9).

Assessment is vital in ensuring that a correct diagnosis and appropriate management can be developed and achieved. Any assessment must take into consideration how the person communicates their symptoms, their health history, a physical examination and a baseline assessment. Furthermore, it is essential that support staff are knowledgeable of the full range of interventions that can be employed. These include consideration of diet and nutrition, hydration, positioning, physical activity, medications and appropriate referral to continence advisors and physiotherapists. Appropriate interventions developed by knowledgeable support staff can lead to increased independence and limited reliance on incontinence aids for those with a learning disability thus improving the individual's quality of life.

Intervention plans are multi-factorial and should include some or all of the following aspects, beginning with increasing fibre and fluid in the diet and correct positioning as this is required to ensure comfort, full emptying of the bladder and bowel. In the event that incontinence aids such as incontinence pads are required, it is advisable to liaise with a continence advisor in relation to the selection of the appropriate pads to be used and the correct disposal of them. Additionally, physical activity and the use of medications also need to be addressed as part of the intervention.

Fibre and fluid in the diet

The cultural beliefs of each person needs to be considered as each culture has its own standardised food behaviours that dictate what is edible, the role of certain foods in the diet and how food is prepared. A high-fibre and fluid diet suitable for all the family should be encouraged with regular meal patterns and appropriate frequency of meals. The goal of increasing fibre in the diet applies to all meals as fibre absorbs water thus increasing the water content of stool, making them softer and easier to pass.

The average recommended daily intake of fibre for adults varies from 25 g per day for women to 38 g per day for men (Ramont et al 2010). Children's fibre requirement is calculated as the age of the child plus 5 g in children older than 2 years. For example, if a child is 7 years old, the calculation would be $7 + 5 =$ 13 g per day. Remember, fibre portions should be increased gradually as, if increased too quickly, it is counterproductive resulting in constipation.

Increasing fibre

Try to include some of the following fibre-containing foods at each meal/snack time:

- Breakfast cereals with a high wheat, oats and bran content.
- Wholemeal bread and products made with wholemeal flour – scones, muffins, cakes and pastries.
- Wholemeal pasta and brown rice.
- High-fibre biscuits are good snack choices but care needs to be taken with salt and sugar content.
- Fruit and vegetables (five portions per day).

- Pulses, e.g. baked beans, kidney beans, chickpeas and lentils. These can often be added to a meal or added into stews and casseroles.
- Jacket potatoes with the skin left on.
- High-fibre bread.

Increasing fluids

It is also important to ensure that individuals have an adequate fluid intake of at least 2 litres per day. Additional fluids may be needed during exercise or if the weather is hot.

- Encourage plenty of non-fizzy drinks, e.g. water, squash and fruit juice. Aim for 8–10 glasses of fluid each day. Give after a meal or snack rather than before so they do not reduce appetite.
- Avoid excessive milk consumption as milk can be filling resulting in poor dietary intake.
- For those who find it difficult to increase the amount they drink, try to include foods that contains high fluid level, e.g. gravy, sauces, soups, custard, jelly, ice lollies, fruit, vegetables and salad.

Breakfast ideas

- Bran sprinkled with raisins with milk.
- Wheat with chopped banana and milk.
- Cereal bar and banana.
- Wholemeal toast with margarine and marmalade.

Lunch ideas

- Wholemeal roll/bread with tuna and sweetcorn or egg and salad, yoghurt or fromage frais and an apple.
- Wholemeal pitta bread with ham or turkey and tomato, muesli bar/slice of fruit cake or wholemeal muffin and small bunch of grapes or tangerine.
- Baked beans on toast.
- Vegetable pizza and salad.
- Lentil soup with wholemeal bread/roll.

Main meal ideas

- Fish fingers, mashed potatoes and peas.
- Bean casserole with wholemeal pitta bread.
- Jacket potato and beans.
- Chilli con carne with brown rice.
- Spaghetti bolognaise with wholemeal pasta.
- Stir fry chicken and vegetables with rice/noodles.
- Meat casserole with vegetables and jacket potato.
- Sausage casserole with mashed potato and beans.
- Fish, chips and beans/peas.

Snack ideas

- Fresh fruit/dried fruit.
- Digestive biscuits/hobnobs/fig roll.
- Wholemeal scone.
- Flapjack.
- Fruit cake/malt loaf.

(Adapted from IMPACT 2004)

The above suggested diet can also be adapted for use in the adult population but bearing in mind the higher fibre requirements of adults. Information pertaining to adult dietary requirements is available at the Irish Nutrition and Dietetic Institute (see Useful addresses).

Physical activity

Sedentary lifestyles in people with learning disability have an adverse effect on health, and considering that over half of people with learning disability take little or no exercise, this is a cause for concern (Draheim et al 2002). Consequently, a lack of exercise slows the natural movement of faeces in the bowel resulting in constipation. Therefore, the development of social activities to include sports or physical activity should form an integral part of the intervention cognisant of individuals' coexisting conditions. For example, those with Down syndrome have poor muscle tone (hypotonia) thus impacting on their ability to participate in physical activity. However, this should not prevent them from being able to participate and programmes need to be adjusted to reflect individual needs and abilities.

Medications

It is clear that many medications including iron supplements, tranquillisers, anti-depressants, calcium channel blockers, anti-emetics and anti-epileptic drugs used routinely frequently cause constipation. Notably, iron supplements also alter the colour and consistency of the stool turning it hard and black. As a consequence, medications should be reviewed routinely and appropriate action taken if side effects are noted. Conversely, certain medications which range in action from stool softeners to stimulants (which stimulate the bowel) help alleviate constipation, however long-term use of any of these medications can lead to dependence and loss of bowel function.

Developing a toileting programme

A baseline assessment should be undertaken with the individual's consent to identify current skills in relation to toileting through observation before, during

Reader activity 14.4

Brian is a 26-year-old man with a moderate learning disability and Down syndrome. He lives in a community home with three of his peers with the support of health care workers. He has good communication skills and enjoys interacting with people. Brian has poor muscle tone (hypotonia), is slightly overweight and does not like to participate in regular exercise. In relation to his diet, he needs encouragement to eat fruit and vegetables as part of a balanced diet. In addition, he has a poor fluid intake and needs to be reminded to take drinks during the day. Recently it has been noted that Brian is spending a lot of time in the bathroon and has reported difficulties opening his bowels and feeling uncomfortable. This is proving to be stressful for Brian as he is reluctant to leave the house unless assured he can access a bathroom.

- How would you minimise the effects of constipation?
- How would you ensure adequate food and fluid intake?
- What other actions might you consider to support Brian?
- What factors have influenced your decision?

and after the activity. This information should be used to develop a toileting programme which may need to address some or all of the following:

- Privacy and dignity.
- Communication.
- Toileting pattern.
- Understanding of wet/dry.
- Ability to dress/undress.
- Positioning on toilet.
- Use of continence aids.
- Personal hygiene.

Specific guidance with respect to the different activities that can support toilet use for an individual are included in Table 14.9.

Conclusion

Physical disabilities impact significantly on the lives of people with learning disabilities. This chapter has sought to raise the overall awareness of the reader of the key issues relating to physical disabilities and has offered guidance to support people who experience difficulties relating to disorders of movement, eating and swallowing and nutritional difficulties as well as issues relating to the bladder and bowel. The provision of appropriate person-centred supports identified in this chapter can positively impact on an individual, not only by minimising the impact of physical disabilities on the person's physical, mental and social wellbeing, but by significantly improving their overall quality of life.

References

Aldridge, J., 2009. Assessment. In: Gates, B., Barr, O. (Eds.), Oxford handbook of learning and intellectual disability nursing. Oxford University Press, Oxford.

Batshaw, M.L., 2002. Children with disabilities, fifth ed. Brookes, Maryland.

Batshaw, M.L., Pellegrino, L., Roizen, N., 2007. Children with disabilities, sixth ed. Brookes, Maryland.

Beacroft, M., Dodd, K., 2009. Pain in people with learning disabilities in residential settings – the need for change. British Journal of Learning Disabilities 38, 201–209.

Benninga, M., 2004. Children with constipation: what happens to them when they grow up? Scand. J. Gastroenterol. 39 (Suppl. 241), 23–26.

Berman, A., Snyder, S.J., Kozier, B., Erb, G., 2008. Fundamentals of nursing. Concepts, process and practice, eighth ed. Pearson Prentice Hall, New Jersey.

Bodfish, J.W., Harper, V.N., Deacon, J.R., Symons, F.J., 2001. Identifying and measuring pain in persons with developmental disabilities: a manual for the Pain and Discomfort Scale (PADS). Western Carolina Center Research Reports, Morganton, NC.

Bohmer, C.J.M., Taminiau, J.A.J.M., Klinkenberg-Knol, E.C., Meuwissen, S.G.M., 2001. The prevalence of constipation in institutionalized people with intellectual disabilities. J. Intellect. Disabil. Res. 45 (3), 212–218.

Braden, B., Bergstrom, N., 1989. Clinical utility of the Braden scale for predicting pressure sore risk. Decubitus 2, 44–51.

Bradley, S., 2005. Tackling obesity in people with learning disability. Learning Disability Practice 8 (7), 10–14.

British Association for Parenteral and Enteral Nutrition (BAPEN), 2003. Malnutrition Universal Screening Tool (MUST). BAPEN, Redditch.

British Dietetic Association, 2009. National descriptors for texture modification in adults. British Dietetic Association and the Royal College of Speech and Language Therapists, Birmingham.

Brown, M., 2009. Physical health and well being. In: Gates, B., Barr, O.

(Eds.), Oxford handbook of learning and intellectual disability nursing. Oxford University Press, Oxford.

Cassidy, G., Martin, D.M., Martin, G.H.B., Roy, A., 2002. Health checks for people with learning disabilities – community learning disability teams working with general practitioners and primary health care teams. J. Learn. Disabil. 6 (2), 123–136.

Chadwick, D., Jolliffe, J., Goldbart, J., Burton, M., 2006. Barriers to caregiver compliance while eating and drinking. Recommendations for adults with intellectual disabilites and dysphagia. J. Appl. Res. Intellect. Disabil. 19, 153–162.

Clark, J., 2009. Physical health and well being. In: Gates, B., Barr, O. (Eds.), Oxford handbook of learning and intellectual disability nursing. University Press Oxford, Oxford.

Commission for Healthcare Audit and Inspection, 2007. Investigation into the services for people with learning disabilities by Sutton and Merton Primary Care Trust. Commission for Healthcare Audit and Inspection, London.

Dalton, C., 2009. Physical health and well being. In: Gates, B., Barr, O. (Eds.), Oxford handbook of learning and intellectual disability nursing. Oxford University Press, Oxford.

Dougherty, L., Lister, S., 2008. The Royal Marsden Hospital manual of clinical nursing procedures. Wiley, Oxford.

Doyle, S., Dalton, C., 2008. An action research approach to the development of clinical guidelines for the promotion of oral heath in people with an intellectual disability. Learning Disability Practice 11 (2), 12–15.

Draheim, C.C., Williams, D.P., McCubbin, J.A., 2002. Prevalence of physical inactivity and recommended physical activity in community based adults with mental retardation. Ment. Retard. 40, 436–444.

Dyspraxia Foundation, 2010. Dyspraxia at a glance. Available at:http://www.dyspraxiafoundation.org.uk/services/dys_glance.php (accessed 15.04.10.).

Ebersole, P., Hess, P., Touhy, T., et al., 2008. Towards healthy ageing. Human needs and nursing responses, seventh ed. Mosby, Philadelphia.

Folden, S., Backer, J., Gilbride, J., et al., 2002. Practice guidelines for the management of constipation in adults. Rehabilitation Nursing Foundation. Available at:http://www.rehabnurse.org/pdf/BowelGuideforWEB.pdf (accessed 15.04.10.).

Freshwater, D., Maslin-Prothero, S.E., 2005. Blackwell's nursing dictionary. Blackwell, Oxford.

Hong, C.S., 2005. Assessment for and provision of positioning equipment for children with motor impairments. International Journal of Therapy and Rehabilitation 12 (3), 130–131.

Hopkins, S.J., 2005. Drugs and pharmacology for nurses, thirteenth ed. Churchill Livingstone, London.

IMPACT, 2004. Tips on increasing fibre and fluid in your diet. Paediatric bowel care pathway. Royal College of Nursing, London.

Kozier, B., Erb, G., Berman, A., et al., 2008. Fundamentals of nursing. Concepts, process and practice. Pearson Education, New Jersey.

Kyle, G., 2006. Assessment and treatment of older patients with constipation. Nurs. Stand. 21 (8), 41–46.

Lennox, N., Beange, H., Parmenter, T., et al., 2002. Health guidelines for adults with an intellectual disability. International Association for the Scientific Study of Intellectual Disabilities. Available at:http://www.iassid.org/pdf/healthguidelines-2002.pdf (accessed 15.04.10.).

Lewis, S.J., Heaton, K.W., 1997. Stool form scale as a useful guide to intestinal transit time. Scand. J. Gastroenterol. 32 (9), 920–924.

Lohiya, G.S., Tan-Figueroa, L., Iannucci, A., 2004. Identification of low bone mass in a developmental centre: finger bone mineral density measurement in 562 residents. J. Am. Med. Dir. Assoc. 5, 371–376.

Marsh, L., Caples, M., Dalton, C., Drummond, E., 2010. Management of constipation. Learning Disability Practice 13 (4), 26–28.

McCaffery, M., 1968. Nursing practice theories related to cognition, bodily pain and man environment. Student store, UCLA, Los Angeles.

Melville, C.A., Hamilton, S., Hankey, C.R., et al., 2007. The prevalence and determinants of obesity in adults with intellectual disabilities. The International Association for the Study of Obesity. Obes. Rev. 8, 223–230.

Mencap, 2004. Treat me right! Better healthcare for people with a learning disability. Mencap, London.

Mencap, 2007. Death by indifference. Mencap, London.

National Institute for Clinical Excellence, 2007. Faecal incontinence. The management of faecal incontinence in adults. NICE, London.

National Institute of Diabetes and Digestive and Kidney Disease, 2007. Urinary retention. United States Department of Health and Human Services, USA.

National Institutes of Health, 2000. Consensus Development Conference on Osteoporosis Prevention, Diagnosis, and Therapy. 27–29 March 2000. United States Department of Health and Human Services, USA.

Northumberland Tyne & Wear NHS Trust and St Oswald's Hospice, 2008. Disability Distress Assessment Tool (DisDat). Northumberland Tyne & Wear NHS Trust and St Oswald's Hospice, UK.

Pawlyn, J., Carnaby, S., 2009. Profound intellectual and multiple disabilities. Wiley-Blackwell, Oxford.

Purves, W., 2007. Life: the science of biology, fourth ed. Sinauer, Massachusetts.

Ramont, R., Niedringhaus, D., Towle, M.A., 2010. Comprehensive nursing care, second ed. Pearson, New Jersey.

Royal College of Physicians and British Society of Gastroenterology, 2010. Oral feeding difficulties and dilemmas. A guide to practical care, particularly towards the end of life. Report of a working party. Royal College of Physicians and British Society of Gastroenterology, London.

Rubin, L., Crocker, A., 2006. Medical care for children and adults with developmental disabilities. Paul H Brookes, Canada.

Seeley, R., VanPutte, C., Reagan, J., Russo, A., 2010. Seeley's anatomy and physiology, ninth ed. McGraw Hill, New York.

Sharma, M., 2006. International school-based interventions for preventing obesity in children. Obes. Rev. 8, 155–167.

Stenson, A., Danaher, T., 2005. Continence issues for people with learning disabilities. Learning Disability Practice 8 (9), 10–14.

Telch, J., Telch, F.E., 2003. Practical aspects of nutrition in the disabled pediatric patient. Clin. Nutr. 3, 1–6.

Wallace, R.A., 2007. Clinical audit of gastrointestinal conditions occurring among adults with Down syndrome attending a specialist clinic. J. Intellect. Dev. Disabil. 32 (1), 45–50.

Walsh, M., 2002. Watsons clinical nursing and related sciences, sixth ed. Baillière Tindall, Edinburgh.

Waterlow, J., 2005. The Waterlow Score. Available at:http://www.judy-waterlow.co.uk/waterlow_score.htm (accessed on 15 April 2010).

William, K., Purves, David Sadava, Gordon, H., Orians, and Craig Heller, H., 2007. Life: The Science of Biology, 4th Edition, by Sinauer Associates (HYPERLINK "http://www.sinauer.com/"www.sinauer.com) and WH Freeman (HYPERLINK "http://www.whfreeman.com/"www.whfreeman.com).

World Health Organization, 2004. Diet and physical activity: a public health priority. World Health Organization, Geneva.

Yoshihara, T., Morinushi, T., Kinjyo, S., Yamasaki, Y., 2005. Effects of periodic preventative care on the progression of periodontal disease in young adults with Down's syndrome. J. Clin. Periodontol. 32 (6), 556–560.

Further reading

Berman, A., Snyder, S.J., McKinny, D., 2011. Nursing basics for clinical practice. Pearson, New Jersey.

Brown, I., Percy, M., 2007. A comprehensive guide to intellectual and developmental disabilties. Paul Brookes, London.

Cambridge, P., Carnaby, S., 2005. Person centred planning and care management with people with learning disabilities. Jessica Kingsley, London.

Prasher, V.P., Janicki, M.P., 2002. Physical health of adults with intellectual disabilities. Blackwell, Oxford.

Useful addresses

Irish Nutrition and Dietetics Institute http://www.indi.ie

NHS Evidence- Learning Disabilities http://www.library.nhs.uk/learningdisabilities

Dyspraxia Foundation http://www.dyspraxiafoundation.org.uk

National Institute on Deafness and Other Communication Disorders http://www.nidcd.nih.gov/health/voice/dysph.html

Understanding Intellectual Disability and Health: http://www.intellectualdisability.info

British Institute of Learning Disabilities http://www.bild.org.uk

Inclusive Solutions. Making inclusion happen: http://www.inclusive-solutions.com

15

Sensory awareness

Debbie Crickmore

CHAPTER CONTENTS

KEY ISSUES

- Impairments of vision and hearing are common in people with learning disabilities, sometimes associated with particular syndromes or other frequently experienced conditions. As life expectancy for people with learning disabilities increases, so will the likelihood of age-related sensory disabilities
- Difficulties in relation to the commonly identified five senses of sight, hearing, smell, taste and touch may occur singly or in combination
- In common with many health issues, sensory disabilities may not be recognised, the effects may be attributed to the individual's learning disability and access to services may be poor
- Sensory conditions can benefit from access to routine screening, primary, secondary and tertiary interventions
- Strategies in relation to sensory disabilities may be preventative, restorative or compensatory
- Supporting people with learning disabilities using sensory channels can be both stimulating and pleasurable

Introduction

> *Consider ... if you could not see an oncoming car, hear a baby's cry, smell smoke, taste your favourite dessert ...*
>
> (Tortora & Derrickson 2010:297)

Tortora & Derrickson (2010) suggest the inability to 'sense' your environment and make the necessary adjustments might mean you could not survive very well on your own. If impairments to the senses are in addition to, or indeed associated with the cause of, a learning disability, then the implication is – at best – of a double disadvantage. Add to this well-documented difficulties experienced by people with learning disabilities in not only identifying health issues, but in having them met (e.g. Disability Rights

Commission 2006, Mencap 2007, Michael 2008), and the role for knowledgeable supporters is clear. A further important consideration is sensory deterioration associated with advancing age (Age Scotland 2010) now that people with learning disabilities are enjoying increased life expectancy (Emerson & Hatton 2008). Declining sensory responses may contribute to anxiety and depression in a population already overburdened with mental health problems (see Chs 17 and 29).

Drawing upon the content of chapters from the previous edition of this book (Ferris-Taylor 2007, Manners et al 2007, Wake 2007, Wray & Paton 2007), this new chapter brings together key information in relation to the commonly identified five senses: sight, hearing, smell, taste and touch; how things work, what can go wrong and how supporters can help. It will identify difficulties individuals may have been born with (congenital) or acquired, those that persist (chronic) or worsen over time (progressive) and those that may occur periodically (acute or transient). It will focus on practical strategies for prevention, assessment, promoting and maximising the senses at individual and environmental levels to achieve both remedial and therapeutic benefit.

The information provided here is not intended to meet the needs of all those interested in the senses; further, more detailed or technical, material can be easily sourced from specialist websites (see Useful addresses) and literature (e.g. Tortora & Derrickson 2010). Rather, it is intended to give a helpful level of understanding, so those supporting people with learning disabilities can more confidently give explanations to those affected, carers and colleagues. This chapter should be read with reference to Chapter 6.

While the chapter will inevitably focus on the distance senses of vision and hearing, people with learning disabilities may also display varied responses to smell (olfactory), taste (gustatory) and touch (tactile) sensations. This may be particularly the case in those experiencing an aura preceding a seizure, as epilepsy is highly associated with learning disability (see Ch. 16). Epilepsy Action (2005) gives the following example of types of aura experienced, related to the five senses discussed here:

> a change in body temperature . . . a strange taste or smell, even musical sounds or visual disturbance.

Although the senses are largely discussed sequentially for clarity, it is acknowledged they are not mutually exclusive, existing in combination and relation to each other. Neither are they fixed; an individual should be seen as having a particular sensory profile at a given point in their life, rather than being in possession of an artificially separate collection of (mal)functions. The reader is directed to Chapter 20 for further discussion of the proprioceptive and vestibular senses, how abnormalities may be addressed, for example by therapy, and the concept of a 'sensory diet'. A summary of sensory integration in relation to learning disability, including therapy to ameliorate dysfunction, is provided by Bell (2009a).

While it is difficult to establish the true extent to which people with learning disabilities experience additional sensory problems, information is easier to elicit on visual and hearing impairment than the more subjective and anecdotal experiences of taste, touch and smell. However, in common with learning disability itself, the terminology used tends to be indeterminate. For sight/vision and hearing there may be *problems*, *losses*, *impairments* and *disabilities* compounded by additional descriptions of severity including *mild*, *partial*, *moderate*, *significant*, *severe*, *profound*, and so on. As a starting point, however, The Foundation for People with Learning Disabilities (FPLD 2007) presents one in three people with learning disabilities as likely to have problems with their sight or hearing, or both.

Dual/multi-sensory impairment

Sense (2010a), a national charity supporting and campaigning for children and adults who are deafblind, describes *deafblindness* as comprising a visual and hearing impairment, of any type or degree, which may also be referred to as dual sensory loss (Deafblind UK 2007). Robertson & Emerson (2010), despite being commissioned by Sense, adopted the term *co-occurring vision and hearing impairments* for their recent research estimating current and projected numbers of people affected in the UK. In addition to findings suggesting the population experiencing deafblindness has been significantly underestimated and is set to rise dramatically (in line with projections for people entering older age), this research seeks to collate information on the nature and severity of individuals' difficulties, identifying lists of conditions suggestive of *more severe impairment* of both vision and hearing, making a distinction between them and *less severe impairment* of both vision and hearing. The headline figure of 356 000 deafblind people in the UK, of which 132 000 are believed to be severely affected, includes some variations in data for age and gender across the devolved administrations of Northern Ireland, Scotland and Wales.

In the report based on Robertson & Emerson's (2010) findings, Sense (2010b) recognised the real figure of deafblind people in the UK may well be higher than 356 000 as it was calculated using information from self-reporting surveys that many older people may not complete. Also, older people may discount any difficulties they are experiencing with their sight and vision as attributable to the ageing process and therefore not worthy of report. This potential for diagnostic overshadowing (when a person's presenting symptoms are assumed to be part of another condition) is similar to that experienced by people with learning disabilities. Data contained within the report *Sense of Urgency* (Sense 2010b), including age and gender of those affected by deafblindness, are aimed at providers of health and social care services, particularly local authorities that have responsibility to register, assess and provide services for people who have dual impairment. Sense (2010b) calls upon services to offer adequate proactive support in deafblindness to avoid expensive – financial and personal – crisis situations occurring later.

When someone is born with combined sight and hearing difficulties, this is called *congenital* deafblindness. This can be caused by conditions associated with learning disability such as congenital rubella syndrome (CRS), where the developing baby, if not miscarried or stillborn, is affected by their mother contracting the German measles virus (see Ch. 2). Maternal infection with cytomegalovirus or toxoplasmosis during pregnancy is also associated with sensory impairment and learning disability (Higgins & O'Toole 2008). Babies born with CRS may have sensorineural (relating to nerve cells associated with hearing) deafness in one or both ears and cataracts in one or both eyes (Sense 2008a). These conditions (discussed later) may worsen progressively; diabetes is also associated with CRS, with attendant potential for eye problems. When Sense started its work in 1955, rubella in pregnancy was the main cause of congenital deafblindness, although this is much less common since combined measles, mumps and rubella (MMR) vaccination was introduced in childhood. Later unproved links to autism threatened uptake of the vaccination in the last decade (Cole 2005).

Hearing and sight problems developed in child or adulthood are called *acquired* deafblindness. This may be due to an accident, illness or as a result of ageing in later life. A wealth of information is shared between the websites of Sense England, Northern Ireland, Scotland, Wales and Deafblind UK and Ireland (see Useful addresses). Deafblind UK has also created a permanent exhibition showing the history and heritage of deafblindness in its national centre in Peterborough where visitors can investigate a broad spectrum of topics related to the condition.

Deafblindness is considered a distinct impairment that is more than just a loss in vision plus hearing loss. This combination will multiply the difficulties an individual experiences as they will be unable to compensate for the lack of one sense with another. For example, children affected by the CHARGE syndrome (Sense 2008b) will experience multi-sensory impairment in its most extreme form, being likely to experience difficulties not only with hearing and vision but also with balance, smell, touch, pain, pressure and temperature. Box 15.1 illustrates features of this condition, associated with developmental delay, relevant to the exploration in this chapter.

Box 15.1

Features of CHARGE syndrome relevant in a multi-sensory context

- More than 60% of affected people are deafblind:
  - temporary or permanent, conductive and sensorineural* hearing loss
  - cataracts, glaucoma, retinal detachment.*
- Reduced motivation to lift head and explore beyond immediate body space.
- Facial palsy leads to difficulties eating.
- Absent or reduced balance.
- Low muscle tone.
- Delayed/abnormal mobility/walking with frequent falls.
- Sensory defensiveness:
  - tactile: e.g. dislike of soft toys
  - visual: e.g. dislike of bright lights
  - auditory: e.g. dislike of certain sounds.
- Can lead to 'shutting down', seeking solitude, self-stimulation.

*see Sight and Hearing sections
(Sense 2008b)

Sight

According to Vision Matters (2010:2), "sight is the sense that we fear losing the most". This appears feasible when considering how sight helps us maintain our independence; communicate with others; develop and maintain relationships; move safely around; and make sense of our world. Difficulties are likely to encroach on areas of life including leisure, recreation, skills, education and work. A study on the prevalence and costs of sight loss (Access Economics PTY Ltd 2009), commissioned by the Royal National Institute of Blind people (RNIB), found 8 million people in the UK of an estimated population of 61.8 million (Office for National Statistics 2010) are living with *sight loss*; around half could benefit from a simple sight test and new glasses. Yet it is stated that one in three people with a learning disability has a *sight problem* (many of which may also be correctable), with up to 90% of people with Down syndrome experiencing significant *sight impairments* and an estimated 70% of people with cerebral palsy and learning disabilities with a *significant impairment of vision* (SeeAbility-Look Up undated). Additionally, the FPLD (2007) claims problems with sight are more common among people with severe learning disabilities. While these descriptions may not be directly comparable, and are discussed further in the section on Registration, the differences between the general and learning disability figures are notable. Other general risk factors for eye disease include advancing age (over 60), being a member of a minority ethnic group (because access to eye care services is lower and undetected eye conditions more likely to be severe) (Access Economics PTY Ltd 2009) and being a member of a family with a history of eye disease (Vision Matters 2010).

The eyes are the organs of the sense of sight; while eye tests are typically associated with identifying visual problems, the eyes might also be described as 'windows to health'. Vision Matters (2010) explains it is easy to neglect eyes because they do not usually hurt when something is wrong. A sight test not only identifies the need for glasses but also provides a vital health check following which an individual can be directed to their GP if there are concerns. Using an opthalmoscope to shine a small beam of light into the eye, it is possible for an eye care professional to examine different parts of the eye, including the retina and the surfaces of the cornea and lens (see Fig. 15.1). The surface of the retina is the only place in the body where blood vessels can be viewed directly and checked for changes, such as those that occur with hypertension (high blood pressure) or diabetes (Tortora & Derrickson 2010). Diabetes is a condition five times more common in people with learning disabilities (Lindsey & Burgess 2006) and can lead to diabetic retinopathy, where blood vessels leak into the retina or are destroyed causing vision to become patchy. Of course, it is also possible to observe, without the use of equipment, indicators of a developing problem, such as sore, blood-shot or cloudy eyes and changes in behaviour or response to activities (SeeAbility 2007). Oculogyric crises (where the eyes roll up in the head so that only the whites can be seen) occur when the muscles controlling the eyes go into spasm, a side effect associated with older anti-psychotic medications that requires treatment with an antidote and review of dose (Healy 2003).

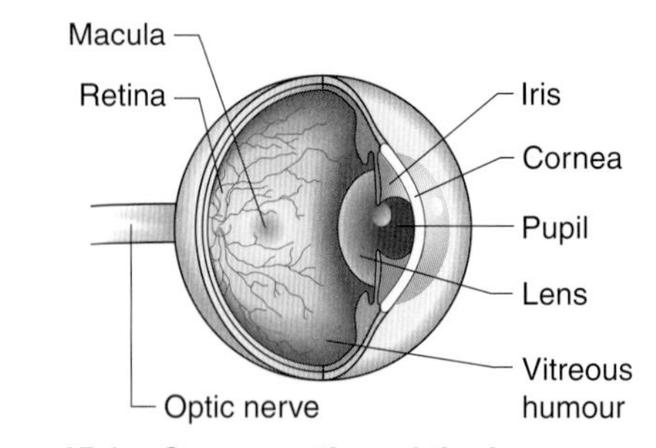

Figure 15.1 • Cross-section of the human eye

As each eye is connected to the brain by an optic nerve, degeneration of the brain caused by conditions like multiple sclerosis, Alzheimer's and Parkinson's disease can also damage cells along the nerve and in the retina which can be tracked using an optical version of ultrasound (Graham-Rowe 2009). Linking eye nerve cell death and brain cell death led recently to media claims that 'a simple eye test could detect Alzheimer's disease'. This could be of future relevance to people with learning disabilities who experience a higher rate of this form of dementia (see Chs 17 and 29). The test would involve instilling drops of a harmless fluorescent dye into the eyes to seek out and chemically mark affected nerve cells that could then be photographed using an infrared camera. However, the research on which the claim was based (Cordeiro et al 2010) has not progressed to humans and is not yet able to differentiate between *causes* of nerve cell death in the eyes and brains of animals.

How the eyes work

The eye is a complex part of the body and knowing how it works can make it easier to appreciate what happens when something goes wrong (RNIB 2010a). Some awareness of the experience of people with particular visual difficulties can be gained by the use of simulation glasses in training events and by viewing modified photographs, for example those at the National Council for the Blind of Ireland website (NCBI; see Useful addresses). It could also be useful to experience both guiding, and being guided; Action for Blind People's *Top 10 Tips to Guiding Visually Impaired People* (see Useful addresses) would be a good place to start.

Structurally, each eye is separate, being almost spherical in shape and about 2.5 cm in diameter, but they are designed to function as a pair, enabling binocular (literally meaning two-eye) vision. For example, while it is possible to *see* with only one eye (monocular vision), three-dimensional vision is impaired, especially in relation to judgement of distances. The external parts of the eye (Fig. 15.1) are:

- The pupil – the 'black hole' in the centre of the eye that adjusts the amount of light passing through to the internal workings, normally becoming smaller in bright light (constricting) and bigger (dilating) in dim light
- The iris – the ring surrounding the pupil that provides the colour of our eyes (the white of the eye is known as the sclera)
- The cornea – the transparent membrane (in front of the iris and pupil and merging into the sclera) through which light passes to reach the retina at the back of the eye.

The externally visible accessory structures of eyebrows, eyelashes and eyelids have important protective functions with each eye sitting in a bony socket (known as the orbit) occupied by fatty tissue designed to reduce the risk of injury. The hairs comprising brows and lashes shade the eyes and protect from foreign bodies. Eyelids are folds of skin that meet at the corner of the eye by the nose (the medial canthus) and the outer corner (the lateral canthus). The epicanthic folds that are cardinal features of Down syndrome (see Ch. 2) mean a fold of skin is additionally vertically present across the inside corner of the eye. The inner side of each lid is covered by mucous membrane called conjunctiva (the pink area you see if you pull your eyelids up or down) which becomes inflamed in the common condition of conjunctivitis. Blinking cleans and lubricates the eye using fluid secreted by glands including the tear (lacrimal) glands. Internal narrowing between the corner of the eye and the back of the nose (nasolacrimal duct) in Down syndrome can impede drainage with resultant stickiness, irritation and tendency to become infected (Crofts 2008).

Directly behind the structures we can see externally is the lens (Fig. 15.1). This has the ability to adjust to bend (refract) light bouncing off objects and entering the eye. Light passes in this way through the vitreous humour to the retina at the back of the eye where two types of specialised cells (rods and cones) begin the process of converting light rays into impulses that travel via the optic nerve to the brain for interpretation of the image. The macula, at the centre of the retina, contains the highest concentration of cones, with rods increasing in number towards the edges of the retina. Rods allow sight of shades of grey in dim light, for example moonlight, whereas cones are sensitive to blue, green and red light, combining to produce different colours. An absence or deficiency in one of the three types of cones leads to inability to distinguish some colours from others, known as colour blindness (Tortora & Derrickson 2010).

The complex process of sight is shown as a simple visual in Figure 15.2. It has been likened to taking pictures with a camera onto film that then must be developed. The retina represents the camera film, storing an image of what we are looking at. The image directed onto the retina is then sent along to the brain

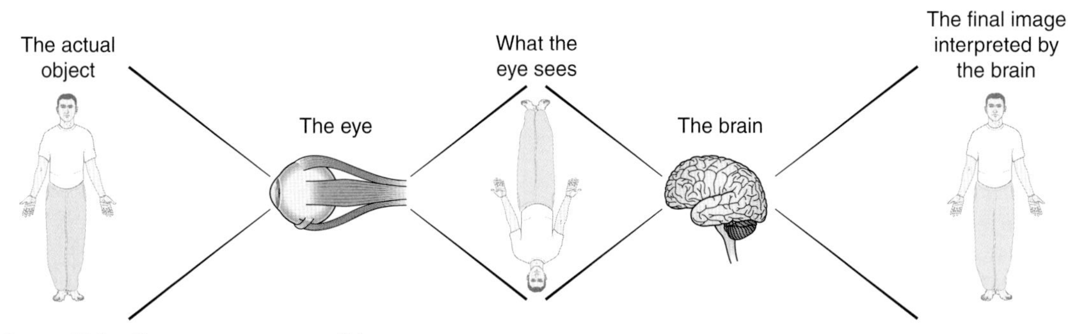

Figure 15.2 • How your eye sees things

where it is processed, like developing a camera film. So, we 'see' in our brain using the light information sent from our eyes (RNIB 2010b). With the advent of digital photography, there may be readers who have little, or no, experience on which to base this analogy, but the speed and cleverness of the process may still be – if not better – appreciated.

A further mechanical process involving the function of the eye relates to the action of six muscles that coordinate the eyeball in vertical, horizontal and rotational movements. This is important to enjoy the benefits of binocular vision described earlier, and to adjust to seeing things at different distances. Imbalance in the eye muscles manifests as strabismus (squint) that can be bilateral (affecting both eyes), unilateral (affecting one), divergent or convergent ('crossed eyes'). Around 20% of children with Down syndrome have a squint (Crofts 2008).

Eye health

Having established the basic structures of the eye and how they work, it is important to promote eye health. Action for Blind People (see Useful addresses) and Vision Matters (2010) both give helpful tips for protecting your eyes. Some of these are listed in Box 15.2.

These tips help supporters of people with learning disabilities understand the roles they might need to adopt, for example ensuring details of eye tests, known conditions and family history are collected and recorded as part of the health action planning process (see Ch. 13). Conditions including retinitis pigmentosa (RP) and colour blindness (or, more accurately, colour vision deficiency) can be hereditary (British Retinitis Pigmentosa Society 2010). Eye tests may need to be facilitated on the High Street, at hospital or community clinic or in the home. Helping to choose, and giving encouragement to wear, good quality sunglasses (check for UV factor rating and CE quality mark) and taking care with cosmetics (e.g. keeping shampoo out of the eyes when hair washing) are components of a competent and sensitive approach to the delivery and support of personal care. From work, leisure and health perspectives, accessible educative material and support relating to screen breaks (at least one an hour), use of safety goggles, smoking cessation, alcohol use, healthy diet and exercise can be provided. While smoking is less prevalent in people with learning disabilities than the general population (Taylor et al 2004), those who smoke are more likely to develop age-related macular degeneration (AMD) and cataracts (where the lens becomes opaque, affecting the passage of light) than those who do not. Foods containing lutein or zeaxanthin, found in fruit and vegetables including mango, broccoli, green beans and spinach, can also guard against these conditions. Regular exercise helps because it ensures eyes get a good supply of oxygen (Vision Matters 2010). Reader activity 15.1 is designed to help you promote eye health in your local area.

Vision 2020 (see Useful addresses) is the global initiative for the elimination of avoidable blindness, a joint programme of the World Health Organization (WHO) and the International Agency for the Prevention of Blindness (IAPB) with an international membership of non-government organisations (NGOs), professional associations, eye care institutions and corporations. The UK Vision Strategy is a devolved initiative of Vision 2020, led by the RNIB (see Useful addresses), an example of a UK-wide charitable organisation. Other sources of support are specific to

Box 15.2

Top tips for looking after your eyes

- Have an eye test every 2 years (or as recommended for known conditions).
- Wear sunglasses to protect from ultraviolet (UV) damage.
- Take regular breaks from your computer screen.
- Eat healthily and don't drink too much alcohol.
- Know your family health history.
- Use safety glasses.
- Take care with cosmetics.
- Stop smoking.
- Take regular exercise.
- Never guess the severity of an eye injury; always seek medical attention.

(Action for Blind People and Vision Matters 2010)

Reader activity 15.1

Conduct a scoping exercise in the area around where you live or work. With reference to the text, including the top tips in Box 15.2, identify services available that promote eye health. How accessible might they be (physically and in terms of information provided) for people with varying abilities? Are they services available to all, or directed at particular groups; are they provided by the government, private or charitable organisations; are there costs associated with their use?

people with learning disabilities, for example SeeAbility, with many generic learning disability (for example, Enable) or condition specific (for example, Diabetes UK, Down's Syndrome Association (DSA), National Autistic Society (NAS)) websites also carrying useful information.

Eye testing

Children with learning disabilities should access the universal Child Health Surveillance Programme that begins with a physical examination within the first 72 hours of life and continues at intervals through childhood. While we may be heartened that Emerson & Hatton (2008) report more than half of almost 3000 people surveyed for *People with Learning Difficulties in England* had an eye test in the last year, without understanding the process and outcome it is difficult to judge benefits. Eyesight testing may be provided on the High Street, at the local hospital or community clinic or by a domiciliary (home visiting) service, and is free in Scotland (Vision Matters 2010). In other parts of the UK, being in receipt of particular benefits entitles individuals to a free NHS-funded sight test and a voucher towards the cost of glasses. Box 15.3 shows titles and descriptions of people who specialise in eye conditions.

SeeAbility (2007) has produced a resource, *You and Eye* (film accompanied by a book), about eye care for people with learning disabilities. It emphasises (p. 2) "No one is too disabled to have his or her eyes tested" and "You don't have to be able to read or talk to have an eye test", providing encouragement to both people with learning disabilities and those supporting them to routinely access eye care. This is in respect not only of the test, but the potential consequences from prescription of glasses to surgery to remove cataracts. The resource includes useful prompts and templates to prepare for the eye test, any subsequent action and aftercare. Undertaking a *Functional Vision Assessment for People with Learning Disabilities* (SeeAbility 2010) provides a useful starting point for supporters of people with learning disabilities who are concerned regarding someone's eye health and sight.

See Reader activity 15.2 on the Evolve website.

Eye tests may include some, or all, of the following

1. Taking a history, to include symptoms and medication:
   - important to have support from someone who knows the individual well and has prepared with them.
2. Eye health check:
   - torch shone into the eye, possibly in darkened room
   - use of eye drops to widen (dilate) the pupil
   - pressure test (see Table 15.1; glaucoma)
   - photograph of retina
   - eye movement check
   - field of vision test.
3. Level of vision test:
   - Snellen chart (traditional letter chart with largest letters at top)
   - Kay Picture Test (see Case illustration 15.1)
   - Cardiff Acuity Test.
4. Prescription of glasses:
   - use of trial frames and lenses.
5. Referral to GP:
   - potential health problem detected
   - referral to hospital eye clinic indicated.

Box 15.3

People who specialise in eye conditions

- *Optometrist*: trained to test for glasses, other aspects of visual function, recognises ocular abnormalities, able to dispense glasses.
- *Optician*: trained to fit spectacle frames, arranges to have glasses made with appropriate measurements and lenses for individual people.
- *Orthoptist*: trained in assessment of vision in people of all ages and abilities, recognises squints and disorders of eye movements, treats squints and related disorders.
- *Ophthalmologist*: doctor specialising in eye conditions.

Registration

If a person is diagnosed as having an eligible degree of sight loss, they can choose to be registered. Depending on their sight problem, they will be registered as *severely sight impaired* (blind) *or sight impaired* (partially sighted). Detailed statistics on persons registered with Councils with Adult Social Services Responsibilities (CASSRs) in England as being blind or partially sighted (Information Centre for Health

Table 15.1 Examples of eye conditions with suggested requirement for accompanying skills

Conditions experienced by individual	Accompanying skills required
• Blepharitis, inflammation of the eyelids, particularly the edges. • Stye, abscess in the follicle of an eyelash.	• Bathing of eyes, using cooled boiled water, cotton or gauze pads. Each eye swabbed once from inside corner to outside edge, using each pad once then discarding. Same pad never used for both eyes. Cotton wool not recommended as tiny fibres can get into eye, cause irritation, place for germs to grow. • Application of ointment, instillation of drops, good standards of hygiene (see Mason & Stevens 2010 for technique).
• Long sight (hypermetropia), affects ability to see close-up objects. • Short sight (myopia), distant objects appear blurred, close objects can still be seen clearly. • Presbyopia (lens loses elasticity, 'reading' glasses may be required after age 40).	• Persistence while becoming accustomed to wearing glasses. • Keeping glasses clean, grease and scratch free. • If more than one prescription required, understanding which glasses are needed in which situations, differentiating between them.
Nystagmus, eyes make small, involuntary, jerky movements, often more noticeable when looking sideways.	Acceptance that • compensatory head posture may be adopted to minimise movements • items may be held very close to optimise vision.
Retinal detachment, where the retina separates from the inner wall of the eye.	Awareness of increased risk of retinal detachment where there has been self- or non-accidental injury (NAI).
Glaucoma, disease associated with increased pressure within the eye, leads to retina being damaged causing tunnel vision and sometimes total blindness.	• Preparation for assessment using a machine that fires a puff of air against the eye. • Awareness of family history as can be hereditary. • If identified, may be managed by daily use of eye drops (Sense 2008a).

Case illustration 15.1

Several years ago, when Sammy-Jo was a child, I accompanied her and her mum to a hospital eye clinic appointment in my role as a community learning disability nurse. Sammy-Jo has Down syndrome and had been prescribed glasses from an early age, which she became accustomed to. At the appointment, black and white cards carrying line drawings were used. When shown the card bearing a fish, Sammy-Jo enthusiastically signed 'chips'. Her mum and I were delighted that she could not only identify the picture, but could also link it with a favourite meal *and* clearly produce the sign! However, the orthoptist was less enthused, insisting that unless Sammy-Jo could *tell* her what the picture was, in terms of administration of that part of the test, she had failed.

It is heartening, therefore, to read the DSA's current position on this which states (Crofts 2008:12)

> *Some children with Down's syndrome prefer to sign to identify them* rather than say what the pictures show.*

*The standardised black and white Kay pictures held a measured distance away.

and Social Care 2008) display figures of 153 000 and 156 300 respectively. The age profile is that 64% of blind and 66% of partially sighted people are aged 75 or over (this is above the mean life expectancy for those with mild, moderate and severe learning disabilities, estimated to be 74, 67 and 58 respectively in an Australian study by Bittles et al 2002). Where councils reported additional disabilities, 8% of those registered as blind and 4% of those registered as partially sighted had a learning disability. Diagnoses including *cerebral/cortical blindness/visual impairment* have been attributed to the difficulties experienced by some people with learning disabilities, whose eyes appear normal but who are believed to have damage to the visual area in the occipital lobe at the rear of the brain; it is the impact rather than the cause of difficulties that triggers eligibility to register. It seems possible, given the higher numbers of people with learning disabilities experiencing sight problems, that not only are there those where the severity of their difficulties is not recognised, but also those who may be able to register, but have not. Given that many people with learning disabilities may be socioeconomically disadvantaged (Emerson et al 2009), potential opportunities for additional benefits should not be disregarded, for example Blind Person's Allowance (Directgov 2010).

Awareness of sight in your work

Where visual impairment could not be prevented, people with learning disabilities can be introduced to alternative leisure activities to replace, or enhance, existing favourites. For example, audio description is available for television, magnifiers for screens, large-print books and magazines, talking books and newspapers. Equipment and adaptations can be provided following assessment, often by an occupational therapist (OT), in relation to retaining independence in everyday living skills wherever possible. Other chapters in this book, for example 6 and 13, stress the importance of accessible information for people with learning disabilities. Where there is visual impairment, it is also possible to customise websites according to personal need, for example by changing the size of the text, the colour and the background, to create high contrast. The importance of good lighting for those with some useful sight should not be underestimated (Sense 2010c).

Management of eye health should be a partnership between people with learning disabilities and their supporters. Table 15.1 gives examples of eye conditions with accompanying skills that could be required of either, or both, parties.

Hearing

As the Royal National Institute for Deaf people (RNID; see Useful addresses) asserts:

> The thought of losing your hearing can be worrying. The largest charity working on behalf of the UK's estimated 9 million deaf and hard of hearing people, the RNID (2006) reports about 698 000 of these are *severely* or *profoundly deaf*. In common with statistics for visual impairment and ageing, this figure is rising. For the population of people with learning disabilities, the FPLD (2007) suggests about 40% have *moderate* or *severe hearing loss*, particularly common in people with Down syndrome and occurring more frequently as people grow older. While recognising persistent differences in description, there remains a significant gap between the 1 in 7 rate in the general population (Deafness Research UK 2009) and the learning disability figures. As with visual impairment, hearing impairment can be congenital (present at birth) or occur early in life. This will have an impact upon the ability to acquire language and is described as prelingual deafness, often considered profound in nature. *Deafened* is a term used to refer to people whose hearing loss was acquired after speech develops, possibly as a result of illness, disease or older age (Scottish Council on Deafness 2008).

There are two main types of hearing loss. Sensorineural loss accounts for over 80% of deafness and is caused by damage to (sensory) hair cells in the ears and/or damage to the auditory nerve (neural) pathway to the brain. In conductive loss, sounds are unable to pass freely to the inner ear. It is possible to have mixed loss where both sensorineural and conductive hearing losses are present at the same time. More rarely, hearing loss can result from damage to the brain in the primary auditory area (see How the ears work, below, and Table 15.2). Although age (over 50) is a risk factor for hearing loss, research has shown it tends to halt around the age of 70 (Deafness Research UK 2010a). Other risk factors for hearing loss include prolonged or repeated exposure to loud noise, being a member of a minority ethnic group (RNID 2006) and having a history of middle ear disease. Age-related hearing loss (presbyacusis) can also run in families and be related to a high-fat diet that impairs the blood flow to the ears (Age Cymru 2010).

How the ears work

Tortora & Derrickson (2010) recognise the sensitivity of the receptors in the ear to convert sound vibrations into electrical signals 1000 times faster than photoreceptors in the eye respond to light. In addition, the ear also contains receptors for balance

Table 15.2 Characteristics of hearing loss

Type	Possible causes	Effect	Management
Sensorineural			
Damage to (sensory) hair cells and/or damage to auditory nerve (neural).	• Age related. • Noise related. • Genetic.	Changes ability to hear quiet sounds, reduces quality of sound, will often struggle to understand speech.	Currently irreversible, use technological/ augmentative support, e.g. • hearing aids • objects of reference.
Conductive			
Sounds unable to pass freely to the inner ear.	Blockage or abnormality in outer or middle ear, e.g. • excess ear wax • fluid from infection • ruptured eardrum.	Sounds become quieter, although not usually distorted.	Can be temporary or permanent Medical management, e.g. • drops • minor surgery.

(equilibrium). The structure of the ear is divided into three main regions, shown in Figure 15.3:

1. Outer ear: collects sound waves and passes them inward.
2. Middle ear: carries sound vibrations to the oval window (see below).
3. Inner ear: contains receptors for hearing and balance.

The part of the ear that is external to the head is known as the auricle or pinna. Its shape (like the flared end of a trumpet) is designed to collect sound waves and pass them into the ear canal, a curved tube extending from the side of the head toward the eardrum. The ear canal contains hairs and ceruminous glands that secrete wax (cerumen) to help prevent dust and dirt from entering the ear. The eardrum (tympanic membrane) is a thin, semitransparent partition between the outer and middle ear that vibrates when sound waves enter the ear.

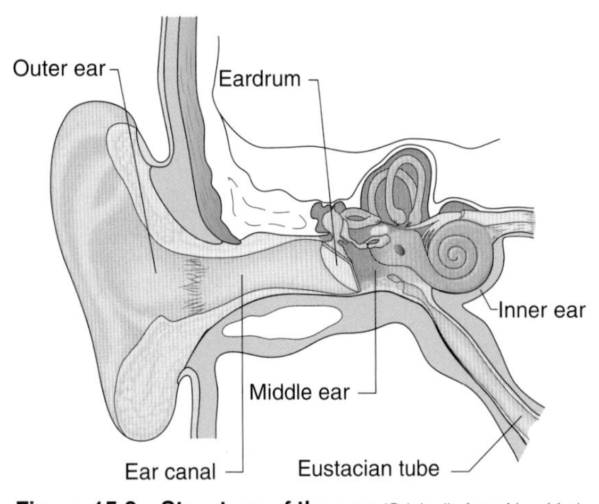

Figure 15.3 • Structure of the ear (Originally from New York State Department of Health 2000. Available at: http://www.tutorvista.com/biology/ear-structures-involved-with-balance)

The middle ear is a small, air-filled cavity between the eardrum and inner ear. An opening leads directly to the eustachian tube (see Fig. 15.3) connecting with the upper part of the throat. Its function is to allow air into the middle ear to keep pressure even on both sides of the eardrum so the risk of rupture is reduced. Infection or trauma, for example caused by self- or non-accidental injury, can also cause tearing of the eardrum, known as perforation. Three tiny bones are attached to and extend across the middle ear, taking their names from their shapes – hammer (malleus), anvil (incus) and stirrup (stapes). Together they are known as ossicles. Equally tiny muscles control the amount of movement of these bones to prevent damage from excessively loud noises. The stirrup bone fits into a small opening between the middle and inner ear known as the oval window. The condition, otosclerosis, can cause severe conductive hearing loss as excess bone growth prevents the ossicles in the middle ear from moving freely.

The inner ear contains semicircular canals and the cochlea (appearing in Fig. 15.3 resembling a snail's shell). The semicircular canals are the sense organs for balance (also referred to as the vestibular apparatus) and the cochlea is the sense organ for hearing. When sound waves enter the ear canal, they cause the ear drum to vibrate. In turn, this vibration is passed to the hammer, anvil and stirrup bones to the oval window. Fluid in the cochlea carries waves of pressure that are transmitted into nerve impulses by hair cells and carried to the primary auditory area in the temporal lobe of the brain. In addition to detecting sound, the cochlea can produce sounds (otoacoustic emissions) that can be recorded by a sensitive microphone placed next to the eardrum. This vibration of the hair cells is absent or greatly reduced in deaf babies and can be detected quickly and non-invasively by a screening test (Tortora & Derrickson 2010). A cochlear implant, often referred to as a bionic ear, is a surgically implanted electronic device that provides a sense of sound to a person who is profoundly deaf or severely hard of hearing.

As people grow older, hair cells naturally die off, the eardrum loses its elasticity and the tiny bones stiffen, leading to deterioration in hearing. Exposure to excessive noise can also distort and damage hair cells, so they become unable to transmit incoming sound to the brain resulting in permanent hearing impairment. Mammals, including humans, lose the ability to create new hair cells before birth, unlike birds. Amphibians and fish have been found to have very similar cells produced throughout life, providing rich research material in the quest for future treatment of hearing loss (Deafness Research UK 2010b).

The semicircular canals are responsible for two types of balance

1. Static equilibrium: maintenance of the body (mainly the head) relative to the force of gravity.
2. Dynamic equilibrium: maintenance of body position (mainly the head) in response to rotational acceleration or deceleration.

As with hearing, a combination of fluid and hair cells in the vestibular apparatus carry information from the inner ear to the brain where it is translated into actions to maintain balance, for example head, neck and eye movements.

Ear health

Having established the basic structures of the ear and how they work, it is important to promote healthy ears. The RNID (see Useful addresses) and Deafness Research UK (2010c) both give helpful tips for protecting your ears. Some of these are listed in Box 15.4.

Box 15.4

Top tips for looking after your ears

- Remember wax is there for a reason; ears are normally self-cleaning.
- Don't poke anything into your ears.
- Avoid loud noise, or wear earplugs or defenders.
- Don't rinse your hair in the bath (bacteria could get trapped behind ear wax).
- Don't ignore an ear or hearing problem.

(RNID and Deafness Research UK 2010c)

These top tips help supporters of people with learning disabilities understand the roles they might need to adopt, for example teaching, facilitating or delivering personal care that takes them into account. In work environments and leisure pursuits, information, strategies and protective equipment to reduce excess noise must be offered.

Hearing tests

The Newborn Hearing Screening Programme (National Health Service 2010) aims to identify moderate, severe and profound hearing impairment in newborn babies. The programme automatically offers all parents in England the opportunity to have their baby's hearing tested shortly after birth. It employs the technique discussed in 'How the ears work'. All babies who record 'no clear response' to the initial screening are referred for further audiological assessment, with the aim of identifying all children born with moderate to profound permanent bilateral deafness within 4–5 weeks of birth.

Emerson & Hatton (2008) found significantly lower rates (21% overall) of people with learning disabilities having their hearing tested in the last year than sight. With suspected – previously undetected – hearing difficulties, a visit to the GP would be a good place to start to rule out or identify and treat infection or wax build up contributing to conductive loss. The GP can then refer to a community or hospital audiology clinic for a hearing test. High Street and domiciliary (in the home) testing may also be available. The test is likely to involve

- looking into your ears using an otoscope
- asking a number of questions about your ears, hearing problems, family history of hearing problems and your health in general

- testing your hearing
- explaining the results and, if required, which hearing aid(s) is/are most suited to you
- taking an impression of your ear if needed for the type of hearing aid(s) indicated
- coming back for a second appointment to have your hearing aid(s) fitted
- coming back for a third appointment to have your hearing aid(s) checked and adjustments made if required.

Referral to an ear, nose and throat (ENT) clinic can be made by the GP for other ear problems, such as glue ear (serous otitis media) that may previously have been routinely treated by surgical insertion of grommets (tubes in the eardrum to drain the thick, sticky fluid from the middle ear). A Cochrane Systematic Review by Lous et al (2005) suggested 'watchful waiting' might be an appropriate management strategy for most children with glue ear as the beneficial effect of grommets on hearing diminished during the first year, during which time most grommets come out. The review did not find any evidence that grommets help speech and language development.

Registration

As with sight loss, if a person is diagnosed as having an eligible degree of hearing loss, they can choose to register with the social services department of their local council. For example, the Greater London Authority (2010) has published data showing the number of people registered with councils with social services responsibilities (CSSRs) as being deaf or hard of hearing by age group (0–17, 18–64, 65–74, 75 and over) and borough.

Awareness of hearing in your work

Some prescribed medications are known to have potentially damaging effects on the ears. They are known as ototoxic and include some antibiotics, some chemotherapy drugs and some anti-inflammatory drugs. It is important that people with learning disabilities – and those who support them who may be administering medication – are aware of potential side effects and can make an informed decision about their use, using best interests where capacity to consent is lacking according to the Mental Capacity Act 2005.

Tinnitus refers to a ringing, roaring or clicking in the ears (Tortora & Derrickson 2010). It is experienced by an estimated 7 million people in the UK at some time, having various causes. Individuals experience tinnitus in many different ways but some understanding of the condition could be gained from listening to the MP3 sample file and reading or watching people's stories via the RNID website (see Useful addresses).

There are a variety of types of hearing aid and people with learning disabilities may require support to use and maintain them optimally. Good quality information regarding the aid in relation to the individual, including arrangements for follow up, should be recorded in an appropriate format, for example health action plan, and acted upon.

If you are supporting someone with a hearing loss, approach from the side or front to avoid startling them, use their name and make sure you have their attention before you speak. Turn the radio or the television off before you start a conversation (RNID 2008). Be aware that some voices may be easier to hear than others; the individual who apparently 'responds best to men' may do so simply because they can hear a lower voice better.

Sense of smell

As the eyes are the organs of the sense of sight, so the nose is the organ of the sense of smell (olfaction). Odorous materials give off chemical particles that are carried into the nose with inhaled air and stimulate the nerve cells. Just as optic nerves carry nerve impulses from the eyes to the brain, olfactory nerves extend from the nose terminating in olfactory bulbs below the frontal lobes of the brain. From here, the olfactory tract carries information to other areas of the brain; the primary olfactory area in the temporal lobe where conscious awareness of smell begins and the limbic system and hypothalamus, accounting for emotional and memory-evoked responses to odours. Tortora & Derrickson (2010) suggest it is possible for humans to recognise about 10 000 different odours in this way. The nose is also the beginning of the upper respiratory tract and it has been recognised that respiratory disease is the main cause of death in people with learning disabilities (Royal College of Nursing 2006). Gatcum & Jacob (2001) suggest we take our sense of smell for granted, relegating it to the 'forgotten sense'.

Awareness of the sense of smell in your work

With ageing, the sense of smell deteriorates. Hyposmia is a reduced ability to smell, affecting half of those over 65, and 75% of those over 80. However, as hyposmia can also be caused by neurological changes, such as a head injury or Alzheimer's disease, certain drugs such as anti-histamines, analgesics or steroids, and the damaging effects of smoking (Tortora & Derrickson 2010), it can be seen as a condition that those supporting people with a learning disability should be aware of.

Anosmia is loss of the sense of smell and can have a detrimental effect on the ability to taste leading to potential loss of appetite or seeking out highly flavoured foods. In those living alone, inability to detect rotten food could lead to food poisoning. A sense of smell can enhance quality of life for an individual, particularly where fragrances are emotionally associated with particular events, people or memories; conversely, loss of smell can bring anxiety and lead to depression (Gatcum & Jacob 2001).

Aromatherapy, using pure essential oils from fragrant plants such as peppermint, sweet marjoram and rose (Aromatherapy Council 2009), commonly uses the inhalation route, by warming oil in a burner (although there is agreement that robust research evidence is required before firm conclusions are reached about the therapy's effectiveness in improving physical and emotional wellbeing; see, for example, Holt et al 2003). Alternative, less systematic ways of introducing relaxing or stimulating smells to people with learning disabilities (requiring care but not necessarily qualifications) include use of scented candles and joss sticks. Flowers and toiletries may be more acceptable in some areas in relation to assessment of risk and local policy. Cleaning and laundry products, possibly selected more for their properties, and air fresheners (to mask less desirable smells) can be overpowering or clash, anecdotally leading to streaming eyes, sneezing and tingling lips, a challenge for individuals who have no verbal way to express. Staff should therefore maintain awareness of physical and emotional effects of smells – both intentionally introduced and incidentally present – on individuals, taking appropriate action where distress or pleasure is expressed. The sense of smell can be positively harnessed to assist people who are visually impaired, for example by staff who always use the same perfume to aid recognition. Fragrant objects of reference (see Ch. 6), for example soap or shampoo, can be offered to indicate bath or shower time and the opportunity can be provided to make menu choices by smelling food and drink.

Reader activity 15.3

To retrieve smell from its position as the 'forgotten sense' (Gatcum & Jacob 2001) and illustrate that the sense is not just about detection of odour, try to identify your most favourite and least favourite smells. Are they present in your life today or are they from another time, perhaps childhood? When you recall – or actually smell – them, do they evoke memories? If you had hyposmia or anosmia, do you think you could as easily summon up any memories and emotions associated with them?

Community practitioners should be aware that adaptation (decreasing sensitivity to odours) occurs rapidly (Tortora & Derrickson 2010). This is apparent when the curry we cooked last night 'hits' us when we open the front door arriving home from work, yet we were (relatively) unaware of it at breakfast. So, people living with particular smells, for example blocked drains or local industry, may become accustomed to them, not identifying them as potentially detrimental to health. In some cases this may have been perceived as indicative of individuals lacking skills to keep themselves healthy and safe.

Sense of taste

Taste is a sense difficult to separate from others; food has texture, stimulating tactile sensations, and aroma. When affected by a cold, it is actually the blocked nose that makes food seem tasteless. As the eyes are the organs of the sense of sight, the nose is the organ of the sense of smell, the tongue is the organ of taste (gustation). As food is dissolved in saliva, nerve cells are stimulated. Just as optic and olfactory nerves carry impulses from the eyes and nose to the brain, impulses from the taste buds traverse cranial nerves to the medulla oblongata in the brain. From here, the gustatory pathway carries information to other areas of the brain; the primary gustatory area in the parietal lobe where conscious perception of taste arises, the limbic system, hypothalamus and thalamus (Tortora & Derrickson 2010). Taste is considered much simpler than smell, as only five primary tastes can be distinguished; sour, sweet, bitter, salty and umami (described as 'meaty' or 'savoury'), with all other flavours being a combination of these and accompanying smells and tactile sensations. A young adult will have nearly 10 000 taste buds, predominantly situated on the tongue, but also on the roof of the mouth, throat and epiglottis (cartilage lid over the voice box).

Awareness of the sense of taste in your work

As the number of taste buds declines with age, older people might derive less enjoyment from foods they previously favoured. They may indicate a preference for more seasoned foods. Complete adaptation (loss of sensitivity) to a specific taste can occur in 1–5 minutes of continuous stimulation (Tortora & Derrickson 2010), possibly contributing to continuing ingestion by some people with learning disabilities of substances others might find noxious (for example pica, see Ch. 18, and the voracious appetite associated with Prader-Willi syndrome). Conversely, there may be occasions where we are encouraging people to take substances they find unpleasant, for example medication. Practitioners should be guided by their professional codes, the Mental Capacity Act 2005 and the invaluable support of their local pharmacist in addressing this.

Like smell, taste has links to pleasant and unpleasant emotions (you may have discovered this in Reader activity 15.3), with even babies reacting positively to sweet foods and expressing disgust at bitter tastes (Tortora & Derrickson 2010). Evidence suggests people with a learning disability are especially vulnerable to some types of cancer (Patja et al 2001). Drugs and radiation treatments used to combat cancer often cause nausea and gastrointestinal upset regardless of what the individual tries to eat, leading to loss of appetite due to development of taste aversion. So people can learn to avoid food if it has previously made them unwell, even if the root cause is the treatment. This can be hugely difficult for carers, where food represents nurture, and can engender similar emotions to those experienced where oral nutrition is no longer advisable, as with those having enteral feeds due to aspiration (see Ch. 14).

Sense of touch

As the eyes are the organs of the sense of sight, the nose is the organ of the sense of smell and the tongue is the organ of taste, so the skin is the organ for tactile sensations. Components of these include touch, pressure, vibration, tickle and itch. They are referred to collectively with thermal, pain and proprioceptive sensations as somatic (literally, of the body) senses, activating a variety of types of receptor, information from which is then carried to the brain.

Proprioception refers to the sense we have of the position and movement of our bodies – where our head and limbs are located and how they are moving, even if we are not looking at them – created by information derived from a variety of different receptors, including the sense organs for balance (vestibular apparatus; see 'How the ear works', above), receptors in the skin, joints, muscles and tendons. Proprioception is important in posture and movement, with difficulties experienced by many people with learning disabilities. The physiotherapist and occupational therapist have key roles in working with individuals, their carers and supporters to improve this area of functioning.

Awareness of the sense of touch in your work

The ability to tolerate human touch is clearly important for the development of relationships and promotion of holistic health. From self-care and examination, personal care delivered by others through to the attentions of dentist, doctor and hairdresser, its significance can be seen. Chapters 12 and 28 remind us of the touch of the abuser and the lover. Where there is loss of movement and sensation in the legs (paraplegia), arms and legs (quadriplegia) or one side of the body (hemiplegia), individuals may rely on supporters to anticipate potential effects of impaired somatic senses. For example, the temperature of bath water should be checked, positions should be altered to reduce pressure, particular care should be taken where skin is breached. Emphasising the significance of touch in multi-sensory impairment, Sense (2010d) says of Kiera:

> As a deafblind child, touch is both her eyes and her ears . . . However, touch alone can be scary.

Aromatherapy, mentioned in the earlier section on smell, is often administered in conjunction with massage (Wray 2009) and abdominal massage is increasingly being used as part of total bowel management, both requiring skilled, purposeful touch. However, touch should not be something supporters simply 'administer' to people with learning disabilities during delivery of care; it should be (appropriately) reciprocated. For example, it may be used by children and adults who are deafblind to identify

Case illustration 15.2

Keith had an ingrowing toenail. His doctor referred him to a chiropodist. When he first met the chiropodist, her light touch caused him to withdraw his foot from her attention, saying "it tickles". This sensation typically occurs only when someone else touches you. While it is possible the chiropodist's apparent apprehension related to the pain Keith was expressing, the soles of the feet are abundant in touch receptors so reasonably firm handling is generally tolerated better than trying to be gentle.

A course of treatment was indicated. Keith prepared for each visit (occurring on the same day, Monday, at the same time) with a combination of discussion, questions and answers, role play and familiarisation with both the chiropodist and the environment, including the treatment chair and equipment that would be used. While he expressed some mild anxiety, it was insufficient to warrant intensive, structured desensitisation; education, information and reassurance were enough.

Unfortunately, the treatment was unsuccessful and Keith ultimately needed to have the toenail removed. This called for use of a further technique – auditory distraction. The treatment had been taking place during the Formula One World Championship, of which Keith was a great fan. It provided an ongoing topic of conversation between him and the chiropodist, his Monday appointments tending to follow weekend Grand Prix. So, Keith's appointment for minor surgery was kept to the regular slot and the procedure was successfully completed while he reclined, eyes closed, listening to the previous day's Brazilian Grand Prix via headphones.

supporters (perhaps by a watch or a more intentional identifier, for example a particular key fob around their neck), to seek and give reassurance, convey emotion and so on. In Case illustration 15.2, touch as part of a physical health treatment was used alongside other approaches, including auditory, to achieve a successful outcome.

Combining awareness of the senses in your work

Roberts (2010) suggests using a sensory room to help assess when a child with learning disabilities reacts to visual and auditory stimulation as it could allow for control of sight and sound experiences. The history in learning disability services of multi-sensory rooms is reported by Bell (2009b) as emerging in the 1970s and 1980s from the Dutch form of sensory intervention Snoezelen (meaning to sniff and to doze). As is the case with aromatherapy, successive investigations (for example, Kwok et al 2003) recommend more research on the impact and therapeutic value of their use. The senses of hearing, sight and touch may be used in therapies including music and art, and taste and smell in the formal teaching of cookery skills. Rebound therapy (in this context, the use of trampolines to promote balance and sensory integration) and hydrotherapy may have formal (i.e. intended) and informal (extra) therapeutic benefit, perhaps derived from the company and relationships. However, opportunities for stimulating, calming or enjoyable sensory activities should enrich the everyday lives of people with learning disabilities. This may be via activities in the home or outside. Days can be themed around a colour or country, including dress and decoration, or a world menu or different kinds of music offered. Any inclination to stay in when the weather is less than clement should be resisted, so people (accounting for health and personal choice) can experience wind and rain, see and feel snow, have sand trickle between their fingers and toes, hear the crunch of autumn leaves beneath their feet or wheels and smell the forest or the sea.

Conclusion

This chapter has considered the range of functioning of the five commonly identified senses – sight, hearing, taste, smell and touch – in relation to people with learning disabilities. It has recognised the frequency with which sight and hearing impairments occur in relation to causes of learning disability, associated conditions (for example cerebral palsy) and ageing. Possible variations in the lesser discussed senses of smell, taste and touch have been explored and the likelihood recognised of difficulties coexisting. Explanations have been provided for the structure and workings of the senses, on which to base discussion of the issues that may then arise. A model for practice that promotes the senses is offered, ranging from top tips for looking after your eyes and ears, through testing and provision of treatment or aids. Supporters of people with learning disabilities are urged to develop their sensory awareness to enable natural access to stimulating, relaxing and pleasurable activities.

References

Access Economics PTY Ltd, 2009. Future sight loss UK (1): the economic impact of partial sight and blindness in the UK adult population. RNIB, London.

Age Cymru, 2010. Hearing. Available at: http://www.ageuk.org.uk/cymru/health–wellbeing/conditions-illnesses/hearing-/ (accessed 01.08.10.).

Age Scotland, 2010. At home with Scotland's older people: facts and figures 2009–2010. Age Scotland, Edinburgh.

Aromatherapy Council, 2009. About aromatherapy. Available at: http://www.aromatherapycouncil.co.uk/index_files/Page390.htm (accessed 18.07.10.).

Bell, M., 2009a. Sensory integration. In: Gates, B., Barr, O. (Eds.), Oxford handbook of intellectual and learning disability nursing. Oxford University Press, Oxford, pp. 300–301.

Bell, M., 2009b. Multisensory rooms. In: Gates, B., Barr, O. (Eds.), Oxford handbook of intellectual and learning disability nursing. Oxford University Press, Oxford, pp. 298–299.

Bittles, A.H., Petterson, B.A., Sullivan, S.G., et al., 2002. The influence of intellectual disability on life expectancy. J. Gerontol. 57 (7), 470–472.

British Retinitis Pigmentosa Society, 2010. About RP. Available at: http://www.brps.org.uk/index.php?tln=aboutrp (accessed 17.07.10.).

Cole, A., 2005. Japanese study is more evidence that MMR does not cause autism. Br. Med. J. 330, 558.

Cordeiro, M.F., Guo, L., Coxon, K.M., et al., 2010. Imaging multiple phases of neurodegeneration: a novel approach to assessing cell death in vivo. Cell Death and Disease e3, 1.

Crofts, B., 2008. Eye problems in children with Down's syndrome. Down's Syndrome Association, London.

Deafblind UK, 2007. Cause and cure: deafblind people's experience of the NHS. Deafblind UK, Peterborough.

Deafness Research UK, 2009. Deafness – the facts. Deafness Research UK, London.

Deafness Research UK, 2010a. Age-related hearing loss. Available at: http://www.deafnessresearch.org.uk/1618/about-deafness/agerelated-hearing-loss.html (accessed 01.08.10.).

Deafness Research UK, 2010b. Hearing loss research. Available at: http://www.deafnessresearch.org.uk/3395/research/hearing-loss-research.html (accessed 01.08.10.).

Deafness Research UK, 2010c. 10 top tips for healthy ears. Available at: http://www.deafnessresearch.org.uk/factsheets/top-tips-healthy-ears.pdf (accessed 01.08.10.).

Directgov, 2010. Blind person's allowance. Available at: http://www.direct.gov.uk/en/MoneyTaxAndBenefits/Taxes/BeginnersGuideToTax/IncomeTax/Taxallowancesandreliefs/DG_078319 (accessed 01.08.10.).

Disability Rights Commission, 2006. Equal treatment: closing the gap: a formal investigation into physical health inequalities experienced by people with learning disabilities and/or mental health problems. DRC, London.

Emerson, E., Hatton, C., 2008. People with learning difficulties in England. Centre for Disability Research, Lancaster.

Emerson, E., Madden, R., Robertson, J., et al., 2009. Intellectual and physical disability, social mobility, social inclusion and health. Centre for Disability Research, Lancaster.

Epilepsy Action, 2005. Auras and warnings. Available at: http://www.epilepsy.org.uk/info/aura (accessed 21.07.10.).

Ferris-Taylor, R., 2007. Communication. In: Gates, B. (Ed.), Learning disabilities: toward inclusion. fifth ed. Churchill Livingstone, Edinburgh, pp. 333–338.

Foundation for People with Learning Disabilities, 2007. More on health needs of people with learning disabilities. Available at: http://www.learningdisabilities.org.uk/information/issues/rights-and-values/heath-needs/more-on-health-needs/?locale=en (accessed 20.07.10.).

Gatcum, H., Jacob, T., 2001. Anosmia: a resource for those who have lost their sense of smell and taste. Available at: http://www.cardiff.ac.uk/biosi/staffinfo/jacob/Anosmia/anosmia.html (accessed 18.07.10.).

Graham-Rowe, D., 2009. Eyes reveal health secrets of the brain. New Sci. 201 (2691), 20–21.

Greater London Authority, 2010. Number of people registered deaf or hard of hearing by age group, borough. Available at: http://data.london.gov.uk/datastore/package/number-people-registered-deaf-or-hard-hearing-age-group-borough (accessed 01.08.10.).

Healy, D., 2003. Psychiatric drugs explained, third ed. Churchill Livingstone, Edinburgh.

Higgins, S., O'Toole, M., 2008. Meeting the needs of people with intellectual impairment. In: Clark, L., Griffiths, P. (Eds.), Learning disability and other intellectual impairments. Wiley, Chichester, pp. 15–40.

Holt, F.E., Birks, T.P.H., Thorgrimsen, L. M., et al., 2003. Aroma therapy for dementia. Cochrane Database Syst Rev. (3). Art. No.: CD003150. doi: 10.1002/14651858.CD003150.

Information Centre for Health and Social Care, 2008. Registered blind and partially sighted people, year ending 31 March 2008. NHS Information Centre, England.

Kwok, H.W.M., To, Y.F., Sung, H.F., 2003. The application of a multisensory Snoezelen room for people with learning disabilities – Hong Kong experience. Hong Kong Med. J. 9 (2), 122–126.

Lindsey, P., Burgess, D., 2006. Care of patients with intellectual or learning disability in primary care: no more funding so will there be any change? Br. J. Gen. Pract. 56 (523), 84–86.

Lous, J., Burton, M.J., Felding, J., et al., 2005. Grommets (ventilation tubes) for hearing loss associated with otitis media with effusion in children. Cochrane Database Syst Rev. (1). Art. No.: CD001801. doi:10.1002/14651858.CD001801.pub2.

Manners, R., Stevens, G., Chaplin, E., 2007. Art, drama and music therapies. In: Gates, B. (Ed.), Learning disabilities: toward inclusion. fifth ed. Churchill Livingstone, Edinburgh, pp. 507–526.

Mason, I., Stevens, S., 2010. Instilling eye drops and ointment in a baby or young child. Community Eye Health Journal 23 (72), 15.

Mencap, 2007. Death by indifference. Mencap, London.

Michael, J., 2008. Healthcare for all: report of the independent inquiry into access to healthcare for people with learning disabilities. Department of Health, London.

National Health Service, 2010. Newborn hearing screening programme. Available at: http://hearing.screening.nhs.uk/ (accessed 02.08.10.).

Office for National Statistics, 2010. Population estimates. Available at: http://www.statistics.gov.uk/cci/nugget.asp?id=6 (accessed 21.07.10.).

Patja, K., Eero, P., Iivanainen, M., 2001. Cancer incidence among people with intellectual disability. J. Intellect. Disabil. Res. 45 (4), 300–307.

Roberts, B., 2010. Addressing the physical and sensory needs of children with profound and multiple learning disabilities. In: Grant, G., Ramcharan Flynn, M. (Eds), Learning disability: a life cycle approach. second ed. McGraw Hill, Maidenhead.

Robertson, J., Emerson, E., 2010. Estimating the number of people with co-occurring vision and hearing impairments in the UK. Centre for Disability Research, Lancaster.

Royal College of Nursing, 2006. Meeting the health needs of people with learning disabilities: guidance for nursing staff. RCN, London.

Royal National Institute of Blind people, 2010a. How the eye works. Available at: http://www.rnib.org.uk/eyehealth/eyeconditions/Pages/how_eye_works.aspx (accessed 17.07.10.).

Royal National Institute of Blind people, 2010b. Eye health. Available at: http://www.rnib.org.uk/eyehealth/Pages/eye_health.aspx (accessed 17.07.10.).

Royal National Institute for Deaf people, 2006. Facts and figures on deafness and tinnitus. RNID, London.

Royal National Institute for Deaf people, 2008. Living with someone who has gradual hearing loss. RNID, London.

Scottish Council on Deafness, 2008. Defining deafness. SCOD, Glasgow.

SeeAbility, 2007. You and eye. Look Up, Epsom.

SeeAbility, 2010. Functional vision assessment for people with learning disabilities. SeeAbility eye 2 eye, Epsom.

SeeAbility-Look Up. undated. The eye care needs of people with learning disabilities. Available at: http://www.lookupinfo.org/carers_supporters/default.aspx (accessed 17.07.10.).

Sense, 2008a. The delayed effects of congenital rubella syndrome. Factsheet 19. Sense, London.

Sense, 2008b. CHARGE and multi-sensory impairment. Factsheet CG03. Sense, London.

Sense, 2010a. What is deafblindness?. Available at: http://www.sense.org.uk/what_is_deafblindness (accessed 20.07.10.).

Sense, 2010b. A sense of urgency. Sense, London.

Sense, 2010c. Lighting. Available at: http://www.sense.org.uk/help_and_advice/people_who_are_deafblind/equipment_and_accessibility/lighting (accessed 20.07.10.).

Sense, 2010d. Kiera. Available at: http://www.sense.org.uk/support/who_we_help/kiera (accessed 20.07.10.).

Taylor, N.S., Standen, P.J., Cutajar, P., et al., 2004. Smoking prevalence and prevalence of associated risks in adult attenders at day centres for people with learning disabilities. J. Intellect. Disabil. Res. 48 (3), 239–244.

Tortora, G., Derrickson, B., 2010. Essentials of anatomy and physiology, eighth ed. John Wiley & Sons, Chichester.

Vision Matters, 2010. A sight test is a vital health check. Vision Matters, UK.

Wake, E., 2007. People with profound and multiple disabilities. In: Gates, B. (Ed.), Learning disabilities: toward inclusion. fifth ed. Churchill Livingstone, Edinburgh, pp. 243–280.

Wray, J., 2009. Complementary and alternative therapies. In: Gates, B., Barr, O. (Eds), Oxford handbook of intellectual and learning disability nursing. Oxford University Press, Oxford, pp. 308–309.

Wray, J., Paton, K., 2007. Complementary therapies in learning disability settings. In: Gates, B. (Ed.), Learning disabilities: toward inclusion. fifth ed. Churchill Livingstone, Edinburgh, pp. 483–506.

Further reading

Waite, L., 2002. Sight problems and people with intellectual disabilities. Available at: http://www.intellectualdisability.info/physical-health/sight-problems-and-people-with-intellectual-disabilities#drops (accessed 20.07.10.).

Useful addresses

Action for Blind People's Top 10 Tips to Guiding Visually Impaired People: *http://www.actionforblindpeople.org.uk/help-advice/top-ten-tips-to-guiding,520,SA.html*

Deafblind UK: http://www.deafblind.org.uk/

Deafblind Ireland: http://www.deafblindireland.org/

Diabetes UK: http://www.diabetes.org.uk/

Down's Syndrome Association: http://www.downs-syndrome.org.uk/

Enable: http://www.enable.org.uk/

National Autistic Society: http://www.autism.org.uk/

National Council for the Blind of Ireland: http://www.ncbi.ie/

Rebound Therapy: http://www.reboundtherapy.org.uk

Royal National Institute for Blind people: http://www.rnib.org.uk/Pages/Home.aspx

Royal National Institute for Deaf people: http://www.rnid.org.uk/

Scottish Council on Deafness: http://www.scod.org.uk/

SeeAbility: http://www.lookupinfo.org, Tel: 01372 755066

Provided by SeeAbility (Royal School for the Blind), Look Up advocates 'seeing beyond disability' and provides information and advice to eye care and vision professionals on the needs of people with learning disabilities and those who support people with learning disabilities on the importance of eye care and vision.

Sense: http://www.sense.org.uk/

Vision 2020 (global initiative): http://www.vision2020.org/main.cfm

Vision 2020 UK: http://www.vision2020uk.org.uk/: incorporating UK Vision Strategy, transforming the UK's eye health, eye care and sight loss services: http://www.vision2020uk.org.uk/ukvisionstrategy/

Vision Matters: http://www.visionmatters.org.uk

Epilepsy

16

Heather Gregory

CHAPTER CONTENTS

KEY ISSUES

- Epilepsy is the oldest and most common form of neurological condition known to man and is signified by the presence of recurrent unprovoked seizures
- Seizures are a symptom of underlying brain dysfunction the cause of which is multi-factorial
- All manifestations of epileptic activity are idiosyncratic as the contributing factors are pertinent to individuals
- An accurate assessment of seizure type experienced by an individual is vital if the effectiveness of treatment is to be optimised
- Treatment interventions must suit the needs of the individual and range from the prescription of anti-epileptics through to vagus nerve stimulation and a ketogenic diet

- Sometimes the epilepsy of people with learning disabilities is very difficult to both detect and treat and requires specialist skills to ensure maximum health gain

Introduction

Epilepsy is the oldest and most common neurological condition known to man. Hippocrates, born 460 BC, may have been the first to write about epilepsy at a time when people believed in its association with possession. The term 'epilepsy' is used to indicate the presence of recurrent unprovoked epileptic seizures. In normal brain activity there is a balance between the actions of neurones that ensures that neither the excitatory or inhibitory functions become overwhelming. A seizure occurs as a result of excessive firing and synchronisation of neurones (Jefferys 2002) with the imbalance between excitation and inhibition occurring in either specific areas of the cerebral cortex or over the entire cerebral cortex (Hickey 2003). The manifestation of a seizure depends on the part of the brain where the neuronal discharge originates and its presence should be seen as a symptom of underlying brain dysfunction rather than a condition in itself.

Epilepsy is a common condition with a prevalence rate of between 5 and 10 per 1000 people in the general population (Shorvon 2000). However, among those with a learning disability, the reported incidence is higher and is estimated to be 3.7 per 1000 of the population (Morgan et al 2000), affecting 15% of people with mild to moderate learning disabilities and 30% of people with severe learning disabilities across the course of a lifetime. Such figures serve to illustrate a positive correlation between the prevalence of epilepsy and the severity of the learning disability.

For people with learning disabilities, prognosis for seizure control has been found to be poorer than for those experiencing epilepsy in the general population (Sillanpaa 2004) and with this come increased mortality rates within this group (Nashef et al 1995). People with a learning disability are already known to have lower life expectancy but this is further compromised for those who have the additional diagnosis of epilepsy. In a Swedish study of over 1400 people with learning disabilities followed up for 7 years, the standardised mortality ratio (SMR) for those with a learning disability without epilepsy was 1.6 but the SMR increased to 5.0 in those with a dual diagnosis of learning disability and epilepsy (Forsgren et al 1996). It is also recognised that this client group have more admissions to accident and emergency departments (Clinical Standards Advisory Group 2000) and a higher risk of fractures.

Because of the complexities of such issues, the provision of good quality, evidence-based care for people with a dual diagnosis of a learning disability and epilepsy is imperative. Indeed, because the epilepsy of people with learning disabilities is so notoriously difficult to treat effectively, specialist skills are required to ensure maximum health gain. Indeed, many individuals are resistant to treatment and may experience more than one seizure type. It is therefore essential to make an accurate diagnosis with careful consideration of suitable treatment regimes. Assessing the impact of epilepsy goes beyond assessing the impact of the seizures or the anti-epileptic medication, while care consists of more than just controlling seizures and considering the impact on the person with learning disabilities but extends to its effect on friends and relatives. Indeed, the stresses on family members may be extreme and long lasting and may influence their approach to new treatments (Farnalls & Renwick 2003). The aim of this chapter therefore is to provide a comprehensive overview of such issues and evidence best practice in meeting the needs of this group. In particular, it considers the role of the specialist epilepsy nurse in working with individuals and their families in facilitating the achievement of an optimum health status.

Causation and classification

With advances throughout the 20th century in diagnostic techniques such as magnetic resonance imaging (MRI), computerised tomography (CT) and electroencephalography (EEG), it has been possible to identify underlying causes of epilepsy. Epilepsy is a group of disorders known as epilepsy syndromes which have an onset in childhood. A number of these syndromes are benign whereas others are malignant and are often associated with significant learning disabilities. The disability may be present at the onset of seizures or may develop as a result of prolonged seizures; the evolution of a syndrome related to frequent clinical seizures and abnormal inter-ictal activity (Appleton cited in Trimble 2003). It is also important to consider the aetiology of the epilepsy syndrome and that it may have arisen from a number of different causes. Some will have arisen from a defined cause as in an early brain injury such as severe birth hypoxia or meningitis. Other epilepsy syndromes may be as a result of genetic syndromes such as Angelman or Rett syndrome or a chromosomal syndrome such as Down syndrome. However, a number of the epilepsy syndromes have no known cause.

The nature of seizure activity is also now better understood and epilepsy has been reclassified to include seizure types and epilepsy syndromes. The International League against Epilepsy (ILAE) developed a universally accepted classification of seizures in 1986 (Commission on Classification and Terminology of the International League Against Epilepsy 1989), classifying seizures according to their presentation and EEG recording but not taking into account the cause. Within this classification, seizures are classified as to whether they are *generalised*, affecting the whole cortex of the brain with loss of consciousness, or *partial*, affecting one part or associated parts of the brain where consciousness is not lost but may be altered. If a partial seizure leads immediately to a generalised seizure, the term used is *secondary generalised*; this is an important distinction as it has implications for treatment. Generalised seizures without partial seizure may be termed *primary generalised*. Figure 16.1 illustrates the different seizures types within this classification and the presentation of each will now be discussed

Seizure types

All manifestations of epileptic activity are idiosyncratic as the contributing factors are pertinent to that individual. There are various seizure types that may be preceded by a prodrome and these are discussed below

Prodrome and auras

A prodrome can be described as a seizure warning and manifests itself as distinct changes in mood or behaviour before the seizure commences. Symptoms of depression and irritability may occur and may last any length of time, sometimes up to a few days before the seizure. A prodrome is not part of the actual epileptic activity and the emotional disturbances usually cease when the seizure occurs but may re-emerge prior to the next seizure event.

An aura is a partial seizure and is a direct result of electrical activity, usually lasting a few minutes, at which point the person can experience intense fear, dizziness or any partial seizure experience. Where people with a learning disability are unable to communicate their experience of, for example, this intense fear, they may present with significant changes in behaviour. Fear and anxiety may provoke unsettled behaviour. It is possible for partial seizures to persist so becoming partial status (see section on prolonged seizures) when a range of psychiatric and emotional states can occur, including confusion, psychotic experiences and irritability (Ring 2009). Again this can be difficult to accurately diagnose in people with learning disabilities where the presenting behaviour may be related to anxiety, autistic traits or communication of pain or fear.

Partial seizures

Simple partial seizure

This form of seizure originates from an isolated part of the brain and the person will remain conscious throughout its duration. Sensory or motor functioning may be affected depending on where the seizure originates in the brain (see Fig. 16.2). People may feel a tingling sensation, numbness or twitching in a limb or limbs. They may experience an odd taste or smell. These seizures may occur as an aura and then develop into a generalised seizure. If people are unable to communicate their experience due to cognitive impairment, these seizures may go undetected.

Complex partial seizures

In a complex partial seizure, consciousness is not lost but may be affected and can lead to the person becoming confused and disorientated. Complex partial seizures usually originate from the temporal or frontal lobes of the brain which are involved

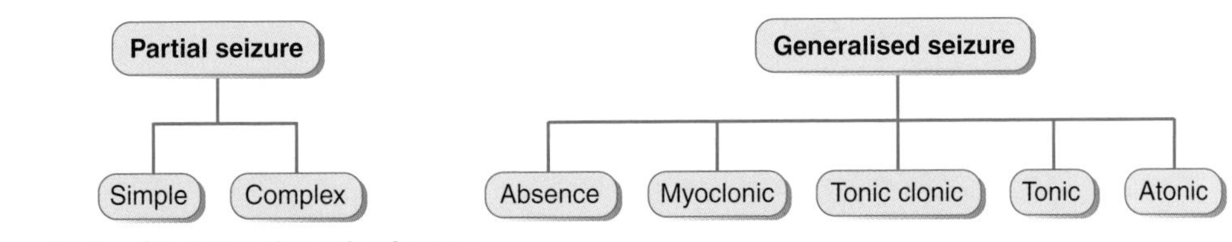

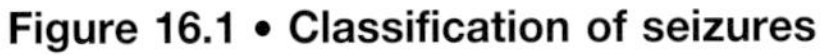
Figure 16.1 • Classification of seizures

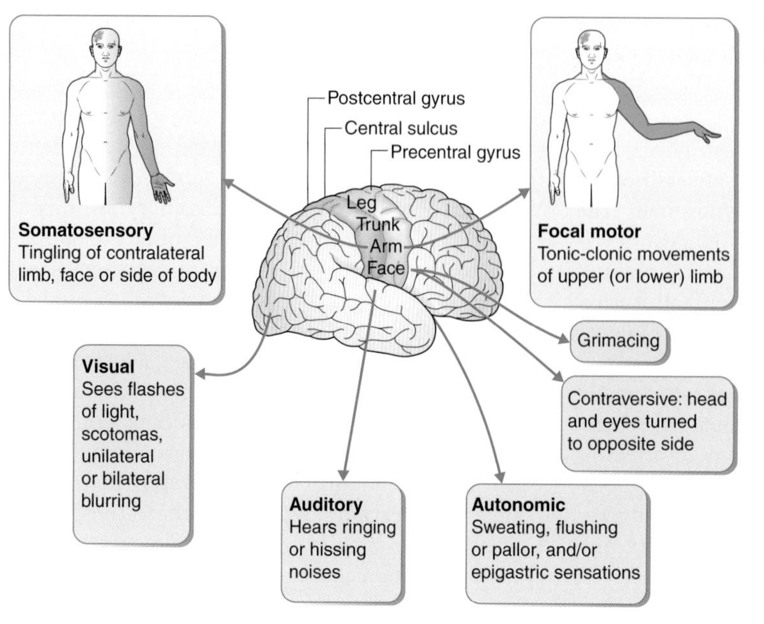

Figure 16.2 • Simple partial seizures

in complex functioning such as emotion, communication, memory, sense of smell and taste. Complex partial seizures may take many different forms (see Fig. 16.3). People may experience a strange smell or taste. They may have auditory or visual hallucinations and/or experience feelings of déjà vu. Some may fiddle with objects or their clothes and undress, or may present with lip smacking or chewing movements. They may wander around aimlessly, become agitated and behave strangely. Others may experience strong emotional states such as paranoia and be unfamiliar in familiar surroundings. These presentations don't appear as epileptic seizures so are often misinterpreted or not recognised and recorded as seizures by carers. This is particularly the case for people with learning disabilities where they are often misdiagnosed as features of autism or behavioural problems. Support advised for those experiencing complex partial seizures can be found in Box 16.1.

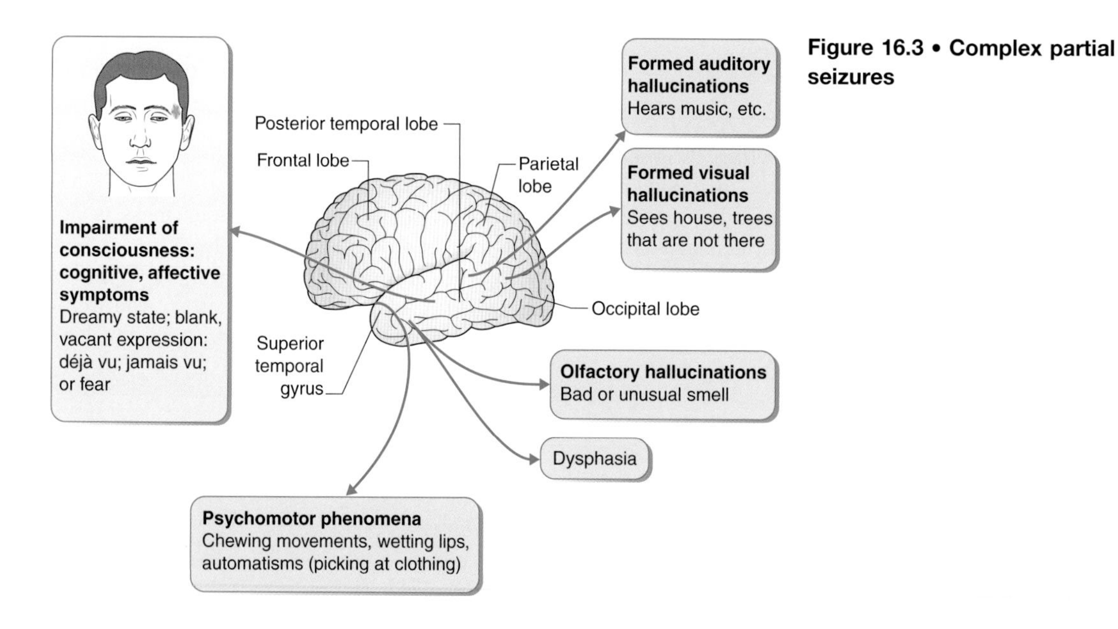

Figure 16.3 • Complex partial seizures

Box 16.1

Support advised for complex partial seizures

- Stay with the person.
- Give reassurance and support.
- Speak gently and clearly to the person.
- Guide them away from danger.
- The seizure may develop into a secondary generalised seizure; ensure safe environment, check epilepsy management plan.
- Do not leave them until they have returned to their usual self.
- Inform them what has happened.
- Record details of the seizure (see section on recording).

Generalised seizures

Absence seizures

An absence is a brief momentary loss of consciousness. The person may look blank with a fixed stare for a few seconds. These are commonly seen in children and can be mistaken for day dreaming. Some children experience hundreds of absences a day. People with learning disabilities and epilepsy may experience atypical absences which may be more prolonged, lasting minutes rather than seconds, and may include some slight facial twitching.

Myoclonic

Myoclonic seizures often occur in the morning. The person will present with a brief, sudden jerk of the upper or lower trunk and consciousness is briefly lost. If standing, the person may lose balance. These can often occur in clusters where a person experiences frequent myclonic jerks over a short period of time.

Tonic–clonic

This is the seizure type typically recognised as epilepsy by the general public and, contrary to partial seizures, the person will be unconscious. The seizure may start with a loud, often distinctive cry, caused by air in the lungs being forced out through the larynx; it does not indicate pain but may seem alarming when first heard. During the next phase (tonic phase), all the muscles in the body will tighten, then relax and tighten in rapid succession causing the convulsive (clonic) phase. Excess saliva may be produced and, if this is forced through tightly closed teeth, it may be perceived as 'foaming at the mouth'. During the convulsive phase the person may also bite their tongue. Breathing will be laboured, cyanosis (bluish colouration) around the lips may be present due to lack of oxygen and the person may be incontinent. Following the seizure they may experience post-epileptic automatisms including confusion. People often experience muscle aches and headaches and are quite tired, some needing to sleep for several hours. Most tonic clonic seizures last between 2 and 3 minutes (not including recovery time). The seizure may be primary or secondary generalised, although partial onset can often be difficult to identify in people with learning disabilities as so few partial seizures have an observable presentation. Support advised for those who experience tonic–clonic seizures can be found in Box 16.2.

Tonic

In a tonic seizure, consciousness is lost and the body will stiffen as muscles tighten. If the person is standing, they will fall backwards and, as such, injuries to the back of the head are common. There are no convulsions and these seizures are usually quite brief lasting between 20 seconds to a minute.

Box 16.2

Support advised for tonic–clonic seizure

- Note the time of onset.
- Make the environment safe.
- Protect head and limbs from danger.
- Remove glasses, high heel shoes, loosen tight clothing.
- Stay with the person until consciousness has returned.
- Maintain clear airway.
- Check for injuries.
- Reassure the person, inform them what has happened.
- Place them in the recovery position and wipe away any saliva.
- Note the time of recovery.
- Respect the person's dignity; they may have been incontinent.
- Record the details of the seizure (see section on recording).
- Allow the person to sleep.

Do not:

- Put anything in the person's mouth.
- Give anything to eat or drink.
- Restrain or restrict movements in a seizure.
- Move the person, unless they are in danger.

Atonic

In this type of seizure there is a sudden loss of all muscle tone and strength causing a sudden fall; consciousness is briefly lost with a quick recovery. Due to the sudden onset and rapid fall, injuries to the face, head, collar bone, hips and limbs are quite common. Where treatment hasn't yet controlled the seizures and where frequent atonic seizures occur, personal protective equipment may be an option to discuss with the clinician to reduce impact of injury. Support advised for those with tonic and atonic seizures can be found in Box 16.3.

Prolonged seizures (status epilepticus) and rescue medication

Shorvon (2000) describes status epilepticus as prolonged or recurrent tonic–clonic seizures persistent for 30 minutes or more. Partial status can also occur where partial seizures are prolonged or recurrent. Anti-epileptic drug (AED) changes, particularly drug withdrawal, or concurrent illness may be a cause. Prior to the occurrence of the condition, usual seizure patterns may become more frequent or intense. Shorvon refers to this as the premonitory stage which, if not rectified, can result in status epilepticus. Generalised tonic–clonic epilepticus is a medical emergency as it is associated with significant morbidity and mortality if not treated promptly (Stokes et al 2004). The aim of treatment is to stop seizure activity and prevent irreversible cerebral, systemic, metabolic, autonomic and cardiovascular changes.

For many years, the only rescue treatment for prolonged seizures administered in the community was rectal diazepam. Changing attitudes and reticence about the invasive and undignified nature of this treatment provoked the search for an alternative rescue medication that was as effective and more acceptable. Buccal midazolam provided an acceptable alternative for use in the community care setting. It is administered into the buccal cavity, a small area inside the mouth in front of the gum and behind the cheek. The drug is administered into the buccal cavity by means of a syringe, drawing up a measured amount as directed by the doctor and outlined on the emergency epilepsy management plan (Fig. 16.4). The main advantage of using buccal midazolam is that it offers a more convenient route of administration. It is also as effective as rectal diazepam in rapidly aborting prolonged seizures (Ariano et al 1994, Scott et al 1999).

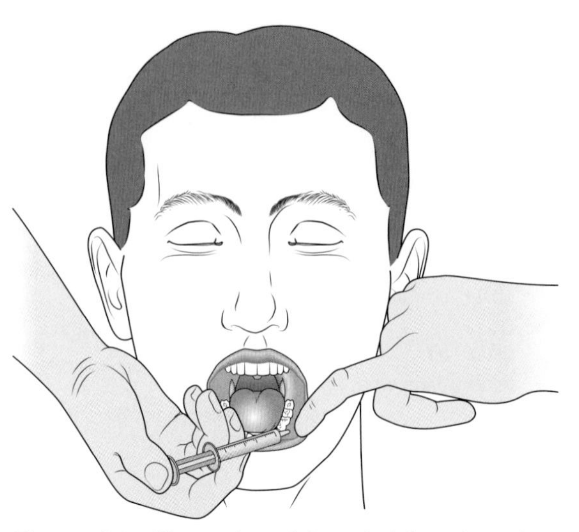

Figure 16.4 • Illustration of the administration of buccal midazolam (Image from: www.medicinesforchildren.org.uk)

Box 16.3

Support advised for tonic and atonic seizures

- Check for injuries.
- Attend to injuries.
- Reassure the person and remain with them until they appear their usual self.
- Inform them what has happened.
- Record all details (see section on recording).

Reader activity 16.1

A person with learning disabilities is prescribed buccal midazolam as a rescue treatment for prolonged tonic–clonic seizures.

- What information should be included in their emergency epilepsy management plan to ensure the appropriate safe administration of this medication?
- Who should provide training to carers on the administration of this drug?
- What should the training include?

Assessment and diagnostic process

The assessment of epilepsy in people with learning disabilities may be complicated by other co-morbid conditions such as communication difficulties, medical problems, mental health issues and challenging behaviour. The National Institute for Clinical Excellence (NICE) guidelines (Stokes et al 2004) and Working Group of IASSID (2001) outline the need for clear assessment and diagnostic process for this population. A comprehensive epilepsy learning disability assessment (Gregory cited in Trimble 2003) can inform this process and should include the following:

- Information relating to the onset of epilepsy and any identified causes.
- Eyewitness accounts of the seizure with an accurate description.
- An evaluation of the individual's experience of the seizure to determine any warning signs and precipitating factors in its development.
- A record of any suspicion that an episode may not be epileptic in origin.
- A list of possible trigger factors such as stress, infection, constipation, etc.
- A description of the behavioural presentation.
- The results of seizure recording methods and investigative results, EEG, MRI or CT scans or medical investigations.
- A list of medications including current and previous anti-epileptic drugs and reasons for discontinuing medication. Any other medication, preparation and administration.
- The needs of the individual and carers.
- Quality of life issues, e.g. seizure impact on sleep, mood, social and leisure activities.

Differential diagnosis

The misdiagnosis rate is quite high, with an estimated 50% of patients referred to specialist care in the UK with suspected epilepsy then identified not to have this condition, and 20% of people being actively treated for epilepsy subsequently found to be misdiagnosed (Morrow 2007). Some of the conditions leading to a misdiagnosis can be found in Box 16.4.

The co-terminosity of learning disability and epilepsy together with communication difficulties and additional health needs can cause considerable problems in diagnosis, as well as confusing accurate seizure monitoring and therefore obtaining appropriate treatment.

It is recognised that people with learning disabilities often present with several different seizure types, which are commonly refractory to treatment. The presentation of these can hamper correct diagnosis as they may present in a way that could be misinterpreted as a number of possible differential diagnoses including syncope, non-epileptic attack disorder, psychosis and sleep apnoea. These differential diagnoses occur both in the general population with epilepsy and in people with learning disabilities with the condition, however they are less likely to be recognised in the latter group because of assumptions made regarding the way this population may present. Moreover it can be immensely problematic to differentiate between epileptic-induced abnormal behaviours and environmentally-influenced behaviours or indeed partial epilepsy in someone who routinely presents with unusual movement disorders. In addition, involuntary movements, such as orofacial dyskinesia, may be a consequence of treatment with anti-psychotic or anti-convulsant medication and/or seizure activity.

While the process of diagnosing epilepsy relies in part on an eyewitness account of the episode, diagnostic overshadowing can complicate differentiation between seizures and behaviour. The description of the episode can be influenced by an expectation for the episode to be either epilepsy or behaviour. It is therefore helpful to investigate with routine and ambulatory electroencephalograms with telemetry, although it is recognised that some people with learning disabilities may refuse waking EEG. In addition, the accuracy of classification may be limited by communication abilities which may make the recognition of aura and post-ictal phenomena difficult; the prevalence of partial seizures may be underestimated due partly to carers' inability to recognise these subtle seizures and, as such, carer training is essential.

Box 16.4

Some conditions misdiagnosed as epilepsy

- Syncope.
- Panic attacks.
- Psychoses.
- Autistic traits.
- Challenging behaviour.
- Transient ischaemic attacks.
- Startle response.
- Non-epileptic seizures.

Reader activity 16.2

Peter is 20 years of age and lives with his parents. He attends a local college where he is studying a life skills course. He enjoys an active social life including swimming, playing football and drinking alcohol with his fiends at his local pub. He had been diagnosed as a child with a mild learning disability and he has difficulty communicating and comprehending complex information. As a child, he had episodes where he became vacant; these were not investigated. He remains in good health but has lately experienced recurrent ear infections.

His parents recently witnessed Peter present with an episode where he lost consciousness and his limbs became rigid followed by slight rhythmical jerking. The episode lasted approximately 2 minutes. Afterwards Peter appeared confused and then slept for a few hours. His parents have become extremely anxious and have suggested to Peter that he should not go swimming or go drinking with his friends. He has been seen by his GP who has referred him to a neurologist specialising in epilepsy and to the learning disability epilepsy specialist nurse for support and assessment.

- What information should be collated by the epilepsy specialist nurse prior to the neurology appointment?
- What investigative procedures may be used as part of the assessment and diagnostic procedure
- What support and advice should be given to Peter and his family at this stage?

Treatment and management

Pharmacological

Anti-epileptic drugs (AEDs) are the mainstay of the management of epileptic seizures. The overall aim is the achievement of seizure freedom with minimal adverse drug reactions (ADRs). This has been widened to include optimal outcomes of health-related quality of life with regard to physical, mental, educational, social and psychological functioning of the person with epilepsy (Panayiotopoulos 2008). Seizure freedom with minimal ADRs is achieved in approximately 50–70% of people with epilepsy with one AED. This seizure freedom varies significantly with seizure type, causation, age of onset and epilepsy syndrome.

Seizure control should not be pursued at the expense of ADRs. Total seizure control may be important for family members because of their anxieties, but the occasional partial seizure is relatively unimportant compared with the side effects of medication which may jeopardise the quality of life of the person with a learning disability and epilepsy.

People with learning disabilities often experience refractory epilepsy where seizures are treatment resistant and three or more AEDs have failed (Kwan & Brodie 2000). Uncontrolled seizures have a profound impact on the life of individuals with epilepsy and learning disabilities. Conflicting concerns regarding ADRs and seizure impact are further compounded by complex problems of communication and care provision. In addition, people with learning disability have difficult epilepsy syndromes that provide a significant therapeutic challenge.

National guidelines

The National Institute for Clinical Excellence (NICE) guidelines (Stokes et al 2004) and the Scottish Intercollegiate Guidelines Network (SIGN) guidelines (SIGN 2003) are the present 'benchmarks' for providing advice on the principles of initial AED therapy for all countries within the UK. Additional guidelines on the management of epilepsy in adults with learning disabilities (Working Group of IASSID 2001) and consensus guidelines of the management of epilepsy in adults with an intellectual disability (Kerr et al 2009) highlight the following good practice principles in the use of AEDs:

- Ensure that the person has received appropriate first-line treatment for their seizure type, syndrome and aetiology and has knowledge of the side effect profile of the AED.
- Where people continue to have seizures, despite appropriate first-line treatment:
  - review diagnosis
  - review treatment adherence
  - ensure the maximum tolerated dose has been used.
- If the first AED continues to be ineffective, an alternative AED should be introduced slowly. If effective then consider withdrawing the first AED gradually.
- Where reasonable options for monotherapy have been explored without acceptable seizure control, long-term polytherapy may be considered.

There is no evidence from randomised controlled trials that informs AED choices for refractory epilepsy as outlined by a recent Cochrane review (Beavis et al 2007). Selection of the appropriate AED for a given individual must be based on an understanding of that individual, each drug's pharmacology, spectrum of action, drug interactions, availability of varying preparations and likely side effect profile, in particular cognitive, behavioural and mobility side effects (Kerr et al 2009).

AEDs work by raising seizure threshold. They either increase the brain's inhibitory mechanism or reduce the tendency for neurones to fire excessively which causes seizures to occur. The AED needs to build up to a certain level in the bloodstream and then be maintained at that level through regular intake, known as a 'steady state'. Most AEDs are introduced at a low dose and increased very slowly as this reduces the likelihood of side effects. The AED should become effective once the steady state has been achieved. If the seizures are not controlled, the AED may be increased until seizures are controlled or side effects are experienced. Some people experience more seizures if the dose of the AED is too high. It is difficult to predict an individual's responses to AEDs until they have tried the medication. There is an element of trial and error in this process and it is important to balance seizure control with undesirable side effects. Table 16.1 provides a list of commonly used anti-epileptics, their indications and possible side effects.

It is important to recognise that the majority of people with learning disabilities are unable to self-report side effects. Some subtle side effects such as dizziness and double vision may be undetected and only obvious ones such as ataxia may be noted. People who are unable to communicate and present with non-compliance, behavioural problems or where they become withdrawn may be experiencing side effects such as nausea, double vision or headaches. Being aware of any changes in behaviour at times when AEDs are increased or changed will help identify any side effects. If an allergic reaction is suspected, for example presence of a skin rash, this should be reported immediately to the doctor, as this may represent a severe allergic drug reaction such as Stevens Johnson syndrome which could be life-threatening. Most side effects of AEDs are dose related and disappear once the drug level has been reduced or stopped. Baseline assessments should be considered before introducing AEDs as outlined in Figure 16.5.

Seizure recording methods

Accurate seizure recording is an essential component of seizure management. People with learning disabilities frequently rely on carers to observe and record seizures. This recording needs to include seizure type, duration, levels of consciousness, recovery period, including post-ictal automatisms, and if rescue medication was administered. Where seizure types are recorded, the specialist can determine type of AED to use and discuss the effect of these seizures on quality of life: for example, five brief myoclonic jerks a month may not affect someone's quality of life as much as three tonic–clonic seizures a month. It is also important to include precipitating factors or seizure triggers (see later section on types of seizure trigger) as, where these are managed more effectively, seizure occurrence will reduce. The record should also include when AEDs are introduced or withdrawn, including dates of titration increase or decrease, and when any other medication was introduced or withdrawn such as anti-psychotics or anti-biotics as these can affect some AEDs and increase seizure frequency. This record can then be discussed at the epilepsy review to determine future management. This may include management of seizure triggers where identified, adjustments in AEDs or the introduction of rescue medication.

Drug interactions

People with learning disabilities, difficult to control epilepsy and comorbid disorders (e.g. psychiatric illness, cardiovascular disease, mobility disorders, gastrological disorders or even simple infections) are at risk of drug interactions. Possible interactions with AEDs should always be explored at the time of prescription but must be seen as a likely cause of any emerging symptoms after new treatments are introduced. Long-term conditions such as those mentioned above require people to take medication over a long period of time and these medications may interact with AEDs. Other medications may increase or lower the concentrations of the AED thus causing toxicity or reducing the effectiveness of the AED and provoking increased seizures. The measurement of concentrations of an AED, if available, together with a clinical assessment of the individual should be made at the time the person presents with possible dose-related adverse effects (see Fig. 16.5). There is information on all AEDs in the *British National Formulary* and advice can be sought from the hospital or community pharmacist.

Assessment of treatment outcomes

When considering the effects of treatment, several factors need to be considered by the clinician, the person with learning disability and carer, including

Table 16.1 Individual drug characteristics

AED	Main adverse effects	Seizure type
Carbamazepine	Rash, sedation, headache, ataxia, nystagmus, diplopia, tremor, hyponatraemia, cardiac arrhythmia.	• Partial seizures. • Secondary generalised tonic–clonic seizures. • Primarily generalised tonic–clonic seizures.
Gabapentin	Weight gain, oedema, behavioural change.	Partial seizures with or without secondary generalisation.
Lamotrigine	Rash, weight gain, tics, insomnia, dizziness, headache, ataxia, asthenia.	• Partial seizures. • Primary and secondary generalised tonic–clonic seizures.
Levetiracetam	Irritability, behavioural and psychotic changes, dizziness, somnolence, headache.	Partial with or without secondary generalisation, myoclonic and primarily generalised tonic–clonic seizures.
Oxcarbazepine	Rash, headache, dizziness, nausea, somnolence, ataxia.	Partial with or without secondary generalised tonic–clonic seizures.
Phenytoin	Rash, ataxia, drowsiness, lethargy, sedation, gingival hyperplasia, hirsutism.	Tonic–clonic and partial seizures.
Pregabulin	Weight gain, myoclonus, dizziness, somnolence, ataxia, confusion.	• Partial with or without secondary generalisation. • Generalised anxiety disorder.
Topiramate	Somnolence, anorexia, fatigue, difficulty with concentration/attention, weight loss, renal calculi, language dysfunction.	Generalised tonic–clonic seizures, partial seizures with or without secondary generalisation.
Valproate	Nausea, vomiting, weight gain, tremor, hair loss.	Primary generalised epilepsy, absences and myoclonic seizures.
Vigabatrin	Irreversible visual field defects, fatigue, weight gain.	Partial seizures with or without secondary generalisation.
Zonisamide	Drowsiness, anorexia, irritability, weight loss, renal calculi.	Refractory partial seizures with or without secondary generalisation.

This table is based primarily on information obtained from the British National Formulary (BNF) September 2009

whether seizure control is acceptable, potential lifestyle implications (e.g. pregnancy), and whether side effects are tolerable. In order to accurately analyse any seizure change in terms of frequency and severity, accurate seizure charts are necessary. Developing high quality seizure data can be long term and clients and carers will need careful guidance in differentiating varying seizure types. It will also be necessary to determine any negative effects of treatment change such as behaviour change. This may be difficult, especially for those people with communication difficulties where other illnesses may present symptoms not unlike those of AED side effects. It is essential to ensure people with learning disabilities and their carers are fully involved in the decision-making process including risks of long-term seizures and AED side effects.

Vagus nerve stimulation

People with learning disability and pharmacoresistant or refractory epilepsy are at risk of significant mortality, morbidity and psychosocial disability. Pharmacoresistant epilepsy affects approximately 30% of people with epilepsy (Kwan & Brodie 2000). Once pharmacoresistant epilepsy has been recognised and epilepsy surgery is not a feasible

Client's name: D.O.B:

Observational/assessment	Baseline date:	3 months date:	6 months date:
Body mass index **Weight loss/increase**			
Blood pressure			
Ataxia			
Alopecia			
Condition of skin			
Appetite			
Nausea/vomiting Abdominal pain/discomfort			
Communication/changes in expressive communication			
Levels of alertness Concentration/lethargy			
Sleep pattern/ disturbed sleep			
Behaviour/recommended assessment			
Problems with previous medications			
Newly prescribed medications			
Number/type of seizures			
Other			

Name:	Signature:	Date:

Figure 16.5 • Observational nursing assessment/checklist for adverse effects of antiepileptics

option, other treatments such as vagus nerve stimulation (VNS) therapy may be explored as suggested by NICE guidelines (Stokes et al 2004).

VNS therapy delivers mild, intermittent electrical stimulation to the brain via a device implanted under the skin in the left chest area (see Fig. 16.6). It involves:

- an operation under general anaesthetic, which lasts 1–2 hours
- an incision on the left side of the neck for the lead
- an incision on the left upper chest or armpit for the generator
- a stay in hospital of around 1 or 2 days.

Two small scars will be evident after surgery; these are usually not noticeable or fade with time. There may also be a small bulge on the left upper chest where the generator is positioned. Clients are reviewed at a VNS clinic where the output current, signal frequency and pulse can be adjusted dependent on seizure frequency and any adverse

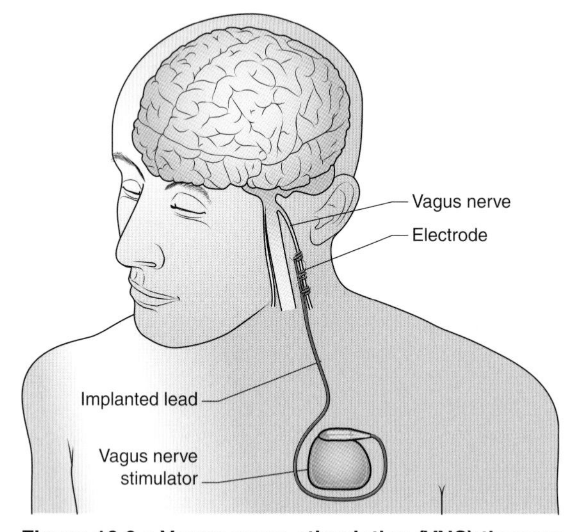

Figure 16.6 • Vagus nerve stimulation (VNS) therapy

effects. In addition, a magnet is available to use to boost the stimulation by passing the magnet over the device when the person starts to experience a seizure. This will provide additional stimulation to abort the seizure quickly. The VNS has an anti-epileptic effect which is comparable in efficacy to the most effective AED regimen with no interactive toxicity (Henry 2003). The most common side effects include temporary hoarseness and changes in voice tone, cough, tickling in the throat and shortness of breath. Reducing the output current, signal frequency and pulse can help eliminate these discomforts.

VNS was first licensed in the UK for epilepsy in 2001. For people with learning disabilities, the efficacy of VNS therapy has been described in the literature (Andriola et al 2001, Huf et al 2005).

Ketogenic diet/modified Atkins diet

The ketogenic diet, which is high in fat and low in carbohydrates, is believed to reduce seizures by promoting neuronal stability through increasing cerebral energy reserves. The diet has been used as a treatment in epilepsy for 80 years. It was originally determined that starvation was effective in the management of seizures. This diet is high in fat where ketone bodies become the primary source of energy for the brain in the absence of adequate glucose. This diet proved effective and was widely used. As anti-convulsants came onto the market, the diet became less popular, however its popularity has recently returned with the realisation that not all people respond to AEDs (Cross 2006). Companies have now developed the ketogenic diet in liquid form which may be helpful for people fed by enteral feeding methods. There is also evidence that a modified Atkins diet can be effective; although the foods contained in each are very similar, there are key differences between the two diets. In the Atkins diet, there is no fluid or calorie restriction and, although fats are strongly encouraged, there are no restrictions on proteins. In addition, foods are not weighed and measured, but carbohydrate counts are monitored by patients and carers and foods can be eaten more freely in restaurants and outside the home.

Prevention and management of seizure triggers

Some seizures occur with no obvious trigger factors, but a number of seizures are triggered by specific precipitants. Recognising and managing these seizure triggers can have a significant impact on overall seizure management and lead to reduction in AEDs and increased quality of life.

Seizure triggers

- Missed or incorrect dose of AED medication.
- Raised temperature (due to infection or environment).
- Lack of sleep.
- Stress (significant trigger factor).
- Excitement (celebrations, holidays, etc.).
- Boredom.
- Alcohol and illicit drugs (only 1.5 units of alcohol per 24 hours recommended; check strength).
- Photosensitivity.
- Startle response (people with cerebral palsy more vulnerable to this).
- Missed meals.
- Constipation.
- Hypoglycaemia.
- Hormones:
  - puberty/menarche
  - menstruation
  - hormone replacement therapy
  - pregnancy.

- Drug interactions:
  - anti-biotics
  - anti-histamines
  - anti-psychotics
  - anti-depressants.

Epilepsy and the individual

This section considers the complexity of epilepsy management in relation to specific groups of people.

Autistic spectrum condition

Autism is associated with epilepsy; however it is difficult to establish the association between autism and specific epilepsy manifistations. Gabis et al (2005) suggests epilepsy should be suspected in children in the autistic spectrum who have paroxysmal events. Studies have shown that nearly all children with autism and seizures also exhibit epileptiform activity on electroencephalograms (Hughes & Melyn 2005, Lewine et al 1999). Careful diagnostic caution is needed in assessing whether behaviour associated with autism might be due to epilepsy.

Down syndrome

Epilepsy occurs in 88% of people with Down syndrome and dementia (Dalton & Crapper-McLachlan 1986). Möller et al (2001) have identified a phenomenon of late-onset myoclonic epilepsy in people with Down syndrome. This condition presents in people with Down syndrome in later adulthood with the onset of myoclonic epilepsy, associated tonic–clonic seizures and progressive dementia. People with Down syndrome and dementia who develop epilepsy require careful and sensitive management due to other possible health-related issues such as dysphagia which can lead to aspirational pneumonia and exacerbate seizure clusters.

Women

There are issues around epilepsy and its treatment that are specific to women. For example, many anti-epileptic drugs may interfere with the contraceptive pill, some may affect fertility, some may be teratogenic and there is a recognised higher incidence of osteoporosis in women with epilepsy later in life. Women with epilepsy, both with and without learning disabilities, therefore require specific individual consideration when prescribing anti-convulsant therapy.

Anti-epileptic drugs and the contraceptive pill

Recognition of the right to relationships means women with learning disabilities and epilepsy may increasingly seek contraceptive advice or plan families. Those AEDs that are hepatic enzyme inducers, namely phenobarbital, primidone, phenytoin, topirimate, carbamazepine and oxcarbazepine, will increase the metabolism of oestrogens and progesterones, rendering the combined pill or progesterone-only pill unreliable as a means of contraception. Special consideration needs to be taken here and referral to a consultant specialist in women's sexual health is appropriate for assessment and advice. Some AEDs are affected by the contraceptive pill, for example lamotrigine serum levels fall with the introduction of the combined oral contraceptive pill.

Adolescence and puberty

Epilepsy can often first present at the time of puberty while puberty itself can exacerbate pre-existing epilepsy in young women. It is recognised that social and psychological factors associated with adolescence and puberty together with non-compliance of AEDs will further increase seizure frequency. One particular type of epilepsy that develops around puberty is juvenile myoclonic epilepsy. It usually presents with early morning myoclonic jerks which can be ignored until they later develop as tonic–clonic seizures occurring in the morning on rising. There should also be consideration made regarding the negative cognitive and unacceptable cosmetic effects of some AEDs on young people at this time such as weight gain, facial hair, acne and gum overgrowth.

Hormones and seizures

It is recognised that sex hormones have an effect on seizure control with some women having more seizures peri-menstrually or at ovulation. Studies have shown that oestrogen makes seizures worse while progesterone has an anti-convulsant effect. Where seizure records indicate increase in seizures peri-menstrually or at ovulation, it is suggested that clonazepam or clobazam can be effective when administered before their anticipated onset and continued for 5–7 days (Taylor 2000). There has been some suggestion that polycystic ovary syndrome (PCOS) may be higher in women with epilepsy taking anti-convulsants, in particular sodium valproate (Isojarvi et al 1996), however this remains controversial with Bauer et al (2000) finding similarities in the occurrence of PCOS between women taking carbamazepine or valproate and those with epilepsy taking no AEDs.

Epilepsy, pregnancy and pre-conceptual counselling

Most women who have epilepsy will have a normal pregnancy. It is recognised that there is potential teratogenic effects of AEDs taken in pregnancy, and evidence from the UK Epilepsy and Pregnancy register (Morrow et al 2006) has highlighted major congenital malformations seen in association with AEDs. Preconceptual advice from a health professional is essential and a number of epilepsy specialist nurses may develop specialist clinics in this area. Re-evaluating the diagnosis and the need for continuing AED therapy may be considered at this time; however this requires specialist consideration from consultant neurologists as abrupt discontinuation of AEDs may lead to uncontrolled seizures.

Epilepsy and menopause

For some women, the menopause has no effect on seizure frequency but others may find an increase or recurrence of seizures. Some women with epilepsy are at risk of bone demineralisation and, while there are conflicting reports regarding the effects of hormone replacement therapy (HRT) on seizures, it is recommended that HRT should be offered to post-menopausal women where it is clinically indicated due to the benefits of HRT on bone density.

Epilepsy and mental health

Earliest writings of neuropsychiatrists highlight that epilepsy is associated with disturbances in behaviour and in mental state. It has been difficult to identify what is neurological, what is seizure-related changes in behaviour, and what is psychiatric, namely those inter-ictal conditions of depression, anxiety, personality disorder and psychosis. While the former may seem obviously related to a seizure, the cause of the latter may prove more difficult to determine. For example, where people with a learning disability and epilepsy develop psychosis, it may not be seen as being the result of the neurophysiological disturbances of the epilepsy but may be related to other social pressures, chronic brain lesions or prescription of anti-convulsant medication (Krishnamoorthy & Trimble 2002). One of the most striking aspects of the psychiatric symptomatology associated with epilepsy is the range of emotional and cognitive symptoms that present themselves. Research has demonstrated that lifetime rates of anxiety, depression and suicidal ideation are all at least twice as high for those with epilepsy as in the population as a whole (Tellez-Zenteno 2008) and more prevalent again in the learning disability population.

Forced normalisation

There are clear accounts in which symptoms of irritability, depression and psychosis occur in association with seizure reduction. This is an EEG phenomenon and it was Landolt (1958) who developed the term 'forced normalisation'. Landolt noted that certain patients became psychotic when prescribed AEDs which stopped their seizures. During the period of psychosis, the EEG normalised, but when the seizures started again, the psychosis stopped and the EEG became abnormal. This phenomenon has been observed more frequently in recent times with the introduction of newer AEDs, effective in controlling seizures in people with intractable epilepsy.

People with a learning disability can often present with states of dysphoria, irritability and clinical withdrawal. Ring et al (2007) suggests that this relationship between seizure control and psychiatric symptoms occurs more frequently in people with learning disabilities and epilepsy.

Post-ictal psychosis

This needs to be distinguished from the post-seizure automatisms that can occur immediately post seizure. These automatisms last for approximately 20 minutes or more and the person may seem confused and present unusual, sometimes agitated, behaviour, but this will stop spontaneously. Post-ictal psychosis is more complex to recognise as it doesn't occur directly before or following the actual seizure. Trimble (2003) suggests the following operational criteria for post-ictal psychosis:

1. Onset of confusional psychosis within a week of the return of apparently normal mental function.
2. Duration of between 1 day and 3 months.
3. A mental state characterised by a) clouding of consciousness, disorientation or delirium; b) delusions, hallucinations in clear consciousness; c) a mixture of a and b.
4. No evidence of factors which may have contributed to the abnormal mental state: a) anti-convulsant toxicity; b) a previous history of inter-ictal psychosis; c) EEG evidence of status epilepticus; d) recent head injury, or alcohol or drug intoxication.

Post-ictal anxiety and depression is not uncommon and can often be related to temporal lobe syndromes.

These seizure-related psychiatric disorders can cause significant diagnostic challenges which are further complicated for those with learning disabilities. Where seizure freedom then leads to unmanageable behaviour then the balance may not be an acceptable one. Where emotional symptoms arising during the prodrome, aura, ictal and post-ictal appear to be related to epilepsy brain activity, clinical interventions to improve seizure control would seem necessary. Inter-ictal depressive states together with the higher rates of suicidal thoughts in those with epilepsy should lead clinicians to consider the use of anti-depressant medication.

There is evidence that stress provokes an increase in seizures (Haut et al 2003), a claim broadened by Moshe et al (2008) that intense physical and mental stress can also provoke seizures. Clinicians need to make a careful assessment of these possible triggers in the management of each individual's epilepsy. Anxiety and depression appear to be the most commonly reported psychological problems among people with epilepsy (Baker & Eatock 2007). Both issues would require further investigation to untangle the biological and psychosocial aspects of them in relation to epilepsy and learning disability; this could be achieved most effectively by utilising a multidisciplinary approach. It is worth noting that some pharmaceutical companies are responding to available research in the development of AEDs with dual action of seizure control and anxiety management, such as pregabalin.

In monitoring the complexities of epilepsy and altered mental state, an initial clear description of any behavioural presentation should be made by carers and needs to include any possible cause or trigger, a detailed behavioural presentation and any past history of similar behaviour, for example is the pattern of behaviour stereotypical? Any physical illness such as pain or urinary tract infections should be excluded as a cause of the behaviour, irrespective of any apparent association with changes in medication. The majority of behaviour problems presented in people with learning disabilities represent long-standing problems relating to their disability such as cognition, communication difficulties, environmental issues or autistic traits. Clinical psychological assessment needs to be considered to assist in determining the causation and therapeutic strategies (Kerr et al 2009).

Meeting the health needs of those with epilepsy

The health surveillance of this client group is often sadly neglected, yet it is recognised that this population often has increased health care needs. One-third of people with learning disabilities have associated physical disabilities, usually cerebral palsy. It is essential that these health needs are carefully assessed from a coordinated multi-disciplinary approach involving speech and language therapists, dieticians, GPs, neurologists and physiotherapists to identify treatment regimes. The problems associated with neglected health care needs further compound the dual diagnosis of epilepsy and learning disabilities. For example, recurrent chest infections provoking seizure clusters are often caused by unidentified aspiration pneumonia as a result of dysphagia. Similarly, episodes of recurring urinary tract infections provoking seizure clusters are often provoked by problems associated with poor hygiene care in people with double incontinence.

Working in a person-centred way

Person-centred planning is now the mainstay of learning disability services yet there is no reason why epilepsy services should not reflect this. We need to enable individuals to consider how their epilepsy affects their life while utilising creative and imaginative methods in providing information on all aspects of the condition. Individuals need to be enabled to make choices and that their priorities are reflected in a bespoke treatment plan which should be part of the individual's health action plan (see Ch. 13). The following suggestions highlight areas where person-centred approaches can be utilised in terms of epilepsy management for people with learning disabilities:

- Providing information specifically for that service user. The individual's ability to manage and cope with their epilepsy may be influenced through their knowledge and understanding of their condition. It is essential to identify methods of communicating and creating information that is meaningful for service users. Information packs illustrating the local epilepsy services can be developed to include photographs of these departments and professionals involved together with the process of assessment and investigation including EEG, MRI or CT scans.
- Promoting control through recording systems in easy read. Video recordings of seizures can help people to understand the various seizure types and practical ways of managing seizures.
- Encouraging self-administration of medication, through use of dossettes and careful supervision. Medication information sheets could be modified and include symbols or photographs to illustrate possible side effects among other things.
- Engaging the service user to the limit of their ability when developing individual epilepsy management plans or hospital patient passports.
- Empowering the service users and their families by using their expertise. A useful resource is a book entitled *Epilepsy* from the series *Books Beyond Words* as it facilitates an exploration of service users' feelings about their epilepsy. Many will have had their condition for many years and may not have had the opportunity to discuss their personal fears and beliefs about their condition. They may have developed inappropriate preconceived ideas about restricting their lifestyle because of their epilepsy or conversely they may be at risk of inducing seizures through lack of knowledge of triggers.
- Developing risk assessments with the service user (see Ch. 11). Lifestyle issues need to be explored with service users in a meaningful way to develop support systems which will promote life experiences through careful risk management. Other resources specifically designed for people with moderate learning disabilities have been published by the National Society for Epilepsy Action.
- Developing educational resources to meet individual needs.

A study undertaken by Clarke et al (2001) which evaluated a video-assisted educational pack for adults with mild learning disabilities and epilepsy entitled *Epilepsy and You* (Paul 1996) found this package to be suitable for a wide range of individuals and demonstrated significant gains in knowledge. They identified that, while knowledge about medication wasn't poor, there were deficits in knowledge regarding why it was important to visit doctors, what an EEG is and how medication works. In addition, they also found that, while some individuals had some knowledge about safety issues, there was little known about the use and importance of seizure diaries. Results also indicated that individuals enjoyed taking part in the training and that it may offer individuals more control over their health, encourage medication compliance and minimise secondary psychological consequences of epilepsy.

There is anecdotal evidence that easy-read documentation generally prepared for people with learning disabilities is of great use to people from different cultures where oral rather than written language is the norm. If easy-read material is made available, the result can be improved communication with all clients, whatever their intellectual or cultural background.

As Cunningham (2000:16–19) suggests:

> We should place clients at the centre of care planning, give them ownership of their epilepsy and create a collective approach in minimising the impact the epilepsy has on their quality of life. We should foster the growing momentum away from practices that exclude clients and their perspective and develop methods that forge alliances and inclusive frameworks.

Role of the epilepsy learning disability nurse

Types of intervention

The epilepsy management in people with learning disability is complex and the issues for this group are often sadly neglected and rarely featured as a priority on local hospital and primary care trust service development agendas, although this has improved since the introduction of the Disability Discrimination Act 2005, the Michael Report (Michael 2008) and the subsequent enforcement of the Care Quality Commission's core standards for better health. The epilepsy learning disability nurse (ELDN) is in a key position, through clinical audit, to highlight the needs of this client group and contribute to the development of local meaningful services (Table 16.2).

The ELDN is also able to facilitate a coordinated approach to aid the correct diagnosis of epilepsy with the following considerations:

- Accurate history taking, careful consideration of medical history (detailed audit of medical notes, psychiatric notes) can often identify initial diagnosis or previous neuroimaging investigations.
- A number of adults with epilepsy and a learning disability may not have had their epilepsy reviewed by neurology services. For this client population, it is essential that a detailed review of the diagnosis of their epilepsy be evaluated.
- People may have been mistakenly diagnosed with epilepsy following one seizure event, and have remained on high doses of mixed polypharmacy unnecessarily. Conversely people with frontal lobe epilepsy may have been inappropriately treated with tranquillisers, anti-psychotic medication, and been mismanaged through challenging behaviour services, as their partial complex epilepsy has not been identified or has been misdiagnosed.
- Historically, due to the inherent difficulties in identifying frontal and temporal lobe seizures and inter-ictal epileptic activity within this client population, many people have been treated inappropriately and will require a full reassessment of their condition. These people may not be referred to neurology or psychiatry for review of their epilepsy as their generalised seizures, which are easily identifiable, may be controlled.

Establishment of epilepsy management plans

Bespoke epilepsy management plans to determine when and how 'rescue medication' such as buccal midazolam should be administered to prevent seizure clusters and prolonged seizures; these have proved essential in the prevention of acute hospital admission. Special consideration needs to be given when developing emergency protocols, as frequently benzodiazepines such as rectal diazepam and buccal midazolam are prescribed as standard practice for those whose seizures are not always self-limiting. Constraints in some social care settings such as day and respite services, where carers are unable to carry out care proceedings considered by their policy as 'invasive', may lead to conflict. It is important to recognise that many carers may feel uneasy at the thought of carrying out a procedure which they perceive to be medical. The ELDN, through a collaborative approach, should establish a clear concise

Table 16.2 Interventions provided by the epilepsy learning disability nurse

Assessment	Planning and implementation	Evaluation
• Completing epilepsy assessments. • Determining the correct diagnosis and assisting in the detailed investigation of differential diagnosis. • Defining seizure type and syndrome. • Identifying health problems and physical difficulties affecting behaviour and epilepsy.	• Ensuring appropriate treatment, including correct dose and administration of medication. • Providing support and advice to clients and carers through complex medication titration regimes. • Investigating difficulties in compliance issues related to, for example, swallowing difficulties, metabolism. • Developing epilepsy management plans. • Ensuring accurate seizure monitoring including type, frequency and intensity. • Advising on measures to reduce seizures through management of 'triggers'.	• Participating in clinical reviews of clients. • Evaluating quality of life and other clinical outcomes. • Reviewing epilepsy management plans.

(Adapted from Gregory, cited in Trimble 2003)

individual management plan which recognises these limitations. Carers need to know when, what and how to administer rescue medications. Often people with learning disabilities receive care from a wide range of service providers; where continuity of treatment is essential, the individual epilepsy management plan provides essential information for the service provider in what to do in the emergency situation or how to manage and prevent clusters of seizures. Through careful monitoring, the effectiveness of managing seizures in this manner can be established.

Epilepsy awareness training

Effective assessment is dependent to a great extent on history provided by carers (see section on epilepsy assessment). Carers, whether paid or family, hold all of the information that the ELDN and neurologist need to complete an effective assessment of the individual's epilepsy, however they are unlikely to know the value of their information. Carers tend to provide only edited highlights, the information they deem to be relevant. To improve the information they are able to provide and to maximise the efficiency of the care they give, training is essential. Understanding breaks down resistance to changes in treatment and promotes shared decision making which is particularly relevant when clients lack capacity to make decisions regarding treatment choices. The ELDN will have a key role in this process.

It is essential that paid carers are also adequately equipped to meet the needs of people with complex epilepsy and learning disabilities. Where organisations place the value of the individual with these needs at the core of an organisational structure, this will be reflected in the value of the support staff employed to provide care and management. A poor value base is often reflected in high staff turnover, poor pay and conditions, sickness and inadequate training. These organisations often support the most vulnerable people with learning disabilities and complex needs. Through the provision of epilepsy awareness training, the ELDN can support these organisations to enrich staff development, and include them in developing epilepsy management plans, seizure recordings, risk assessments and care plans and in minimising seizure triggers. The complex information needs to be assimilated in a way that is understood and maintained. The training programme should be designed to be flexible and adaptable in meeting the needs of people with epilepsy, families and paid carers.

Conclusion

Epilepsy is a common condition in people with learning disabilities and is often refractory and complex to treat. The management of epilepsy in this client group is challenging as it can be more complex due to the severity and impact of the epilepsy, diagnostic difficulties, additional health care needs and communication issues. This is further compounded by the complexities of clinical presentation, difficult epilepsy syndromes and care provision. While specialist epilepsy knowledge is required, a multi-disciplinary approach is essential in the diagnostic process.

Recent advances in the form of new imaging techniques to identify abnormalities of the brain structure and function along with the development of new AEDs to help control seizures have provided wider options in the management of this condition. Recognition of seizure-related behavioural syndromes challenge our concepts of what is seizure presentation in people with learning disability and how this might integrate with psychiatric treatments, for instance.

The use of AEDs remains the most significant option to reduce the impact of epilepsy in people with learning disabilities. For people with intractable epilepsy where AEDs fail to provide adequate control, other treatments may be available such as VNS, surgery or the ketogenic diet. High clinical skill and competency are needed to optimise treatments, particularly where people are unable to communicate their own experience.

For people with learning disability, epilepsy can have a significant impact on cognition, social integration, injury, hospital admission and life-expectancy. Individual management strategies should be focused on reducing these negative impacts, ensuring unwanted side effects of treatments thus promoting improved quality of life. Those involved in this therapeutic pathway are clients, families, carers and health professionals; the ELDN is in a key position to coordinate epilepsy care for this client group

People with learning disability and epilepsy can provide significant complex clinical challenges. Improving knowledge of treatments by developing specialist skills in all service provision will ensure maximum health gain is ensured.

Glossary of terms

The terms used in the text are commonly found in specialist literature and clinical reports. This glossary attempts to provide some explanation for the terms used.

Aetiology The cause of a medical condition or disease; the study of factors involved in causing a condition

Ambulatory EEG A mobile EEG enabling prolonged monitoring over several days

Aspirational pneumonia Inflammation of the lungs due to inhalation of foreign materials such as food or vomit

Anti-epileptic drug concentrations The therapeutic range of AEDs is the optimal AED concentration range at which most patients achieve desired therapeutic effect with no undesirable side effects

Benign A relatively mild form of a disease that will not become progressive or malignant

Computerised tomography (CT) A CT scan of the brain using computerised X-ray techniques to identify any obvious structural abnormality

Diagnostic overshadowing The description of the episode is influenced by preconceived belief or expectation that it is related to one specific cause, e.g. to either behaviour or to epilepsy

Differential diagnosis Conditions of intermittent episodes of altered consciousness or seizure-like activity that are not epileptic in origin and can be misdiagnosed as seizures

Dysphagia Swallowing difficulty possibly due to nerves and muscles affecting the swallowing process

Electroencephalogram (EEG) The EEG records the minute electrical impulses produced by the activity of the brain and will indicate if the neurones in the brain are 'firing' in a normal manner or if there is any 'misfiring' of activity related to seizure activty

Epileptiform Presentation of motor and sensory abnormalities related to epileptic activity

Hepatic enzyme inducers These drugs stimulate the production and increase the amount of cytochrome P450 enzymes, this in turn increases the metabolism of the drug resulting in lower concentration levels

Hypoxia An inadequate supply of oxygen to the tissues

Inter-ictal This refers to the period of time between seizures. The inter-ictal period is often used by neurologists when diagnosing epilepsy since an EEG trace will often show small inter-ictal spiking and other abnormalities known by neurologists as sub-clinical seizures. Inter-ictal EEG discharges are those abnormal waveforms not associated with seizure symptoms

Magnetic resonance imaging (MRI) MRI is a diagnostic technique that provides high quality cross-sectional or three-dimensional images of the brain using short bursts of powerful magnetic fields and radiowaves. It can provide greater detail than the CT scan and identify small lesions and scarring in the brain

Malignant A condition that tends to become progressively worse and can be fatal

Menarche The onset of puberty

Monotherapy One type of drug or treatment

Neuroimaging Imaging techniques including MRI and CT scans of the brain to detect structural abnormalities

Non-epileptic attack disorder (NEAD) This is the occurrence of paroxysmal attacks which resemble epileptic attacks but are devoid of clinical features associated with epilepsy and usually have a psychological cause

Orofacial dyskinesia Abnormal facial muscular movements, including twitching or jerking movements

Panic attacks A brief period of acute anxiety, dominated by intense fear, hyperventilation, chest pains, palpitations, trembling and faintness

Paroxysmal events Short, sudden, frequent and stereotyped symptoms such as a spasm or possible seizure

Post-ictal The altered state of consciousness that a person enters after experiencing a seizure

Peri-menstrually The time period around menstruation

Pharmacoresistant Where medical therapy such as AEDs fail to control seizures

Resective epilepsy surgery Surgical removal of all or part of a diseased or abnormal structure

Stevens Johnson syndrome This is sometimes a life-threatening condition affecting the skin and mucous membranes. It can present with a flu-like prodrome and is characterised by severe mucocutaneous lesions; pulmonary, gastrointestinal, cardiac and renal involvement may occur. It may occur as a severe adverse reaction to medication

Syncope This is an episode of brief loss of consciousness with possible micturition and jerking movements due to cardiovascular causes and can be mistaken for a generalised seizure

Telemetry Simultaneously recording the EEG with a video of the person

Teratogenic A drug that causes an increased risk of physical abnormalities in the developing embryo or fetus

Transient ischaemic attack A brief interruption of the blood supply to part of the brain, resulting in temporary impairment of vision, speech, sensation or movement lasting several minutes or a few hours.

References

Andriola, M.R., Susan, A., Vitale, N.P., 2001. Vagus nerve stimulation in the developmentally disabled. Epilepsy and Behaviour 2, 129–134.

Ariano, R.E., Kassum, D.A., Aronson, K. J., 1994. Comparison of sedative recovery time after midazolam verses diazepam administration. Crit. Care Med. 22, 1492–1496.

Baker, G., Eatock, J., 2007. Epilepsy and Anxiety. Epilepsy Professional 6, 30–33.

Bauer, J., Jarred, A., Klingmuller, D., Elger, C., 2000. Polycystic ovary syndrome in patients with focal epilepsy: a study in 93 women. Epilepsy Res. 41, 163–167.

Beavis, J., Kerr, M., Marson, A.G., 2007. Pharmacological interventions for epilepsy in people with intellectual disabilities. Cochrane Database Syst. Rev. (3), Art. No.: CD005399.DOI: 10.1002/14651858.CD005399. pub2.

British National Formulary, 2009. British Medical Journal and Royal Pharmaceutical Society, London.

Clarke, A.J., Espie, C.A., Paul, A., 2001. Adults with learning disabilities and epilepsy: knowledge about epilepsy before and after an educational package. Seizure 10, 492–499.

Clinical Standards Advisory Group, 2000. Services for patients with epilepsy. Department of Health, London.

Commission on Classification and Terminology of the International League Against Epilepsy, 1989. Proposal for revised classification of epilepsies and epileptic syndromes. Epilepsia 30, 389–399.

Cross, H., 2006. Guide to the ketogenic diet. Epilepsy Professional 3, 10–12.

Cunningham, O., 2000. Person centred planning. Learning Disability Practice 3, 16–19.

Dalton, A.J., Crapper-McLachlan, D.R., 1986. Clinical expression of Alzheimer's disease in Down's syndrome. Psychiatric Perspectives on Mental Retardation 9, 659–670.

Farnalls, S., Renwick, J., 2003. Parent's care giving approaches: facing a new treatment alternative in severe childhood epilepsy. Seizure 12, 1–10.

Forsgren, L., Edvinsson, S.O., Nystrom, L., Blomquist, H.K., 1996. Influence of epilepsy on mortality in mental retardation: an epidemiologic study. Epilepsia 37, 956–963.

Gabis, L., Pomeroy, J., Andriola, M.R., 2005. Autism and epilepsy: cause, consequence comorbidity or coincidence? Epilepsy and Behaviour 7, 652–656.

Haut, S., Vouyiouklis, M., Shinnar, S., 2003. Stress and epilepsy: a patient perception survey. Epilepsy and Behaviour 4 (5), 511–514.

Henry, T.R., 2003. Vagus nerve stimulation for epilepsy: anatomical, experimental and mechanistic investigations. In: Schachter, S.C., Schmidt, D. (Eds.), Vagus nerve stimulation. second ed. Martin Dunitz, London and New York, pp. 1–31.

Hickey, J.V., 2003. The clinical practice of neurological and neurosurgical nursing. Lippincott, Williams & Wilkins, Philadelphia.

Huf, R.L., Mamelak, A., Kneedy-Cayem, K., 2005. Vagus nerve stimulation therapy: 2-year prospective open-label study of 40 subjects with refractory epilepsy and low IQ who are living in long term care facilities. Epilepsy and Behaviour 6, 417–423.

Hughes, J.R., Melyn, M., 2005. EEG and seizures in autistic children and adolescents: further findings with therapeutic implications. Neuroscience 36, 15–20.

Isojarvi, J., Laatikainen, T., Pakarinen, A., et al., 1996. Polycystic ovaries and hyperandrogenism in women taking valproate for epilepsy. N. Engl. J. Med. 329, 1383–1388.

Jefferys, J., 2002. Basic mechanisms of epilepsy. In: Duncan, J.S., Siodiya, S.M., Smalls, J.E. (Eds.), Epilepsy: from science to patient. International League Against Epilepsy, Bristol.

Kerr, M., Scheepers, M., Arvio, M., et al., 2009. Consensus guidelines into the management of epilepsy in adults with an intellectual disability. J. Intellect. Disabil. Res. 53, 687–694.

Krishnamoorthy, E.S., Trimble, M.R., 2002. Neuropsychiatric disorders in epilepsy – epidemiology and classification. In: Trimble, M.R., Schmitz, B. (Eds.), The neuropsychiatry of epilepsy. Cambridge University Press, Cambridge, pp. 5–17.

Kwan, P., Brodie, M.J., 2000. Early identification of refractory epilepsy. N. Engl. J. Med. 342, 314–319.

Landolt, H., 1958. Serial electroencephalographic investigations during psychotic episodes in epileptic patients and during schizophrenic attacks. In: Lorenz De Haas, A.M. (Ed.), Lectures on epilepsy. Elsevier, Amsterdam, pp. 91–133.

Lewine, J.D., Andrews, R., Chez, M., 1999. Magnetoencephalographic patterns of epileptiform activity in children with regressive autism spectrum disorders. Paediatrics 104, 405–418.

Michael, J., 2008. Healthcare for all: report of the independent inquiry into access to healthcare for people with learning disabilities. Available at:http://www.dh.gov.uk/en/Publicationsandstatistics/Publications/PublicationsPolicyAndGuidance/DH_099255 (accessed on 1 February 2010).

Möller, J.C., Hamer, H.M., Oertel, W. H., Rosenow, F., 2001. Late-onset myoclonic epilepsy in Down's syndrome (LOMEDS). Seizure 10, 303–306.

Morgan, C.L., Ahmed, Z., Kerr, M.P., 2000. Healthcare provision for people with learning disability. Record-linkage study of epidemiology and factors contributing to hospital care uptake. Br. J. Psychiatry 176, 37–41.

Morrow, J., 2007. The XX factor: treating women with anti-epileptic drugs. Nuffield Press, Essex.

Morrow, J., Russell, A., Guthrie, E., et al., 2006. Malformation risk of antiepileptic drugs in pregnancy: a retrospective study from the UK Epilepsy and Pregnancy Register. J. Neurol. Neurosurg. Psychiatry 77, 193–198.

Moshe, S., Shilo, M., Chodick, G., et al., 2008. Occurrence of seizures in association with work-related stress in young male army recruits. Epilepsia 49 (8), 1451–1456.

Nashef, L., Fish, D., Garner, S., Sander, J., Shorvon, D., 1995. Sudden death in epilepsy – a study of incidence in a young cohort with epilepsy and learning difficulty. Epilepsia 36, 1187–1194.

Panayiotopoulos, C.P., 2008. A clinical guide to epileptic syndromes and their treatment, second ed. Springer, Heidelberg, Germany.

Paul, A., 1996. Epilepsy and you. Pavillion, Brighton.

Ring, H., 2009. Epilepsy: an emotive issue. Seizures and emotions and the links between them. Epilepsy Professional 13, 18–21.

Ring, H., Zia, A., Lindeman, S., Himlock, K., 2007. Interactions between seizure frequency, psychopathology and severity of intellectual disability in a population with epilepsy and learning disability. Epilepsy and Behaviour 11 (1), 92–97.

Scott, R.C., Besag, F.M., Neville, B.G.R., 1999. Buccal midazolam and rectal diazepam for the treatment for prolonged seizures in childhood and adolescence: a randomised trial. Lancet 20 (353), 623–626.

Scottish Intercollegiate Guidelines Network (SIGN), 2003. Diagnosis and management of epilepsy in adults. SIGN, Edinburgh.

Shorvon, S., 2000. Handbook of epilepsy treatment. Blackwell, Oxford.

Sillanpaa, M., 2004. Learning disability: occurrence and long term consequences in childhood-onset epilepsy. Epilepsy and Behaviour 5, 937–944.

Stokes, T., Shaw, E.J., Juarez-Garcia, A., et al., 2004. Clinical guidelines and evidence review for the epilepsies: diagnosis and management in adults and children in primary and secondary care. Royal College of General Practitioners, London.

Taylor, M.P., 2000. Managing epilepsy: a clinical handbook. Blackwell Science, Oxford.

Tellez-Zenteno, J.F., 2008. Psychiatric comorbidity in epilepsy: a population-based analysis. Epilepsia 48 (12), 2336–2344.

Trimble, M.R., 2003. Learning disability and function: an integrative approach. Clarius Press, Guildford.

Working Group of IASSID, 2001. Clinical guidelines for the management of epilepsy in adults with an intellectual disability. Seizure 10, 401–409.

Further reading

Kerr, M., et al., on behalf of the Guidelines Working Group, 2009. Consensus guidelines into the management of epilepsy in adults with an intellectual disability. J. Intellect. Disabil. Res. 53 (8), 687–694.

Martin, J.P., Brown, S.W., 2009. Best clinical and research practice in adults with an intellectual disability. Epilepsy and Behaviour 15 (Suppl. 1), 64–68.

Trimble, M.R., 2003. Learning disability and function: an integrative approach. Clarius Press, Guildford.

Working Group of IASSID, 2001. Clinical guidelines for the management of epilepsy in adults with an intellectual disability. Seizure 10, 401–409.

Useful addresses

The National Society for Epilepsy: www.epilepsysociety.org.uk

Epilepsy Action: www.epilepsy.org.uk

National Institute for Clinical Excellence: http://guidance.nice.org.uk/CG/WaveR/52 and http://guidance.nice.org.uk/TA76

Mental health problems in people with learning disabilities

17

Laurence Taggart

CHAPTER CONTENTS

KEY ISSUES

- Readers will be introduced to a systematic and structured approach to the gathering of the typical and atypical signs and symptoms of mental health
- The inter-related risk factors of mental health will be explored using the bio-psycho-social model as identified by the International Association for the Scientific Study of Intellectual Disability (IASSID 2001)
- Greater credence will be given to a multi-professional approach in the mental health assessment process
- A range of evidence-based bio-psycho-social interventions will be shown to be effective with people with learning disabilities
- The importance of mental health promotion and prevention will be highlighted from an early age and throughout the lifespan of people with learning disabilities

Introduction

Mainstream mental health has dramatically shifted from the custodial hospitalised medical model of 100 years ago to a holistic model of care in the community with a greater focus on community-based policies of inclusion and recovery. There has also been a significant increase and recognition across the Western world that people with learning disabilities can develop mental health problems. This growing momentum has now led to a number of governments developing specific learning disability policies and documents that highlight and target the mental health needs of this population (Department of Health (DH) 2001, Department of Health, Social Services and Public Safety (DHPSS) 2005). These policies target the mental health needs of this population as well as promoting positive mental health or emotional wellbeing.

Mental health is a subjective state that can be observed to be based upon a fluctuating continuum where each person assesses their own internal strengths against the external events/stressors/demands placed upon them. However, for some people, their feelings or emotions, thoughts or perceptions, way of thinking or reasoning, memory and behaviours are affected for an extended period of time affecting their daily activities of living. Therefore, when the person reports these signs and symptoms to their health care professional, they may be diagnosed with a psychiatric disorder. The person therefore moves along to the opposite end of the mental health continuum.

This chapter provides the reader with a discussion of the advancements and achievements that have occurred in the care of people with learning disabilities who have mental health problems. Read Case illustration 17.1 of Joan and reflect upon this

Case illustration 17.1

Joan

Joan is a 24-year-old woman with mild learning disabilities. She lives with her mother and father and has three sisters; all are now married, have children and live locally. At the strong request of Joan's parents, she attended a mainstream primary school and was supported to attend a mainstream secondary school. Her parents found it difficult to accept Joan had a learning disability and was different from her three sisters although were contented with her progression through school. However, Joan recalls numerous accounts of being bullied and having no friends.

It was not until Joan's late teens that her behaviour changed. Joan became uncommunicative, isolating herself from her family, wanting to remain in her bedroom and not wanting to go out of the house. Joan's weight was increasing. Her parents would describe some of her behaviours as bizarre; washing her hands continuously, she made strange noises and paced up and down in her bedroom frequently.

As a result of these behaviours she was referred to mainstream psychiatry, where upon identification that she had a learning disability she was referred to the local learning disability inpatient psychiatry team. Upon admission to hospital, the multi-disciplinary team gathered information from a wide range of sources. Joan was assessed by a medical practitioner who discovered that there was an undersecretion of her thyroid gland. The nurses on the ward also discovered that around the time of Joan's menstrual cycle her behaviours intensified. Within the interview with both parents, it was identified that there was a history of mental illness in the mother's family. Both parents were not accepting that their daughter could have a mental health problem as well as a learning disability.

Joan was also approached and questioned about her mental health. The nurses on the ward undertook an unstructured interview with Joan using the Mini PAS-ADD Interview (this will be discussed later in this chapter). From careful interviewing with Joan, she reported to the psychiatrist that she heard a man and woman's voice talking to each other and telling her what to do: she did not know either person but they strongly influenced her behaviours.

From this information, she was diagnosed with paranoid schizophrenia with an associated contamination phobia. Working with Joan, her parents and members of the multi-disciplinary team a bio-psycho-social package of care was developed and agreed upon by all. Joan was prescribed Depo-Provera to regulate her menstrual cycle and chlorpromazine to manage her auditory hallucinations. By using flash cards, headphones, word searches and other diversional activities initiated by Joan, her community learning disability nurse was able to work with Joan to manage but also live with her auditory hallucinations. Socially, Joan's week was structured; she attended a local drop-in centre for people with learning disabilities 2 days a week and participated with a college of further education programme 1 day a week. Joan also now has a befriender; they go out every Saturday into her local town.

woman's story as you will be asked to answer a number of questions throughout this chapter regarding her mental health problem.

What do we mean by the term 'mental health problems'?

The Mental Health Foundation (2010) defined mental health as:

> A state of well-being in which the individual realises his or her own abilities, can cope with the normal stresses of life, can work productively and fruitfully, and is able to make a contribution to his or her community.

The terms 'mental health problems', 'mental illness' and 'psychiatric disorders' have been used within society interchangeably to cover a wide range of feelings and behaviours from those that can be described as normal (i.e. feeling low or sad) to chronic and enduring feelings (i.e. thought disturbance, ideas of self-harm, feelings hopeless). These feelings and behaviours can last for a few hours or days through to more negative feelings and behaviours that last over weeks and months and can lead to a diagnosis of a psychiatric condition such as an affective disorder or otherwise known as a group that includes depression. The person then moves along to the opposite end of the mental health continuum. Nevertheless, for many people diagnosed with a psychiatric disorder, they can also report feeling well and healthy.

As many people with learning disabilities have limited communication skills as well as cognitive deficits, making verbal reports of internal states (i.e. emotions, perceptions, reasoning and memory) and how these affect their behaviours may be difficult. As a consequence, many people with learning disabilities may not receive a clinical diagnosis or label. Although some people with learning disabilities may not receive a psychiatric diagnosis they may still have 'mental health problems'

Reader activity 17.1

Identify a person with learning disabilities with whom you have contact who has a diagnosis of a mental health problem. Identify the type of disorder they have, list the medication(s) they are taking and what the medication is for, and the other interventions the person is receiving. Also, list the signs and symptoms they display. You may need to speak with other people to gather this information. You will need this information to undertake further Reader activities later within this chapter. Keep your answer safe.

Types of mental health problems

Like non-disabled people, people with learning disabilities can also develop an array of mental health problems. Each of these groups of disorders are made up of a number of core signs/symptoms contained within the *International Classification of Diseases-10* (*ICD-10*) (World Health Organization (WHO) 1992).

Affective disorders

This group contains disorders in which the main sign is a change in mood. The mood change is usually associated with a change in the overall level of emotion, perception and activity. Most affective disorders tend to be recurrent and the onset of individual episodes can often be related to stressful events or situations. Disorders within this group include bipolar affective disorder, depressive disorder, recurrent depressive disorder, persistent mood disorder and dysthymia disorder.

Neurotic or stress-related disorders

A group of disorders in which anxiety-related symptoms are the core sign, for some people this can occur in certain well-defined situations. As a result, these situations are avoided or endured with dread. Physical or somatic symptoms like palpitations, feeling faint, trembling and muscular tension are often associated with secondary fears of dying, losing control or going mad. Other disorders in this group include agoraphobia, social phobias, specific phobias, panic disorder, generalised anxiety disorder, mixed anxiety and depressive disorder, obsessive-compulsive disorder, adjustment disorders and post-traumatic stress disorder.

Schizophrenia disorders

This group brings together a range of psychotic disorders with schizophrenia being the most common condition. Schizophrenia is characterised by distortions of thinking and perception, and emotions that are inappropriate or blunted. Other disorders include paranoid schizophrenia, hebephrenic schizophrenia, catatonic schizophrenia, schizotypal disorder, persistent delusional disorders, acute and transient psychotic disorders and schizoaffective disorders. An example of this condition is illustrated in Case illustration 17.1.

Organic disorders

This group of disorders comprises a range of conditions that are grouped together on the basis of their having in common a demonstrable aetiology in brain injury/disease. Dementia is a syndrome due to disease of the brain in which there is disturbance of memory, thinking, orientation, comprehension, language and judgement. Other disorders in this group include dementia in Alzheimer's disease with early and also late onset, vascular dementia and multi-infarct dementia.

Other groups of mental health conditions included within the *ICD-10* (WHO 1992) include:

- mental and behavioural disorders due to psychoactive substance use
- behavioural syndromes associated with physiological disturbances and physical factors
- disorders of adult personality and behaviour
- disorders of psychological development
- unspecified mental disorder.

See Reader activity 17.2 on the Evolve website.

Prevalence of mental health problems

Mental health problems can occur across the lifespan of the person, whether they have a disability or not. Young people, adults and older people can and do experience the same range of mental health problems as people with learning disabilities. However, not only does this population experience the same types of clinical conditions but there is an increasing body of evidence to illustrate that specific groups within it have higher rates of these disorders. Readers should note that there is considerable variance in the prevalence rates reported (Devine et al in press). There are a number of inter-related reasons why prevalence rates vary and these include the following:

- According to Allen (2009), diagnostic overshadowing, behavioural overshadowing (i.e. presence of challenging behaviour) and psychiatric overshadowing (i.e. the person using psychotropic medication) may make obtaining an accurate diagnosis more difficult. For example, behaviours that are part of the person's learning disability may be mistaken as symptoms of a mental health problem such as talking to oneself, solitary fantasy play, stereotypical movements, bizarre language, poor social skills and withdrawal; all symptoms that can be associated with schizophrenia (Taggart & Slevin 2006). These 'atypical' behaviours could lead to 'diagnostic confusion' and the rejection of a mental health problem existing at all.
- Many people with mild learning disability may be able to verbally report how they feel regarding their subjective internal mental health (i.e. emotions, perceptions, reasoning and memory) and their behaviours with minimal assistance. However, many other people with limited communication and moderate to severe/profound learning disability will have difficulty expressing how they feel. Consequently, how this group of people express themselves may be through behaviours that are not identified as typical signs/symptoms of a specific condition such as an affective disorder like depression. This manifestation or expression can be described as 'atypical symptomology' or also 'challenging behaviours'.
- There are difficulties in defining what is and what is not a psychiatric disorder, as some prevalence studies have excluded those with a personality disorder, autistic spectrum conditions (ASCs) or a behavioural disorder.
- Higher prevalence rates are reported in hospital settings and community-referred psychiatry clinics compared to lower prevalence rates found in community samples of people with learning disabilities (Bouras & Holt 2007).
- Different screening instruments also reflect variation in prevalence rates. For example, information can be collected based upon questionnaires developed for adults without learning disabilities who can self-report (i.e. Beck's Depression Inventory (Beck et al 1961), Hamilton Anxiety Scale (Hamilton 1959)). Such instruments can be used with adults with mild learning disabilities but are less reliable for

adults with moderate to profound learning disabilities. Other screening instruments have been developed for front-line staff to complete on behalf of people with learning disabilities (i.e. PAS-ADD Schedules (Moss 2002), Reiss Scale (Reiss 1988) and the Psychopathology Instrument for Mentally Retarded Adults (PIMRA) (Matson 1988)). In addition, differences also occur as a result of self-report from the person with learning disabilities compared with family/front-line staff report.

Prevalence rates of mental health problems in young people

Meltzer et al (2000), in a large national survey in England, Scotland and Wales, found that 13% of boys and 10% of girls aged between 11 and 15 years without learning disabilities had mental health problems. Emerson (2003), using secondary analysis of the Meltzer et al (2000) sample, found that children and adolescents with learning disabilities were four times more likely to have a mental health problem compared with their non-disabled peers. Similar international studies have reported that children and adolescents with learning disabilities are also more likely to have mental health problems ranging between 30% and 50% (Einfeld & Tonge 1996a, 1996b, Hoare et al 1998, Molteno et al 2001). Furthermore, Taggart et al (2007a), in a study that examined the mental health status of young people with learning disabilities living in state care (i.e. children's home, foster care) in Northern Ireland, found over three-quarters of these young people had a mental health problem.

Prevalence rates of mental health problems in adults

Affective disorders have been reported to be more common in people with learning disabilities than the general population; rates of bipolar disorders have also been reported to be higher compared to adults without disabilities (Cooper et al 2007, Hurley 2006). Likewise, people with learning disabilities are more likely to develop anxiety disorders, including an adjustment disorder and post-traumatic stress disorder, as a result of major life event(s) or trauma compared to their non-disabled peers (Masi et al 2000, Turk et al 2005).

Studies also report higher prevalence rates of psychosis. A small number of studies have examined schizophrenia in people with mild/moderate learning disabilities and have reported that prevalence rates are four to six times higher than reported in the non-disabled population (Hemmings 2006), ranging from 1.3% to 5.2%. Difficulties occur in receiving a diagnosis of schizophrenia for people with severe/profound learning disabilities.

Higher rates of eating disorders such as binge eating, pica, anorexia nervosa, bulimia nervosa, food refusal and psychogenic vomiting (i.e. patients vomit in the absence of any physical cause) have been found to exist in adults with learning disabilities. However, unlike the non-disabled population, no gender differences were found in these eating disorders (Gravestock 2003, Hove 2004). In relation to substance misuse in people with learning disabilities, this has been reported to be lower compared to the non-disabled population, although it is purported that this population is at a higher risk of abusing such substances in order to 'fit in' within society (Taggart et al 2006, 2007b). But as more people with learning disabilities are supported to live in the community, the prevalence rate of substance misuse is expected to continue to increase (Hassiotis et al 2008).

Prevalence rates of mental health in older people

Older people with learning disabilities also develop mental health problems in addition to the recognised dementias. A number of studies have reported higher rates of affective disorders, anxiety disorders, bipolar disorder and schizophrenia (Cooper & Holland 2007). Prevalence rates of these clinical conditions again have been reported to be higher compared with older people without learning disabilities. Nevertheless, it is the dementias that have been reported to be significantly higher compared to this population's non-disabled peers (Kannabiran & Deb 2010). A more detailed exploration of this issue can be found in Chapter 29.

Recognising the signs/symptoms of mental health

In order for health care professionals to recognise the signs/symptoms of mental ill health in the general population, classification systems are used. There are two classification systems: the first is called the *ICD-10* (WHO 1992); this is developed for practitioners in the UK and Europe. The second is called the *Diagnostic Statistical Manual* (*Version 4*) (*DSM-4*) (American Association of Psychiatry (APA) 1994) developed for practitioners in the USA.

Both classification systems undertake a similar task, that is to define the clinical picture of the person in order to provide an accurate diagnosis. These two systems provide a clinical psychiatric diagnosis based upon a range of signs/symptoms, or a cluster of these, as verbally reported by the person via a clinical interview. Furthermore, verbally reporting these signs/symptoms will aid the health care professional in attempting to understand the nature of the mental illness, the potential causes of the illness and also to develop an effective treatment package. Case illustration 17.1 highlights the importance of the patient's verbal reports, as Joan's behaviours may have been associated with being bullied at school and/or watching her sisters moving on with their lives such as getting a boyfriend, getting married, moving out of the family home and having children.

A more recent development has been the publication of the *DC-LD: Diagnostic Criteria for Psychiatric Disorders for Use with Adults with Intellectual Disabilities/Mental Retardation*, by The Royal College of Psychiatrists (RCP 2001). The aim of this classification system is "to improve upon existing general population psychiatric diagnostic classificatory systems" for the learning disability population (RCP 2001).

Typical clusters of signs/symptoms of mental ill health

Current classification systems attempt to list the typical signs/symptoms described by the person using six main categories or clusters, although some of these may fall into more than one of these categories. Typical signs/symptoms within these clusters include:

1. somatic (or physical symptoms)
2. emotional
3. behavioural
4. thought/cognition/perception
5. attention or motivation
6. activities of daily living (ADL).

On the basis of the signs/symptoms listed above, the health care professional also needs to know the length of time the person has been experiencing them (i.e. 2 weeks, 1 month, 6 months). In order to identify a correct diagnosis, the person with learning disabilities has to display a number of identified signs/symptoms for these clusters for a specified period of time.

Atypical clusters

Many people with mild learning disabilities will probably display many of the typical signs/symptoms of mental ill health as above. Some of these signs/symptoms may be more marked, such as agitation, crying, short-temperedness or being withdrawn. Other signs/symptoms may not be directly observable to family carers or front-line staff (i.e. loss of confidence or low self-esteem) and are more difficult to identify. Such signs/symptoms will, however, be displayed via behaviours.

For those people with a moderate to severe/profound learning disability and additional problems (i.e. limited communication skills, sensory disabilities and ASCs), they may display signs/symptoms that can be described as 'atypical', that is they are not normally recognised as characteristic for that specific condition.

From the information you gathered in Reader activity 17.1 earlier, compare and contrast the signs/symptoms you collated with Reader activity 17.3. In Reader activity 17.1, you may have randomly listed the signs/symptoms, whereas using the seven clusters as identified above provides a systematic and structured approach to gathering evidence. This evidence is based upon a very similar structured approach a psychiatrist or psychologist would employ within the *DSM-4* (APA 1994), *ICD-10* (WHO 1992) or *DC-LD* (RCP 2001) as described above.

Using a bio-psycho-social model to understand mental health

In attempting to understand why people with learning disabilities are more likely to develop mental health problems as compared to the non-disabled population, the International Association for the Scientific Study of Intellectual Disabilities (IASSID 2001), in a report to the WHO, proposed adopting a framework that examined the whole person. This was in comparison to the medical/biological model

Reader activity 17.3

Identify two people with learning disabilities with whom you have contact who are considered to have a possible mental health problem: one should have a mild learning disability and the other should have a severe learning disability. Think about their signs and symptoms that they are displaying. Use the following structure to identity each person's signs/symptoms and try to identify if the person is displaying any or all of these signs/symptoms:

- **Somatic (or physical symptoms)**: palpitations, feeling faint, trembling, muscular tension, dizziness, dry mouth, gastric problems, sickness and vomiting.
- **Emotional**: feeling down, sad, weepy, short-tempered, frustrated, low self-esteem, lack of confidence.
- **Behavioural**: idleness, increases or decreases in appetite and subsequent weight change, increases or decreases in sleeping, self-harm, suicidal ideation (i.e. thoughts about planning the suicide act but not actually carrying it out), lethargy, listlessness, disinterest.
- **Thought/cognition/perception**: feeling worried, anxious, apprehensive and nervous, thought disturbance, ideas of self-harm, concentration, orientation, feelings of guilt, remorse, worthlessness, hopeless.
- **Attention or motivation**: lethargy, withdrawal, loss of interest in life, negativity, lack of interest in normal routines, inattention.
- **Activities of daily living (ADL)**: changes in routine, loss of self-care skills and appearance, loss of social skills, disinterested in work, family, life or hobbies.
- **Atypical**: changes in facial expression, biting (self and others), grinding teeth, increase in repetitive hand movements, increase in sexual behaviour, changes in posture, lack of responsiveness, increase or decrease in vocalisation, disruptive behaviour, thumb-biting, self-injurious behaviour, increased agitation, screaming, spontaneous crying, stereotypical behaviours, non-compliance, seeking greater reassurances and increase in seizure activity.

that had been traditionally employed across medicine, psychiatry and nursing where the mental health problem was viewed as organic and based within the person. This model, taken from a health psychology perspective, provided a holistic proactive approach to understanding how mental health problems develop, but also how such problems can be prevented, if possible (see Fig. 17.1). The model identifies the key risk factors for developing mental health problems in four inter-related segments: biological, developmental, psychological and social. For the purposes of application to practice, this model will be applied to understanding the specific risk factors for the development of mental health problems in three client groups: young people, women and people from ethnic backgrounds.

Young people with learning disabilities

Researchers have identified a number of risk factors for why young people with learning disabilities are more likely to develop mental health problems compared to their non-disabled peers:

Biological

Having a specific genetic condition (e.g. Fragile X, fetal alcohol syndrome, Prader–Willi syndrome) or ASCs, having a severe/profound learning disability, having sensory and communication problems, gender (i.e. males are more likely to develop attention deficit hyperactivity disorder (ADHD) and conduct disorders whereas females are more likely to develop affective and anxiety disorders).

Developmental and psychological

The primary care giver(s) having a mental health problems(s), history of family mental health problems and/or substance abuse, presence of negative role model(s) and the employment of punitive child management practices within the family home.

Social

High levels of social deprivation, poverty, family composition (i.e. single parent), little opportunities for education and recreation, excessive amounts of free time, limited friends, lack of meaning in life, social exclusion (Emerson 2003, Emerson et al 2005, Hassiotis & Barron 2007, Stromme & Diseth 2000).

Women with learning disabilities

Women without learning disabilities are more likely to develop specific mental health problems compared to men (i.e. affective disorders, bipolar disorder, anxiety disorders, eating disorders, borderline personality disorder and pre-/peri-menstrual disorders). Likewise it could be argued that women with learning disabilities are also more likely to develop mental health problems (Taggart et al 2008, 2009a, 2010). Common identified risk factors include the following:

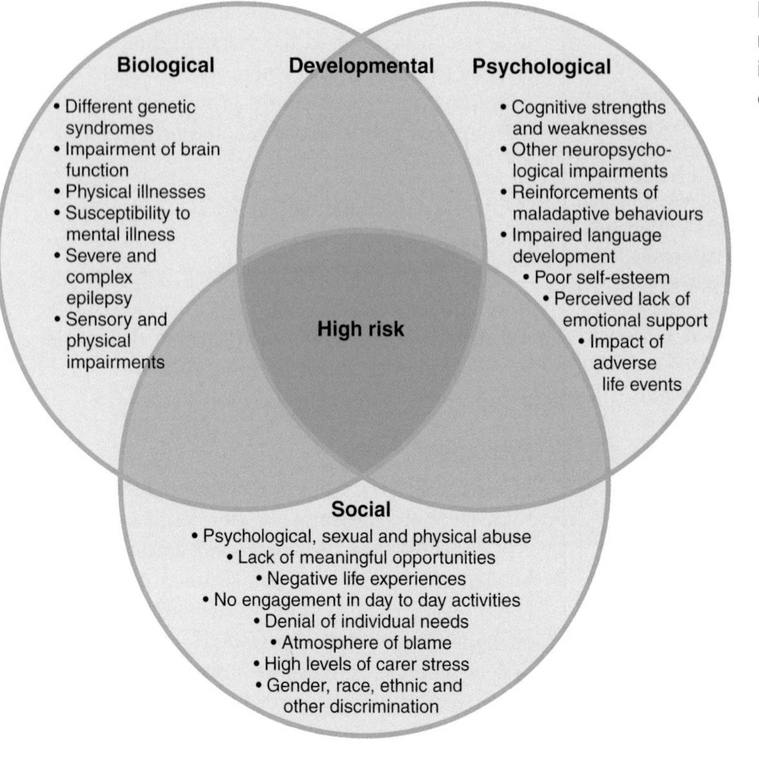

Figure 17.1 • Bio-psycho-social model of mental health problems in people with learning disabilities (IASSID 2001)

Case illustration 17.2

Vidusha is a 28-year-old Asian woman who has mild learning disabilities; she has good communication skills and lives in a flat by herself supported by her 71-year-old mother and older sister who is about to get married and leave the local area. She works at her local supermarket 3 days a week and attends the local college of further education 1 day a week. There is no history of mental health problems within her family. Recently, her attendance at work and college has been sporadic, and when she has attended she has often argued with staff, customers and students. Using the model presented in Figure 17.1, identify the potential risk factors for Vidusha.

(Compare your answers to those at the end of this chapter.)

Biological

Pl... issues related to hormonal changes, ...n, sexual health including contraception, ...psychotropic medication associated with

Psychological

Juggling multiple roles (i.e. caring for children, caring for family members, looking after the household), negative life events, sexual abuse, domestic violence, having a learning disability and how this affects the woman and her identity, relationships, loss of children and loneliness.

Social

Poverty, inequality, social isolation, restricted social support networks, lack of employment, education and recreation (O'Hara 2008, Taggart et al 2008, 2009a, 2009b, 2010).

Ethnicity and learning disability

Research shows that people from ethnic backgrounds are also more likely to have a severe learning disability. A number of other studies have reported that people from different ethnic groups were more likely to be admitted to hospital and community psychiatric clinics compared to their white counterparts: the majority of admissions were found to be for underlying mental health issues (Healthcare Commission 2007). However, evidence is less clear regarding the prevalence rates of mental health problems among people with learning disabilities from ethnic backgrounds although it can be purported they may be higher as a result of a range of psycho-social risk factors. There is growing evidence that people from ethnic communities are more likely to live in poverty, be unemployed, live in poor social housing, be socially isolated and are more likely to be exposed to more negative life events. In addition, people from ethnic communities may not have health information in a format that they can access/understand and also may not utilise health services (Raghavan & Waseem 2007).

Assessing mental health problems

When undertaking a comprehensive mental health assessment of a person with learning disabilities, care must be undertaken to collate various information from multiple informants in order to ensure the accuracy of the data collected as identified within Case illustration 17.1. The sharing and testing of this information will help the health care professional to formulate a working hypothesis of the possible underlying mental health condition. On the basis of this information, a clinical diagnosis can be made, and a multi-element intervention package then developed. The European Association for Mental Health for People with Intellectual Disabilities (EAMHID) (Deb et al 2001) has developed a structured approach to the assessment of mental health problems in people with learning disabilities. Box 17.1 identifies the key sources of information that can be gathered about the factors that predispose, precipitate and/or maintain the person's behaviours.

Use of rating scales

The Department of Health, in *Signposts for Success* (1998), identified the early use of rating scales for the detection of both challenging behaviour and mental health problems as 'good practice'.

Using screening tools will provide further objective evidence and also support the family carer, front-line staff and clinician in identifying that there is a problem(s) by collecting evidence via a structured framework (see Box 17.1). Screening tools are part of the comprehensive assessment process involving information from other sources, as identified within Box 17.2. Screening tools should be used to collect data on the person's baseline behaviours in four core areas and can identify the interplay between the risk factors as demonstrated within the bio-psycho-social model above:

1. Physical health (i.e. OK Health Checklist) (Matthews & Hegarty 1997).
2. Functioning ability (i.e. Adaptive Behaviour Scale) (Nihra et al 1993).

Box 17.1

Framework for assessment of mental health problems in people with learning disabilities

- Developmental, family and social history.
- Medical and psychiatric history, including a full blood count (i.e. red blood cells, white blood cells, platelets, haemoglobin, etc), to examine for infection and also blood toxicology.
- Medication and side effects investigation.
- Forensic history (if required).
- History of presenting complaint.
- Interview with carers.
- Direct observation/functional behavioural analysis.
- Unstructured psychiatric interview.
- Use of standardised rating scales.

Box 17.2

Examples of mental health specific screening tools

- Dementia Scale for people with Down syndrome (Deb & Braganza 1999).
- Mental Retardation Depression Scale (Meins 1996).
- PAS-ADD Checklist (Moss 2002).
- PAS-ADD Interview (Moss 2002).
- Reiss Scale for Children's Dual Diagnosis (Reiss 1988).
- Self-report depression questionnaire (Reynolds & Baker 1988).
- The Diagnostic Assessment for the Severely Handicapped (Part 11) (Matson et al 1999).
- The Psychopathology Instrument for Mentally Retarded Adults (Matson 1988).
- The Reiss Screen (Reiss 1988).
- Yale-Brown OCD Scale (Goodman et al 1989).

3. Challenging behaviours (i.e. Aberrant Behaviour Checklist) (Aman et al 1986).
4. Mental health (i.e. PAS-ADD Checklist or Interview) (Moss 2002).

These screening tools will help to build an established record of the person's physical health, inventory of functioning skills, levels of challenging behaviour and mental health status. In addition, the tools can be used to monitor changes in the person's treatment and also evaluate the impact of the intervention package, thereby ensuring the person returns to their optimal level of physical health and functional ability. Given the bio-psycho-social model in the possible aetiology of the person's mental health problem, utilising such screening tools can help unscramble the various other potential causes for the person to display such signs/symptoms and behaviours.

The application of the structured framework as identified by the EAMHID (Deb et al 2001) in Box 17.1 will be applied to assessing the mental health of young people with learning disabilities and women with learning disabilitie,s although it can be used for a range of other groups.

Assessing young people with learning disabilities

Assessing children and young people with learning disabilities should be based upon the risk factors identified for young people with learning disabilities earlier in this chapter. Read Case illustration 17.3 and undertake the activities.

A number of mental health screening tools have been developed for recognising potential problems in young people; conversely some of these tools have been used with young people with learning disabilities and have been found to be reliable. One example is the Strengths and Difficulties Questionnaire (SDQ) (Goodman 1999). The SDQ has been successfully employed with young people with mild learning disabilities to assess their emotions, behaviours and functional impairment. The SDQ consists of five subscales (emotions, conduct, inattention–hyperactivity, peer problems and pro-social (positive) behaviour). The SDQ has been reported to have moderate to strong reliability and validity properties when used with parent, teacher and as a self-rating. Emerson (2005) reported that the extended SDQ was a simple and robust tool to also measure the mental health of young people with learning disabilities. This scale is freely available to download and use (see Useful addresses).

More recently, a specific screening tool has been developed for young people with learning disabilities. The Cha-PAS (Moss et al 2007) is part of the PAS-ADD Schedules identified above. The Cha-PAS is a 97-item screening instrument that assesses mental health. This tool examines depression, anxiety, ADHD, compulsions, conduct issues, psychotic disorders and the autistic spectrum. Specific training is required to use this tool.

Assessing women with learning disabilities

In assessing the mental health of women with learning disabilities, again the bio-psycho-social model (see Fig. 17.1) should be an underpinning guide.

Case illustration 17.3

John is a 13-year-old boy with moderate to severe learning disabilities. He has Prader–Willi syndrome and is extremely hyperactive. John lives with his single mother and three younger siblings, one of whom has ADHD, in a council estate in an inner city area. John's mother has a history of depression dating back 3 years after his father left the family home. She receives all benefits and the children get free school meals. Since his father left home, John's mother heavily uses alcohol: although there is also a history of substance abuse and domestic violence when his father was at home. John's family is well known to social services and all the children are judged to be at continuing risk of significant harm (on the 'at-risk register'). John's mother has attended several courses ran by the school and Sure Start on positive parenting and behaviour management: it was reported that she did not complete any of these courses. Frequent complaints are made by the school that John displays a range of disruptive and challenging behaviours, he isolates himself and his verbal requests/demands are not typical of young people his age.

From this case study, identify how you would undertake an assessment of John using the model in Figure 17.1:

- Biological.
- Psychological.
- Social.

(Compare your answers to those at the end of this chapter.)

> **Reader activity 17.4**
>
> Based upon the Case illustration 17.2 of Vidusha, can you list how you would undertake a structured assessment of Vidusha again using the model identified within Figure 17.1?
>
> - Biological.
> - Psychological.
> - Social.
>
> (Compare your answers to those at the end of this chapter.)

In addition, a gender-sensitive approach to assessment and intervention should also be undertaken recognising the specific risk factors that women face regarding the development of mental health problems as undertaken within Case illustration 17.1. This assessment should include a greater recognition of the obstetric (i.e. pregnancy) and gynaecological issues (i.e. hormonal, peri-and post-menstrual health, contraception, sexual health care issues) that many women experience and its link with behavioural and mental health problems (Eogan & Wingfield 2010).

Interventions for mental health problems

In keeping with a focus on the bio-psycho-social model, this chapter has shown the reader that there is no one singular cause for the development of mental ill health in people with or without learning disabilities, but a cumulative number of risk factors must be examined in greater detail. In an attempt to fully understand the predisposing, precipitating and/or maintaining factors, a bio-psycho-social assessment must therefore be undertaken. Likewise, in treating the person's underlying mental health problem, then a bio-psycho-social approach should also be employed in order to develop an effective range of interventions. The need for individualised assessments and person-centred planning of interventions also needs to be core to any multi-element intervention package.

Psycho-pharmacology

Aman et al (2000) highlighted that medication remains the first line of defence in managing both mental ill health and challenging behaviours in this population. However, psychotropic or anti-psychotic medications for people with learning disabilities have been purported to be morally and also ethically questionable, as such medications have been too frequently prescribed without the appropriate evidence base and clearly identified psychiatric condition and/or specified targeted challenging behaviour (Devine & Taggart 2008).

Chyka (2000) claims that many of the drugs used to manage mental ill health in people with learning disabilities score highly in the league tables of deaths caused by their side effects, including:

- a range of somatic or physical symptoms
- cholinergic effects (i.e. dry mouth, increase in heart rate, increase in blood pressure, blurred vision, memory problems, loss of coordination, sensitivity to heat), dyskinetic movement disorders (i.e. involuntary repetitive writhing or jerking movements)
- neuroleptic malignant syndrome (i.e. fever, severe muscle rigidity, altered consciousness, automatic arousal and can lead to death)
- memory impairment
- pseudo-parkinsonian symptoms (i.e. unsteady gait, bent posture, expressionless face and tremors).

Despite these serious side effects, medication prescribed within strict guidelines can serve a clinical purpose. Deb et al (2006) provide detailed guidelines on the use and management of psychotropic medication for this population. The use of medication must be a therapeutic treatment component that is part of a larger package and not a tool to create a convenient short-term respite for medical personnel or for care givers. Case illustration 17.1 shows that although Joan was diagnosed with paranoid schizophrenia, part of her treatment package was medication but there was a strong psycho-social intervention package as well. Medication was not the only treatment employed to manage her auditory hallucinations; in addition, medication was also used to regulate her menstrual cycle.

Cognitive behavioural therapy

Cognitive behavioural therapy (CBT) challenges the way an individual thinks about certain situations and helps the individual cope better when negative thoughts arise. CBT has been found to successfully treat the following conditions in people with learning disabilities:

- Anxiety management (Dagnan & Jahoda 2006, Douglass et al 2007).
- Anger management (Rose et al 2008).
- Bereavement (Summers 2003).
- Depression (Jahoda et al 2006).
- Low self-esteem (Whelan et al 2007).
- Management of auditory hallucinations in psychosis (Kirkland 2005).
- Obsessive compulsive disorder (Willner & Goodey 2006).
- Sex offenders (Keeling & Rose 2006).

CBT is not suitable for all people with learning disabilities, and each individual should be assessed to determine their suitability. Dagnan et al (2000) outline several components that will determine suitability, which include assessment of general language, level of learning ability, ability to recognise and understand emotions, and ability to link events to emotion. Case illustration 17.1 clearly illustrates the success of a number of cognitive and behavioural strategies to manage Joan's auditory hallucinations: flash cards, headphones, word searches and other diversional activities such as brisk walks, activities that both Joan and her parents were trained in, thereby supporting Joan to live within her family and remain in her local community.

Psycho-dynamic psychotherapy

Trained psychotherapists help an individual to understand and/or modify feelings, thoughts, attitudes and behaviour that cause distress to themselves. The emphasis is on changing the individual's unconscious conflicts by developing a therapeutic relationship, or working alliance, with the therapist (Beail et al 2005). There is growing evidence in the literature of psychotherapeutic approaches being used successfully to address emotional difficulties, such as poor self-esteem, psychotic behaviour, anxiety and sexually inappropriate behaviour among people with learning disabilities (RCP 2004).

Family therapy

Considering the central and key role that good family life plays in maintaining positive mental health (see Health promotion, below), it is surprising how little family therapy appears to be used in the field of learning disabilities. The most likely constant in the individual's life is the family, while professional personnel and systems of care delivery are likely to frequently change. Therefore, alongside individual therapeutic work, it makes sense that more targeted intervention is directed at working with families. It is also important to recognise that many people with learning disabilities live in 'family' groups and can be supported by staff teams. Family therapy can be successfully applied to help address emotional issues, such as loss, isolation, anxieties about sexuality and concerns about failure, whereby the issues can be fully explored with all members of the family participating and helping each other (Baum 2007).

Solution-focused brief therapy

While solution-focused brief therapy (SFBT) has become a widely used form of psychotherapy in the UK, there is little published on its use in services for people with learning disabilities. Smith (2005) discusses SFBT's potential uses with people with learning disabilities and provides a case illustration of its application with a man with mild learning disabilities referred to clinical psychology services for 'anger management'. The author reports the effectiveness of SFBT in diminishing this man's anger issues.

Psycho-educational interventions

One of the first key elements considered necessary for early intervention in mental health has been engagement and psycho-education, either in groups or individually with people with learning disabilities. Group programmes usually include education about the mental illness, medication and the role of biological, psychological and social risk factors linked to a stress vulnerability model. Again, Case illustration 17.1 illustrates the success of these ranges of psycho-educational interventions. The aims and objectives of these groups have varied from trying to improve members' self-esteem, empowerment, medication compliance to increasing understanding about their illness, improving levels of managing their positive and negative symptoms, and empowering the client to develop and maintain self-management and access to services (Crowley et al 2008).

Social interventions

It is important to remember that for many individuals with learning disabilities:

> . . . it is the specific handicaps they experience in housing, employment, income, social networks, leisure opportunities, and so on, which gives them their greatest frustrations, and their greatest sense of alienation.
>
> (Fryers 1997)

In addition to those shown in Figure 17.1, other factors that enhance susceptibility in the learning disabled population include their experiences of stigma. Consequently, following assessment, it may be determined that one or any number of social factors might have contributed significantly to the development of mental ill health. In such circumstances, it is important to intervene through manipulating or changing the environment and/or situation (Dagnan 2007).

Social interventions can address issues such as mental ill health as well as poverty, communication skills, access to leisure, employment, family relationships and education (Hatton 2002). They are focused on providing for the individual or groups, the opportunity to have a meaningful life, to make choices, to have adequate leisure opportunities and to be free from the constraints of social exclusion. Social interventions require adopting a more proactive, public health-based approach which focuses on prevention.

Health promotion

Promoting mental health involves any action that enhances the wellbeing of individuals, families and also communities. Taggart (2009) identifies three barriers to health promotion for people with learning disabilities:

1. **Individual barriers**: people with learning disabilities may lack the knowledge required of what to do when feeling unwell, where to go to get help.
2. **Carer barriers**: many people with learning disabilities are dependent upon family carers and front-line staff to identify symptoms when they are unwell and make a prompt referral to a GP. However, many of these carers may not recognise the early indications/triggers of mental ill health.
3. **Professional barriers**: primary health care professionals (e.g. the GP) may have limited experience in working with people with learning disabilities and have less knowledge about the needs of this population who have mental health problems.

The Department of Health (2001) highlighted a two-stage model of promoting mental health:

1. **Reducing risk factors**: poverty, deprived communities, high unemployment, financial difficulties, poor educational opportunities, high crime rates, emotional/physical/sexual abuse, high stress levels, social exclusion, bereavement, family break up, long-term caring, gender.
2. **Increasing protective factors**: quality environments, increasing self-esteem and empowerment, self-management skills, social participation.

Reader activity 17.5

In what activities do you engage that keep you emotionally well? Keep a record of your answers.

Health promotion for young people with learning disabilities

Black & Devine (2008) developed a mental health promotion booklet for parents, teachers and front-line staff, entitled *Head Start* (see Useful addresses) who care for children and young people with learning disabilities. The booklet targets those factors that make these young people resilient or protect against them developing mental ill health, as well as highlighting potential risk factors. Below is a list of a number of key factors to help build resilience; although each factor is important in itself, they all overlap, interact and reinforce each other:

- Good physical health.
- Exercise and activity.
- Success and achievement.

Reader activity 17.6

With regards to people with learning disabilities with whom you have contact, what activities do they engage in that keep them emotionally well? Compare with your previous answer on what keeps you healthy. What barriers might exist for people with learning disabilities accessing the same opportunities?

- Self-awareness.
- Positive family connections.
- Friendships and relationships.
- Meaningful social activity.
- Support during changes and transitions.
- Involvement in making choices and decisions.
- Care and support.

In *Head Start* (Black & Devine 2008), each one of these 10 factors is discussed individually and practical tips are offered for the carer to achieve this optimal goal. For example, young people with a learning disability who have some understanding and awareness of themselves and the challenges they face are more likely to have stronger emotional resilience. It is important that, from an early age, children and young people are helped to see and regard their learning disability as being only one aspect of themselves. This is about helping to build confidence and enabling them to recognise their strengths as much as their limitations. Examples include the following:

- Children and young people should be given opportunities to talk about the limitations imposed by their disability.
- It is important to be open and honest about the disability and to help them understand more about their particular condition. Many organisations provide useful leaflets, videos and DVDs to explain particular conditions and the likely effects on living and lifestyle.
- Group work with peers is one way of helping children and young people with learning disabilities understand that everyone is unique and that everyone has their own limitations.
- Involve the young person in activities and pursuits that provide the best match with their abilities. Focus on activities where participation is not going to draw attention to their disability.
- Emphasise and focus your energy on their talents and abilities.

Taggart & McKendry (2009) indicated that little has been published about mental health promotion literature for young people with learning disabilities. The authors developed a mental health promotion booklet with young people with learning disabilities. Focus groups with young people with learning disabilities were employed and the participants identified the six key themes to be addressed in the booklet with accompanying colourful and energetic pictures. This lively booklet is a valued resource for practitioners in the field of learning disabilities (see Health promotion literature in Useful addresses).

Interprofessional working

Throughout this chapter, clear evidence has been shown that to obtain an accurate clinical picture of the person with learning disabilities, information has to be gathered from a range of sources. Such sources of information include family carers, teachers, day-care staff, residential staff, nurses, social workers, psychiatrists and speech and language therapists.

Costello et al (2007) reported that front-line care staff play a key role in identifying people with learning disabilities and mental ill health. Yet few staff have received training in mental health, and evidence about the effectiveness of training is scant. Using a pre–post study design, significant improvements in staff knowledge, attitudes and referral decisions were observed. Costello and colleagues (2007) concluded that brief training interventions may improve awareness of mental health problems. Recently, a number of credited and non-credited training packs, modules, short courses and Master programmes have been developed across the UK for staff supporting people with learning disabilities who have mental health problems, for example:

- a distance learning course on significant and complex health needs in people with learning disabilities at Post-graduate Certificate, Diploma and MSc level (University of St Andrews, Scotland)
- a specialist module on assessment in mental health in people with learning disabilities (University of Ulster, Northern Ireland)
- an MSc in Mental Health Studies (Estia Centre, London).

Conclusion

This chapter has shown that in order to address the person's mental health problem, readers need to have a clear understanding of the typical and atypical signs/symptoms of the presenting problem as well as the risk factors. Collating this information together is fraught with difficulty in people with learning disabilities and even more complicated with people with limited or no communication. Multiple informants are required to gather this information so an accurate diagnosis can be made and a multimodal intervention package of care can be developed. Utilising the bio-psycho-social framework as proposed within this chapter will offer readers a more holistic approach to addressing the person's mental health problem and will provide a more effective and efficient intervention. Although the chapter has emphasised the importance of recognising the signs/symptoms of mental ill health and developing an intervention package, this chapter has also highlighted the importance of mental health promotion and prevention in attempting, where possible, to avoid such problems from developing, starting with people with learning disabilities themselves.

References

Allen, D., 2009. The relationship between challenging behaviour and mental ill-health in people with intellectual disabilities: a review of current theories and evidence. J. Intellect. Disabil. 12, 267–294.

Aman, M.G., Singh, N.N., 1986. Aberrant behaviour checklist manual. Slossom, New York.

Aman, M.G., Alvarez, N., Benefield, W., et al., 2000. Special issue. Expert consensus guideline series: treatment of psychiatric and behavioural problems in mental retardation. American Journal on Mental Retardation 105, 159–228.

American Association of Psychiatry, 1994. Diagnostic statistical manual of mental disorders, 4th edn (DSM-4). American Psychiatric Association, Washington, DC.

Baum, S., 2007. The use of family therapy for people with learning disabilities. Advances in Mental Health and Learning Disabilities 1 (2), 8–13.

Beail, N., Warden, S., Morsley, K., Newman, D., 2005. Naturalistic evaluation of the effectiveness of psychodynamic psychotherapy with adults with intellectual disabilities. J. Appl. Res. Intellect. Disabil. 18 (3), 245–252.

Beck, A.T., Ward, C., Mendelson, M., 1961. Beck Depression Inventory (BDI). Arch. Gen. Psychiatry 4, 561–571.

Black, L.A., Devine, M., 2008. Head Start: promoting positive mental health for children and young people with a learning disability. South Eastern Health and Social Care Trust, Belfast.

Bouras, N., Holt, G. (Eds.), 2007. Psychiatric and behavioural disorders in development disorders in development disabilities and mental retardation. Cambridge University Press, Cambridge.

Chyka, C., 2000. How many deaths occur annually from adverse drug reactions in the United States? Am. J. Med. 109 (2), 122–130.

Cooper, S.A., Holland, A., 2007. Dementia and mental ill health in older people with intellectual disabilities. In: Bouras, N., Holt, G. (Eds.), Psychiatric and behavioural disorders in development disabilities and mental retardation. Cambridge University Press, Cambridge.

Cooper, S.A., Smiley, E., Finlayson, J., et al., 2007. The prevalence, incidence, and factors predictive of mental ill-health in adults with profound intellectual disabilities. J. Appl. Res. Intellect. Disabil. 20 (6), 493–501.

Costello, H., Bouras, N., Davis, H., 2007. The role of staff training in improving community care staff awareness of mental health problems in people with intellectual disabilities. J. Appl. Res. Intellect. Disabil. 20, 228–235.

Crowley, V., Rose, J., Smith, J., Hobster, K., Ansell, E., 2008. Psycho-educational groups for people with a dual diagnosis of psychosis and mild intellectual disability. J. Intellect. Disabil. 12 (1), 25–39.

Dagnan, D., 2007. Psychosocial interventions for people with intellectual disabilities and mental ill health. Curr. Opin. Psychiatry 20 (5), 456–460.

Dagnan, D., Jahoda, A., 2006. Cognitive-behavioural intervention for people with intellectual disability and anxiety disorders. J. Appl. Res. Intellect. Disabil. 19 (1), 91–98.

Dagnan, D., Chadwick, P., Proudlove, J., 2000. Toward an assessment of suitability of people with mental retardation for cognitive therapy. Cognitive Therapy and Research 24, 627–636.

Deb, S., Braganza, J., 1999. Comparison of rating scales for the diagnosis of dementia in adults with Down's syndrome. J. Intellect. Disabil. Res. 43, 400–407.

Deb, S., Matthews, T., Holt, G., Bouras, N., 2001. Practice guidelines for the assessment and diagnosis of mental health problems in adults with intellectual disability. Pavilion, Brighton.

Deb, S., Clarke, D., Unwin, G., 2006. Using medication to manage behaviour problems among adults with a learning disability. University of Birmingham, Birmingham.

Department of Health, 1998. Signposts for success. NHS Executive, London.

Department of Health, 2001. Valuing people: a new strategy for learning disability for the 21st century. A White Paper. The Stationery Office, London.

Department of Health, Social Services and Public Safety (N. Ireland), 2005. Equal lives: review of policy and services for people with a learning disability in Northern Ireland. DHSSPS (N.I.), Belfast.

Devine, M., Taggart, L., 2008. Improving practice in the care of people with learning disabilities and mental health problems. Nurs. Stand. 22 (45), 40–48.

Devine, M., Taggart, L., McLorinan, P., (in press). Prevalence of psychiatric disorders in people with intellectual disabilities. British Journal of Learning Disabilities..

Douglass, S., Palmer, K., O'Connor, C., 2007. Experience of running an anxiety management group for people with a learning disability using a cognitive behaviour intervention. British Journal of Learning Disabilities 35 (4), 245–252.

Einfeld, S., Tonge, B.J., 1996a. Population prevalence of psychopathology in children and adolescents with intellectual disability: 1. Rationale and methods. J. Intellect. Disabil. Res. 40, 91–98.

Einfeld, S., Tonge, B.J., 1996b. Population prevalence of psychopathology in children and adolescents with intellectual disability: 2. Epidemiological findings. J. Intellect. Disabil. Res. 40, 99–109.

Emerson, E., 2003. The prevalence of psychiatric disorders in children and adolescents with and without intellectual disabilities. J. Intellect. Disabil. Res. 47, 51–58.

Emerson, E., 2005. Use of the Strengths and Difficulties Questionnaire to assess the mental health needs of children and adolescents with intellectual disabilities. J. Intellect. Dev. Disabil. 30 (1), 1–10.

Emerson, E., Robertson, J., Wood, J., 2005. Emotional and behavioural needs of children and adolescents with intellectual disabilities in an urban conurbation. J. Intellect. Disabil. Res. 49 (1), 16–24.

Eogan, M., Wingfield, M., 2010. Obstetric and gynaecological disorders. In: O'Hara, J., McCarthy, J., Bouras, N. (Eds.), Intellectual disability and ill health. Cambridge University Press, Cambridge.

Fryers, T., 1997. Impairment, disability, and handicap: categories and classifications. In: Russell, O. (Ed.), Seminars in the Psychiatry of Learning Disabilities. Royal College of Psychiatrists, London, pp. 16–30.

Goodman, R., 1999. The extended version of the Strengths and Difficulties Questionnaire as a guide to child psychiatric cases and consequent burden. J. Child Psychol. Psychiatry 40, 791–799.

Goodman, W.K., Price, L.H., Rasmussen, S.A., et al., 1989. Yale–Brown Obsessive Compulsive Scale: I. Development, use and reliability. Arch. Gen. Psychiatry 46, 1006–1111.

Gravestock, S., 2003. Diagnosis and classification of eating disorders in adults with intellectual disability: the 'Diagnostic Criteria for Psychiatric Disorders for use with Adults with Learning Disabilities/Mental Retardation' (DC-LD). J. Intellect. Disabil. Res. 71 (Suppl. 1), 72–83.

Hamilton, M., 1959. The assessment of anxiety states by rating. Br. J. Med. Psychol. 32, 50–55.

Hassiotis, A., Barron, D.A., 2007. Mental health, learning disabilities and adolescence: a developmental perspective. Advances in Mental Health and Learning Disabilities 1 (3), 32–39.

Hassiotis, A., Strydom, A., Hall, I., et al., 2008. Psychiatric morbidity and social functioning among adults with borderline intelligence living in private households. J. Intellect. Disabil. Res. 52 (2), 95–106.

Hatton, C., 2002. Psychosocial interventions for adults with intellectual disabilities and mental health problems. A review. J. Ment. Health 11, 357–1353.

Healthcare Commission, 2007. A life like no other: a national audit of specialist inpatient healthcare services for people with learning difficulties in England. Healthcare Commission, London.

Hemmings, C.P., 2006. Schizophrenia spectrum disorders in people with intellectual disabilities. Curr. Opin. Psychiatry 19 (5), 470–474.

Hoare, P., Harris, M., Jackson, P., Kerley, S., 1998. A community survey of children with severe intellectual disabilities and their families: psychological adjustment, carer distress and effects of respite care. J. Intellect. Disabil. Res. 42, 218–227.

Hove, O., 2004. Prevalence of eating disorders in adults. American Journal on Mental Retardation 109 (6), 501–506.

Hurley, A.D., 2006. Mood disorders in intellectual disability. Curr. Opin. Psychiatry 19 (5), 465–469.

International Association for the Scientific Study of Intellectual Disability, 2001. Mental health and intellectual disabilities: addressing the mental health needs of people with intellectual disabilities. IASSID. http://www.iassid.org.

Jahoda, A., Dagnan, D., Jarvie, P., Kerr, W., 2006. Depression, social context and cognitive behavioural therapy for people who have intellectual disabilities. J. Appl. Res. Intellect. Disabil. 19 (1), 81–90.

Kannabiran, M., Deb, S., 2010. Diseases of the nervous system 2: neuro-degenerative diseases including dementia. In: O'Hara, J., McCarthy, J., Bouras, N. (Eds.), 2010 Intellectual disability and ill health. Cambridge University Press, Cambridge.

Keeling, J.A., Rose, J.L., 2006. The adaptation of a cognitive-behavioural treatment programme for special needs sex offenders. British Journal of Learning Disabilities 34 (2), 110–116.

Kirkland, J., 2005. Cognitive-behaviour formulation for three men with learning disabilities who experience psychosis: how do we make it make sense? British Journal of Learning Disabilities 33 (4), 160–165.

Masi, G., Favilla, L., Mucci, M., 2000. Generalized anxiety disorder in adolescents and young adults with mild mental retardation. Psychiatry 63 (1), 54–64.

Matson, J.L., 1988. The PIMRA manual. International Diagnostic Systems, Orland Park, IL.

Matson, J.L., Rush, K.S., Hamilton, M., et al., 1999. Characteristics of depression as assessed by the Diagnostic Assessment for the Severely Handicapped-II (DASH-II). Res. Dev. Disabil. 20 (4), 305–313.

Matthews, D.R., Hegarty, J., 1997. The 'OK' Health Check: a health assessment checklist for people with learning disabilities. British Journal of Learning Disabilities 25 (4), 138–143.

Meins, W., 1996. A new depression scale designed for use with adults with mental retardation. J. Intellect. Disabil. Res. 40, 220–226.

Meltzer, G., Gatward, R., Goodman, R., Ford, T., 2000. The mental health of children and adolescents in Great Britain. Office for National Statistics, London.

Mental Health Foundation, 2010. Availabe at: http://www.mentalhealth.org.uk/information/wellbeing-podcasts/?locale=en.

Molteno, G., Molteno, C.D., Finchilescu, G., Dawes, A.R.L., 2001. Behavioural and emotional problems in children with intellectual disability attending special schools in Cape Town, South Africa. J. Intellect. Disabil. Res. 45, 515–520.

Moss, S., 2002. PAS-ADD schedules. Pavilion, Brighton.

Moss, S., Friedlander, R., Lee, P., 2007. The Cha-PAS interview. Pavilion, Brighton.

Nihra, K., Leland, H., Lambert, N., 1993. AAMR Adaptive Behaviour Scale, second ed. Harcourt Brace, New York.

O'Hara, J., 2008. Why should I care about gender. Advances in Mental Health and Learning Disabilities 2, 9–18.

Raghavan, R., Waseem, F., 2007. Services for young people with learning disabilities and mental health needs from South Asian communities. Advances in Mental Health in Learning Disabilities 1 (3), 27–31.

Reiss, S., 1988. Reiss Screen for maladaptive behaviours. IDS, Worthington, OH.

Reynolds, W.K., Baker, J.A., 1988. Assessment of depression in persons with mental retardation. American Journal of Mental Retardation 93, 93–103.

Rose, J., Dodd, L., Rose, N., 2008. Individual cognitive behaviour intervention for anger. Journal of Mental Health Research in Intellectual Disabilities 1 (2), 97–108.

Royal College of Psychiatrists, 2001. Diagnostic Criterion for people with Learning Disabilities (DC-LD). Royal College of Psychiatrists, London.

Royal College of Psychiatrists, 2004. Psychiatric services for children and adolescents with learning disabilities. Royal College of Psychiatrists, London.

Smith, I.C., 2005. Solution-focused brief therapy with people with learning disabilities: a case study. British Journal of Learning Disabilities 33 (3), 102–105.

Stromme, P., Diseth, T.H., 2000. Prevalence of psychiatric diagnoses in children with mental retardation: data from a population based study. Dev. Med. Child Neurol. 42, 266–270.

Summers, S.J., 2003. Psychological intervention for people with learning disabilities who have experienced bereavement: a case illustration. British Journal of Learning Disabilities 31, 37–41.

Taggart, L., 2009. Promoting emotional well-being. In: Gates, B., Barr, O. (Eds.), Oxford handbook of intellectual disability nursing. Oxford University Press, Oxford, pp. 216–217.

Taggart, L., McKendry, L., 2009. Developing a mental health promotion booklet for young people with learning disabilities. Learning Disability Practice 12 (10), 27–32.

Taggart, L., Slevin, E., 2006. Care planning in mental health settings. (Chapter 8). In: Gates, B. (Ed.), Care planning and delivery in intellectual disability nursing. Blackwell, Oxford.

Taggart, L., McLaughlin, D., Quinn, B., Milligan, V., 2006. An exploration of substance misuse in people with intellectual disabilities. J. Intellect. Disabil. Res. 50 (8), 588–597.

Taggart, L., Cousins, W., Milner, S., 2007a. Young people with learning disabilities living in state care: their emotional, behavioural and mental health status. Child Care in Practice 13 (4), 401–416.

Taggart, L., Mc Laughlin, D., Quinn, B., Mc Farlane, C., 2007b. Listening to people with intellectual disabilities who abuse substances. Journal of Health and Social Health Care 15 (4), 360–368.

Taggart, L., Huxley, A., Baker, G., 2008. Alcohol and illicit drug misuse in people with learning disabilities: implications for research and service development. Advances in Mental Health in Learning Disabilities 2 (1), 11–21.

Taggart, L., McMillan, R., Lawson, A., 2009a. Women with intellectual disabilities: risk and protective factors for psychiatric disorders. J. Intellect. Disabil. 13 (4), 321–340.

Taggart, L., McMillan, R., Lawson, A., 2009b. An exploration of the characteristics of women with learning disabilities and psychiatric disorders admitted into a specialist hospital. Advances in Mental Health in People with Learning Disabilities 3 (1), 30–41.

Taggart, L., McMillan, R., Lawson, A., 2010. Staffs' knowledge and perceptions of working with women with intellectual disabilities and psychiatric disorders. J. Intellect. Disabil. Res. 54 (1), 90–100.

Turk, J., Robbins, I., Woodhead, M., 2005. Post-traumatic stress disorder in young people with intellectual disability. J. Intellect. Disabil. Res. 49, 11.

Whelan, A., Haywood, P., Galloway, S., 2007. Low self-esteem: group cognitive behaviour therapy. British Journal of Learning Disabilities 35 (2), 125–130.

Willner, P., Goodey, R., 2006. Interaction of cognitive distortions and cognitive deficits in the formulation and treatment of obsessive-compulsive behaviours in a woman with intellectual disability. J. Appl. Res. Intellect. Disabil. 19 (1), 67–74.

World Health Organization, 1992. ICD-10: international statistical classification of diseases and related health problems, 10th revision. WHO, Geneva.

Further reading

Advances in Mental Health and Learning Disabilities. http://www.pavpub.com.

Journal of Mental Health Research in Intellectual Disabilities. http://www.thenadd.org.

Useful addresses

International Association for the Scientific Study of Intellectual Disabilities. http://www.iassid.org.

This is an international and interdisciplinary scientific non-governmental organisation with official relations with the WHO. It promotes worldwide research and exchange of information on learning disabilities.

The Foundation for People with Learning Disabilities. http://www.learningdisabilities.org.uk.

This provides a range of resources centred on meeting the emotional needs of children and young people with a learning disability.

The Mental Health and Growing Up series. http://www.rcpsych.ac.uk/mentalhealthinformation/mentalhealthandgrowingup.aspx

This contains 36 leaflets on a range of common mental health problems encountered by children and young people.

Assessment tools

Strengths and Difficulties Questionnaire. http://www.sdqinfo.com/b1.html.

PAS-ADD schedules. http://www.pasadd.co.uk/.

Health promotion literature

Head Start. Promoting positive mental health for children and young people with a learning disability. http://www.wellnet-ni.com/publications.php.

'How are you today?' Health promotion leaflet for young people with learning disabilities. http://www.howarewetoday.com.

Training materials for staff

Dodd, K., Turk, V., Christmas, M., 2002. Down's syndrome and dementia resource pack. British Institute of Learning Disabilities, Kidderminster.

Foundation for People with Learning Disabilities, 2006. Well-being workshop: recognising the emotional and mental well-being of people with profound and multiple learning disabilities. Foundation for People with Learning Disabilities, London.

Gregory, M., Newbigging, K., Cole, A., Pearsall, A., 2003. Working together: developing and providing services for people with learning disabilities and mental health problems. Mental Health Foundation, London.

Hollins, S., Curran, J., 1997. Understanding depression in people with learning disabilities. Pavilion, Brighton.

Holt, G., Hardy, S., Bouras, N., 2005. Mental health in learning disabilities: a training resource. Pavilion, Brighton.

Olsen, K.M., Hellings, J.A., Black, P.A., 2003. Dual diagnosis: mood disorders and developmental disabilities (video). Paul Brookes, Baltimore.

Olsen, K.M., Hellings, J.A., Black, P.A., 2003. Dual diagnosis: schizophrenia and other psychotic disorders and developmental disabilities (video). Paul Brookes, Baltimore.

Answers to Case illustration 17.2

Vidusha

- The woman's physical health and her weight should be examined to identify how this may have contributed to her developing low self-esteem and a potential mental health problem. Attention should be paid if the woman is prescribed psychotropic medication as there has been a correlation between this and abdominal obesity and reproductive complications.
- The assessment should explore the woman's psychosocial world in relation to how the mental health problem has developed. Staff could explore how the woman feels about having a learning disability and how this has affected her self-esteem and confidence about being 'female' and a 'woman'.
- For those women not in a relationship, issues of feeling lonely, not having a boyfriend, not getting married and not having a husband could also carefully be explored to identify if these are underlying areas of emotional pain and conflict.
- Staff could also examine how the woman who is in relationship is managing and coping with multiple roles/demands requested of her (i.e. undertaking household chores, caring for an older family member and/or children, being in an abusive relationship, suffering domestic violence, etc.).
- Focus should also be on identifying whether the woman has been physically, emotionally and/or sexually abused and obtaining the facts of this abuse and how this has affected the woman's health. Such disclosure could require passing this information onto the Safeguarding/Vulnerable Adult Team and/or the police for a full investigation.
- Another area to investigate is the woman's life events (e.g. death and/or illness of family members, move into residential care and loss of children into care), lack of employment/routine and little contact with family and friends and how these have affected her health; many issues that may not have been identified as problems by carers before.

Answers to Case illustration 17.3

John

- Comprehensive developmental history using parental/carer interview exploring the mental health of the primary care giver(s), history of family mental health and/or substance abuse, whether parent(s) are negative role models and if punitive child management practices are used. In addition, information will be collated with reference to the young person's signs/symptoms, life events and possible causation.
- Physical/neurological examination to dismiss if physiological or neurological factors are potential other causes for the young person's signs/symptoms.
- Genetic screenings to identify if the young person has 1) a genetic condition such as Prader–Willi syndrome and the potential for behavioural phenotypes, and 2) previous psychiatric consultations/diagnosis/treatments/use of services.
- Interview with the young person exploring his/her view of the cause for their distress including life events, and their perspective on their signs/symptoms using the identified clusters above.
- Behavioural observations undertaken by both parent and teachers across home and school to dispel other possible causes (i.e. environmental, frustration, loneliness, attention) for the young person's behaviour, as well as a functional analysis of behaviour.
- Use of rating scales by parent, teacher and,where possible, self-ratings by the young person to provide further objective evidence to support the health professionals' clinical judgement.

Challenging behaviour

18

Michael Wolverson

CHAPTER CONTENTS

KEY ISSUES

- Definitions and associated aspects including labelling and stigma
- The prevalence and manifestations of challenging behaviour and of self-injurious behaviour
- Self-injurious behaviour and its association with challenging behaviour
- The spectrum of causations – organic, behavioural and psycho-social and appropriate interventions
- The assessment of challenging behaviour to include process and assessment tools
- Working within an ethical and legal framework

Introduction

The subject of challenging behaviour encompasses a wide spectrum of presentations and outcomes which represent some of the greatest challenges to carers and service providers across a range of settings. The understanding and interpretation of challenging behaviour has evolved over time and recent developments in social policy have affected ways in which the label of challenging behaviour has impacted upon the lives of people so labelled and the configuration of services. Examples are provided throughout to demonstrate how the reality of practice is influenced by key issues.

Definitions and associated issues

The term 'challenging behaviour' has become an accepted and much used label to refer to people with learning disabilities who present with behaviours that other people including family carers, paid care workers and professionals involved with this client group find problematic. Wolverson (2003) discussed how there are several potentially useful definitions that are still worthy of consideration. Such definitions ascribe different meaning to the existence of challenging behaviour and hence direct the type of intervention employed in its management. The first is that of Blunden & Allen (1987:14):

> We have decided to adopt the term challenging behaviour rather than problem behaviour or severe problem behaviour since it emphasises that such behaviours represent challenges to services rather than problems which individuals with learning difficulties in some way carry around with them. If services could rise to the 'challenge' of dealing with these behaviours they would cease to be problems.

This definition of challenging behaviour places the focus of discussion on services rather than the individual showing the behaviours. Another intention is to shift the interpretation of the presenting behaviour from the individual displaying it, for whom the behaviour may not be a problem, to the care giver/service provider. In essence, this had the commendable intention of encouraging care givers to interpret behaviour as a 'challenge' to them and not the individual displaying it and one which they had an obligation to explore constructive ways of managing. This is most important as, prior to this definition, some care givers often interpreted presenting behaviours in a range of negative ways. One dominant interpretation originating from the medical/'deficit' model was that challenging behaviour was an innate part of the personality of the individual who displayed it, an inevitable consequence of their learning disability or associated condition, and as something in need of dehumanising control (Bilton et al 2002, Thomas & Woods 2003). The consequence of this was that people with learning disabilities and challenging behaviour were often viewed with a sense of 'therapeutic pessimism' and subjected to controlling patterns of care in institutionalised settings.

It is likely that the most often used definition of challenging behaviour is that of Emerson et al (1988:16):

> Severe challenging behaviour refers to behaviour of such an intensity, frequency or duration that the physical safety of the person or others is likely to be placed in serious jeopardy, or behaviour that is likely to seriously limit or deny access to the use of ordinary community facilities.

This is also a useful definition as its emphasis on duration, intensity and frequency should encourage care givers to realise that, just like any other individual, a person with learning disabilities who displays infrequent, low-intensity and short-lived episodes of problematic behaviour should not necessarily be labelled as having challenging behaviour. Furthermore, Emerson et al's (1988) definition also includes the issue of social and community involvement. Evidently, many behaviours displayed by some people with learning disabilities will not result in them being unable to access community facilities and if this is the case then careful consideration should be given before a person is labelled as having challenging behaviour. The Mansell Report (Department of Health (DH) 1992:3) broadened the definition of challenging behaviour by stating that it can apply to a diverse range of people with a learning disability, including:

> ... people with mild or borderline learning disability who have been diagnosed as mentally ill and who enter the criminal justice system for crimes such as arson or sexual offences: as well as people with profound learning disability, often with sensory handicaps and other physical problems who injure themselves for example by repeated head banging or eye poking.

Whereas there is a consensus that this is a useful interpretation, and an acceptance that such categories of behaviour should be included in a comprehensive definition of challenging behaviour, there may be potential problems with such an all-encompassing definition. This broad definition in combination with the indiscriminate use of the term 'challenging behaviour' can potentially lead to more people with learning disabilities being so labelled than is necessary. This can render the term challenging behaviour almost functionally meaningless as it is now used to cover such a wide spectrum of behaviour (Naylor & Clifton 1993). It is also worthy of note that this situation can also apply to conditions that are often associated with challenging behaviour and learning disabilities. One such condition is autism or rather 'autistic spectrum condition' with an apparent trend in learning disability services to apply this term arbitrarily in describing almost any behaviour displayed by a person with a learning disability (Anderson 2007).

This discussion of the term challenging behaviour indicates that those using this term need to be specific as to what they are defining (Gates 1996) and when they use it. Lists of specific behaviours have often been proposed that may be useful in enabling care staff to reach a decision as to whether a person's behaviour is challenging or not and also whether it is

Box 18.1

A behavioural checklist and a list of common forms of self-injurious behaviours

Behavioural checklist

- Violence.
- Destructiveness.
- Rebelliousness.
- Untrustworthiness.
- Stereotyped behaviour.
- Peculiar mannerisms.
- Inappropriate interpersonal manners.
- Unacceptable or eccentric habits.
- Hyperactivity.
- Sexually aberrant behaviour.
- Self-injury.
- Psychological disturbances.

(Adapted from Nihira et al 1993)

Common manifestations of self-injurious behaviour in people with learning disabilities

- Trichillotomania (pulling out own hair).
- Eating inedible substances (pica), eating faeces (coprophagia).
- Gouging of ears, mouth, eyes, nose, sexual organs and rectum.
- Head hitting/face slapping/striking face and chest with knees.
- Self-induced vomiting/vomiting and re-ingesting.
- Skin picking/picking at wounds.
- Hand biting.
- Kicking, or hitting body parts against, hard surfaces.

(Wolverson 2006)

a form of self-injurious behaviour. Box 18.1 gives an example of a 'behavioural checklist' developed by Nihira et al 1993 and also a list of the common forms of self-injurious behaviour displayed by people with a learning disability. Whereas checklists may be useful, it should be noted that all behaviours are open to subjective interpretation and situational and contextual 'triggers'.

These considerations about the definition of challenging behaviour are necessary as it is now likely that the original intention of Blunden & Allen (1987) has been corrupted through overuse and misuse and that it is now often used pejoratively thus increasing the stigmatisation of those so labelled. This can have the paradoxical effect of increasing rather than decreasing the likelihood that a person will display challenging behaviour as a result of treatment regimes and it can have a direct impact on the design of services.

Prevalence and demography

Research that has attempted to ascertain the prevalence of challenging behaviour displayed by people with a learning disability has produced a variation in incidence among people with learning disabilities of between 8% and 38% (Chung et al 1996). While it is acknowledged that findings vary, there is consensus that the prevalence of challenging behaviour is between 10% and 17% (Emerson et al 2001, Quereshi & Alborz 1992). The variation in prevalence is attributable to the demographics associated with learning disabilities as follows:

- Challenging behaviour increases with age during childhood and peaks between the ages of 15 and 34 after which it declines (Moss et al 2000).
- If it involves aggression, destruction of property and self-injury, this is positively correlated to the severity of learning disability (Moss et al 2000).
- Males are more likely than females to display challenging behaviour (Moss et al 2000).
- Challenging behaviour is more common if the individual with learning disability has an additional impairment, reduced mobility, communication difficulties and certain behavioural phenotypes (Borthwick-Duffy 1994).
- Challenging behaviour is more prevalent if there is the coexistence of learning disability and mental ill health (Priest & Gibbs 2004).
- Challenging behaviour is more common in institutional settings (Bruininks et al 1995).

The prevalence and demographics of self-injurious behaviour

The necessity of discussing self-injurious behaviour within this chapter is reinforced by the fact that self-injurious behaviour is relatively common within the learning disability population, with Borthwick-Duffy (1994) reporting that as many as 10–50% of people with learning disabilities may at some point display self-injurious behaviour. As with other forms of challenging behaviour, self-injurious behaviour can be influenced by situational factors that increase the likelihood of it occurring. It has been reported that the rate of self-injurious behaviour in institutionalised settings is as high as 41% (Cooper et al 2008) compared with generally lower rates for those living in other environments such as segregated day centres (3–10%), special schools (3–12%) and people living at home (1–4%) (Gates 2007). Individual characteristics can also influence prevalence with people with learning disabilities who also have sensory deficits, autistic spectrum conditions, ambulatory difficulties, limited expressive communication skills, undiagnosed pain and profound learning disabilities being more likely to engage in self-injurious behaviour (Heslop & Macauley 2009).

This brief overview of the prevalence of challenging behaviour and self-injurious behaviour indicates not only that these are significant issues in learning disabilities but that services should base their delivery of care on its key demographics.

Causation

This section of the chapter will explore the multifaceted causative factors of both challenging behaviour and self-injurious behaviour. There are many similarities between these categories of behaviour; however, important differences in their causation will be explored. It is vitally important that attempts are made to accurately identify the causation of an individual's challenging or self-injurious behaviour in order that appropriate interventions can be offered. This individual consideration of causation should result in constructive person-centred approaches and specifically targeted interventions. Wolverson (2003) suggested that the causations of challenging behaviour can be categorised into three areas: organic/biological, psychological and environmental. Although it may be useful to discuss causation within these domains, it should be noted that very often the causation of an individual's challenging and/or self-injurious behaviour can be attributed to more than one category of causation and that an initial causation may well create situations that will maintain this behaviour. An example of this can be explored by use of the electronic resource 18.1. See electronic resource 18.1 on the Evolve website.

Organic and biological dysfunction

It is often the case that some people consider challenging and/or self-injurious behaviour to be an inevitable outcome of a person having a learning disability or an associated condition. This may result in diagnostic overshadowing whereby people are expected to exhibit certain behaviours as a result of an original label or diagnosis often leading to failure to identify the actual causation of the behaviour. It is in fact almost always the case that a condition associated with a learning disability will not necessarily give rise to challenging behaviour or self-injurious behaviour in the affected person. Indeed, Murphy (1994:39) has stated that "there are only two known conditions which can be biologically defined and which always lead to a specific behavioural difficulty". One of these conditions is Lesch–Nyhan syndrome which invariably results in self-injurious behaviour whereby those affected will often bite at both their lips and hands. The other is Prader–Willi syndrome which involves an inability to suppress appetite, resulting in desperate attempts to get food, resulting in behaviours that are perceived as challenging, and 85% of people with this condition will display self-injurious behaviour (Didden et al 2007).

It is most important to understand that these two conditions are very rare and that if these are the only two conditions that inevitably result in challenging behaviour (and often self-injurious behaviour) then biological dysfunction is not usually the sole reason why a person will display challenging behaviour. The discussion will now focus on associated conditions that can lead to challenging behaviour if they remain undiagnosed and therefore untreated. Behaviours are often compounded by psychological, environmental and organisational issues. An example of such a condition is phenylketonuria (PKU) that results from an inborn error of metabolism. PKU increases the likelihood that those affected will display frequent and repetitive behaviours such as scratching, hair pulling and slapping and often self-injurious behaviour (Yannicelli & Ryan 1995). Fortunately PKU is easily identified at birth by the Guthrie test and it is subsequently controlled by diet. It should also be noted that Tourette's syndrome and Smith–Magenis syndrome can, but not inevitably, be causative factors in self-injury (Gates 2007, Heslop & Macauley 2009).

Some people, often those with complex needs, may have neurological dysfunctions (Reeves 1997) which may be left untreated because carers are unaware of their existence. This is because the affected person may lack expressive language and cannot describe the symptoms; resulting in behaviours being simply attributed to 'attention seeking'. Reeves (1997) suggested that these dysfunctions include apraxia (the inability to engage in purposeful voluntary movement without losing muscle power), visual agnosia (the inability to recognise objects and their shapes) and problems with proprioception (difficulty in judging the position of limbs and the body in space).

There are three conditions which are disproportionately associated with learning disabilities and may result in challenging behaviour. First, it is widely accepted that epilepsy affects approximately 0.5% of the general public yet it is far more commonly associated with learning disability (see Ch. 16). Epilepsy can be a complex condition with varied presentations involving altered states of consciousness. During these transient periods, usually associated with the pre- and post-ictal phases of a tonic–clonic seizure and with temporal lobe epilepsy, those affected may display strange, bizarre and dangerous behaviours over which they have no control or recollection.

Second, Lindsay & Burgess (2006) discuss how diabetes is five times more likely to affect people with learning disabilities than the general population. Hypo- or hyperglycaemia can result in impaired consciousness during which time an individual could display behaviours such as disorientation and being uncooperative that are perceived as challenging.

Third, another condition that is commonly associated with learning disabilities is autistic spectrum conditions (ASC). For a full exploration of ASC, readers should see Chapter 20, however it is worthy of consideration in this section because ASC is often strongly correlated with challenging and self-injurious behaviour. ASC is often characterised by ritualistic, repetitive and stereotypical behaviours, described as challenging because they appear bizarre, meaningless or likely to result in harm to self and others. This situation can often be exacerbated if attempts are made to alter rituals and routines. ASC is also believed to result in those affected 'objectifying' care givers and viewing them as inanimate objects without emotion or feeling (Baron–Cohen 2004). This can account for the occasions when an individual with ASC may physically harm a care giver and fail to respond empathically to the harm caused. ASC can also result in self-injury, and Hare & Leadbeater (1998) have suggested that this may be because some people with the condition are obsessional about routine, have a higher pain threshold than others and view their body as a machine and so may harm themselves to see 'how it works'. There is also much research (Gates 2007) that indicates that some people with ASC have heightened or different levels of sensory perception. This may result in them displaying challenging behaviour in order to 'escape' from environments or situations that have created an intolerable 'sensory overload'.

Endogenous opiates and self-injurious behaviour

There is much evidence that 'addictive' chemical changes can take place in the body as a result of self-injurious behaviour (Murphy 1999). Wisely et al (2002) have identified how the release of endogenous opiates when engaging in self-injurious behaviour can produce a morphine-like effect. There are two hypotheses that are linked to how these naturally occurring chemicals can lead to the development and maintenance of such behaviours. First, that self-injury (such as head slapping) stimulates the production of endogenous opiates, creating an analgesic effect on pain. Second, self-harm produces pleasurable feelings of euphoria so that the individual engaging in self-injury will repeat it in order to experience these feelings of euphoria and analgesia (Gates 2007, Winchel & Stanley 1991).

It should be noted that there are some conditions such as urinary tract infections that are equally prevalent among the general population and those with a learning disability which may result in challenging behaviour. Others include dementia and degenerative conditions which result from organic changes within the brain and can result in marked changes in behaviour. It is important to note that Down syndrome can result in dementia developing at a younger age than the general population. Behaviours that result from this such as disinhibition are initially misinterpreted and not attributed to dementia because of the age of onset (Stanton & Coetzee 2004).

Western industrialised societies have tended to develop organisational patterns of care of people with learning disabilities and challenging behaviour based on the medical model of care. This interpretation of learning disability was based on an overemphasis on the organic causation of learning disabilities resulting in the institutionalisation of many people with learning disabilities within medical settings. Because of the depersonalisation associated with institutionalisation and other negative consequences of these regimes, the focus of care has shifted towards a social model of care based upon the principles of person-centredness. A result of this paradigm shift is that care givers are encouraged not to focus on the categorisation of people with learning disability by labels or syndromes. Although there is consensus that this is a positive approach, it is nevertheless vitally important to realise that care services need an understanding of how some organic dysfunctions, which may historically have been associated with negative labelling, can lead to challenging behaviour if misunderstood or left untreated. An understanding of how a condition may result in challenging behaviour and person-centred approaches are not mutually exclusive. It is often the case that the individualised care of a person with an organic condition that could result in challenging behaviour can only be effective if there is both an understanding of the nature of that condition and a broader person-centred approach.

Environmental and psychological causation

It can be convenient to explore environmental and psychological issues in discrete sections, however these areas of study are very closely linked in relation to challenging behaviour and to self-injurious behaviour. This section will therefore offer an overview of how powerful 'psycho-social' issues can lead to challenging behaviour and how this behaviour is often the result of emotional distress and/or psychological disturbance that has been created by environmental factors. In practice, these issues should be seen to be indivisible if holistic, person-centred care is to be achieved.

Stigma and labelling

To some extent challenging behaviour is a social construct (DH 2007). The central principle of social constructionism is that an individual's interpretation of reality is a subjective conglomeration of perceptions derived from language and cultural perceptions. Foucault (1990) extended this concept to explain how negative labelling in relation to stigmatised groups can lead to them being treated in controlling and other unacceptable ways. The terms challenging behaviour and self-injurious behaviour are associated with many negative assumptions about an individual or group so labelled. Pilgrim & Rogers (1999) have discussed the concepts of primary and secondary labelling and the powerful effect this can have on a person's life. Primary labelling is the process of giving a label in the first instance and secondary labelling explains how once a person has been given a negative label they will seem to exhibit the expected symptoms associated with the condition. This can result in care staff viewing a person as a 'label' which (in this case) is challenging behaviour. Care staff might then expect behaviours to occur as an inevitable consequence of the label (Wilner & Smith 2008). It may also be the case that a person labelled as having a challenging behaviour may internalise the label and its negative connotations and 'act out' the behaviours expected as a result of the label. Although attempts have been made to avoid challenging behaviour and self-injurious behaviour from becoming altogether negative labels, they are often associated with a degree of pathology and therapeutic pessimism, some of which is as a consequence of the label, resulting in poor expectations, leading to self-fulfilled prophecies (Bicknell & Conboy- Hill 1992). Wolfensberger (1975:2) summarised these concepts thus:

> It is a well established fact that a person's behaviour tends to be profoundly affected by the role expectations that are placed upon him. Generally, people will play the roles that they have been assigned. This permits those who define social roles to make self-fulfilling prophecies by predicting that someone cast into a certain role will emit behaviour consistent with that role. Unfortunately, role appropriate behaviour will then often be interpreted to be a person's 'natural' rather than elicited mode of acting.

Wolfensberger also extended these concepts to explain how they can, often subconsciously, lead to a variety of perceptions of a person with a learning disability and how these can then heavily influence the configuration of services. Although Wolfensberger first outlined this in 1975, Mansell's report for the Department of Health (2007) demonstrates how, in many instances, specialist challenging behaviour provision is still heavily influenced by these perceptions.

Services based on these negative perceptions can result in an individual with challenging behaviour spending much of their time exposed to the powerful forces of institutionalisation which can compound existing patterns of challenging behaviour or create conditions that maintain it (DH 2007, Wolverson 2003). Much government legislation and resulting social policy over the past 40 years has been developed in order that the pernicious effects of institutionalisation can be eradicated and the large Victorian institutions have been closed. There was an expectation that the closure of the large institutions in combination with philosophies of care based on the four key principles of *Valuing People* (DH 2001) (inclusion, rights, choice and independence) would result in a reduction in levels of challenging behaviour. However, Mansell for DH (2007) has reported that in general the closure of the long-stay institutions has not resulted in a reduction in challenging behaviour and that increases may be expected in some instances. The DH (2007) has outlined how the development of specialist contemporary challenging behaviour services has resulted in the re-institutionalisation of many people with challenging behaviour (see Box 18.2). It is also the case that newer specialist services may be subdivided by labels so that, within one service, there are units for personality disorder, autistic spectrum conditions, self-injurious behaviour and assessment and treatment thus potentially further pathologising individuals.

Self-injurious behaviour offers examples of how controlling regimes and consequent disempowerment can cause or maintain behavioural distress. People with learning disabilities who display self-injurious behaviour may do so as part of a power struggle (Heslop & Macauley 2009). The 'expert' power of doctors and care staff (Buchanan 1997) can be seen to be challenged by people who display self-injurious behaviour and the power struggle that ensues can become increasingly disempowering for the person with self-injurious behaviour as a consequence of controlling, isolating, 'narrow' systems of care that interpret their purpose to be the elimination of self-injurious behaviour. This 'power struggle' can paradoxically reinforce the self-injurious behaviour rather than alleviate it and all too often a negative cycle is created. Within such systems, individuals may feel that the only thing over which they have any control is their body and self-injury is employed to exert some limited form of control. This may also serve the function of drawing attention to the individual's predicament, as a protest at being controlled or as an expression of anger against a body that may not conform with society's expected 'norms' (Favazza & Rosenthal 1993, Halliday & Mackrell 1997). Specialist care provision for people with a learning disability who self-injure has often been predicated on controlling behavioural and/or the bio-reductionist medical approaches (Heslop & Macauley 2009). These approaches are influenced by the medicalisation of emotional distress and treatments that are often aimed at correcting some perceived organic causation or chemical imbalance. The medical model can pathologise individuals by assuming the cause of the self-injury as being innate rather than seeking to identify powerful psychosocial 'setting conditions'. In effect, this model treats the symptoms of self-injury and not the causation.

Box 18.2

Environmental risk factors of contemporary challenging behaviour

- Poorly organised and trained staff.
- Unskilled 'caring' and 'minding'.
- Little interaction between staff and clients (approximately 9 minutes each hour).
- Substantial turnover of staff with poor continuity of care.
- Demoralisation of staff.
- Poor provision of psychotherapeutic interventions.
- Lack of choice and control.
- Crisis intervention and placement breakdowns and out of areas placements.
- Increased risk of abuse.
- Bad care practices.
- The 'silting up' of specialised services.
- Re-institutionalisation.

(Mansell for the DH 2007)

Reader activity 18.1

Think about the places where people live or are treated in if they have challenging behaviour. Use Box 18.2 to consider whether the characteristics listed can be seen in the environments that you are familiar with. Think about how these factors might influence challenging behaviour. Next try to identify ways in which you could support a person with challenging behaviour who is living in that environment.

Parenting and family issues

The perception that children with learning disabilities are different from other children can lead to 'faulty' parenting that often results in behaviour that is perceived to be challenging. Rolland (1993) has discussed the concept of centripetal forces (those that push family members together) and centrifugal forces (those that force family members apart) in relation to caring for a child with chronic care needs. Centripetal forces can result in challenging behaviour with McConachie (1986) suggesting that children with learning disabilities are overprotected and thus discouraged from reaching their full potential. In such situations, behaviours associated with early stages of child development are maintained into adulthood when they are viewed as challenging. Vetere (1993) has discussed how children

Reader activity 18.2

Consider and list the possible differences in the early life experiences of children with learning disabilities. Try to explain how these differences can lead to the development of challenging behaviour and the possible effects of this on the lives of people labelled as having challenging behaviour.

with learning disabilities can be 'infantilised'. This is a process in which those with a learning disability are treated as 'eternal children' and therefore expected to display some of the often difficult behaviours associated with childhood. Centrifugal forces can result in the child with a learning disability being blamed for family disintegration and discord resulting in problems with attachment such as psychological abuse or emotional abandonment and consequently resulting in challenging behaviour.

Self-injurious behaviour associated with abuse and attachment

People with learning disabilities are more at risk of abuse than the general population (Cambridge 1999). Challenging behaviour may develop as an attempt to draw attention to the fact that an individual has been abused or it could be a manifestation of socially learned behaviour that can develop as a result of consistent exposure to environments in which abuse and aggression are accepted forms of behaviour (Hepworth & Wolverson 2006). Research suggests that people with a learning disability will experience more psychological distress than the general population and this will often be manifested as challenging behaviour (Sequeira et al 2003).

These are important factors to consider as it is proposed that self-injurious behaviour may serve several functions that develop as a consequence of these. Examples include how care staff may fulfil a 'pseudo' paternal or maternal role and individuals may perceive negative responses to self-injury as perversely rewarding as any attention is more rewarding than none. Some self-harm involves damage to the skin (scratching, cutting, burning, picking). Babiker & Arnold (1997) discuss how the skin is used throughout life particularly by mothers to communicate attachment, love, to bond and to soothe by patting, stroking and kissing. This is significant when the histories of people who self-injure are explored as often the attachment between mother and the infant with a learning disability has been to some extent dysfunctional, broken or damaged and self-injurious behaviour related to damaging the skin can be a physical representation of the associated emotional distress. Self-injury may serve a purpose of engendering a particular response that is not usually expected in their relationship with care staff. If care staff are perceived to be indifferent to them, then the individual might self-injure to engender a more caring response. The 'soothing' action and the immediate attention of the first aid and treatment of wounds may demonstrate this. Self-injury can also serve the function of being a psychological defence mechanism. Malin & Birch (1998) explain how self-harm can be a manifestation of psychological transference. This is a process in which a range of emotions previously associated with, for example, an abuser or an abandoning parent is transferred onto a professional carer. Another defence mechanism is projection and some people with a learning disability who self-injure may find their thoughts and feelings too overwhelmingly distressing, unacceptable or inadmissible and may 'project' them onto care staff. Self-injurious behaviour may also serve as a regulatory function within the individual allowing them to cope with feelings of distress and anxiety (Babiker & Arnold 1997). Some individuals may find that the trauma of the abuse they have endured causes them to 'dissociate' and the only way they can return to 'reality' is by injuring themselves in order to feel the sensations which arise. Dissociation is the psychological process associated with experiences of trauma whereby the only way a person can manage the emotional distress is to mentally distance themselves from it by replacing it by inflicting physical pain (Klonsky 2007).

Behaviourist interpretations

The behaviourist interpretation of challenging behaviour is based on the assumption that behaviour is learned and maintained as a response to a range of positive and negative reinforcers (Pavlov 1927, Skinner 1953). In order to explain how behaviour can be learned, theorists have developed and used what has become known as the antecedent, behaviour, consequence sequential triad (McBrien & Felce 1995, McCue 2000). The outcome of this process is that there is a likelihood that an individual will repeat behaviours if they result in some form of reward or reinforcement. Whereas this behavioural interpretation of the development of appropriate behaviour seems entirely plausible, it can, at least superficially, appear less plausible when applied to the development of challenging behaviour as responses to it can seem to have negative consequences. The sequential triad in Case illustration 18.1 demonstrates how a challenging behaviour can develop in an attempt to gain attention. Every human being requires attention, however it is often the case that some people with a learning disability have been compelled to seek attention in challenging ways as this is possibly the only way that attention has been given. Theorists also postulate that even if the response to challenging behaviour appears to have a negative outcome for the individual (e.g. physical restraint), it is still reinforcing as any attention is more reinforcing than none.

There is also an assumption that behaviour can be learned vicariously. Bandura (1977) postulated that individuals can learn to behave in certain ways by observing the behaviour of others; this he termed 'social learning theory'. It has been historically the case, and it remains so in contemporary practice, that people with learning disability and challenging behaviour are often treated together in specialist units (DH 2007). It is entirely feasible that individuals being cared for in specialist units can develop a repertoire of challenging behaviours developed as a consequence of observing others.

Assessment of challenging behaviour

The preceding exploration of the causation of challenging behaviour and self-injurious behaviour explained how complex and multi-factorial their development can be. It is therefore imperative that care planning and interventions designed to deal with challenging behaviour reflect the eclectic nature of causation by offering a range of specific and person-centred strategies. This section of the chapter will outline the key elements of good practice in relation to assessment of challenging behaviour and appropriate assessment tools will be identified.

It is imperative that the assessment process includes a wide ranging contextual analysis of a person's challenging behaviour. Depending on the individual, this is likely to include the involvement of both direct and indirect care givers within a multi-disciplinary and mult-agency context. Assessment should be person-centred and the person being assessed and their family members should contribute as much as possible to the process. This involves an extensive exploration of the person's past and current experiences within a variety of environmental contexts that may have contributed or continue to contribute to the causation and maintenance of the challenging behaviour. The section on causation

Case illustration 18.1

A sequential triad demonstrating the development of challenging behaviour

Antecedent

David, who has difficulties with verbal communication, would try to gain the attention of care staff in appropriate ways such as using gestures, making noises and 'leading' staff by the hand or their clothing to areas where his needs could be met. Often these attempts were ignored, misinterpreted or responded to inadequately. Care staff would also sometimes describe the behaviour as being 'attention seeking' or 'manipulative'.

Behaviour

In response, David would bite his hands and knees and then 'pick' at the resulting wounds.

Consequence

Staff would give attention to David by attempting to stop the behaviour by distraction and the administering of 'soothing' first aid thus reinforcing the behaviour and increasing the likelihood of it being repeated.

A functional analysis of David's behaviour was conducted by care staff using antecedent, behaviour, consequence (ABC) recording charts. This process identified that David's behaviour had a communicative function and that it served a variety of other functions. Although it was discussed that David's behaviour may have a self-stimulatory function, the ABC recording strongly indicated that David's behaviours were displayed most when he wanted:

- a physical need to be met such as needing to use the toilet, have a drink or engage in a physical activity
- human contact with peers and care staff.

In order to alter David's patterns of behaviour, care staff were encouraged to meet David's needs when he was calm and before he resorted to challenging behaviour thus altering the antecedents. In effect, the consequences were also altered as he was now being 'rewarded' when displaying appropriate behaviour.

explained how challenging behaviour can be caused by organic, environmental and psychological factors and that it can be caused by a complex combination of these. There are specific assessment tools that focus on each of these three areas.

Assessment of organic causation

A 'global' assessment of a person's health should be undertaken to ascertain if there are any underlying and previously unknown conditions that may account for the challenging behaviour. An example of this is the widely used *'OK' Health Check* (Matthews 2004). A preliminary global assessment can be used to screen for conditions such as epilepsy and sensory deficits that may account for or contribute to the challenging behaviour. If specific conditions are identified then more specific and detailed assessments should be undertaken. An example of this is the *Dementia Scale for Down Syndrome* (Gedye 1995). This assessment tool could be used to verify the causation of the behaviour so that appropriate care planning can take place (see Ch. 29).

Behavioural checklists and rating scales

A wide range of behavioural checklists have been developed to target and prioritise specific behaviours for consequent intervention. These are often used in the preliminary stages of the assessment process. Although they can be used generically, they are most often utilised if it is suspected the challenging behaviour has an environmental causation and that behaviour has evolved as a functional response. In the USA and Britain, one of the most widely used tools is the Aberrant Behaviour Checklist (ABC) (Aman & Singh 1986). This is a generalised rating scale that categorises behaviours into the subscales of lethargy, irritability, stereotypy, hyperactivity and inappropriate speech. Originally developed for the assessment of self-injurious behaviour and stereotypical behaviour, the Behaviour Problems Inventory (BPI) is another frequently used checklist that has been expanded to also assess for aggressive/destructive behaviour (Rojahn et al 2001). Although there are differences between these two tools, research suggests that both of these are valid and reliable assessment checklists (Hill et al 2008). It is worthy of note that the Aberrant Behaviour Checklist has been identified by a panel of experts in the USA as the 'gold star' of rating scales for the assessment of both behavioural and psychiatric issues (Taggart & Slevin 2006). An extensive list of behavioural assessment tools can be seen in Box 18.3.

Box 18.3

Behavioural assessment tools

- Aberrant Behaviour Checklist (Aman & Singh 1986).
- Reiss screen for maladaptive behaviour (Reiss 1988).
- Adaptive Behaviour Scale (Nihira et al 1993).
- Behavioural and Emotional Rating Scale (BeERS).
- Diagnostic assessment of severely handicapped (DASH -11).
- Motivation Assessment Scale (MAS) (Durand & Crimmins 1988).
- Functional analysis of problem behaviour (O'Neil et al 1997).

Assessment of mental ill health

It is widely acknowledged that people with a learning disability also experience mental ill health and can do so more frequently than other groups of people (Priest & Gibbs 2004). The symptomologies associated with mental illness are often conflated with challenging behaviour and this can cause significant problems when assessing and planning care. Studies have demonstrated that a wide range of challenging behaviours displayed by people with learning disability including self-injury can be an atypical feature of mental ill health within this client group (Emerson et al 1999, Taggart & Slevin 2006). Assessment tools have been developed to screen for the existence of psychiatric disorders in people with a learning disability. These should be used to ascertain if an individual with challenging behaviour has a coexisting psychiatric disorder. Assessment should also allow for an exploration of the inter-relationship between challenging behaviour and psychiatric disorder and whether they exist independently of each other. In the UK, the PAS-ADD (Psychiatric Assessment Schedule for Adults with Developmental Disabilities) is widely used (Moss 2002). Other screening tools are available and some of these are listed in Chapter 17.

Interventions

This section of the chapter will outline a range of interventions with some discussion as to how their effectiveness can depend on the individual nature of the person displaying the behaviour and the reality of practice. Interventions should be based on the assessment processes and tools outlined in the previous section. This can enable interventions to be individualised and to target specific behaviours. Interventions will be explained in discrete sub-sections of this chapter although it is vitally important to emphasise that, in practice, a combination of interventions can be used. Increasingly interventions for people with challenging behaviour are integral parts of a systemic approach that offers a global therapeutic approach to challenging behaviour in all aspects of a person's life (Heslop & Macauley 2009, Kaur et al 2009). It should be noted that individualised intervention within a systemic approach is recommended as best practice in challenging behaviour services in Mansell's report (DH 2007). The following interventions can, depending on circumstances, be used for both challenging and self-injurious behaviour.

Chemotherapeutic and physical interventions

It has been discussed how the medical model can overemphasise the importance of organic causations in the development of challenging behaviour. This can lead to physical interventions being used as a primary response to manage challenging behaviour even when there is no organic condition present. Although there may be an over-reliance on the use of medication to manage challenging behaviour (Tyrer et al 2008), it is the case that some of the conditions associated with challenging behaviour are responsive to its use. Examples of this include the use of the opiate blockers naltrexone and naxolone in the treatment of self-injurious behaviour (Murphy 1999). Oliver (1995) has discussed how naltrexone, which is an opiate antagonist, specifically targets self-injury that is a consequence of the individual self-harming to release the body's natural endogenous opiates. The use of the endogenous opiates dopamine and serotonin can also result in a reduction in self-injurious behaviour in people with learning disabilities (Clarke 1997). However, it is also the case that a mainstay of clinical intervention in challenging behaviour is the prescription of anti-psychotic/psychotropic drugs that are used almost arbitrarily to control behaviours where no specific causation has been identified and where there is little proof of efficacy (Tyrer et al 2008). Whereas these drugs can be effective if there is an underlying psychiatric disorder, there are concerns that they can be used instead of adequate staffing (DH 2001) and more appropriate behavioural support (Emerson et al 2000). It has been suggested that the following principles of good practice should apply in relation to medication:

- Medication should be used alongside a range of other therapeutic interventions.
- Whenever possible, the use of medication should be time limited and regularly reviewed.
- Specific conditions should be treated by the appropriate medication.
- Consent and compliance should be sought.
- Potential side effects should be identified and care staff should be vigilant in noticing these.

(Wolverson 2003)

In addition to chemotherapeutic interventions, physical interventions including physical restraint and time out from positive reinforcement are accepted forms of behavioural management. Time out from positive reinforcement is a behavioural approach based on the idea that some people gain positive reinforcement from being in a social environment and that temporary removal from such an environment will discourage the challenging behaviour that resulted in time out because the individual learns that such behaviour results in time out and the associated loss of positive reinforcement. These are generally used in specialist inpatient units and physical restraint should only be used as a last resort by staff properly trained to use it. Care staff should only use these procedures as directed by appropriate policies and legislation such as the Mental Health Act Code of Practice (DH 2008) and the Mental Capacity Act 2005 Deprivation of Liberty Safeguards (MCA DOLS; see later in this chapter). These interventions can have a hugely negative and disempowering effect on individuals that can paradoxically increase the likelihood of challenging behaviour recurring. Care staff and services should be aware of this area of practice and develop processes for the monitoring of the side effects of medication and the implementation and review of care plans that include the use of physical interventions.

Behavioural approaches and functional analysis

Behaviour modification is an approach that is based on the premise that if behaviour can be learned, equally it can be 'unlearned' and people with challenging behaviour can learn adaptive ways of functioning. A further key tenet of the behavioural approach is that all behaviour has meaning and a communicative function regardless of how challenging and meaningless it may appear. McBrien & Felce (1995) have explained how this approach is firmly based on the antecedent, behaviour, consequence triad and functional analysis is the process by which attempts are made to identify the potential reasons why a person may display challenging behaviour and which factors serve to reinforce the behaviour (thus making it more likely to be repeated). Functional analysis is conducted by using charts that accurately record the three stages of the antecedent, behaviour, consequence triad. Once these charts have been completed, hypotheses are made as to what purpose the behaviour serves for the individual and what may reinforce it. Care plans can then be devised that alter the reinforcement of the challenging behaviour (Case illustration 18.1 illustrates this process). Behaviour modification has been criticised as follows:

- The recording of the antecedent, behaviour, consequence triad can be extremely inaccurate.
- Rewards and reinforcers aimed at altering behaviours may be meaningless to the individual.
- It is too simplistic and can ignore emotional and cognitive causations of behaviour.
- Care givers lack the knowledge and skills to apply it adequately.
- It can be seen to be aversive, controlling and mechanical and therefore potentially ethically questionable.
- It can be inconsistently applied.
- The focus for the behaviour is heavily placed on the individual and environmental factors can be overlooked.

Because of these criticisms, attempts have been made to make the process more person-centred and behavioural approaches are now more commonly known as positive behavioural support (PBS). Allen et al (2005) and McCue (2000) have argued that behaviour modification/positive behavioural support can be effective and the above criticisms addressed if the following concepts are considered:

- Interventions should be designed to alter systems and not individuals.
- Behavioural approaches should seek to improve the quality of life of individuals and not merely attempt to eradicate challenging behaviour.
- Some behaviours may have more than one function and they may operate differently in different contexts.
- Detailed functional assessment must be conducted prior to intervention.

It has been demonstrated that PBS can be effective in the management of challenging behaviour across a wide range of service settings (McClean et al 2005).

Gentle Teaching

Gentle Teaching evolved as a rejection of the chemotherapeutic, physical and behavioural approaches due to their potentially 'aversive' nature and the criticisms of them outlined above. Both behaviour modification and physical approaches can be criticised for the perception that they are controlling and not person-centred. The proponents of Gentle Teaching assert that its goal is not only to eradicate the symptoms of challenging behaviour but also to encourage valued and meaningful life changes. This is achieved by the development of a rapport between client and carer while engaged in a range of purposeful activities. These activities can be developed to offer a functional and communicative alternative to challenging behaviour (O'Rourke & Wray 2000). Components of Gentle Teaching that underpin the process are:

- unconditional positive regard – even when the individual is displaying challenging behaviour
- equity – the development of an equal relationship between carer(s) and the individual with challenging behaviour
- mutual change – care giver(s) and client develop mutual coping strategies.

(McGee et al 1987)

These three central principles of Gentle Teaching represent laudable goals; however potential problems have been identified with its use:

- The suggested ways of engaging in Gentle Teaching are poorly defined and difficult to implement.
- Is it merely a variation of the behavioural approach because it is an attempt to control and alter behaviour?

- It lacks an evidence base.
- It can 'trigger' challenging behaviour as the function of some challenging behaviours are to 'escape' from proximity to care staff who may be attempting to engage the client in Gentle Teaching.

(O'Rourke & Wray 2000)

The term 'teaching' implies that there must be a didactic element to Gentle Teaching and some care staff have made the mistake of implementing this approach on a sessional basis as one would for teaching. The central principles of Gentle Teaching should be interpreted as an underpinning philosophy of any human service or care regime and, as such, they can contribute to supporting people with challenging behaviour in person-centred ways.

Cognitive behavioural therapy

Priest & Gibbs (2004) have discussed how people with learning disabilities experience significantly more mental illness than the general population and that this is often associated with challenging behaviour. Theorists postulate that many manifestations of challenging behaviour and self-harm are the consequence of errors in thinking and 'faulty' cognition (Turnbull 2007, Wilberforce 2003). It is also plausible to suggest that these, often unconscious negative cognitions are attributable to the life experiences, environmental and social 'setting' conditions discussed by Wolverson (2003). In recent years there has been an increase in the use of cognitive approaches in alleviating challenging behaviour and self-harm. Cognitive behavioural therapy (CBT) and other 'talking therapies' are now employed by therapists in learning disability services. The use of these non-aversive approaches has been met with a degree of scepticism because of the following points:

- There is a presupposition that the client must have adequate cognitive ability and expressive language skills to benefit.
- The client must be willing to engage in the process.
- They require conformity to a 'normal' world view rather than an acceptance that some people with learning disability may interpret their existence in different ways.

In spite of these criticisms, Wilberforce (2003) has identified that there are some universal benefits of therapy that can help to lessen challenging behaviour as follows:

- A relationship based on person-centredness, trust, mutual respect and genuineness.
- The offer of support and reassurance.
- A working alliance in which client and therapist work in partnership.
- The client develops insight into their patterns of behaviour.
- Healthy and positive responses are reinforced by the therapist.
- The client feels empowered and listened to.

Thus it can be seen that the process of therapeutic interventions can be as important as the content. It should also be noted that attempts have been made to adapt CBT to suit the requirements of people with learning disabilities by simplifying language and ideas and by the use of materials such as plasticine and dolls (Hurley et al 1998). It has been reported that CBT can have encouraging results when used with people who have challenging behaviour and a mental health problem (Oathamshaw & Haddock 2006). Case illustration 18.2 gives an example of how CBT can be applied.

Other therapeutic approaches

There is a range of other therapeutic approaches that embrace the assumption that person-centredness and individual care planning are prerequisites of constructive interventions. These interventions should be used selectively depending on the needs of each individual and with consideration of potential causations. Readers can explore these interventions in depth by accessing the sources listed after each intervention:

- Family therapy (Wolverson 2003).
- Structured teaching (Barr et al 2000).
- The arts therapies (Liebmann 2000).
- Complementary therapies (Wray & Paton 2007).
- Intensive interaction (Caldwell 1999).

The intervention(s) selected for use with people with learning disabilities should be chosen because they can effectively offer solutions to the causative factors that have led to the challenging behaviour or self-injury displayed in individual circumstances. Whereas this may seem self-evident, it is often the case that the reality of practice may compromise this process (DH 2007). It is also commonly the case that individuals who could benefit from a range of interventions may be denied access to some of these.

Case illustration 18.2

The use of cognitive behavioural therapy within a broader therapeutic context

Jane, who is 28, has had involvement with specialist challenging behaviour services from the age of 13. This was because of her challenging and self-injurious behaviours. Jane had been referred because she would physically assault the care staff in the treatment and assessment unit where she was staying. She would also display sexually promiscuous behaviour and attempt to mutilate her genitals. Initially behavioural attempts had been made to help Jane manage her behaviour. This involved Jane being 'rewarded' with trips out and material 'treats' when she had displayed appropriate behaviours for a specified time. The behavioural approach had limited success and Jane would always return to displaying her challenging behaviour. She had a known history of sexual and emotional abuse. Because of this there was an assumption that her behaviours were attributable to the emotional distress caused by the abuse and the development of entrenched negative patterns of thought (schema). These included very low self-esteem, feelings of worthlessness and guilt. After a thorough assessment it was decided by the multi-disciplinary team that Jane might benefit from cognitive behavioural therapy (CBT). This involved attempting to encourage Jane to understand how her history of abuse had led to the development of her negative thoughts and how these could be changed. This process also enabled Jane to begin to understand the causal links between her negative self-image and her behaviours. Over a period of time, this process helped Jane to develop a more positive self-view and acceptable behaviours.

Jane engaged with her CBT within a broader person-centred context in which she exerted as much choice as possible over key aspects of her life. In an attempt to improve her self-image and self-esteem, complementary therapies such as aromatherapy and hand massage were used as these both soothed her when stressed and helped her to feel more feminine and attractive. Jane also was encouraged to engage in creative art activities as a cathartic process and, in doing so, she improved her feelings of self-worth.

Emerson et al (2000) have demonstrated how medication is often the only intervention available in some circumstances. This may be attributable to the dominance of the medical model in challenging behaviour services or the lack of resources precluding access to other interventions. Further practice complications can arise from hierarchical structures in which certain powerful professional groups can dictate that their preferred intervention is the one most used. This can be influenced by professional training courses and potentially result in, for example, psychologists and nurses favouring behavioural approaches and occupational therapists advocating for activities such as engaging in drama and music. The development of integrated multi-disciplinary teams and shared care planning processes can alleviate some of these potential difficulties. There is also a historical dimension to interventions and challenging behaviour that can affect the reality of practice. There can be seen to be a 'timeline' of interventions that began in the 1960s with the advent of the benzodiazepines and the resulting dominance of medication as an intervention. This was gradually supplemented by the development of behaviour modification in the 1970s, Gentle Teaching in the 1980s and the 'talking therapies'/complementary therapies from the 1990s. Each intervention along this 'timeline' can be seen to be a positive development and to some extent a 'rejection' of the earlier interventions because of their perceived failings in the management of challenging behaviour. Practitioners should be aware of these trends in intervention because, while each intervention has at some time been criticised, all have both positive and negative elements and all of them can have some degree of success. The major consideration that will influence the potential for the success of the chosen intervention(s) is whether or not causative factors can be addressed within an overall system that is person-centred and empowering.

Working within an ethical and legal framework

Wolverson (2004) has explained how one of the most contentious areas that influences the support of people with a learning disability and challenging behaviour is the use of restrictive physical interventions including the deprivation of liberty and the ethical dilemmas associated with them. This section of the chapter will offer an overview of how current legislation can guide practice within an ethical framework. It is recognised that the challenging behaviour and/or self-injurious behaviour displayed by some people with a learning disability can present a danger to themselves and to others. If this is the case, a range of physical interventions can be utilised in the individual's best interest to prevent or limit self-harm and/or harm to others. These interventions should only be practised in accordance with the Revised Mental Health Act Code of Practice (DH 2008). Restrictive physical interventions include a wide range of practices, some of which may have been used in an unregulated way within learning disability services. The DH (2002) indicates that restrictive physical interventions range from full-scale physical restraint to any bodily contact such as holding a person's hand to stop them from hitting out. They also explain how other devices that exert control over the person with challenging behaviour and deny them their liberty, such as baffle locks that only staff can unlock, are a form of restrictive intervention. Clarke & Bright (2002) and Horsburgh (2003) comment that there are insidious and subtle ways in which a person's liberty can be interfered with, such as making unavailable to an individual equipment such as walking aids that are necessary for an autonomous lifestyle, and that, in effect, these amount to de facto restraint.

The ethical dilemmas associated with challenging behaviour and the use of restrictive physical interventions and chemical restraint emanate from some complex and potentially conflicting concepts of professional practice. The major area of ethical conflict pivots on the tensions that can arise between duty of care, best interest, individual autonomy, mental capacity and the ability to consent. Care staff are rightly encouraged to seek consent from the people they care for and to allow individuals to exercise free will and to act autonomously. Tensions can occur when a person's free will may result in them self-injuring or harming others. In such circumstances, care staff will often decide that restrictive physical interventions and sometimes the deprivation of liberty are justified because they have a duty of care to both the individual concerned and others they care for who may be harmed as a result of the challenging behaviour. Care staff can also reason that it is in the best interests of the person displaying challenging behaviour or self-injury to use restrictive interventions to prevent harm. It is often the case that an individual whose behaviour may result in a restrictive physical intervention has not consented to this intervention and/or they lack the mental capacity to do so. The important concepts of mental capacity and consent further complicate the legal and ethical context of restrictive physical intervention. Clearly this is a potentially problematic area of practice and one that can result in ethically questionable practices and negative outcomes for both care staff and people with challenging behaviour.

It is crucial that service providers and care staff operate within defined ethical and legal frameworks if restrictive physical interventions, including those that interfere with liberty, are used in the management of challenging behaviour. The ability to provide care within a legal and ethical framework has been greatly improved within the past decade by the introduction of recent legislation and guidance, which will now be discussed.

Mental Capacity Act 2005 Deprivation of Liberty Safeguards, Adults with Incapacity (Scotland) Act 2000

The European Convention on Human Rights (ECHR) forms the basis of the Human Rights Act 1998 which is enforceable by courts within the United Kingdom and which has contributed to the developing 'rights culture' within the field of learning disabilities. The Convention is divided into 15 rights or 'articles'. Article 5 is 'the right to liberty and security' and it is this article that led to current legislation within the United Kingdom that governs the use of restrictive physical interventions. The key resulting legislation in England and Wales is the Mental Capacity Act 2005 Deprivation of Liberty Safeguards (MCA DOLS). In Scotland, the relevant legislation is the Adults with Incapacity (Scotland) Act 2000 which is based on very similar principles; however, there are also differences and therefore interested readers should study the main points of this piece of legislation. The MCA DOLS provide legal protection for vulnerable people, including those with a learning disability who could be deprived of their liberty (in contravention of Article 5 of the ECHR) within a care home or a hospital (other than under a section of the Mental Health Act 1983). They were developed as a result of a legal judgement made by the ECHR, commonly known as the Bournewood Judgement, relating to a man (HL) with autistic spectrum condition and a learning disability who lacked the capacity to consent to admission to a specialist unit and who had self-harmed. It caused much debate within learning disability services because HL's situation was not particularly unusual and it brought into question accepted working practices. HL had been admitted to hospital on an 'informal' basis but was subsequently prevented from leaving hospital for reasons deemed to be in his best interests. This decision was challenged by his carers and the ECHR ruled that there had been a breach of his rights in contravention of Article 5.

The MCA DOLS were developed to prevent any further breaches to the ECHR and to ensure that a vulnerable person can only be deprived of their liberty if it is in their best interests and authorised by a supervisory body. This has had the beneficial effect in learning disability practice of services developing robust processes and guidance that can help care staff to operate within a prescribed legal and ethical framework that clarifies many of the dilemmas and uncertainties outlined above. In a general sense, the MCA DOLS also contribute to a person-centred ethos within environments that can be overly controlling.

The MCA DOLS do not apply to individuals detained under the Mental Health Act (MHA) 1983 (amended 2007). It is the case that sometimes individuals with challenging behaviour and/or self-harm may receive treatment under sections of the MHA 1983 and indeed specialist – often private sector – provision is expanding to provide care for this area of practice. The MHA 1983 provides very clear instruction relating to how treatment is to be provided and how individual rights can be considered. Interested readers should consult the parts of the MHA 1983 that are relevant to their area of practice and/or individuals they are supporting. One provision of the MHA 1983 that applies to many people with challenging behaviour is Section 117, Aftercare, that resulted in the care programme approach (CPA). The CPA encourages a multi-agency and person-centred approach to managing care.

Conclusion

This chapter has discussed a range of issues relating to challenging behaviour within contemporary contexts and the impact of this on the reality of practice. This overview has demonstrated that challenging behaviour remains a hugely problematic area of care that can have a major impact on the people that display it, those who care for them and on the provision of care. The chapter has highlighted how care provision for people with challenging behaviour is often at variance from how other people with learning disability are cared for and treated. This is because the contemporary approaches based on individualised/person-centred care and the key principles of *Valuing People* (DH 2001) are often not being applied within specialist challenging behaviour services resulting in the re-institutionalisation of this group of people with many of its consequent negative effects. The chapter explored possible ways in which appropriate person-centred and therapeutic approaches can be implemented in an attempt to offer individualised care that can help to address some of the negative aspects associated with this shift to 're-institutionalised' practices. It illustrated how the process by which this can be achieved is by identification of the causation of behaviour via a thorough assessment process so that a range of appropriate interventions can be implemented as part of an individualised approach within a systemic life planning process.

References

Allen, D., Evans, J., Hawkins, S., Jenkins, R., 2005. Positive behavioural support: definition, current status and future directions. Learning Disability Review 10 (2), 4–11.

Aman, M.G., Singh, N.N., 1986. Aberrant behaviour checklist manual. Slossom, New York.

Anderson, M., 2007. Autistic spectrum disorder. In: Gates, B. (Ed.), Learning disability: toward inclusion. fifth ed. Churchill Livingstone, Edinburgh.

Babiker, G., Arnold, L., 1997. The language of injury: comprehending self mutilation. British Psychological Society, Leicester.

Bandura, A., 1977. Social learning theory. Prentice Hall, New Jersey.

Baron–Cohen, S., 2004. Autism: research into causes and intervention. Pediatr. Rehabil. 7, 73–78.

Barr, O., Sines, D., Moore, K., Boyd, 2000. Structured teaching. In: Gates, B., Gear, J., Wray, J. (Eds.), Behavioural distress: concepts and strategies. Baillière Tindall, London.

Bicknell, J., Conboy–Hill, S., 1992. The deviancy career and people with mental handicap. In: Waitman, A., Conboy–Hill, S. (Eds.), Psychotherapy and mental handicap. Sage, London.

Bilton, T., Bonnett, K., Jones, P., et al., 2002. Introductory sociology, fourth ed. Palgrave Macmillan, Basingstoke.

Blunden, R., Allen, D., 1987. Facing the challenge: an ordinary life for people with learning disabilities and challenging behaviour. Kings Fund paper No.74. Kings Fund Centre, London.

Borthwick-Duffy, S.A., 1994. Prevalence of destructive behaviours. In: Thompson, T., Gray, D.B. (Eds.), Destructive behaviour in developmental disabilities: diagnosis and treatment. Sage, Thousand Oaks, CA.

Bruininks, R.H., Olson, K.M., Larson, S. A., Lakin, K.C., 1995. Challenging behaviours among persons with mental retardation in residential settings. In: Thompson, T., Gray, D. B. (Eds.), Destructive behavior in developmental disabilities. Sage Focus Edition 170 Sage, Thousand Oaks, CA.

Buchanan, W.F., 1997. Adherence – a matter of self-efficiency and power. J. Adv. Nurs. 26, 132–137.

Caldwell, P., 1999. Person to person: establishing contact and communication with people with profound learning disabilities and extra special needs. Pavilion, Brighton.

Cambridge, P., 1999. The first hit: a case study of the physical abuse of people with learning disabilities and challenging behaviours in a residential service. Disability and Society 14 (3), 285–308.

Chung, M.C., Cummella, S., Bickerton, W.L., Winchester, C., 1996. A preliminary study on the prevalence of challenging behaviours. Psychol. Rep. 79, 1427–1430.

Clarke, D., 1997. Physical treatments. In: Read, S. (Ed.), Psychiatry in learning disability. Saunders, London.

Clarke, A., Bright, L., 2002. Showing restraint: challenging the use of restraint in care homes. Counsel and Care, London.

Cooper, S.A., Smiley, E., Alla, L.M., et al., 2008. Adults with intellectual disabilities: prevalence, incidence and remission of self- injurious behaviour, and related factors. J. Intellect. Disabil. Res. 53 (3), 217–232.

Department of Health, 1992. Mansell report on services for people with learning disabilities and challenging behaviour or mental health needs. HMSO, London.

Department of Health, 2001. Valuing people: a strategy for learning disability. The Stationery Office, London.

Department of Health, 2002. Guidance for restrictive physical interventions: how to provide safe services for people with learning disabilities and autistic spectrum disorder. Available at: http://www.dh.gov.uk/en/Publicationsandstatistics/Publications/PublicationsPolicyAndGuidance/DH_4009673.

Department of Health, 2007. Services for people with learning disabilities and challenging behaviour or mental health needs. Available at: http://www.dh.gov.uk/en/Publicationsandstatistics/Publications/PublicationsPolicyAndGuidance/DH_080129.

Department of Health, 2008. Revised Mental Health Act code of practice. Department of Health, London.

Didden, R., Korzilius, H., Curfs, L., 2007. Skin-picking in individuals with Prader–Willi syndrome: prevalence, functional assessment, and its comorbidity with compulsive and self-injurious behaviours. J. Appl. Res. Intellect. Disabil. 20 (5), 409–419.

Durand, M., Crimmins, D., 1988. The MAS administration guide. Monaco, Topeka, KS.

Emerson, E., Cummings, R., Barret, S., et al., 1988. Challenging behaviour and community services: 2. Who are the people who challenge services? Mental Handicap 16, 16–19.

Emerson, E., Moss, S., Kiernan, C., 1999. The relationship between challenging behaviours and psychiatric disorders in people with severe developmental disabilities. In: Bouras, N. (Ed.), Psychiatric and behavioural disorders in people with severe developmental disabilities and mental retardation. Cambridge University Press, Cambridge.

Emerson, E., Robertson, N., Gregory, N., Hatton, C., Kessissoglou, S., 2000. Treatment and management of challenging behaviours in residential settings. J. Appl. Res. Intellect. Disabil. 13, 197–215.

Emerson, E., Kiernan, C., Alborz, A., et al., 2001. The prevalence of challenging behaviours: a total population study. Res. Dev. Disabil. 22 (1), 77–93.

Favazza, A.R., Rosenthal, R.J., 1993. Diagnostic issues in self-mutilation. Hosp.Community Psychiatry 44 (2), 134–140.

Foucault, 1990. Madness and civilisation: a history of insanity in the age of reason. Routeledge, London.

Gates, B., 1996. Issues of reliability and validity in measurement of challenging behaviour (behavioural difficulties) in learning disability: a discussion of implications for nursing research and practice. J. Clin. Nurs. 5, 7–12.

Gates, B., 2007. Theory and practice of managing self-injurious behaviour in people with learning disabilities. In: Gates, B. (Ed.), Learning disabilities: toward inclusion. fifth ed. Churchill Livingstone, Edinburgh.

Gedye, A., 1995. Dementia scale for Down syndrome. Gedye Research and Consulting, Vancouver, Canada.

Halliday, S., Mackrell, K., 1997. Psychological interventions in self-injurious behaviour: working with people with a learning disability. Br. J. Psychiatry 172, 395–400.

Hare, D.J., Leadbeater, C., 1998. Specific factors in assessing and intervening in cases of self-injury by people with autistic conditions. Journal of Learning Disabilities for Nursing, Health and Social Care 2 (2), 60–65.

Hepworth, K., Wolverson, M., 2006. Care planning and delivery in forensic settings for people with intellectual disabilities. In: Gates, B. (Ed.), care Planning and delivery in intellectual disability nursing. Blackwell, Oxford.

Heslop, P., Macauley, F., 2009. Hidden pain? Self-injury and people with learning disabilities. Bristol Crisis Service for Women, Bristol.

Hill, J., Powlitch, S., Furniss, F., 2008. Convergent validity of the aberrant behaviour checklist and behaviour problems inventory with people with complex needs. Res. Dev. Disabil. 29 (1), 45–60.

Horsburgh, D., 2003. The ethical implications and legal aspects of patient restraint. Nurs. Times 99 (6), 26–27.

Human Rights Act, 1998. The Stationery Office, London. Available at :http://www.dh.gov.uk/en/Publicationsandstatistics/Publications/PublicationsLegislation/DH_4009802.

Hurley, A., Tomasulu, D.J., Pfadt, A.G., 1998. Individual and group psychotherapy approaches for persons with intellectual disabilities and developmental disabilities. Journal of Developmental and Physical Disabilities 10, 365–386.

Kaur, G., Scior, K., Wilson, S., 2009. Systemic working in learning disability services: a UK wide survey. British Journal of Learning Disabilities 37, 213–220.

Klonsky, D., 2007. The functions of deliberate self-injury: a review of the evidence. Clin. Psychol. Rev. 27, 226–259.

Liebmann, M., 2000. The arts therapies. In: Gates, B., Gear, J., Wray, J. (Eds.), Behavioural distress: concepts and Strategies. Baillière Tindall, London.

Lindsay, P., Burgess, D., 2006. Care of patients with intellectual or learning disability in primary care: no more funding so will there be any change? Br. J. Gen. Pract. 56, 84–86.

McBrien, J., Felce, D., 1995. Working with people who have severe learning dificulty and challenging behaviour: a practical handbook on the behavioural approach. BILD, Kidderminster.

McClean, B., Dench, C., Grey, I., et al., 2005. Person focused training: a model for delivering positive behavioural supports to people with challenging behaviours. J. Intellect. Disabil. Res. 49 (5), 340–352.

McConachie, H., 1986. Parents and young mentally handicapped children: a review of research issues. Croom Helm, Beckenham.

McCue, M., 2000. Behavioural interventions. In: Gates, B., Gear, J., Wray, J. (Eds.), Behavioural distress, concepts and strategies. Baillière Tindall, London.

McGee, J., Menolascino, M.D., Hobbs, D., Menousek, P., 1987. Gentle teaching: a non aversive approach to helping persons with mental retardation. Human Sciences Press, New York.

Malin, T., Birch, A., 1998. Introductory psychology. MacMillan Press, London.

Matthews, D.R., 2004. The 'OK' health check: health facilitation and health action planning, third ed. Fairfield, Preston.

Mental Capacity Act, 2005. Deprivation of liberty safeguards. Code of practice to supplement the main Mental Capacity Act 2005 code of practice. The Stationery Office, London. Available at: www.publicguardian.gov.uk.

Moss, S., 2002. PAS-ADD schedules. Pavilion, Brighton.

Moss, S., Emerson, E., Kiernan, C., Turner, S., Hatton, C., 2000. Psychiatric symptoms in adults with learning disability and challenging behaviour. Br. J. Psychiatry 177, 452–456.

Murphy, G., 1994. Understanding challenging behaviour. In: Emerson, E., McGill, P., Mansell, J. (Eds.), Severe learning disabilities and challenging behaviour: designing high quality services. Chapman and Hall, London.

Murphy, G., 1999. Self- injurious behaviour: what do we know and where are we going? Tizard Learning Disability Review 4 (1), 5–12.

Naylor, V., Clifton, M., 1993. People with learning disabilities – meeting complex needs. Health and Social Care in the Community 1 (6), 343–353.

Nihira, K., Leland, H., Lambert, N., 1993. AAMR adaptive behaviour scale – residential and community examiners manual, second ed. Pro ed, Texas.

Oathamshaw, S.C., Haddock, G., 2006. Do people with intellectual disabilities and psychosis have the cognitive skills required to undertake cognitive behavioural therapy? J. Appl. Res. Intellect. Disabil. 19 (1), 35–46.

Oliver, C., 1995. Self-injurious behaviour in children with learning disabilities. J. Child Psychol. Psychiatry 30, 909–927.

O'Neil, R.F., Horner, R.H., Albin, R.W., et al., 1997. Functional analysis and programme development for problem behaviour: a practical handbook, second ed. Brooks Cole, California.

O'Rourke, S., Wray, J., 2000. Gentle teaching: In: Gates B, Gear J, Wray J (eds) Behavioural distress: concepts and strategies. Baillière Tindall, London.

Pavlov, I.P., 1927. Conditional reflexes. Oxford University Press, London.

Pilgrim, D., Rogers, A., 1999. A sociology of mental health and illness. Oxford University Press, Trowbridge.

Priest, H., Gibbs, M., 2004. Mental health care for people with learning disabilities. Churchill Livingstone, Edinburgh.

Quereshi, H., Alborz, A., 1992. Epidemiology of challenging behaviour. Mental Handicap Research 5, 130–145.

Reeves, S., 1997. Behavioural misdiagnosis. Nurs. Times 93 (19), 44–45.

Reiss, S., 1988. Reiss screen for maladaptive behaviours. IDS, Worthington, OH.

Rojahn, J., Matson, J.L., Lott, D., Esbensen, A.J., Smalls, Y., 2001. The behavior problems inventory: an instrument for the assessment of self-injury, streotyped behavior and aggression/destruction in individuals with developmental disabilities. J. Autism. Dev. Disord. 31, 577–588.

Rolland, J.S., 1993. Helping couples live with illness. Family Therapy News (December), 15–26.

Sequeira, H., Howlin, P., Hollins, S., 2003. Psychological disturbance associated with sexual abuse in people with learning disabilities. Br. J. Psychiatry 183, 451–456.

Skinner, B.F., 1953. Science and human behaviour. MacMillan, New York.

Stanton, L., Coetzee, R., 2004. Down's syndrome and dementia. Advances in Psychiatric Treatment 10, 50–58.

Taggart, L., Slevin, E., 2006. Care planning in mental health settings. In: Gates, B. (Ed.), Care planning and delivery in intellectual disability nursing. Blackwell, Oxford.

Thomas, D., Woods, H., 2003. Working with people with learning disabilities: theory and practice. Jessica Kingsley, London.

Turnbull, J., 2007. Psychological approaches. In: Gates, B. (Ed.), 2007 Learning disabilities: toward inclusion. fifth ed. Churchill Livingstone, Edinburgh.

Tyrer, P., Oliver-Africano, P.C., Ahmed, Z., Booras, N., et al., 2008. Risperidone, haloperidol, and placebo in the treatment of aggressive challenging behaviour in patients with intellectual disability: a randomised controlled trial. Lancet 371, 57–63.

Vetere, A., 1993. Using family therapy in services for people with learning disabilities. In: Carpenter, J., Treacher, A. (Eds.), Using family therapy in the 90s. Blackwell, Oxford.

Wilberforce, D., 2003. Psychological approaches. In: Gates, B. (Ed.), Learning disabilities: toward inclusion. fourth ed. Baillière Tindall, London.

Wilner, P., Smith, M., 2008. Attribution theory applied to helping behaviour towards people with intellectual disabilities who challenge. J. Appl. Res. Intellect. Disabil. 21, 150–155.

Winchel, R.M., Stanley, M., 1991. Self-injurious behaviour: a review of the behaviour and biology of self mutilation. Am. J. Psychiatry 148 (3), 306–317.

Wisely, J., Hare, D., Fernandez-Ford, L., 2002. A study of the topography of self-injurious behaviour in people with learning disabilities. J. Learn. Disabil. 6 (1), 61–71.

Wolfensberger, W., 1975. The origin and nature of institutional models. Human Policy Press, Syracuse.

Wolverson, M., 2003. Challenging behaviour. In: Gates, B. (Ed.), Learning disabilities: toward inclusion. fourth ed. Churchill Livingstone, Edinburgh.

Wolverson, M., 2004. Restrictive physical interventions. In: Holland, S. (Ed.), Introducing nursing ethics. APS, Salisbury.

Wolverson, M., 2006. Self-injurious behaviour and learning disabilities. Therapy Weekly August 24, 8–10.

Wray, J., Paton, K., 2007. Complementary therapies. In: Gates, B. (Ed.), Learning disabilities: toward inclusion. fifth ed. Churchill Livingstone, Edinburgh.

Yannicelli, S., Ryan, A., 1995. Improvements in behaviour and physical manifestations in previously untreated adults with pnenylketonuria using a phenylaline-restricted diet: a national survey. J. Inherit. Metab. Dis. 18 (2), 131–134.

Further reading

British Psychological Society, 2004. Challenging behaviours: psychological interventions for severely challenging behaviours shown by people with learning disabilities. British Psychological Society, Leicester.

Emerson, E., 2001. Challenging behaviour, analysis and intervention in people with learning difficulties. Cambridge University Press, Cambridge.

Imray, P., 2007. Turning the tables on challenging behaviour: a practitioner's perspective to transforming challenging behaviours in children, young people and adults with SLD, PMLD or ASD. Fulton, London.

Royal College of Psychiatrists, British Psychological Society, Royal College of Speech and Language Therapists, 2007. Challenging behaviour: a unified approach. Clinical service guidelines for supporting people with a learning disability who are at risk of receiving abusive or restrictive practices. Royal College of Psychiatrists, London.

Stirling, C., Wakefield, M., 2008. Supporting parents and carers: a trainer's guide to positive behaviour strategies. BILD, Kidderminster.

Useful addresses

British Institute of Learning Disabilities, http://www.bild.org.uk.

Department of Health, http://www.doh.gov.uk.

Foundation for People with Learning Disabilities, http://www.learningdisabilities.org.uk.

Guide to the Mental Health Act, http://www.dh.gov.uk/en/Publicationsandstatistics/Publications/PublicationsPolicyAndGuidance/DH_088162.

International Association for the Scientific Study of Intellectual Disabilities, http://www.iassid.org.

National Electronic Library for Learning Disabilities, http://www.bild.org.uk/04projects_eleclib.htm.

Norah Fry Centre, http://www.bristol.ac.uk/norahfry/.

Mental health and learning disabilities portal, http://www.connects.org.uk/index.cfm?js=1@dom=1.

Tizard Centre, http://www.kent.ac.uk/tizard/.

19

Working with offenders

Jenny Talbot

CHAPTER CONTENTS

KEY ISSUES

- Prevalence of people with learning disabilities caught up in the criminal justice system is unclear although between 5% and 10% of the offending population is generally accepted
- There is no routine or systematic procedure for identifying people with learning disabilities at any point in the criminal justice system; consequently their support needs are often left unrecognised and unmet
- While there are a number of safeguards to protect the welfare and legal rights of suspects, defendants and offenders with learning disabilities, evidence suggests these are not always put in place

- There is disagreement among criminal justice and health care professionals about the appropriateness of dealing with people with learning disabilities who are alleged to have offended through the criminal justice system
- Criminal justice staff do not routinely undertake learning disability awareness training

Introduction

This chapter considers particular elements of the criminal justice pathway for individuals with learning disabilities suspected of committing a criminal offence, from the point of arrest through to disposal from the court. Opportunities for diversion away from the criminal justice system are discussed. The experiences of prisoners with learning disabilities are given particular attention.

People with learning disabilities who come into contact with the criminal justice system are generally referred to as being 'vulnerable'. At the police station and in court, the word 'vulnerable' is used to describe people who are less able to cope with the rigors of, for example, police caution and interview, and who are in need of support. In prison, however, 'vulnerable' has a very different meaning and is routinely used to describe the threats posed to certain prisoners, rendering them 'vulnerable', due to the nature of their offending, for example prisoners who are sex offenders.

It is important to note that many disability rights campaigners challenge the use of the term ≈ 'vulnerability': a summary of the argument using the social model of disability is that disabled people are not inherently vulnerable, rather it is the context of a society that has not accepted the adjustments necessary to allow disabled people to participate which lead to them being perceived as vulnerable. While recognising the social model of disability, this chapter uses the term 'vulnerable' to describe people who are less able to cope with the exigencies of the criminal justice system and who are likely to need support. At the time of writing this chapter, public sector services were undergoing a time of uncertainty. In 2010 the new coalition government launched a number of consultations, including the NHS white paper, *Equality and Excellence: Liberating the NHS* (Department of Health, 2010); *Promoting equality through transparency* (Government Equalities Office, 2010), and the justice green paper. These, and an adverse economic climate, will undoubtedly precipitate significant changes for criminal justice, health and social services.

Prevalence and experience of people with learning disabilities in the criminal justice system

It is known that people with learning disabilities enter the criminal justice system; average estimates of prevalence in the UK range from 1% to 10%. Studies in Cambridge and London have suggested that between 5% and 9% of suspects seen at police stations have learning disabilities (Gudjonsson et al 1993, Lyall et al 1995) and 6% of people supervised by probation services on community orders (Mason & Murphy 2002); while 7% of people in prison have an IQ below 70, and a further 25% an IQ between 70 and 79 (Mottram 2007).

In practical terms, almost one-third of offenders have learning disabilities or difficulties that interfere with their ability to cope within the criminal justice system, and which will affect and undermine their performance in both education and work (Loucks 2007:1, Rack 2005:2).

Similarly, McBrien (2003:101) notes:

> One of the most prevalent vulnerable groups amongst offenders comprises those who do not have an intellectual disability [learning disability] as formally defined but who do have much lower cognitive and adaptive abilities than do either the general population or the offending population.

Precise information about prevalence among black and minority ethnic offenders is virtually non-existent, however gender differences are notable. One of the few research projects involving women (Mottram 2007) reports higher proportions of women prisoners with an IQ below 70 (8%) and between 70 and 79 (32%) than among the male prisoners.

While it is generally recognised that between 5% and 10% of the offending population will have learning disabilities and many more will have borderline disabilities or other difficulties that interfere with their ability to cope, precise figures remain vague and further work needs to be undertaken in this area.

Knowing who has a learning disability

The first step in ensuring that people with learning disabilities are appropriately dealt with when they come into contact with the criminal justice system is being able to identify who they are. Some people will be known to local health and social services and, where good links exist, steps can be taken to ensure the most appropriate outcome. There is, however, no routine or systematic procedure for identifying people with learning disabilities at any point in the criminal justice system (Jacobson 2008, Loucks 2007, Talbot 2007).

A number of learning disability screening tools have been developed that may assist in ascertaining how many people are in need of additional support, though none is universally accepted as a 'gold standard'. Results from a recent study undertaken by the Department of Health (DH) (England) established a learning disability screening tool that was effective for use in prisons (DH unpublished). It is expected that the tool will be made available more widely across the criminal justice system during 2010.

Linked to the identification of people with learning disabilities is the sharing of appropriate information. Research shows that information concerning an individual's identified support needs is not routinely shared between different parts of the criminal justice system. Thus information that might usefully inform criminal justice and health care staff is rarely available (Talbot 2007, Loucks 2007).

Particular difficulties faced by people with learning disabilities in the criminal justice system

While some people with learning disabilities are willing to tell criminal justice staff that they have a learning disability and need support, the same cannot be said for all. Many people choose to keep their difficulties to themselves for fear of ridicule or to appear the same as other people, and some may not know that they have a learning disability.

People with learning disabilities may face particular problems in terms of their general welfare and, more fundamentally, the risk of wrongful conviction. Many empirical studies strongly suggest that people with learning disabilities are 'vulnerable' in the sense that, compared to their non-disabled peers, they are:

- less likely to understand information about the caution and legal rights
- more likely to make decisions which would not protect their rights as suspects and defendants
- more likely to be acquiescent . . . [and] more likely to be suggestible.

(Clare 2003:251)

Legal and policy framework

There are various legal and policy safeguards aimed at protecting the general welfare of vulnerable people, facilitating their access to treatment and support where appropriate, and reducing risks of miscarriages of justice that could arise from their vulnerability and, where appropriate, these safeguards are referred to under the different sections in this chapter. Provisions tend to be framed within the language of 'mental disorder' as a broad term encompassing learning disability alongside mental illness. This is problematic to the extent that it masks the more specific needs of people with learning disabilities.

One recent document, which has particular significance for offenders with learning disabilities, is the government's National Delivery Plan (NDP), *Improving Health, Supporting Justice* (HM Government 2009). Published in November 2009, the NDP draws extensively on a review of people with mental health problems or learning disabilities in the criminal justice system, which was commissioned by the government in 2007 and undertaken by Lord Keith Bradley (DH 2009). The aims of the review were:

- to examine the extent to which offenders with mental health problems or learning disabilities could, in appropriate cases, be diverted from prison to other services and the barriers to such diversion
- to make recommendations to government, in particular on the organisation of effective court liaison and diversion arrangements and the services needed to support them.

The NDP incorporates all of Lord Bradley's recommendations and has stated 'key deliverables' and time frames.

Human Rights Act

The Human Rights Act (HRA) 1998 came into force throughout the UK in October 2000 and brings the European Convention on Human Rights (ECHR) into British law. The HRA places an obligation on all public bodies, and on those private bodies that carry out functions previously delivered by the state, to ensure they respect human rights.

The most relevant articles of the HRA for the purposes of this chapter are:

- Article 2: the right to life

- Article 3: the right to protection from torture, inhumane or degrading treatment
- Article 5: the right to liberty and security
- Article 6: the right to a fair trial
- Article 8: the right to respect for private and family life
- Article 14: the prohibition of discrimination.

(Watson 2007)

An important concept introduced through this act is that public bodies have a positive obligation to protect rights – that is they must take active steps to safeguard a person's Convention rights. This is particularly relevant where people are in the care of the state, as are prisoners.

Disability Discrimination Act and the inclusion agenda

Recent years have seen an increasing emphasis upon inclusion as a goal of public policy with respect to people with disabilities, including people with learning disabilities. This principle of inclusion was given legislative force by the 2005 revision of the Disability Discrimination Act (DDA) 1995. The DDA 1995 made it unlawful for public services to discriminate against people with disabilities. The DDA 2005 took this further, by introducing the Disability Equality Duty (DED). The DED requires statutory authorities actively 'to promote equality of opportunity between disabled persons and other persons' and 'to eliminate discrimination'as part of their mainstream work (section 49A DDA 1995, inserted by section 3 of DDA 2005). Thus authorities must work to ensure that discrimination does not occur: for example, by making adjustments to existing service provision and ensuring that future provision is accessible to people with disabilities.

The principle of inclusion promotes the legal and human rights of people with disabilities to live full and active lives in society. As well as rights, the concept of inclusion implies that individuals with disabilities have the same duties and obligations as their fellow non-disabled citizens – in this context, the duty to live a law-abiding life (Talbot 2008:72).

The inclusion agenda thus fosters the presumption that, unless their capacity to participate effectively in the criminal justice process is severely limited, people with learning disabilities should be subject to the same due process as anyone else, with appropriate support.

Diversion away from the criminal justice system

However, there is disagreement among practitioners – including police officers, health care workers and legal practitioners – about the appropriateness of taking formal action against some suspects with learning disabilities. This, to an extent, reflects a lack of clarity in current policy and guidance on the application of the concept of criminal responsibility to these individuals.

On the one hand, the provision of treatment and support for suspects with learning disabilities, rather than prosecution, may help individuals overcome the problems that led them to (allegedly) offend. On the other hand, failure to arrest and prosecute carries its own risks. For example, the individual who has committed a crime but is not prosecuted may not appreciate the gravity of his actions and may reoffend, and possibly commit more serious offences as a result (Murphy et al in press). Another risk is that a suspect may be subjected to compulsory treatment without ever being afforded the opportunity to prove his innocence (Seden 2006, see also Strategic Policy Team 2006:29).

In practice, the paucity of provision towards which a person with learning disabilities may be diverted for treatment and/or support, in particular preventative services and low-level support, often begs the question 'diversion into what?'

Service provision

The move towards deinstitutionalisation for people with learning disabilities has seen an increase in their use of mainstream services, including criminal justice (Carson et al 2010). Over a 13-year period, Lindsay et al (2006) noted that, in later years, a higher percentage of referrals to a community forensic learning disability service came from criminal justice services rather than community services; further, those referred were younger, probably reflecting a trend that "younger offenders with LD [learning disabilities] would not automatically be diverted into institutions, but might rather become involved with criminal justice agencies and the courts" (p. 125).

Carson et al (2010) argue that this will have undoubtedly influenced the profile of services for offenders with learning disabilities as secure health care institutions have closed and different pathways into services have developed. Such services will include, for example:

> entry into the criminal justice system and continuation through trial; some diversion from the court and criminal justice system; entry into statutory services; referral to private secure accommodation for individuals with LD [learning disabilities] and/or severe challenging behaviour; and for some less serious offences, diversion into generic community learning disability services.
>
> (Carson et al 2010:40)

Service provision to help prevent people from engaging in risky or offending behaviour is the ideal but access to such support is not straightforward. Reduced budgets often result in local services targeting people with the most severe or complex needs at the expense of those with milder disabilities. The lack of national criteria for providing support is confusing and means that a person with learning disabilities in one area might receive support, while in another they would not.

The support needs of people with mild learning disabilities are frequently of a relatively low level, for example help with budgeting, paying bills, personal care and friendship networks – but they are long term. Quite low levels of support can make all the difference between a person staying on the right side of the law and getting involved in risky and offending behaviour.

Further, local services are not always willing or able to work with people with offending or challenging behaviour, especially if they are not known, and in many areas there is no learning disability forensic service or forensic expertise. Local drug and alcohol services may not offer programmes designed or adapted for people with low cognitive ability, and multi-agency working between criminal justice, health care and other local services to prevent offending is rare.

Criminal justice liaison and diversion schemes

Criminal justice liaison and diversion schemes work with police and court services to assess suspects and defendants with possible mental health problems and learning disabilities; they provide information about support needs and can refer people to treatment and support services.

The creation of liaison and diversion schemes was stimulated by the 1992 Reed review of health and social services for mentally disordered offenders (DH/Home Office 1992), which called for nationwide provision of properly resourced court assessment and diversion schemes. However, only one-third of magistrates' courts currently have access to such schemes (HM Government 2009).

The purpose of liaison and diversion schemes was originally to identify people whose imprisonment was not in the public interest because, due to their vulnerability, it was likely to be disproportionately harmful, and because prison was an inappropriate setting for the vulnerable offender. For example, research by James et al (2002) showed that timely diversion from the criminal justice system produced better outcomes both in terms of the person's mental health and in reducing the risk of reoffending. However, current practice too often fails to use alternatives that are less damaging than prison for vulnerable offenders. Diversion, properly implemented, would direct vulnerable offenders to support in the community, improve public health and reduce crime.

It is notable that although most existing schemes tend to be multi-disciplinary, the "vast majority ... do not currently have learning disability expertise" (DH 2009:82). However, some schemes explicitly include learning disabilities within their remit; one such scheme, based in Norwich, is described in Jacobson & Talbot (2009).

The National Delivery Plan (HM Government 2009) commits to "promote and stimulate the development of liaison and diversion services" (paragraphs 3.7–3.12). Importantly, Bradley's recommendations (14 and 28) state that all police custody suites and all courts "should have access to liaison and diversion services" (Department of Health, 2009).

Identification of need

One of the most important elements of the work of liaison and diversion schemes is the identification and assessment of an individual's impairments and support needs. Ideally, this would occur prior to the point of charge and inform all subsequent proceedings.

Mental Health Act

Part III of the Mental Health Act (MHA) 1983, as amended by the Mental Health Act 2007, allows people who are mentally disordered to be diverted from the criminal justice system into compulsory treatment by the health care system either before or after conviction. The 2007 Act defines mental disorder as "any disorder or disability of the mind" (section 1(2)). It is

> **Box 19.1**
>
> **Key disposals for mentally disordered defendants**
>
> - Hospital Order: permits court to order defendant's admission to hospital if mental disorder makes detention for medical treatment appropriate, and appropriate treatment available (section 37). Up to 6 months' duration in the first instance can be renewed; thus, unlike most criminal justice disposals, it is essentially indeterminate.
> - Guardianship Order: defendant placed under responsibility of local authority or person approved by local authority (s. 37).
>
> Hospital and Guardianship Orders can be made by magistrates' court or crown court following conviction for imprisonable offence, or by magistrates' court without conviction if the court is satisfied that the defendant committed the act/omission with which they are charged.
>
> - Interim Hospital Order: made by crown court or magistrates' court after conviction when court needs more time to decide whether to impose hospital order or use alternative disposal (s. 38).
> - Restriction Order: imposed by crown court alongside hospital order, where deemed necessary by court to protect public from 'serious harm' (s. 41). Order places limits on individual's discharge from hospital.

specified, however, that for many of the provisions of the Act, including the Part III provisions discussed here, a person with learning disabilities should not be considered mentally disordered unless the "disability is associated with abnormally aggressive or seriously irresponsible conduct on his part" (s. 2(2)). Learning disability is defined in the Act as "a state of arrested or incomplete development of the mind which includes significant impairment of intelligence and social functioning" (s. 2(3)).

The key disposals under the Mental Health Act 1983 for mentally disordered defendants are set out in Box 19.1.

Contact with the police

Legal and policy framework

The statutory framework is largely established by the Police and Criminal Evidence Act (PACE) 1984, and its accompanying codes of practice, particularly Code C (Code of Practice for the Detention, Treatment and Questioning of Persons by Police Officers) (Home Office 2006).

> **Reader activity 19.1**
>
> There is disagreement among and between different professional groups about the appropriateness of subjecting an individual with learning disabilities to the criminal justice system. While some argue for a therapeutic approach to tackling offending behaviour, administered through health care, others consider criminal justice an appropriate response due to the more obvious and direct penalty to be paid for breaking the law. In your view, should people with learning disabilities who offend be subject to the criminal justice system – as are their non-disabled peers – or should they be diverted away from it and into health care? Consider the pros and cons for each approach.

The main policy safeguards for suspects with learning disabilities are the following:

- Diversion away from the criminal justice system.
- An appropriate adult (AA) should be called to the police station if a person who is 'mentally disordered or otherwise mentally vulnerable' has been detained.
- A custody officer has a duty to seek clinical attention for a detainee who appears to be suffering from a mental disorder.
- There are statutory grounds for excluding confession evidence from a trial, where the confession has been obtained under circumstances in which undue pressure was exerted on a vulnerable suspect in a police interview, or the police failed to ensure that the requisite safeguards were in place.

Pre-arrest and arrest

The police have a duty to investigate any criminal offence that is reported to them. That investigation may lead to the arrest of an individual who is suspected of having committed the offence. If the suspect has a learning disability, this is unlikely to have a bearing on how any arrest is carried out (see Murphy & Mason 2007). It might, however, have a bearing on whether the suspect is arrested.

The exercise of discretion by the police

Whatever the suspect's psychological state and capacity, an arrest is only one of several possible outcomes when an offence appears to have been committed by an identifiable individual. Assuming the alleged offence is reported, the police have a substantial degree of discretion in deciding what action to take (see Box 19.2).

> **Box 19.2**
>
> **Potential outcomes other than an arrest include (this is not an exhaustive list):**
>
> - **No further action** taken against the suspect.
> - Police issue **informal warning**.
> - Police deploy **non-judicial criminal punishment** such as fixed penalty notice.
> - Police undertake **civil enforcement** such as anti-social behaviour order (ASBO).
> - Suspect **removed to 'place of safety'** under sections 135 or 136 of Mental Health Act 1983.
> - **Psychiatric assessment** carried out, having been arranged by police, and treatment accordingly put in place.
> - Local agencies, in cooperation with police, introduce or improve **support services** available for suspect, with aim of preventing future offending.
>
> The last three potential outcomes constitute diversion from the criminal justice system.

Factors determining actions taken

A number of factors determine what, if any, action is taken by the police when an offence is believed to have been committed. These factors include the following.

Nature and seriousness of the alleged offence

Whether or not a suspect has a learning disability, the more serious the offence, the more likely it is to be reported, and the more likely the police are to take action following the report. Conversely, if the offence is relatively minor, the police may decide that an arrest and subsequent prosecution is not in the public interest and may take no further action.

Context of the alleged offence

A report by Murphy et al (in press) notes that crimes committed in public places by people with learning disabilities are more likely to be reported than crimes committed in service settings. Research by Lyall et al (1995) and by McBrien & Murphy (2006) found some reluctance among care staff to report crimes committed by people with learning disabilities.

Mental capacity of the offender

Individuals with mild or moderate learning disabilities are more likely to be arrested for an offence than those with more severe learning disabilities. Situations where severely learning disabled suspects come to the attention of the police are relatively unusual. Such individuals are likely to live with carers and have limited ability to go out alone (hence illegal activities would not occur in public). Generally, the milder a learning disability, the more likely that formal action will be taken against a suspect, because the police will be more confident that the suspect can be interviewed and can ultimately be held responsible for his actions.

Caution and legal rights

Individuals who have been arrested have certain rights, which are safeguarded by PACE 1984. In addition to the longstanding right to silence, there are three legal rights which are presented to the suspect in writing in the 'notice of rights and entitlements'; these are:

- right to see a solicitor
- right to have someone told that you are at the police station
- right to look at the police codes of practice (Home Office 2005).

The particular consideration for suspects with learning disabilities is whether they are able to understand and thereby exercise their rights.

The right to silence is expressed in the police caution, which must be given when a suspect is arrested, and at the outset of each police interview:

> You do not have to say anything. But it may harm your defence if you do not mention when questioned something that you later rely on in court. Anything you do say may be given in evidence.
>
> (PACE 1984, Code C, para. 10.5)

Under PACE 1984, minor variations in the wording of the caution are permitted, and "if it appears that a person does not understand the caution, the person giving it should explain it in their own words" (PACE 1984, Code C, notes for guidance 10D).

Research by Clare et al (1998) found limited understanding of the caution not only among the general population and a sample of A-level students, but also among serving police officers – only two-thirds of the officers in the sample provided an adequate explanation of the middle sentence. This clearly suggests that the allowance for officers to explain the caution 'in their own words' may frequently be of little benefit to suspects.

Right to see a solicitor

Section 58 of PACE 1984 gives a detainee the right to consult a solicitor, in private, at any time. Section 6 of PACE 1984, Code C, sets out some of the detail with regard to the right to legal advice. Paragraph 6.8, for example, states that a detainee (with some specified exceptions) "shall be entitled on request to have the solicitor present when they are interviewed".

The critical importance of legal advice to 'mentally disordered' suspects is highlighted by Robertson et al (1996), who argue that the legal rights of such detainees "are best ensured by the presence in the station and at interview of a legal adviser", and that ideally such a person should be a solicitor with experience of working with mentally vulnerable suspects.

Writing more generally about legal advice, Clare (2003:28) notes:

> ... though many criticisms have been made of the competence and effectiveness of legal advisers ... there is overwhelming evidence that suspects who receive such help are less likely to make self-incriminating confessions, and more likely to exercise their right to silence.

Detention at the police station

Following arrest, a suspect must be taken to a police station as soon as is practical. Once there, the suspect can be detained without charge for up to 24 hours in the first instance if the custody officer determines that this is necessary to preserve or obtain evidence relating to the offence (Home Office 2006).The statutory provisions for detainees that have most specific relevance to people with learning disabilities are those relating to medical attention and to the provision of an appropriate adult (AA).

Medical attention

A suspect's identifiable learning disability may or may not, in itself, necessitate clinical attention. Two main issues to be addressed in any medical examination deemed necessary by the custody officer are likely to be whether the detainee is fit to be detained and, if so, whether he is fit to be interviewed. For assessment of fitness for interview, see page 347.

Appropriate adult provision

The role of the appropriate adult (AA), as outlined in Home Office guidance (2003), is:

- to support, advise and assist the detained person, particularly while they are being questioned
- to observe whether the police are acting properly, fairly and with respect for the rights of the detained person and to tell them if they think they are not
- to assist with communication between the detained person and the police
- to ensure that the detained person understands their rights and that they have a role in protecting their rights.

Under PACE 1984, Code C, an AA should be called to the police station if a person who is 'mentally disordered or otherwise mentally vulnerable' has been detained. AAs are also required for detainees under the age of 17. The AA can be a relative or carer of the detainee, an individual with experience of working with mentally disordered or mentally vulnerable people, or any other responsible adult. The AA must not be employed by the police.

Over the past 15 years, extensive research has been conducted into AA provision, which has consistently found provision to be patchy, and that many vulnerable adult detainees do not receive the support of an AA. The shortcomings in AA provision appear to have two main causes:

1. Failures in the identification of vulnerable suspects.
2. Practical problems associated with AA provision.

The failure to identify vulnerable suspects reflects a general absence of routine screening mechanisms and limited awareness training undertaken by the police. The theme of poor identification of vulnerable suspects frequently recurs in both the older and the more recent studies of AA provision (see, for example, Bucke & Brown 1997).

There is no statutory requirement for AA provision. Consequently their availability is patchy – both geographically and at certain times of the day or night – and their effectiveness variable. There is also a lack of awareness on the part of the police of what is available locally (see, for example, Medford et al 2000:19).

Police interview

The police interview with the suspect is very often a critical element of the investigative process. Section 11 of PACE 1984, Code C, contains general provisions relating to the police interview. The particular vulnerability of some suspects in police interviews is explicitly recognised in paragraph 11C:

> Although ... people who are mentally disordered or otherwise mentally vulnerable are often capable of providing reliable evidence, they may, without knowing or wishing to do so, be particularly prone in certain circumstances to provide information that may be unreliable, misleading or self-incriminating.

Therefore, a suspect who is 'mentally disordered or otherwise mentally vulnerable' should only be interviewed in the presence of an appropriate adult (AA). Three further, interlinked issues relating to the police interview are of particular relevance to people with learning disabilities:

1. Assessment of fitness for interview.
2. Interviewing style.
3. Statutory safeguards on the use of confession evidence.

Assessment of fitness for interview

Where a suspect is referred to a health professional because of an apparent physical or mental need or vulnerability, one aim of the medical examination may be to assess the suspect's fitness for interview. Annex G of PACE 1984, Code C, deals specifically with this.

Gudjonsson et al (2000) surveyed a sample of consultant psychiatrists, forensic medical examiners, lawyers and police officers about the psychological factors they considered important in assessing fitness for interview. The factors given the greatest weight were confusion and disorientation, withdrawal from heroin, communication problems, paranoid beliefs and poor understanding of simple questions. Among factors that were not rated highly were apparent suggestibility and eagerness to please. The researchers also found differences of opinion, between and within the different professional groups. This, they argue, suggests that the treatment of potentially vulnerable suspects at police stations is inconsistent – a problem exacerbated by the lack of agreed guidelines on assessment to determine whether a detained suspect is fit to be interviewed. Gudjonsson et al (2000) conclude there is a strong case for development of a clear framework to guide the inevitably complex and challenging process of making these assessments.

Interviewing style

Although, under PACE 1984, police officers are expected to show 'special care' when interviewing a mentally disordered or vulnerable suspect, and the presence of an AA is required in this situation, no specific guidance has been developed with respect to interviewing style. In contrast, Home Office guidance on the interviewing of vulnerable victims and witnesses was developed in the wake of the publication of *Speaking up for Justice* (Home Office 1998) – the publication which led to the establishment of 'special measures' for vulnerable and intimidated witnesses under the Youth Justice and Criminal Evidence Act 1999.

Admissibility of confession evidence

Sections 76–78 of PACE 1984 deal with the admissibility of confession evidence in court – that is, with the circumstances under which evidence in the form of a confession by the suspect can or cannot be used in the case against him. While this issue has more direct relevance to court proceedings than to police investigative work, it has profound implications for police interviewing of suspects with learning disabilities. The exercise of undue pressure on a vulnerable suspect, or the failure to provide the requisite safeguards, such as an AA, when interviewing such a suspect, can lead to a confession being ruled inadmissible.

Disposal

After arresting a suspect and undertaking initial investigative work, the police choose between various courses of action, or 'disposal'. As applies to the initial decision as to whether or not to make an arrest, the police often exercise a considerable degree of discretion in determining the disposal. The major disposal options available to the police are shown in Box 19.3.

The option of diversion is likely to be considered for a suspect who has learning disabilities. Diversion requires collaboration between the police and health and social care agencies. The Home Office circular 66/90 (1990) requires that diversion for mentally disordered offenders be considered before a decision on charging is made, and that mentally disordered offenders should wherever possible receive health and social care as an alternative to being punished by the criminal justice system.

However, the Home Office circular 12/95 (1995) emphasises that: "the existence of mental disorder should never be the only factor considered in reaching a decision about charging. The need to protect the safety of the public may indicate that formal action is needed." (1995:4) Other factors to be taken into consideration may include, for example, whether the incident was an isolated event, the risk to others if it is repeated, and whether it is part of an escalating pattern requiring intervention by the criminal justice system.

See Reader activity 19.2 on the Evolve website.

Box 19.3

Major disposal options

- **Discontinue** investigation because of lack of evidence or because prosecution not believed to be in public interest.
- Release suspect on **police bail** pending further investigation, in expectation that further evidence may be forthcoming.
- Issue **formal caution**, if suspect admits offence and gives informed consent to caution and offence not serious (see DH 2009:37).
- Where sufficient evidence available and prosecution appears in public interest, proceed to **charge**.
- **Divert** away from criminal justice to health and social care.

The criminal courts

Legal and policy framework

There is a general recognition in law that defendants must be able to understand and participate effectively in the criminal proceedings of which they are a part. Two aspects that govern how defendants with learning disabilities, and other vulnerable defendants, are treated are the right to a fair trial and fitness to plead. Another relevant component of the legal framework is that, for a defendant to be convicted, he must not only have committed the criminal act (actus reus) but must also have had a degree of criminal intent or guilty mind (mens rea). If a defendant has learning disabilities, the defence might argue that he lacked mens rea, in which case this question could be addressed by an expert witness.

The right to a fair trial

Article 6 of the European Convention on Human Rights (which was incorporated into British law by the Human Rights Act 1998) sets out the right to a fair trial. It states that everyone charged with a criminal offence should be presumed innocent until proved guilty by law, and establishes five minimum rights for the defendant:

1. To be informed properly, in a language which he or she understands and in detail, of the nature and cause of the accusation against him.
2. To have adequate time and facilities for the preparation of his defence.
3. To defend himself in person or through legal assistance of his own choosing or, if he has not sufficient means to pay for legal assistance, to be given it free when the interests of justice so require.
4. To examine or to have examined witnesses against him and to obtain the attendance and examination of witnesses on his behalf under the same conditions as witnesses against him.
5. To have the free assistance of an interpreter if he cannot understand or speak the language used in court.

The above 'minimum rights' are arguably violated where a defendant's learning disabilities significantly inhibit his understanding and involvement in the trial and where the necessary support is not provided (see Jacobson & Talbot 2009).

Continuing concerns about potential infringement of the right to a fair trial were highlighted by the Joint Committee on Human Rights (JCHR) (2008, para 212).

Fitness to plead

It is a longstanding principle in criminal law in England and Wales that any individual who stands trial "must be capable of contributing to the whole process of his or her trial, starting with entering a plea" (British Psychological Society 2006:68). The HRA 1998 Article 6 enshrinement of the right to a fair trial reinforces this principle. Where there are concerns about a defendant's mental state or capacity, a 'fitness to plead' hearing can be held in the crown court (there is no specific procedure by which fitness to plead can be determined in the magistrates' court). The main criteria used in determining fitness to plead are:

- capacity to plead with understanding
- ability to follow the proceedings
- knowing that a juror can be challenged
- ability to question the evidence
- ability to instruct counsel.

The law on fitness to plead is contained in various statutes, the most recent of which is the Domestic Violence, Crime and Victims Act 2004 (sections 22–25). The prosecution, defence or judge can raise the question of fitness to plead; this is usually done before arraignment. The issue is decided by the judge, without a jury, on the basis of evidence submitted by two or more appropriately qualified medical practitioners.

If a defendant is found to be fit to plead, the case will continue and support may be made available. If a defendant is found to be unfit to plead, a 'trial of the facts' may be held, at which the jury decides whether or not the defendant committed the act or omission of which he has been accused. Under section 24 of the Domestic Violence, Crime and Victims Act 2004, three disposals are available to the court if the jury determines that the accused had committed the act or made the omission: a hospital order under the Mental Health Act; a supervision order which places the individual under the supervision of a social worker or probation officer and may include a treatment requirement; or an absolute discharge.

Concerns have been raised about the broad and somewhat subjective criteria for fitness to plead. The Law Commission has recently launched a review of the current test for determining fitness to plead, noting that the legal principles date back to 1836 when "the science of psychiatry was in its infancy; and that the application of these antiquated rules is becoming increasingly difficult and artificial" (Law Commission 2008).

Box 19.4

How people with learning disabilities described their experiences in court

- *Everyone was talking; I didn't know what was going on.*
- *I just felt sick, you go backwards and forwards. In court, the psychology woman said I was like a kid . . . they said I had learning difficulties.*
- *I couldn't really hear. I couldn't understand, but I said 'yes, whatever' to anything because if I say 'I don't know', they look at me as if I'm thick. Sometimes they tell you two things at once.*
- *They think you can understand because you can speak English.*
- *It was weird. The court was big and there were lots of people, people could just walk in off the streets. I didn't know who they all were.*
- *It was scary because I just see this man and two women sitting on a great big bench and I was in a glass box and there were all these others looking. A man then came over and said he was my solicitor but he was different from the one the night before. I thought to myself, what is going on?*

Appearing in court

The vulnerability of a defendant with learning disabilities can be heightened during court proceedings, as illustrated in *Prisoners' Voices* (Talbot 2008:21) (see, for example, Box 19.4)

Support in the courtroom

Protection and support for vulnerable witnesses in court have been significantly enhanced over the past 10 years. Most notably, Part II of the Youth Justice and Criminal Evidence Act 1999 provides for a range of 'special measures' to assist vulnerable and intimidated witnesses – that is, witnesses who are under 17 or have a mental disorder and/or learning disability, or have a physical disability or disorder. However, Section 16 of this Act made it explicit that these measures were not designed to cover vulnerable defendants.

The fact that vulnerable defendants do not have the same statutory entitlement as vulnerable witnesses to the full range of special measures has been a cause of concern. Hoyano (2001), for example, has argued that this asymmetry of provision could contravene the HRA 1998 Article 6 right to a fair trial.

Perhaps in response to these concerns, some steps have been taken towards the extension of special measures to defendants. Section 47 of the Police and Justice Act 2006 amends the special measures provisions to allow a 'vulnerable accused' aged 18 or over to give evidence to the court by a live television link, where certain conditions are met. Under the provisions of the Coroners and Justice Act 2009, the statutory right to support from an intermediary in court has been extended to vulnerable adult defendants whose ability to give evidence is limited.

The Lord Chief Justice issued a practice direction in April 2007, which outlines a range of measures that should be adopted by the criminal courts, where appropriate, "to assist a vulnerable defendant to understand and participate in ... proceedings" (III.30.3). A vulnerable defendant is defined as one who has a mental disorder (according to the MHA 2007 definition) or "some other significant impairment of intelligence and social function" (III.30.1). The practice direction does not have the force of law, but is, in effect, a set of guidelines for the judiciary. It goes so far as to recommend that *the ordinary trial process should, so far as necessary, be adapted* (III.30.3).

Most of the specific measures recommended by the practice direction (paragraphs III.30.9–III.30.18) are aimed at making the court environment less intimidating for vulnerable defendants. However, in terms of statutory provision, there is no parity between vulnerable witnesses and vulnerable defendants.

Court disposals

A vulnerable adult defendant who is convicted of an offence, and is not diverted from the criminal justice system at this stage through a Mental Health Act disposal, faces the same range of possible disposals as any other adult offender. These include custody and the community order; the community order can be passed for an offence that is not so serious as to make custody unavoidable, but which merits a more severe disposal than, for example, a fine or discharge.

The sentencing decision is often informed by a pre-sentence report (PSR) prepared by a probation officer. The PSR contains information about the offence and the background and circumstances of the offender, and includes recommendations for sentence. However, such information is predicated on the probation officer being informed or recognising that an individual might have learning disabilities, and the availability locally of appropriate sentencing options.

Community order

A community order is a generic community-based penalty, to which one or more conditions or requirements can be attached; it was created by section 177 of the Criminal Justice Act 2003. The range of conditions provides scope for addressing the specific needs of vulnerable defendants. Clearly, if a court is to identify appropriate and effective requirements for a community order, it needs good information both about the individual offender's needs and about the availability of local services. Ideally, conditions should be adapted and/or appropriate support given to ensure they are accessible. In practice, however, this does not always happen. One such example is the requirement that entails the offender's participation in a specified programme targeting his offending behaviour. The court cannot make this requirement unless it is satisfied that the programme is suitable for the offender; but most programmes (including those based in prison as well as in the community) are inaccessible to offenders with learning disabilities because of the complexity of the issues addressed and the level of participation required (see, for example, Beech et al (undated) and Talbot (2007)). For Mental Health Act disposal, refer back to page 344.

> **Reader activity 19.3**
>
> In their report, *A Life Like Any Other? Human Rights of Adults with Learning Disabilities* (2008), the UK Joint Committee on Human Rights expressed concern about the rights of people with learning disabilities in connection with Article 6, the right to a fair trial (paragraph 212).
>
> - Visit a magistrates' court during a criminal hearing: what support do you think a defendant with learning disabilities would need to participate effectively in their own trial?
> - Find out what support is available in your area for defendants with learning disabilities: you can do this by contacting your area's Criminal Justice Liaison and Diversion scheme – if there is one – or, if not, try contacting your local community learning disability services and the learning disability partnership board.
> - Speak to people with learning disabilities who have experience of appearing in court and ask what it was like for them. You may find that very little support, if any, exists; in which case what do you think the main risks and implications are for defendants with learning disabilities?

The National Offender Management Service (NOMS)

Established in April 2008, NOMS incorporates HM Prison Service and the National Probation Service. NOMS is responsible for commissioning and delivering adult offender management services in custody and in the community, and works within a policy and regulatory framework set by the Ministry of Justice. NOMS manages around 260 000 offenders a year on custodial and community sentences. There are 135 prisons, 124 run by the public sector and 11 by private contractors; there are 42 probation boards and trusts (Ministry of Justice 2009). The prison population is rising steadily, and during 2009, overcrowding gave cause for grave concern. Prison capacity is set to increase to 96 000 by 2014 (Ministry of Justice 2009). Learning disability awareness training is not routinely available to either prison or probation staff.

The Prison Service

Legal and policy framework

There are a number of rules, regulations and guidelines by which prisons are run. These are outlined in Prison Service Instructions (PSI) and Prison Service Orders (PSO). PSOs are mandatory instructions and PSIs are short-term instructions or amendments to PSOs. These instructions will apply to prisoners with learning disabilities as they would to any other prisoner; there are, however, some that are particularly relevant. For example, PSO 2855, 'Prisoners with Disabilities', states:

> It is Prison Service policy ... that disabled prisoners are not discriminated against in any aspect of prison life and that equality of opportunity in accessing all parts of prison life, and in particular to address their offending behaviour and be resettled is offered to all prisoners.
>
> (p. 4, issue 241)

The same PSO specifies that a disability liaison officer (DLO), generally a prison officer, should be nominated and given sufficient time to fulfill the responsibilities outlined in the order. However, a review by HM Inspectorate of Prisons found that "two-fifths of DLOs did not feel they had enough time to fulfill their role, with many also reporting a lack of training, funding and support" (HM Inspectorate of Prisons 2009).

Other PSOs and PSIs that may be relevant for prisoners with learning disabilities are:

- PSI 31/2008, 'Allocation of Prisoners with Disabilities'
- PSO 3050, 'Continuity of Healthcare for Prisoners'
- PSO 2700, 'Suicide Prevention and Self-Harm'
- PSO 2750, 'Violence Reduction', which covers bullying.

Prisoners with learning disabilities are generally accommodated alongside other prisoners unless particular concerns, for example a prisoner's personal safety or psychological state, are raised, in which case a prisoner may be isolated for a period in the segregation unit or placed in a special unit for vulnerable prisoners.

Recent guidance from the Department of Health notes that learning disability should not generally be 'medicalised' in prison. The guidance goes on to note that:

> Prisoners with learning disabilities, or other similar conditions, are likely to need additional support and reasonable adjustments to allow them to cope with, and understand, the demands of prison life.
>
> (DH 2010:46)

Prisoner health and social care

From April 2006, responsibility for commissioning prison health services was devolved to primary care trusts (PCTs). Prisoners are entitled to access the same quality and range of health care services as the general public. Primary care and mental health trusts in the area that a prison is located are responsible for the physical and mental health needs of prisoners.

The social care needs of prisoners are the responsibility of the local authority where the prisoner lived prior to arriving into prison or, if the prisoner was of 'no fixed abode', the local authority where the court was located from which the prisoner was sentenced. Determining which local authority is responsible is both time-consuming and confusing; consequently very few demands are placed on such services by prison staff. Where local authorities are involved in providing services, for example via learning disability partnership boards, it is often a locally negotiated arrangement.

For some prisoners with learning disabilities, it may be deemed necessary to transfer them away from prison and into health care under the Mental Health Act 1983 (refer back to Criminal Justice Liaison and Diversion, page 342). Most prisoners with learning disabilities will, however, serve their sentence in prison.

The reality of life in prison for people with learning disabilities

How prison staff identify and support prisoners with learning disabilities was the subject of a report by the Prison Reform Trust (Talbot 2007). A number of important findings emerged from the research, which illustrate graphically the difficulties people with learning disabilities, and those who work with them, face within the prison environment:

> People with learning disabilities are not routinely identified prior to arriving into prison and once in prison face a number of difficulties. They are more likely to be victimised than other prisoners and are unable to access prison information routinely. They are likely to receive inadequate levels of support of varying quality and,

> because of their impairments, will be excluded from certain activities and opportunities. Their exclusion from offending behaviour programmes in particular makes it less likely that their offending behaviour will be addressed and more likely that they will return to prison again and again.
>
> (Talbot 2007:45)

While there were many examples of good practice and prison staff 'going the extra mile', often in difficult situations, the overall picture was bleak.

Further research by the Prison Reform Trust (Talbot 2008) involved interviews with 173 prisoners, 154 of whom were identified by prison staff as having learning disabilities or difficulties. Interviewees were asked about their experiences of life in prison, and for many it was 'hard', 'stressful', 'scary', 'depressing' and 'lonely'. Some said they felt unsafe; others made of it what they could, taking each day as it came and some were ambivalent. A small number had more positive things to say and some said they preferred being 'inside' than 'out':

> Sometimes I feel I am better in here than when I'm out. I rely on my family a lot on the outside, so my family aren't under stress when I'm inside.

Other findings from this research are described below under key headings; all quotes are from prisoners with learning disabilities.

Reading and writing

Prisons are largely 'paper-based' regimes – that is, information is disseminated in writing, for example displayed on notice boards or contained in booklets, and information for individual prisoners is often 'posted' under cell doors. To get things done, a form or 'application' generally has to be filled in, for example choosing meals, getting laundry done and arranging visits from family and friends. For prisoners unable to read or write very well, or at all, life is hard. Most prisoners with learning disabilities said they had difficulties reading prison information and filling in prison forms:

> I know 'a' was sandwiches, so I lived off sandwiches.
>
> I can read some things but not others. I skim over the words that I don't know and then it doesn't make sense to me.

When asked how, if he couldn't read, he knew about prison rules, one prisoner said:

> That's easy. You know the rules when you break the rules.

A number of prisoners had, however, learnt to read in prison and many attended education classes.

Understanding and being understood

Adapting and responding to new situations have a particular resonance for people with learning disabilities. Difficulties such as failure to follow instructions and routines in prison are often viewed as non-compliant or manipulative behaviour and punished accordingly. Prison behaviour deemed disruptive, such as misusing in-cell emergency bells, kicking cell doors and shouting, have been linked to prisoners with learning disabilities (Loucks 2007, Bryan et al 2004). Over two-thirds of interviewees experienced difficulties in verbal comprehension skills, including difficulties understanding certain words and in expressing themselves, and over two-thirds said they had difficulties making themselves understood in prison:

> I muddle up words and that causes problems.
>
> I get depressed when people don't understand me so I leave them alone, but then things don't get done.
>
> They say I don't explain properly, well if they gave me more time I would.

Asking for help

Prisoners were asked if they ever asked for help, and while some did, most didn't like to because they felt 'embarrassed', 'ashamed' or 'stupid'. Some said they did ask for help but that it was hard; sometimes other prisoners or prison staff would help and sometimes not:

> If somebody doesn't help me I'm stuck.
>
> Nobody tells you who can help. You've got to find out and because I can't read or write I can't ask anyone and nobody comes.

Being scared and being bullied

Prisons can be intimidating places for the most confident and capable of prisoners, and being scared and bullied is not something that happens just to prisoners with learning disabilities. Estimates of the prevalence of bullying range from 8% to 57% in adult prisons and the broad range suggests they are inherently vague (Ireland 2002). That said, around two-fifths of interviewees said they had been bullied or that someone had been nasty to them, and slightly less than half said they had been scared:

> I am a bit scared in the shower; someone got raped by eight lads and then two days later he killed himself and that scared me.

Prisoners with learning disabilities were more likely to spend time alone in their cell than other prisoners and have fewer things to do. High numbers had clinically significant depression or anxiety. Liebling (1992) identified prisoners who spent most of their time in their cells 'doing nothing' as being at most risk of suicide while in custody.

They were also the least likely to have a job in prison; to know when their parole or release date was; to be in touch with family and friends; to know what to do if they felt unwell; to know how to make a complaint or to have participated in cognitive behaviour treatment programmes, for example to address their offending behaviour. Not being able to address offending behaviour has particular implications, which may result in prisoners spending longer in prison as a result (see, for example, HM Chief Inspectors of Prisons and Probation (2008), JCHR (2008: para. 215), Talbot (2008)).

Although there were a number of occasions when prisoners spoke warmly of prison staff and other prisoners providing much needed support, the overall picture provided by this research was, once again, bleak.

Support upon release from prison

People with learning disabilities are more likely to reoffend, or to be abused or exploited by others upon release from prison if they do not get an aftercare package of health, housing and community care services (Edgar et al 2008).

People being released from prison have the same entitlement to health, housing and community care services as anyone else, however these rights are often not met. The first step in enforcing prisoners' rights is to have their needs assessed prior to their release from prison. Section 47 of the National Health Service and Community Care Act 1990 requires local authorities to assess the needs of people who appear in need of community care services – this is where prison resettlement officers or probation officers have a role to play. The duty to assess need is triggered when the local authority becomes aware of an individual who might need support, which in the case of a prisoner can come from the prison resettlement unit.

The local authority is the lead and the gateway through which to access support and care services, ideally coordinating with service providers to develop a single integrated care plan.

Additional weight for prisoners' entitlement to assistance is Public Service Agreement (PSA) 16 on socially excluded adults (HM Government 2007). The PSA framework provides a focus for the Government's highest priorities and provides the public and users of services with information with which to hold services to account. PSA 16 sets out a strategy to "increase the proportion of socially excluded adults in settled accommodation and employment, education or training" and identifies four at-risk groups, which include adult offenders under probation supervision and adults with learning disabilities. Although PSA 16 is no guarantee of a home or job, it represents a commitment to increasing support for certain vulnerable groups.

According to PSA 16, the National Offender Management Service expects prison and probation staff to work with commissioners and providers to ensure that offenders' support needs are addressed.

Reader activity 19.4

The governor at your local prison wants to make sure that prisoners with learning and borderline learning disabilities at his prison are identified and receive appropriate support. He has listed a number of areas where he would like input from learning disability services:

- Helping prison staff to recognise when prisoners might have a learning disability.
- Making sure that prisoners with learning disabilities can access prison information, for example prison rules.
- Making prison forms easy to fill in, for example menus for meals and request forms for visitors.
- Ensuring prisoners with learning disabilities know what they should be doing during the day, for example help following routines and knowing where they should be at certain times of the day.
- Preparing a prisoner with learning disabilities for release from prison – what sort of information and/or activities might help to prepare the individual prisoner; which community organisations might be able to help?

Try and develop ideas for discussion. The publications *Positive Practice, Positive Outcomes* (Department of Health 2010) and *Prisoners' Voices* (Talbot 2008:95) may help you. Ideally, invite a member of prison staff, possibly the Disability Liaison Officer, to comment on your plan and to take part in a discussion. You could also ask people with learning disabilities who have experience of being in prison about the sorts of things that might have helped them.

Reader activity 19.5

Refer back to the section in this chapter on the Human Rights Act. Identify where, within this chapter, the different articles listed might apply.

Conclusion

Despite the various legal and policy safeguards described in this chapter, the reality for many people with learning disabilities is that the criminal justice system frequently does not recognise, let alone meet, their particular needs. The lack of routine screening for learning disability, at an early stage in the criminal justice process, and learning disability awareness training for criminal justice staff in large part reflects this. Consequently, people with learning disabilities are unlikely to receive the support of an appropriate adult at the police station and may incriminate themselves during police questioning. In court, their lack of understanding grows as they grapple with opaque court proceedings and legalistic terminology. Once in prison, their situation often goes from bad to worse. Their inability to read or write very well and poor verbal communication skills relegates them to a world of not quite knowing what is going on around them or what is expected of them. They spend more time alone than their peers and have less contact with family and friends. They are more likely to experience high levels of depression and anxiety. They are more vulnerable to ridicule and exploitation. Many will be excluded from programmes to address their offending behaviour, which may mean longer in prison as a result (Talbot 2008).

Lord Bradley's review (Department of Health 2009) has made a number of recommendations which, if put into practice, will make a significant difference to the lives of people with learning disabilities who offend, and of the staff who work with them. While the government must ensure the National Delivery Plan of the Health and Criminal Justice Programme Board (*Improving Health, Supporting Justice*, HM Government 2009) is met, there is much that can be done locally without reliance upon the interventions of central government. Many practitioners – from health, social care and criminal justice agencies – have long known what needs to be done; recent attention to the plight of people with learning disabilities who offend and the two documents cited above provide both clear guidance and the licence to operate.

This chapter has drawn on the work of Jessica Jacobson (Jacobson 2008, Jacobson & Talbot 2009) and Jenny Talbot (Talbot 2007, 2008), which is reproduced with kind permission of the Prison Reform Trust.

References

Beech, A., Oliver, C., Fisher, D., Beckett, R., (undated). STEP 4: The Sex Offender Treatment Programme in prison: addressing the offending behaviour of rapists and sexual murderers. Available at: http://www.hmprisonservice.gov.uk/assets/documents/100013DFSTEP4report(SOTP).doc.

British Psychological Society, 2006. Assessment of capacity in adults: interim guidance for psychologists. British Psychological Society Professional Practice Board, Assessment of Capacity Guidelines Group. British Psychological Society, London.

Bryan, K., Freer, J., Furlong, C., 2004. Speech and language therapy for young people in prison project: third project report. May 2004–October 2004. University of Surrey, Surrey.

Bucke, T., Brown, D., 1997. In police custody: police powers and suspects' rights under the revised PACE codes of practice. Home Office Research Series 174. Home Office, London.

Carson, D., Lindsay, W.R., O'Brien, G., et al., 2010. Referrals into services for offenders with intellectual disabilities: variables predicting community or secure provision. Crim. Behav. Ment. Health 20, 39–50.

Clare, I.C.H., 2003. Psychological vulnerabilities of adults with mild learning disabilities: implications for suspects during police detention and interviewing. Unpublished PhD thesis. Institute of Psychiatry, King's College, London.

Clare, I.C.H., Gudjonsson, G.H., Harari, P.M., 1998. Understanding of the current police caution (England and Wales). Journal of Community and Applied Social Psychology 8, 323–329.

Department of Health, 2009. The Bradley Report: Lord Bradley's review of people with mental health problems or learning disabilities in the criminal justice system. Department of Health, London.

Department of Health, 2010. Positive practice, positive outcomes: a handbook for professionals in the criminal justice system working with offenders with learning disabilities. Department of Health, London.

Department of Health/Home Office, 1992. Review of health and social services for mentally disordered offenders and those requiring similar services ('The Reed Review'). HMSO, London.

Edgar, K., Rickford, D., Talbot, J., 2008. Getting healthcare, housing support, and community care set up for prisoners who will need it on release. Prison Reform Trust, London.

Gudjonsson, G., Clare, I.C.H., Rutter, S., Pearse, J., 1993. Persons at risk during interviews in police custody: the identification of vulnerabilities. The Royal Commission of Criminal Justice, Research Study No. 12. London, HMSO.

Gudjonsson, G.H., Hayes, G.D., Rowlands, P., 2000. Fitness to be interviewed and psychological vulnerability: the views of doctors, lawyers and police officers. The Journal of Forensic Psychiatry 11 (1), 74–92.

HM Chief Inspectors of Prisons and Probation, 2008. The indeterminate sentence for public protection: a thematic review. HMCIP, London.

HM Government, 2007. PSA delivery agreement 16: increase the proportion of socially excluded adults in settled accommodation and employment, education or training. HM Government, HM Treasury, London.

HM Government, 2009. Improving health, supporting justice: the national delivery plan of the Health and Criminal Justice Programme Board. Department of Health, London.

HM Inspectorate of Prisons, 2009. Disablerd prisoners: a short thematic review on the care and support of prisoners with a disability. HM Inspectorate of Prisons, London.

Home Office, 1990. Provision for mentally disordered offenders. Home Office circular 66/90. Home Office, London.

Home Office, 1995. Home Office circular on inter-agency working. Home Office circular 12/95. Home Office, London.

Home Office, 1998. Speaking up for justice: report of the interdepartmental working group on the treatment of vulnerable or intimidated witnesses in the criminal justice system. Home Office, London.

Home Office, 2003. Guidance for appropriate adults. Home Office, London.

Home Office, 2005. Notice of rights and entitlements, issued in accordance with PACE codes of practice. Available at: http://police.homeoffice.gov.uk/news-andpublications/publication/operationalpolicing/notice-of-rights/NOTICES_OF_RIGHTS_ENTITLEMEN.pdf.

Home Office, 2006. Police and Criminal Evidence Act 1984 (s66(1)), Code C: Code of practice for the detention, treatment and questioning of persons by police officers. The Stationery Office, London.

Hoyano, L., 2001. Striking a balance between the rights of defendants and vulnerable witnesses: will special measures directions contravene guarantees of a fair trial? Crim. Law Rev. (December), 948–969.

Ireland, J., 2002. Bullying in prisons. The Psychologist 15 (3), 130–133.

Jacobson, J., 2008. Police responses to suspects with learning disabilities and learning difficulties: a review of policy and practice. Prison Reform Trust, London.

Jacobson, J., Talbot, J., 2009. Vulnerable defendants in the criminal courts: a review of provision for adults and children. Prison Reform Trust, London.

James, D., Farnham, F., Moorey, H., et al., 2002. Outcomes of psychiatric admissions through the courts. RDS Occasional Paper No. 79. The Home Office, London.

Joint Committee on Human Rights (House of Lords, House of Commons), 2008. A life like any other? human rights of adults with learning disabilities. Seventh report of session 2007–08, vol. 1. The Stationery Office, London.

Law Commission, 2008. Unfitness to plead and the insanity defence. Available at: http://www.lawcom.gov.uk/insanity.htm (accessed 25.06.10.).

Liebling, A., 1992. Suicides in prison. Routledge, London.

Lindsay, W.R., Steel, L., Smith, A.H.W., Quinn, K., Allan, R., 2006. A community forensic intellectual disability service: twelve year follow-up of referrals, analysis of referral patterns and assessment of harm reduction. Legal and Criminological Psychology 11, 113–130.

Loucks, N., 2007. Prisoners with learning difficulties and learning disabilities – review of prevalence and associated needs. Prison Reform Trust, London.

Lyall, I., Holland, A.J., Collins, S., 1995. Offending by adults with learning disabilities: identifying need in one health district. Mental Handicap Research 8, 99–109.

McBrien, J., 2003. The intellectually disabled offender: methodological problems in identification. J. Appl. Res. Intellect. Disabil. 16, 95–105.

McBrien, J., Murphy, G., 2006. Police and carers' views on reporting alleged offences by people with intellectual disabilities. Psychology, Crime and Law 12 (2), 127–144.

Mason, J., Murphy, G.H., 2002. Intellectual disability amongst people on probation: prevalence and outcome. J. Intellect. Disabil. Res. 46 (3), 230–238.

Medford, S., Gudjonsson, G., Pearse, J., 2000. The identification of persons at risk in police custody: the use of appropriate adults by the Metropolitan Police. Metropolitan Police Service and King's College, London.

Ministry of Justice, 2009. NOMS annual report and accounts summary 0809. Ministry of Justice, London.

Mottram, P.G., 2007. HMP Liverpool, Styal and Hindley study report. University of Liverpool, Liverpool.

Murphy, G., Mason, J., 2007. People with intellectual disabilities who are at risk of offending. In: Bouras, N., Holt, G. (Eds.), Psychiatric and behavioural disorders in intellectual and developmental disabilities, second ed. Cambridge University Press, Cambridge.

Murphy, G., Shackell, P., (in press). Breaking the cycle: better help for people with learning disabilities at risk of committing offences: a framework for the North-West. North-West Training and Development Team.

Rack, J., 2005. The incidence of hidden disabilities in the prison population. Dyslexia Institute, Egham, Surrey.

Robertson, G., Pearson, R., Gibb, R., 1996. Police interviewing and the use of appropriate adults. The Journal of Forensic Psychiatry 7 (2), 297–309.

Seden, R., 2006. Access to justice for vulnerable defendants. Monthly Journal of the Legal Action Group March.

Strategic Policy Team 2006 Final report of the Strategic Policy Team project on mentally disordered offenders.

Talbot, J., 2007. Identifying and supporting prisoners with learning difficulties and learning disabilities: the views of prison staff. Prison Reform Trust, London.

Talbot, J., 2008. Prisoners' voices: experiences of criminal justice system by prisoners with learning disabilities and difficulties. Prison Reform Trust, London.

Watson, J., 2007. Briefing paper: human rights and offenders with learning difficulties and learning disabilities. Prison Reform Trust, London.

Further reading

This chapter has been adapted from the series of publications from the Prison Reform Trust's *No One Knows* programme, which can be downloaded from http://www.prisonreformtrust.org.uk/nok.

Jacobson, J., 2008. Police responses to suspects with learning disabilities and learning difficulties: a review of policy and practice. Prison Reform Trust, London.

Jacobson, J., Talbot, J., 2009. Vulnerable defendants in the criminal courts: a review of provision for adults and children. Prison Reform Trust, London.

Loucks, N., 2007. Prisoners with learning difficulties and learning disabilities – review of prevalence and associated needs. Prison Reform Trust, London.

Talbot, J., 2007. Identifying and supporting prisoners with learning difficulties and learning disabilities: the views of prison staff. Prison Reform Trust, London.

Talbot, J., 2008. Prisoners' voices: experiences of criminal justice system by prisoners with learning disabilities and difficulties. Prison Reform Trust, London.

Watson, J., 2007. Briefing paper: human rights and offenders with learning difficulties and learning disabilities. Prison Reform Trust, London.

In addition to the above, the following are recommended reading.

Carson, D., Lindsay, W.R., O'Brien, G., et al., 2010. Referrals into services for offenders with intellectual disabilities: variables predicting community or secure provision. Crim. Behav. Ment. Health 20, 39–50.

Department of Health, 2009. The Bradley report: Lord Bradley's review of people with mental health problems or learning disabilities in the criminal justice system. Department of Health, London.

Department of Health, 2010. Positive practice, positive outcomes: a handbook for professionals in the criminal justice system working with offenders with learning disabilities. Department of Health, London.

Useful addresses

Website on the care and treatment of offenders with a learning disability, http://www.ldoffenders.co.uk.

British Institute of Learning Disabilities, http://www.bild.org.uk.

British Psychological Society, http://www.bps.org.uk.

Department of Health – Valuing People Now Team, http://www.valuingpeople.gov.uk.

Foundation for People with Learning Disabilities, http://www.learningdisabilities.org.uk/.

Howard League for Penal Reform, http://www.howardleague.org.

Mencap, http://www.mencap.org.uk.

Nacro, http://www.nacro.org.uk.

National Appropriate Adult Network, http://www.appropriateadult.org.uk.

National Autistic Society, http://www.nas.org.uk.

Prison Reform Trust, http://www.prisonreformtrust.org.uk.

Royal College of Nursing, http://www.rcn.org.uk.

Royal College of Speech and Language Society, http://www.rcslt.org.uk.

Sainsbury Centre for Mental Health, http://www.scmh.org.uk.

Turning Point, http://www.turning-point.co.uk.

Valuing People, http://www.valuingpeople.gov.uk.

See the following for a comprehensive list of helpful contacts and information:

Department of Health, 2010. Positive practice positive outcomes: a handbook for professionals in the criminal justice system working with offenders with learning disabilities. Department of Health, London.

Autism spectrum conditions

20

Tom Berney Lisa Belshaw

CHAPTER CONTENTS

KEY ISSUES

- Our perception of what autism is, what defines it and what causes it is evolving. Diagnosis is a clinical judgement (there is no biological test) and, although most cases have a genetic basis, this appears to vary across families and geographical areas
- There is debate as to whether autism is simply a variation in the range of characteristics that make up the human condition (i.e. autism spectrum condition – ASC) or whether it is a more discrete abnormality that causes a medical disorder (i.e. autism spectrum disorder – ASD)
- Autism tends to be accompanied by other disorders and disabilities making it very difficult for individuals, families and carers to know what to expect and to adjust to it
- There is an increase in the prevalence but this is largely because, with better resources and greater public awareness, more people are being diagnosed. If, over time, there is a real, underlying increase in numbers, it is very small
- Autism covers a wide range of ability and presents a very varied appearance. Common to all its forms are difficulties with coping with people and uncertainty. The importance of sensory issues to the person with ASC has been acknowledged only recently
- Structure and predictability across all areas can reduce stress while a good understanding of the way people with ASC communicate is essential, particularly the frequent difficulty in understanding speech and the relative importance of visual information
- There are many different approaches to treatment; most are based on anecdotal rather than real evidence. The severity of the condition and the limited knowledge about it leaves individuals and families open to exploitation in their search for remedies

Introduction

Our perception of the range of disabilities that make up the autism spectrum is evolving, helped on by research and greater public awareness. The number of scientific papers being published is increasing in an exponential fashion and more professionals are expected to be competent in this field.

This chapter sets out the current concept of autism, what causes it, how it is defined, recognised and some of the approaches that are specific to its management. The limitations of our knowledge leave this fertile ground open to hypothesis and commercial exploitation. Our aim is to give a sufficient introduction to point you at areas that merit further exploration without being too diverted by the more speculative gospels promising relief and cure.

What defines autism?

Specific learning disabilities (as opposed to general learning disabilities) are widespread. They include a variety of difficulties, such as with spelling, mental arithmetic, remembering faces or perhaps some clumsiness but, in most cases, they are so mild or subtle that people are unaware of them or at least they do not interfere with everyday life. In about 5% of the population, the disability is sufficient to require recognition and management. Over the last 60 years we have come to recognise a particular pattern of disabilities that is both sufficiently severe and characteristic as to be identified as autism. This comprises:

1. a real difficulty with reciprocal social relationships (an unwitting unawareness of the needs and views of others which can be misinterpreted as selfishness)
2. difficulties with communication (non-verbal as well as verbal; comprehension as well as expression)
3. poor social imagination (understanding and predicting the behaviour of others; difficulty with 'what if . . .').

This triad of core characteristics has been defined in a variety of ways over time but there is now agreement in identifying a much broader disability, autism spectrum condition (ASC), as part of the yet wider group of 'pervasive developmental disorders'. A fourth criterion is that these characteristics must be present from early childhood, the early onset being an important feature distinguishing it from other disorders, notably schizophrenia. By the 1980s, autism had emerged as one of the most clear-cut biological disorders in psychiatry and yet, the more closely it was examined, the less sharp the definition became. An analogy might be made with looking at the stars in the sky and mapping out constellations; the link between the stars making up Orion's Belt is illusory as it is only from our perspective that we see them as connected to each other. Similarly, when we looked for a particular triad of disabilities, we found it, identifying it as 'autism' and distinguishing it from childhood schizophrenia. However, developmental disabilities come in clusters; the greater your degree of disability, the more specific disabilities you are likely to have. As we widen the definition of ASC, so it becomes clear that an individual will have other disabilities in addition to those making up autism; we speak of comorbid disorder. Further research casts doubt as to whether there is a real link between the disabilities of the triad (Mandy & Skuse 2008, Rapoport et al 2009). However, the diagnosis of autism is useful in identifying a group of people who, among their disabilities, number some which cause them to behave and respond very differently to other people of similar intellectual ability and who need a different approach to help them.

The different disabilities making up this syndrome vary both in their detail and in their intensity. The resultant mix gives a spectrum of disorder which ranges from 'childhood autism' at one extreme, through 'Asperger syndrome' and 'atypical autism', to shade into the wider population, where there is no evidence of biological abnormality (identified as 'neurotypical'). While it has been relatively simple to identify clear-cut, core autism, it is much more difficult to define the position of someone who lies further out, on the fringe of this spectrum; while they might have, for example, only two of the three key disabilities, they may also have other equally severe disabilities such as inattentiveness or tics. It is unclear at what point someone moves from having 'autistic tendencies' (showing itself as some characteristic personality traits), to a 'syndrome' (a recognisable group of symptoms), to a 'disability' (deserving the support of others) or a clear 'disorder' (which interferes substantially with their life) (Fig. 20.1). The distinction is more than semantic for it reflects the extent to which we think that it is up to our society:

- to make adjustments to offset a disability, a normal variation in the human condition (a social model of disability) as against the need
- to treat an individual for a psychiatric disorder (a medical model of disability).

Complicating this picture, autism frequently accompanies a general learning disability; the more severe the degree of disability, the more likely it is that the

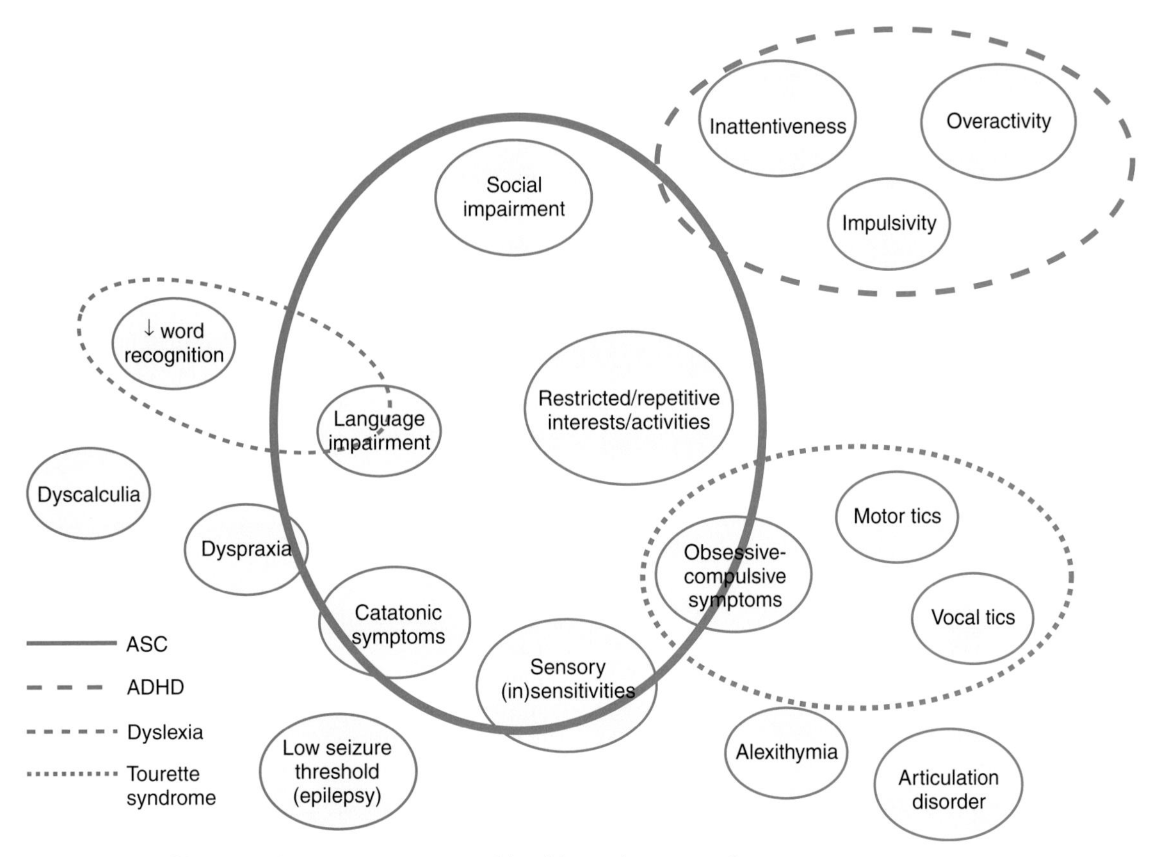

Figure 20.1 • Clusters of symptoms are combined to make up syndromes

person will have autism as well. Still, many people with autism are of normal (or above normal) cognitive ability and, irrespective of their general ability, some will have unusual talents in various cognitive components such as mental arithmetic, dates and memory. The result is that their cognitive profile is jagged, confounding any attempt to categorise their overall ability.

Most attempts to subdivide autism evaporate in the heat of research. The most lasting has been to group people by their social responsiveness into those who are 'aloof', 'passive' or 'active-but-odd' the last group being close to Asperger syndrome.

'Asperger syndrome' was defined as a separate entity in an exploratory move to discover whether those who were of normal ability and with good grammatical speech might have a distinct form of autism. Over time, other characteristics have been proposed as distinguishing Asperger syndrome from the rest of the spectrum. These include the presence of insight, a sense of humour, an interest in social relationships, dyspraxia or a particular cognitive profile; however, none were confirmed on further research. In the end, the lack of any consistent distinguishing characteristic means that Asperger syndrome is likely to disappear from the formal classifications although it will probably live on as a socially useful label, giving an identity to a large group of determined and able people.

The concept of ASC has been developed by a combination of researchers (notably Leo Kanner, Hans Asperger, Lorna Wing, Christopher Gillberg and Michael Rutter) and committees, particularly the World Health Organization (who publish the International Classification of Disease – ICD) (World Health Organization 1992) and the American Psychiatric Association (the Diagnostic and Statistical Manual – DSM) (American Psychiatric Association 1994). The way we see this group of disorders and therefore define and classify them is constantly evolving. This is reflected in successive revisions of the international systems which, at the moment, propose to reduce the defining characteristics from three to two – deficits in social communication, and restricted, repetitive patterns of behaviour, interests or activities. Such shifts in definition mean that the boundary of a particular group will extend and contract over time, including and excluding people on its fringes, obscuring real changes in prevalence and complicating service planning.

The spotlight on diagnosis has put an emphasis on the three areas used as criteria – the triad of impairment – and left all the other characteristics in the shadows. Autism is a much broader disorder than its definitive criteria suggest, affecting the whole body and personality.

Over the last decade we have come to recognise the extent to which problems arise from difficulties in processing and responding to sensory information; so much so that sensory processing disorder (SPD) is now being recognised more formally in diagnostic classifications (Ben-Sasson et al 2009).

Many individuals have difficulties in sensory registration; some will over-register (hypersensitivity) and others under-register (hyposensitivity) sensory stimuli. Individuals can be hypersensitive in one sensory area (e.g. sight) but hyposensitive in another (e.g. smell); some will have fluctuating sensory systems. Most people are sensitive to the sound of chalk on a blackboard or to a baby's cry; however, this hypersensitivity can be painfully distressing in ASC, examples being the flicker of neon lighting, the scratchiness of a woollen jersey, the pungency of a certain perfume or the everyday noise of a street or shop. Unnoticed by those around, these can be severe enough to block listening or thinking and produce agitation and disturbed behaviour. Hyposensitivity might show itself in a lack of awareness of sudden or loud noises, an unusual tolerance of prolonged spinning or an apparent insensitivity to pain with accidental injury passing unnoticed. Sensory abnormalities can occur in any of the seven senses:

1. Visual (sight): includes the perception of movement, colours and particular shapes.
2. Auditory (hearing): includes the ability to analyse and select sounds and the pattern they make so that a song or a baby's cry can be appreciated.
3. Tactile (touch): which can be broken down into information about touch, pressure, temperature, vibration and pain.
4. Vestibular: conveying the sense of balance and movement.
5. Proprioceptive: which, through receptors in muscles and joints, tells us where the parts of our body are in relation to each other and our overall posture.
6. Gustatory (taste): including texture and temperature as well as basic tastes.
7. Olfactory (smell): which also contributes to taste and can also be powerful in awakening memories.

We become aware of and register sensations through the seven senses, balancing the information through modulation. We integrate the information in order to produce an adaptive response to our environment – self-regulation being the nervous system's ability to attain, maintain and change levels of arousal, increasing or reducing our responsiveness to our environment. We can allow ourselves to become more aroused (in terms of alertness) or less aroused to the point of falling asleep using a variety of strategies and activities to alter our levels of alertness. Some activities may be used for both increasing and reducing arousal. For example, chewing gum (a motor oral activity) may be used by some people to help them concentrate and to be more alert or to calm them when they are stressed.

See Reader activity 20.1 on the Evolve website.

Many individuals with ASC have modulation difficulties and some of the behaviours observed may be their attempts to regulate their arousal. Some of the behaviours that might indicate that an individual is trying to regulate their arousal levels include crashing against walls, spinning, biting themselves, masturbating excessively, a spurt of running or chewing their clothing, all forms of behaviour that may be categorised as 'self-stimulatory' and 'without purpose' and result in programmes to extinguish them. It can be more helpful to seek more adaptive ways to adjust their arousal levels such as that described by Temple Grandin who used to seek out deep pressure:

> When I was six, I would wrap myself up in blankets and get under sofa cushions, because the pressure was relaxing.

She developed a squeeze machine that applied pressure to her body and:

> five seconds later I felt a wave of relaxation . . . For an hour afterwards I felt very calm and serene. My constant anxiety had diminished. This was the first time I ever felt comfortable in my own skin.
>
> (Grandin 2006)

Dyspraxia is also associated with ASC, the term becoming extended from describing problems in motor coordination (developmental coordination disorder) to include problems in planning movement. These include difficulties with starting, executing, stopping, combining, sustaining and switching motor actions. Learning new tasks is harder where the processing of information from the tactile, vestibular or proprioceptive systems is impaired. The result affects many areas of the individual's life and may be misinterpreted as a conscious refusal to do something ('they *won't* do it') rather than an inability ('they *can't* do it').

Nor is autism limited to the nervous system; there is no consistent pattern but abnormalities of the immune and autonomic system are frequent while abnormal connective tissue may contribute to problems with joints and heart valves. Gastrointestinal symptoms have been described in anything between 17% and 86% of people with ASC which, besides discomfort, bloating and pain, can range from constipation to diarrhoea (Erickson et al 2005).

Much of the evidence comes from anecdote and case report and may result from other, underlying conditions that can produce autism rather than be symptoms of autism itself. Even when the frequency and intensity of the symptom is defined, there is little information about what might be expected in a comparable neurotypical population. However, the lack of solid research does not hinder the development of fervent belief and charismatically promoted treatment programmes.

Comorbidity

Developmental disabilities, like buses, come in clusters. If someone has autism or a generalised learning disability, they are also more likely to have:

- inattentiveness
- poor impulse control
- overactivity

} the cluster of disabilities that make up attention deficit hyperactivity disorder

- the poor coordination of dyspraxia (developmental coordination disorder)
- tics
- the low seizure threshold that predisposes to epilepsy
- any of many other developmental disabilities.

Psychiatric disorder is more frequent in ASC so that anxiety and/or depression, already common in the general population, occur even more often and are more disabling in this vulnerable group. Is psychosis more likely? People with ASC frequently have difficulty in describing their internal thoughts, emotions and sensations and often fall back on concrete expression. For example, thoughts may be described as voices which the clinician then misinterprets as hallucinations. A person who is unable to describe their feelings, particularly when they also have a fixed facial expression, may be thought to have flattened affect, another potential symptom of schizophrenia. The same impassivity, coupled with an unwitting egocentricity, may lead to the label of dissocial personality disorder.

Overall, people with ASC risk getting an unnecessary psychiatric diagnosis. They are also more likely to have a psychiatric disorder and for it to be missed or misdiagnosed. It has been suggested that 3% of people with Asperger syndrome might develop schizophrenia (Attwood 2007) but this was not confirmed by a follow-up study of 135 people with autism (Hutton et al 2008). Nevertheless, while autism may not predispose to schizophrenia, it is unlikely to protect the individual against it.

A variety of innate behaviours are associated with ASC including sleep problems (particularly an apparent diminished need for sleep), selective feeding and self-injurious behaviour (SIB) (see Ch. 18). The latter, for a number, may stem from a diminished awareness of pain that allows (otherwise normal) self-stimulation to be excessively intense. Greater weight is being given to the problems posed by unusual sensitivity, both increased and decreased, to a variety of stimuli and this is discussed further in the section on sensory integration that deals with their management (below).

The overwhelming need for social care and support (Department of Health 2010) should not overshadow the need for an effective mental health service (Royal College of Psychiatrists 2005).

Developmental change

Starting in early childhood, disabilities change with age and, while the overall tendency is to improve (spurts of improvement are particularly likely in later childhood and early adulthood), symptoms can get worse with adolescence, illness and stress. The last will depend on the setting as, for example, leaving school can be a tremendous relief for some whose difference has been highlighted by teasing and bullying. Others, however, may find the change unwelcome as they go from the predictable certainty of a busy, organised school timetable to the chaotic boredom of unemployment; symptoms improve or intensify accordingly. The result is that behaviour often follows a trajectory typical of many forms of development (Fig. 20.2).

As people with autism get older, they often learn how to cope with (or, at least, hide) their limitations. By adulthood, a mix of growing out of an innate impairment, living in a more tolerant environment and learned compensation, can all combine to transform a clear-cut autism to something more blurred and less disabling. This can make diagnosis in adults difficult, especially if there is no one to describe what the person was like in childhood.

Psychological characteristics

An impaired 'theory of mind' (the ability to recognise that other people might think the way you do), vividly labelled 'mind-blindness', is well known. Although neither specific to ASC nor invariably present, it can explain much of the curious egocentricity in the person's approach to the world and the difficulty in making and maintaining relationships.

'Executive function' is a term for a variety of cognitive functions that include the ability to identify a problem, to work out how to tackle it, then to tackle it, complete it, cope with setbacks and side issues and know when to stop. It involves working memory, impulse control, inhibition and mental flexibility, as well as the initiation and monitoring of action. It is a global concept and, while not specific to ASC, it is a frequent characteristic of developmental disorder in general and often the source of the major difficulties that prevent a person with ASC coping with everyday tasks and with work.

'Weak central coherence' means that, rather than seeing the bigger picture, the individual's mindset tends to see the individual elements, whether looking at a picture or listening to a verbal explanation. Again, as for so many of the characteristics of ASC, not all research studies were able to replicate this. It emerged that the response depended on the instructions as to how the test should be done; given the appropriate directions, people with ASC were able to perform similarly to more neurotypical controls.

The need for a general, stereotypic description of ASC gives a black and white impression that specific abilities are either present or absent. The reality is that, first, an individual's particular ability is less than might be expected *relative* to their age and, second, that both their overall ability and their specific abilities continue to develop over time.

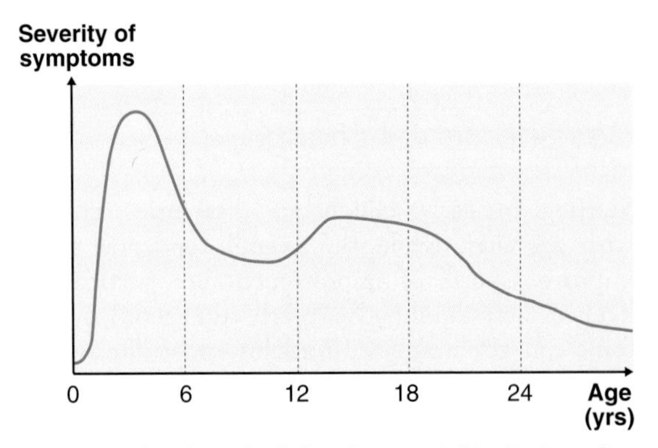

Figure 20.2 • A typical developmental trajectory for someone with ASC

Life with autism spectrum condition

Hidden disability can be more difficult to grow up with than something overt; people are less understanding and individuals sense that, somehow, they are different without knowing how or why. Labels such as 'thick' or 'clumsy' combine with the lack of friends to make people with ASC easy targets to bully and tease. The effect is to erode what self-confidence there is, perpetuating self-isolation and contributing to later underachievement. Unrecognised, the disability is seen as the fault of the individual so that, for example, a wife, initially attracted to the open straightforwardness of her husband, may tire of his lack of intuitive understanding and a failure to respond to her need for romance. In someone less able, episodes of distress may be misinterpreted, being attributed to maladaptive training or communication rather than, for example, to misunderstanding or sensory distress.

The additional disturbance and the non-intuitive responses required make it more stressful to care for a child with ASC compared to a child with a comparable degree of learning disability. Psychiatric conditions are more frequent in the close relatives of people with ASC and are not simply attributable to the stress of looking after them (Daniels et al 2008, Piven & Palmer 1999).

How is autism spectrum condition identified?

With increasing public awareness and readily available lists of alerting characteristics (see Box 20.1), ASC is suspected more frequently; indeed, the label is entering popular use to describe anyone who is slightly unusual.

Diagnosis (as against assessment) requires information that has been gathered systematically so that it can then be matched against the accepted criteria. Whether it comes from questionnaire, rating scale or diagnostic interview, it is important that it is an accurate description of the individual; usually by cross-checking it with a friend or relative who has known the individual for some time and across a number of settings. Box 20.2 provides some examples of diagnostic instruments.

For many, the diagnosis is clear cut. For many more, whose symptoms are less florid, it can be a difficult judgement call, particularly where an adult has settled into a comfortable niche. Here, the clinician needs time to gather sufficient information and to have the background experience of meeting a wide range of people with ASC. There is no laboratory test that helps to determine whether or not someone has ASC; while many physical characteristics have emerged as being associated with ASC, they are of no help to the individual seeking diagnosis or treatment. That someone has a biochemical or physiological abnormality does not mean that it caused their ASC. Unfortunately the lack of solid knowledge has encouraged the growth of laboratories that offer a variety of analyses of doubtful relevance – they suggest tests of blood, hair and urine for a disparate group of metals, amino acids or other metabolites.

Diagnosis is only one element of the broader process of assessment which describes a person, their ability and needs. It also answers the specific questions that led to referral which may, for example, be about the capacity to make a particular decision or the risk of offending.

Box 20.1

Alerting characteristics

Difficulties with social relationships (i.e. social isolation)

- Few or no sustained relationships; those that exist are likely to be either distant or intense.
- Persistent aloofness or awkward interaction with peers (which sometimes may be unduly compliant or passive).
- Unusually egocentric with little concern for others or awareness of their viewpoint and limited empathy or sensitivity.
- Lack of awareness of social rules; prone to social blunders.

Problems in communication

- An odd voice, monotonous and perhaps used at an unusual volume.
- Talking at (rather than to) you with little awareness of your response.
- Language that is superficially good but too formal, stilted or pedantic and with difficulty in catching any meaning other than the literal.
- Limited use of non-verbal expressions so that there is a rather wooden, impassive appearance with few gestures and underused or poorly coordinated gaze. The effect of the last is that the person appears either to be avoiding eye contact (misinterpreted as furtive) or else is looking through you (and appears aggressive).
- An awkward or odd posture and little body language.

Absorbing and narrow interests

- Obsessively pursued interests.
- Unusually circumscribed interests that contribute little to a wider life (for example, collecting facts and objects that have limited practical or social value).
- A set approach to everyday life that may include unusual routines or rituals; change is often upsetting.

What causes autism?

It is clear that autism frequently runs in families; traits, if not the full-blown syndrome, can be seen in parents and siblings. The risk of having a child with ASC is 1% but then the risk of recurrence is at least 3%. An identical twin has a 60% chance of ASC compared to the non-identical twin who is no more likely to have ASC than any other sibling. All this confirms, first, that there is a genetic component to most cases of autism and, second, that the underlying mechanism is complex. Initial studies recognised that there were a number of interacting chromosomal sites but the studies tracking the course of ASC through families homed in on nearly every chromosome; it appeared that the relevant sites might differ for families in different parts of the world, Lately it has been found that ASC is associated with a large number of genetic anomalies, variations in the number of copies of chromosomal material in the

Box 20.2

Some diagnostic Instruments

Questionnaires

- ABC – Autism Behaviour Checklist: a questionnaire to be completed by parents – it has a good statistical basis for identifying ASC in young children (Krug et al 1988).
- AQ – Autism Quotient: a self-report questionnaire giving a summary score that indicates the likelihood of ASC. An effective screening tool from the Autism Research Centre (in Cambridge). Available at: http://www.autismresearchcentre.com/tests/default.asp
- SCQ – Social Communication Questionnaire (previously known as the Autism Screening Questionnaire): a 40-item questionnaire derived from the ADI(R) (see below) and comes in two versions – for people under and over 4 years. It is to be completed by the parent/carer (Chandler et al 2007).
- SRS – Social Responsiveness Scale: a screening questionnaire to be completed by a parent/teacher in less than 20 minutes. It is aimed at young people aged 4–18 years old, grading their behaviour across 65 items to give a total score as well as scoring on five subscales; an adult version is in preparation (Constantino et al 2003).

Interview schedules

All of these are well researched and give numerical scores that can be used in a diagnostic algorithm. Most are complex instruments and require formal training of the user and are complementary to (rather than a replacement for) clinical experience.

- CARS – Childhood Autism Rating Scale: a 15-item scale that organises and grades information gathered from parents, carers and observation. The simplest of the main instruments, it has been updated recently to match the evolving diagnostic criteria (Schopler et al 1988).
- ADI(R) – Autism Diagnostic Interview (Revised): a 96-item interview that takes a developmental history from parents; a substantial part focuses on the presentation in early childhood. It is a diagnostic instrument that only includes items immediately relevant to a diagnosis and takes about 2–3 hours (with an additional 20 minutes for scoring) (Lord et al 1994).
- ADOS-G – Autism Diagnostic Observation Scale (Generic): a subject interview that complements the ADI history (see above). It takes 30–70 minutes (with an additional 20 minutes scoring) and is designed to elicit the symptoms of ASC using a standard kit. Four modules are used to cover the whole range of age and ability (de Bildt et al 2004).
- DISCO – Diagnostic Interview for Social and Communication Disorders: a structured interview that gathers and synthesises information from a variety of informants, including the individual, to give a broad assessment of their developmental disabilities. Favoured for general clinical use, it takes 2–3 hours to administer (Wing et al 2002).
- 3Di – Developmental, Dimensional and Diagnostic Interview: a parent interview that has been developed at Great Ormond Street Hospital for childhood diagnosis. It is briefer than the ADI/ADOS or the DISCO and, using computerised analysis, should take less than an hour (Skuse et al 2004).
- PDD-MRS – a well-validated and reliable structured interview of the carers of people with a learning disability across the whole age range. It is being used as a research tool, particularly in Holland where it was developed (Kraijer & de Bildt 2005).

individual's genome (copy number variations; CNVs), but their exact significance is still unclear (Losh et al 2008).

In about 10% of cases, ASC is secondary to another, underlying medical disorder. While any disorder that disturbs brain function (i.e. causes learning disability) can give rise to ASC, it is particularly likely to occur in tuberous sclerosis (50%) and Fragile X syndrome (20–40%). Poorly controlled epilepsy makes ASC worse and it has been suggested that, occasionally, epilepsy on its own might mimic autism.

The difficulty in saying why a particular person should have developed ASC has left the field open to a wide variety of hypotheses; often assumed to be so self-evident that they must be true. A large number of environmental factors have been proposed to explain an apparent increase in prevalence (Russell et al 2009). At present, it looks as if different mechanisms might operate in different geographical areas and in different families to produce the same common outcome that we recognise as autism (Rutter 2005).

Prevalence

Although there is debate as to whether there has been an increase in the number of people with ASC, it is probable that there has been no substantial change but a steady shift in the way we define, label and view it (Rutter 2005). Everyone is much more aware of ASC and it is more likely now to be

Table 20.1 Prevalence of ASC in 9-year-old children

Overall	1.1%
Normal ability	0.51%
Mild learning disability	0.48%
Moderate/severe learning disability	0.17%

(Baird et al 2006)

Table 20.2 Prevalence of ASC in children and adolescents with a learning disability

All young people with learning disability	8–20%
Mild learning disability	10%
Moderate/severe learning disability	30%

(de Bildt et al 2003)

recognised and diagnosed. We have moved from thinking of autism as a rare condition, occurring in only 0.04% of the population of whom 80% had a substantial learning disability, to seeing ASC as so frequent as to merit its own legislation and specialist services (Department of Health 2010). Recent studies have shown that over 1% of the population has ASC. Of those at school, just over half have a significant learning disability and, the more severe the degree of disability, the more prevalent is ASC (Tables 20.1 and 20.2).

It is less clear what happens as people move into the adult world. The prevalence of ASC is, at 1% of the population living independently, higher than might have been predicted from the childhood studies (Brugha et al 2009). The reason for this discrepancy may be that the population includes a number of people with mild learning disability who, without academic demands, have merged with the general population.

Interventions

Poorly understood, autism offers opportunity for a great range of interventions, many with little to recommend them except the salesman's heartfelt belief in what he has to sell – which probably did work for someone, somewhere, at least once. Interventions variously offer to cure autism, improve the impaired adaptive skills or remove unwanted behaviour. Some treatments target the hypothetical, biological anomalies (medication, diets and supplements) that underlie ASC. It is very difficult to judge how effective an intervention might be for the following reasons:

- Behaviour can change simply because people know they are being studied (the Hawthorne effect); more so if they expect the intervention to be effective (Pygmalion effect). It is difficult and expensive to carry out an objective study in which the individual, those around them and the observers rating the outcome are all unaware as to whether the intervention is being used or not – the requirements of the double-blind trial.
- Even where there is a comparison between two groups, there is the possibility that their allocation has not been random and that any differences are the result of something other than the treatment.
- The symptoms of autism vary over time so any study needs to be long enough to be sure that any change is not simply a natural process that might have happened anyway.
- There is a bias towards only positive results being accepted for publication.

Understanding how ASC affects someone allows us to choose effective interventions. A review found six core components essential to any educational programme (Iovannone et al 2003):

1. Individualised supports and services for individuals and their families.
2. Systematic instruction.
3. Comprehensible and/or structured environments.
4. Specialised curriculum content.
5. A functional approach to problem behaviours.
6. Family involvement.

The first of these points is stressed in the recent English strategy for adult autism (Department of

Reader activity 20.2

Choose a paper reporting a successful intervention. Imagine that it has been handed to you by the parents of someone with ASC; they want to know what you think of it and whether they should get it for their child.

- What would you need to include in your answer?
- How would you decide:
  - whether the programme was likely to help the individual?
  - whether it was worth the cost in time and money?
  - what were its drawbacks?

Health 2010) in its move away from generic planning, based on generalisations about the needs of people with ASC, to an approach that appreciates the abilities and needs of each individual. This means personalised plans to be implemented by services that are sufficiently flexible to accommodate them.

There are many approaches/interventions to draw on in producing such a plan, some with more rigorous evidence to support them than others. The lack of easy, effective treatments opens the door to exploitation in a field that is constantly evolving and dominated by money, miracle cures and enthusiasm. While some charities (such as the National Autistic Society and Research Autism) aim to provide balanced and independent guidance, others promote a particular philosophy.

A key component is the provision of specialist formal education in the areas that most people acquire informally. For example tuition in social skills may need to include training in how to recognise and respond to the viewpoint and feelings of others. Many have to be taught how to understand their own feelings for ASC can bring a lack of both an awareness of the internal state and the language to label it. Teaching this 'emotional literacy' is a specialist task involves both teacher and language therapist, but can be the starting point for learning strategies in emotional management that include both anxiety and anger.

Communication

All individuals with ASC will have some level of difficulty in communication, whether it be their ability to express their needs, to use language in social situations or to understand the language of others; commonly taking the literal meaning of what is said. Some people with autism process auditory information very slowly and need to be given time to respond to a question or request. These communication difficulties are a source of huge frustration and can be a major factor in challenging behaviour. Understanding this gives a guide as to how best to communicate with people on the spectrum (see Box 20.3):

- Use language that is appropriate to the individual's level of understanding.
- Make sure you have their attention. Get them to learn to respond to their name. Even though you are looking and talking to them, do not assume they know this is directed at them.

Box 20.3

Understanding what I'm told

There are some interesting words and it is fascinating how just one word in a sentence can change the whole meaning of that sentence. Even to change an emphasis does that apparently. Here is an example:

- I can't do that ... implies that I can't, but maybe someone else can.
- I can't do that ... implies it is not possible.
- I can't do that ... implies that I can't do that, but may be able to do something else.

I am told that I put an emphasis on the wrong words sometimes and change the meaning when I don't actually want to. This often means that I am misunderstood or misunderstand others.

(Jackson 2002)

- Remember some people find it difficult to listen and look at the speaker at the same time as non-verbal signals can confuse and distract. Don't insist that they look at you.
- Use visual cues (e.g. objects, pictures, symbols or written instruction) to back up verbal communication.
- Keep language brief and clear, focusing on the main message you want to convey rather than lots of woolly, unnecessary language. This becomes even more important when the individual is anxious or distressed.
- Allow extra thinking time so that the individual can process information correctly and repeat the message if necessary. Don't just find different ways of saying the same thing as this can just add to their confusion.
- Use concrete terms, particularly in reference to abstract concepts such as time, and be specific.
- Avoid sarcasm, metaphors or idiosyncratic turns of phrase.
- Be positive when giving instructions. Tell the individual what it is that they should be doing rather than what they should not be doing.

Use of visual supports

We all use, and benefit from, various visual supports; road signs, menus, diaries and shopping lists are just a few which help us to understand the world and to function more easily. Many people with ASC appear

Box 20.4

Thinking visually

I think in pictures. Words are like a second language to me ... when someone speaks to me, his words are instantly translated into pictures ... one of the most profound mysteries of autism has been the remarkable ability of most autistic people to excel at visual spatial skills while performing so poorly at verbal skills.

(Grandin 1995:3)

to be visual learners, more able to process information that comes visually as compared to verbally (Box 20.4).

Visual supports can be objects, photographs, symbols or written words. They are especially useful for people with ASC for the following reasons:

- They help to establish and maintain attention especially where someone is listening selectively. Sometimes people, while apparently attending, are listening to what is happening outside.
- They help someone who has difficulty in filtering out irrelevant information, particularly where there is more information than the person can assimilate and they are struggling to cope with what is important.
- They offset memory problems, for while speech is transient, visual input is more stable. The person can look at visual information for as long as they want and can come back to it as often as required.
- They clarify verbal information.
- They give a structure within which it is easier to understand and accept change.

All people with ASC benefit from some sort of visual support, irrespective of age or ability. What is important is that, whatever aid is used, it is appropriate to the person's specific area of need and that it matches their current level of development.

Augmentative and alternative communication

Augmentative and alternative communication (AAC) is the term used to describe any form of language other than speech that assists a person to communicate. The following are five examples of the ways in which this can be useful to someone with ASC.

Sign language

This comes in a number of different forms, dialects and languages. Irrespective of which is used for someone with ASC, it is worth using a total communication approach, combining speech and sign, so that the same language structure is modelled in two modalities thereby highlighting key word meanings and helping the individual to understand. All of these forms of AAC appear to encourage the development of useful speech.

Picture exchange communication system (PECS)

People are taught to exchange a picture card for a desired item or activity using basic behavioural principles, such as shaping and differential reinforcement. Developed by Frost & Bondy in 1994 for young children with autism who lacked functional speech, it has also proved successful with adolescents and adults.

At first the person is taught to ask for tangible things that they want (e.g. to give a picture in return for the apple) before moving on to more social communicative skills that require them to string together a series of pictures in a 'sentence'. The pictures can be stuck on a board with Velcro® to be used as a vocabulary, sentence or diary. It has the advantage that it requires few complex motor movements on the part of the speaker and does not need the listener to be familiar with an additional language such as sign language. It can be taught relatively rapidly, is portable, suitable for many settings and is relatively inexpensive (Charlop-Christy et al 2002).

Communication cue cards

These are primarily used with individuals who are verbal to remind them what they should do or say and allowing them to become independent of verbal prompts (Fig. 20.3). They are also very useful in enabling someone who is overcome by stressful situations to communicate.

Communication choice boards

Visual supports can be used to help people to make a choice and can help even those with reasonable verbal comprehension and understanding to make up their minds (Fig. 20.4).

Talking Mats

This was developed by Joan Murphy in the late 1990s initially as a means for people with cerebral palsy to express their thoughts and wishes. The framework is based on three sets of picture symbols that are presented to the person:

1. The topic being explored (e.g. activities).
2. The options relating to each topic (e.g. horse riding, swimming, arts and crafts).
3. A visual scale ('happy', 'unhappy' and 'unsure').

The individual might then use the mat to rate how they feel about each of the options within each topic (Fig. 20.5).

Talking Mats is an effective and reliable communication tool for individuals with learning disabilities to express their views (Murphy & Cameron 2008). However, it is also an effective thinking tool, particularly for those that find it difficult to express themselves in words in spite of good verbal and expressive language ability (Bell & Cameron 2007). It takes the pressure off direct interactions and can greatly improve both the quality and the quantity of information given. Its visual format allows individuals to further reflect and alter their views. Talking Mats is also an excellent way of recording a person's thoughts and wishes which can then be used as a central part of a person-centred plan or case conference presentation (Fig. 20.6).

This tool is being used increasingly with individuals with ASC. However, evidence of its effectiveness is still anecdotal and it needs to be subject to objective research.

Figure 20.3 • A cue card used by a middle-aged man with a mild learning disability and ASC who would panic when faced with instructions • It also prevents him from becoming distracted from his work

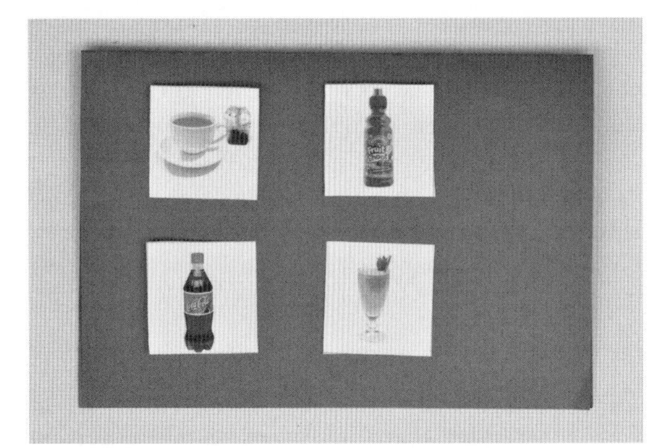

Figure 20.4 • A choice board for a drink

The structured environment

The physical setting

A well structured and supported setting is one of the most effective ways of supporting someone with ASC. Reducing anxiety and challenging behaviour, it allows learning. This is a key component of many recognised programmes including TEACCH (Treatment and Education of Autistic and related Communication-handicapped Children) from the University of North Carolina and SPELL (Structure, Positive (approaches and expectations), Empathy, Low arousal, Links) developed by the National Autistic Society.

HAPPY
(things you like)

UNSURE
(things you are not sure about)

UNHAPPY
(things you do not like)

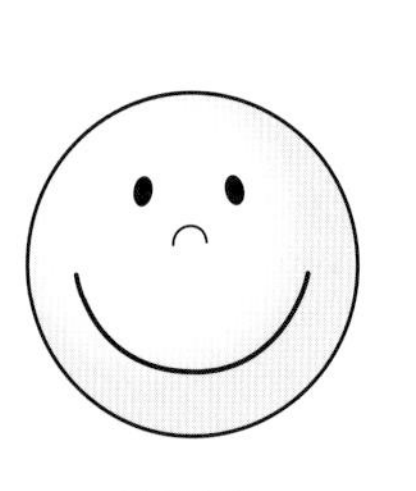

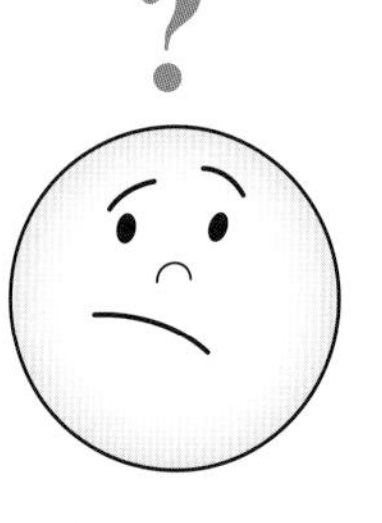

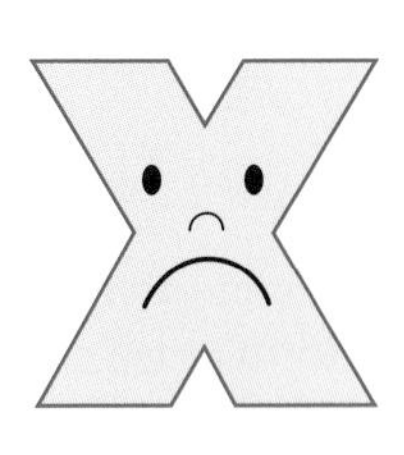

Figure 20.5 • A Talking Mat is built up on this framework

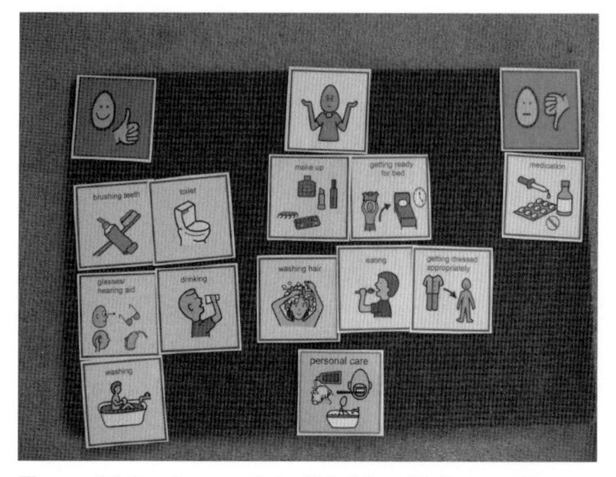

Figure 20.6 • A completed Talking Mat on self-care

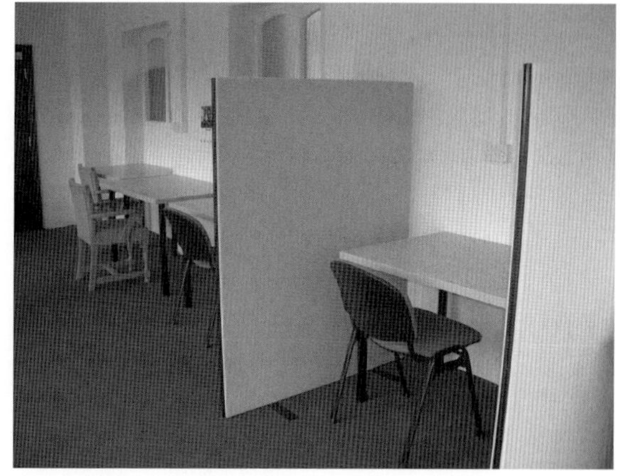

Figure 20.7 • Dividers at a desk where activities are being taught allowing individuals to focus on new and unfamiliar tasks

Distractibility may be an innate part of ASC or part of a co-morbid disorder. The trait will be increased by anxiety and uncertainty and helped by clarity around them including not only the physical layout but also where and how materials are presented. Some individuals need unusually clear, designated areas as, for example, 'this is where I eat', 'this is where I sleep', 'this is where I play', becoming confused and distressed when faced with multi-functional rooms. Sensory distractions must be borne in mind, particularly where the setting is for work or learning. Taking into account the strength of visual information (described earlier), various steps can be taken to create a setting in which people are at their most comfortable and likely to function best:

- A clear, uncluttered, visual environment with well marked and consistent areas and boundaries.
- BLOCK OUT as many distracting sights and sounds as possible. Some may need some form of sensory screen (such as curtains or dividers; Fig. 20.7).
- Mirrors and windows distract.
- Avoid clutter – it too can be very distracting visually.

The temporal setting

Time is an abstract that can be difficult to cope with, particularly if the sense of time is poorly developed. In addition, uncertainty about what the future holds (whether it is the next task or the next day) is distressing. Schedules, in the form of appointment diaries and school timetables, are an everyday tool that can offset these difficulties They help people to understand what will be happening and when; by bringing predictability, they allow people to anticipate events and plan constructively. They can also be used to show that time is passing and where someone is as they progress through their daily programme. In ASC, they are always visual, using physical objects, pictures, text or symbols and covering anything from part of a day to several days or months. For some, they start as simply as 'first this, then that'.

One misconception is that the schedule is a fixed timetable put into visual form and therefore that the sequence of the activities should never change. This reinforces rigidity rather than encouraging people to cope with the change that is, after all, a part of life. The thrust should be towards learning to depend on the schedule rather than on the routine of activities. Used this way, the schedule becomes a means by which people can forewarn the individual about a change and enable a mutually satisfactory programme to be negotiated with them (Fig. 20.8). Although it is sometimes assumed that it is a tool to be used mainly with people of lower ability, it has been shown also to improve the independence of people of normal ability within mainstream settings (Bryan & Gast 2000).

Work systems

Using all of these principles, Eric Schopler and Division TEACCH in North Carolina have developed a system that allows people with ASC to make the most of their ability to function independently. Their work systems guide the individual across a wide range of activities and settings that might include, for example, their work area, bedroom, bathroom, kitchen and dining room (Fig. 20.9).

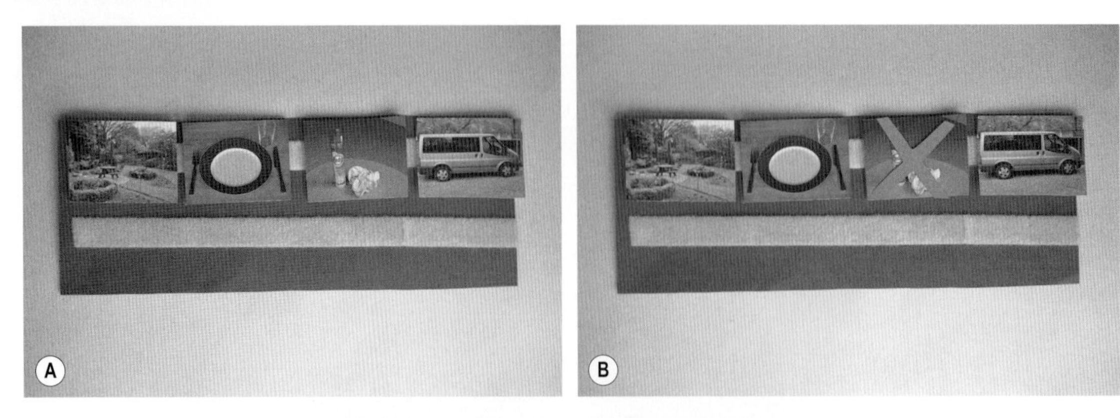

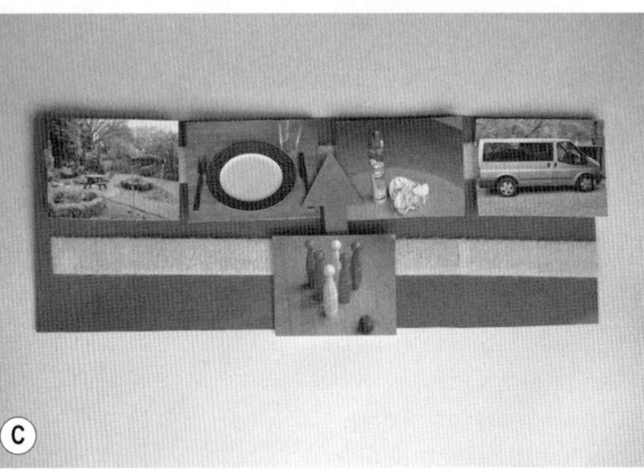

Figure 20.8 • (A) A photograph schedule (B) A change system where an activity has been cancelled (C) A change system where an activity has been added

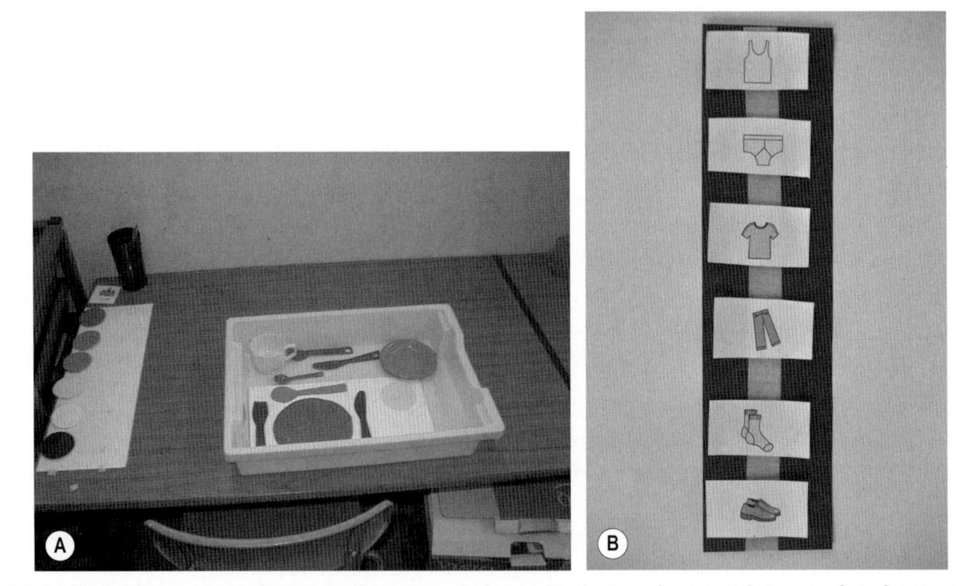

Figure 20.9 • (A) A work system that uses the person's love of colours; she completes each colour-coded task in turn (B) A work system used by an adult to get dressed in the morning. He has organisational and sequencing problems

Continued

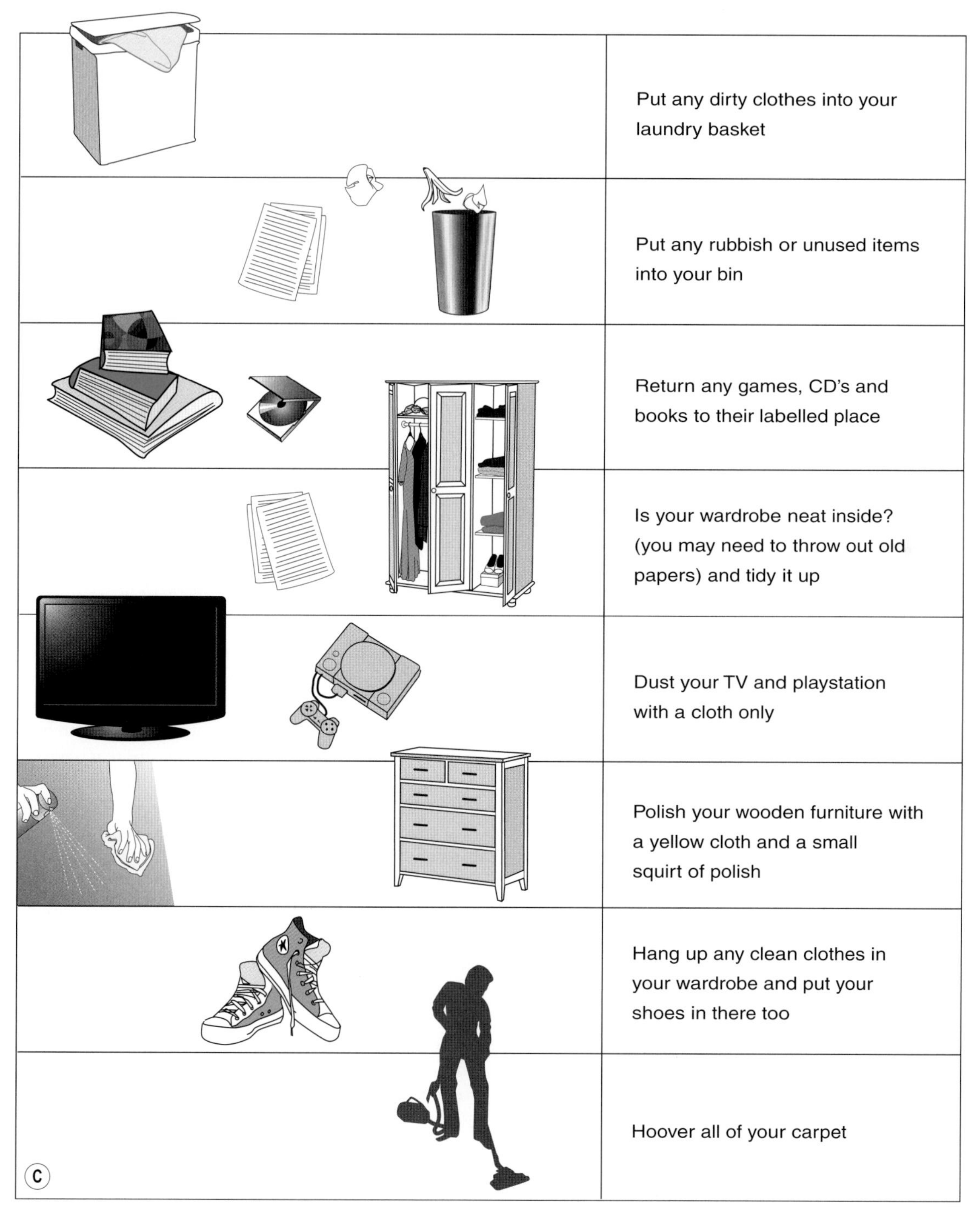

Figure 20.9—cont'd • (C) A work system for room cleaning used by an able individual who lives in a small residential home. • The staff supporting him each had different ideas of what constituted a room clean so it was different each time. Bringing clarity and consistency, the work system helped the individual become more autonomous.

Task organisation

TEACCH uses 'task organisation' to help people with ASC where they have limited organisation and sequencing skills and difficulty in combining and integrating ideas. Tasks are presented visually to show the different components of a task in order. People differ in the amount of structure they need, ranging from a simple written list to a very structured 'shoebox task'. 'Shoebox tasks' visually highlight the relevant details and are constructed as one unit to enable an individual to focus on the intended activity. What is expected is very clear as are the start and finish points (Figs 20.10 and 20.11).

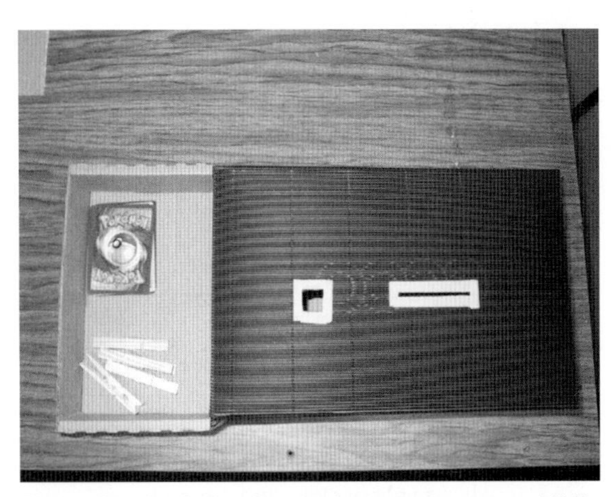

Figure 20.10 • A shoebox task to encourage a child's development of sorting skills engaging him by using his major interest, Pokémon

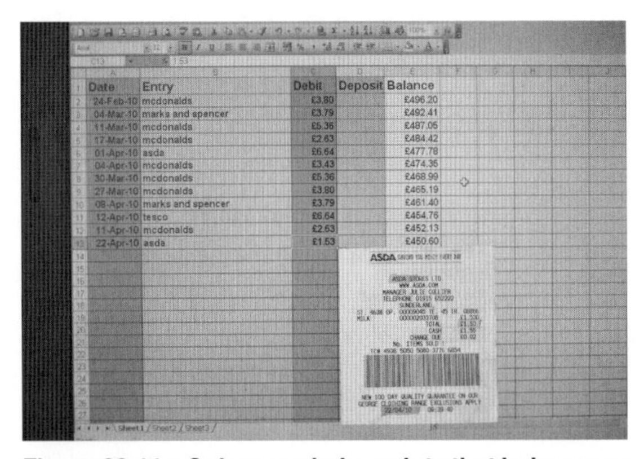

Date	Entry	Debit	Deposit	Balance
24-Feb-10	mcdonalds	£3.80		£496.20
04-Mar-10	marks and spencer	£3.79		£492.41
11-Mar-10	mcdonalds	£5.36		£487.05
17-Mar-10	mcdonalds	£2.63		£484.42
01-Apr-10	asda	£6.64		£477.78
04-Apr-10	mcdonalds	£3.43		£474.35
30-Mar-10	mcdonalds	£5.36		£468.99
27-Mar-10	mcdonalds	£3.80		£465.19
08-Apr-10	marks and spencer	£3.79		£461.40
12-Apr-10	tesco	£6.64		£454.76
11-Apr-10	mcdonalds	£2.63		£452.13
22-Apr-10	asda	£1.53		£450.60

Figure 20.11 • Colour-coded receipts that help a man to keep petty cash accounts

> **Reader activity 20.3**
>
> Samuel is a 26-year-old man with ASD who has recently moved into a small residential home. Staff report that he is constantly asking what is happening and when. He also finds even small changes in his timetable difficult to cope with.
>
> The house is very homely but a little cluttered. The dining room is such a lovely large sunny room that it is used for many different activities, even though there are two other rooms that they could use as well.
>
> - What might you recommend is done to help Samuel understand what is happening better? What systems might you put in place?
> - What environmental changes might you consider?

Intensive interaction

Contrasting with behavioural approaches that aim to teach, train or direct the person with ASC are the approaches that are based on following the individual's lead and seek to enter their world on their terms. The worker copies and follows the actions of the individual in order to build a relationship, treating all their actions as communicative. Used with people who have little functional communication, often having a severe learning disability in addition to their ASC, it focuses on the quality of the interaction itself rather than on a task or outcome (refer to Ch. 6). This approach developed in the UK as 'Intensive Interaction' and in the USA as 'Floortime' (Greenspan 2007) as well as being a central theme of the Son-Rise Program (Autism Treatment Center of America 2008).

It has been questioned whether this is an appropriate approach for people whose social impairment has an innate, biological basis. However, behaviour is the outcome of continuous interaction between innate elements and environmental factors. The real issue is whether this is an effective way of developing a relationship and communication. Here it is important to recognise that there is an effect on both parties, not just the person with ASC. So far, the published evidence of success is limited to a few careful case reports which indicate a fairly global effectiveness (Nind 1999).

Social Stories

These were developed by Carol Gray who recognised that people assimilated ideas more readily when they were given in the form of a story (Gray & Garand

1993). The story is simple, very concrete and gives the student a model of how to think about a very specific piece of social behaviour. Choosing an issue specific to that person, the story is made up of clear, concise and accurate information about that social situation, what is happening, why it is happening and what the typical response might be. The aim is to improve not just behaviour but also the person's understanding of social rules and their basis. Writing a social story first needs the author to make a close study of the piece of behaviour that is to be reinforced or changed. While there is clear guidance and tuition on how to compose Social Stories, they also need practice and experience.

Over the last 20 years, this style of presenting ideas and rules has been successful in helping people with ASC to increase their social understanding and, as a result of this, their social behaviour (Attwood 2007). Like many of the other techniques developed for use with children, it has proved equally successful with adolescents and adults and, while much of the evidence of its effectiveness has been anecdotal, more rigourous research is starting to emerge in its support (Rowe 1999).

See Reader activity 20.4 on the Evolve website.

Sensory Integration Therapy

Sensory Integration Therapy was first developed by Jean Ayres in the late 1960s who attempted to explain the processes by which an individual takes in and responds to the world around them. Her intervention was designed to assist those that have difficulty with sensory processing to organise the sensations from their body and environment better, allowing them to function more effectively. She sought adaptive strategies that would offset difficulties with modulation and the regulation of arousal. For example, she used proprioceptive input and deep pressure for their calming and organising effect on the nervous system, finding that they improved attention and reduced the need for self-stimulatory behaviours.

The concept of a 'sensory diet' has been developed to describe a regular, scheduled set of sensory activities designed for an individual to maintain a level of arousal that is just right for their circumstances. It includes identifying those avoidable activities and sensory environments that trigger negative responses from the individual. Awareness of an individual's sensory sensitivities and preferences can mean that some quite simple environmental modifications can be made that can have quite a dramatic effect for an individual. For example, a sensory diet might include carrying heavy items, swimming and running, pushing a wheelbarrow, digging the garden and pounding clay/Play Dough (Yack et al 2003). Weighted vests and blankets also provide this input and there has been an increase in evidence recently to support their use, with surveys reporting a reduction in repetitive and negative behaviour as well as improved attention (Fertel-Daly et al 2001, Mullen et al 2008, Olson & Moulton 2004).

For those with motor planning difficulties, some strategies that have been found to help are repeated practising of the task, the use of visual cues or talking oneself through the sequence (Box 20.5).

Medication

There is no autism-specific medication available and, so far, what research-based evidence there is comes from the use of medication in childhood. What are open to treatment with medication are all the other disorders that can coexist with ASC and which make the symptoms more pronounced, whether anti-biotics for tonsillitis, anti-histamines for hay fever or a drug to treat anxiety or depression. Anxiety appears to be helped particularly by those drugs that improve serotonin transmission, both the newer antidepressants and the atypical neuroleptics such as risperidone and olanzepine. The risk is that medication may be overused to control disruptive and violent behaviour, assuming that it stems from anxiety. Its adverse effects, often unrecognised, include sedation, obesity and abnormal movements and occur both immediately and in the longer term. It is essential that, whatever medication is prescribed, there is someone who asks constantly whether it is still necessary or, at least, whether a lower dose might work as well.

While it is important to identify and treat additional medical difficulties such as epilepsy, depression and attention deficit, this should be only one part of a wider coordinated approach that includes psychological therapies, education and environmental change (Erickson et al 2007, Myers et al 2007).

Many biological treatments are strongly sold by evangelical advocates, many depending on their pet treatment for their income, to families who feel that,

Box 20.5

The use of a sensory programme

A 17-year-old young man with ASC, severe learning disabilities and no useful speech lives in residential care. The staff, struggling to manage his bouts of extreme overactivity and self-injury, referred him to an occupational therapist for a sensory assessment.

This suggested that he had hyporeactive vestibular and proprioceptive systems; the sensations he was registering were insufficient and, through his disturbed behaviour, he was seeking to increase this input. The staff, concerned that he would become overaroused, blocked this sensory seeking leaving him unable to obtain the stimulus he required to self-regulate and calm himself. This, in turn, led him to try harder, becoming disorganised and overaroused. He appeared to shift abruptly from under- to overarousal. His environment was often unstructured and unpredictable.

The remedy included staff education, the introduction of a sensory diet and modifications to his environment:

- Staff training focused on the ability of motor activities to alter arousal levels as well as the effect of deep pressure and proprioceptive activities on the central nervous system; the basis of self-regulation.
- The sensory diet used a rocking chair, fidget toys and vibrating pillows as well as activities such as tug of war, walking carrying a back pack, sucking thick liquid through straws or from sports bottles, and swimming. As he flipped easily from under- to overarousal, activities that were more likely to alert him, such as spinning and arrhythmic movements, were avoided.
- Environmental modification provided more predictability together with a structured visual timetable. Central were structured sessions within a separate classroom and elimination of long periods of time in the kitchen where much of his self-injurious and overactive behaviour occurred. Classroom activities were structured in a clear and visual way using shoebox tasks. Proprioceptive activities were scheduled prior to work activities to help him organise and calm himself.

Within a month there was less self-injury and he was measurably more able to attend and to engage in table-top activities.

in the absence of anything else, there is little to be lost and much to be gained. The sheer variety of remedies testifies to the lack of any all-round winner. In their time, there was strong evidence of the effectiveness of both fenfluramine and secretin only for it to evaporate in the heat of more rigorous research methodology. What did emerge from the secretin trials (where saline was as effective as secretin) was the power of a placebo (which presumably altered the way the family behaved towards the individual) as well as the difficulty of measuring outcome in a condition such as autism which fluctuates from day to day.

Conclusion

While ASC is frequent in the general population, it is even more so in those with a learning disability adding an extra layer of disability that has to be recognised and managed in its own right. If missed, it blocks the more standard approaches to learning disability, leaving not just the individual but also their family and professionals thwarted and disheartened. It is an exciting time across the whole of the United Kingdom, as new strategies are developing both to identify people and to provide more effective support.

References

American Psychiatric Association, 1994. Diagnostic and Statistical Manual of Mental Disorders (DSM-IV). American Psychiatric Association, Washington, DC.

Attwood, T., 2007. The complete guide to Asperger's syndrome. Jessica Kingsley, London.

Autism Treatment Center of America, 2008. Son-Rise Program. Available at: http://www.autismtreatmentcenter.org/.

Baird, G., Simonoff, E., Pickles, A., et al., 2006. Prevalence of disorders of the autism spectrum in a population cohort of children in South Thames: the Special Needs and Autism Project (SNAP). Lancet 368, 210–215.

Bell, D., Cameron, L., 2007. From dare I say ...? to I dare say: a case example illustrating the extension of the use of Talking Mats to people with learning disabilities who are able to speak well but unwilling to do so. British Journal of Learning Disabilities 36, 122–127.

Ben-Sasson, A., Hen, L., Fluss, R., et al., 2009. A meta-analysis of sensory modulation symptoms in individuals with autism spectrum disorders. J. Autism Dev. Disord. 39, 1–11.

Brugha, T., Mcmanus, S., Meltzer, H., et al., 2009. Autism spectrum disorders in adults living in households throughout England: report from the Adult Psychiatric

Morbidity Survey 2007. A survey carried out for the NHS Information Centre for health and social care by the National Centre for Social Research, the Department of Health Sciences, University of Leicester, and the Autism Research Centre. University of Cambridge, London.

Bryan, L.C., Gast, D.L., 2000. Teaching on-task and on-schedule behaviors to high-functioning children with autism via picture activity schedules. J. Autism Dev. Disord. 30, 553–567.

Chandler, S., Charman, T., Baird, G., et al., 2007. Validation of the social communication questionnaire in a population cohort of children with autism spectrum disorders. J. Am. Acad. Child Adolesc. Psychiatry 46, 1324–1332.

Charlop-Christy, M.H., Carpenter, M., Le, L., LeBlanc, L.A., Kellet, K., 2002. Using the picture exchange communication system (PECS) with children with autism: assessment of PECS acquisition, speech, social-communicative behavior, and problem behavior. J. Appl. Behav. Anal. 35, 213–231.

Constantino, J.N., Davis, S.A., Todd, R.D., et al., 2003. Validation of a brief quantitative measure of autistic traits: comparison of the social responsiveness scale with the autism diagnostic interview – revised. J. Autism Dev. Disord. 33, 427–433.

Daniels, J.L., Forssen, U., Hultman, C. M., et al., 2008. Parental psychiatric disorders associated with autism spectrum disorders in the offspring. Pediatrics 121, e1357–e1362.

de Bildt, A., Sytema, S., Ketelaars, C., et al., 2003. Measuring pervasive developmental disorders in children and adolescents with mental retardation: a comparison of two screening instruments used in a study of the total mentally retarded population from a designated area. J. Autism Dev. Disord. 33, 595–605.

de Bildt, A., Sytema, S., Ketelaars, C., et al., 2004. Interrelationship between Autism Diagnostic Observation Schedule-Generic (ADOS-G), Autism Diagnostic Interview-Revised (ADI-R), and the Diagnostic and Statistical Manual of Mental Disorders (DSM-IV-TR) classification in children and adolescents with mental retardation. J. Autism Dev. Disord. 34, 129–137.

Department of Health, 2010. Fulfilling and rewarding lives. The strategy for adults with autism in England (2010). Department of Health, London.

Erickson, C.A., Posey, D.J., Stigler, K.A., Mcdougle, C.J., 2007. Pharmacotherapy of autism and related disorders. Psychiatric Annals 37, 490–500.

Erickson, C.A., Stigler, K.A., Corkins, M.R., et al., 2005. Gastrointestinal factors in autistic disorder: a critical review. J. Autism Dev. Disord. 35, 713–727.

Fertel-Daly, D., Bedell, G., Hinojosa, J., 2001. Effects of a weighted vest on attention to task and self-stimulatory behaviors in preschoolers with pervasive developmental disorders. Am. J. Occup. Ther. 55, 629–640.

Grandin, T., 1995. Thinking in Pictures. Vintage Press (Division of Random House), New York, p. 3.

Grandin, T., 2006. Thinking in pictures: and other reports from my life with autism. Bloomsbury, London, pp. 58–59.

Gray, C.A., Garand, J.D., 1993. Social stories: improving responses of students with autism with accurate social information. Focus on Autistic Behavior 8, 1–10.

Greenspan, S., 2007. Initiative: a floortime essential and a must for children's emotional and intellectual growth. Interdisciplinary Council on Developmental and Learning Disorders (ICDL), Bethesda MD. http://www.icdl.com

Hutton, J., Goode, S., Murphy, M., le-Couteur, A., Rutter, M., 2008. New-onset psychiatric disorders in individuals with autism. Autism 12, 373–390.

Iovannone, R., Dunlap, G., Huber, H., Kincaid, D., 2003. Effective educational practices for students with autism spectrum disorders. Focus on Autism and Other Developmental Disabilities 18, 150–165.

Jackson, L., 2002. Freaks, geeks and Asperger syndrome: A user guide to adolescence. Jessica Kingsley, London.

Kraijer, D., de Bildt, A., 2005. The PDD-MRS: an instrument for identification of autism spectrum disorders in persons with mental retardation. J. Autism Dev. Disord. 35, 499–513.

Krug, D.A., Arick, J.R., Almond, P.J., 1988. The autism behavior checklist. ASIEP Education Company, Portland, OR.

Lord, C., Rutter, M., le-Couteur, A., 1994. Autism Diagnostic Interview-Revised: a revised version of a diagnostic interview for caregivers of individuals with possible pervasive developmental disorders. J. Autism Dev. Disord. 24, 659–685.

Losh, M., Sullivan, P.F., Trembath, D., Piven, J., 2008. Current developments in the genetics of autism: from phenome to genome. J. Neuropathol. Exp. Neurol. 67, 829–837.

Mandy, W.P.L., Skuse, D.H., 2008. Research review: what is the association between the social-communication element of autism and repetitive interests, behaviours and activities? J. Child Psychol. Psychiatry 49, 795–808.

Mullen, B., Champagne, T., Krishnamurty, S., Dickson, D., Gao, R.X., 2008. Exploring the safety and therapeutic effects of deep pressure stimulation using a weighted blanket. Occupational Therapy in Mental Health 24, 65–89.

Murphy, J., Cameron, L., 2008. The effectiveness of Talking Mats with people with intellectual disability. British Journal of Learning Disabilities 36, 232–241.

Myers, S.M., Johnson, C.P., Council on Children with Disabilities, 2007. Management of children with autism spectrum disorders. Pediatrics 120, 1162–1182.

Nind, M., 1999. Intensive Interaction and autism: a useful approach? British Journal of Special Education 26, 96–102.

Olson, L.J., Moulton, H.J., 2004. Use of weighted vests in pediatric occupational therapy practice. Phys. Occup. Ther. Pediatr. 24, 45–60.

Piven, J., Palmer, P., 1999. Psychiatric disorder and the broad autism phenotype: evidence from a family study of multiple-incidence autism families. Am. J. Psychiatry 156, 557–563.

Rapoport, J., Chavez, A., Greenstein, D., Addington, A., Gogtay, N., 2009. Autism spectrum disorders and childhood-onset schizophrenia: clinical and biological contributions to a relation revisited. J. Am. Acad. Child Adolesc. Psychiatry 48, 10–18.

Rowe, C., 1999. Do Social Stories benefit children with autism in mainstream primary schools? British Journal of Special Education 16, 12–14.

Royal College of Psychiatrists, 2005. Psychiatric services for adolescents and adults with Asperger syndrome and other autistic-spectrum disorders. Royal College of Psychiatrists, London.

Russell, G., Kelly, S., Golding, J., 2009. A qualitative analysis of lay beliefs about the aetiology and prevalence of autistic spectrum disorders. Child Care Health Dev. 36, 431–436.

Rutter, M., 2005. Incidence of autism spectrum disorders: changes over time and their meaning. Acta Paediatr. 94, 2–15.

Schopler, E., Van Bourgondien, M.E., Wellman, G.J., Love, S.R., 2010. The Childhood Autism Rating Scale-Second Edition (CARS2). Western Psychological Services, Los Angeles.

Skuse, D., Warrington, R., Bishop, D., et al., 2004. The developmental, dimensional and diagnostic interview (3Di): a novel computerized assessment for autism spectrum disorders. J. Am. Acad. Child Adolesc. Psychiatry 43, 548–558.

Wing, L., Leekam, S.R., Libby, S.J., Gould, J., Larcombe, M., 2002. The Diagnostic Interview for Social and Communication Disorders: background, inter-rater reliability and clinical use. J. Child. Psychol. Psychiatry 43, 307–325.

World Health Organization, 1992. The ICD-10 classification of mental and behavioural disorders: clinical descriptions and diagnostic guidelines. World Health Organization, Geneva.

Yack, E., Aquilla, P., Sutton, S., 2003. Building bridges through sensory integration: therapy for children with autism and other pervasive developmental disorders. Sensory Resources, Las Vegas.

Useful addresses

There are websites covering most aspects of ASC. Some of those that are more reliable are the following.

The National Autistic Society: http://www.nas.org.uk/ is the largest representative charity in the UK. It reviews a number of approaches at: http://www.autism. org.uk/living-with-autism/approaches-therapies-and-interventions.aspx

Research autism: http://www.researchautism.net provides an objective and up-to-date database.

The Autism Society of America: http://www.autisticsociety.org/index.php

The Texas Autism Resource Guide for Effective teaching (TARGET): http://www.txautism.net/manual.html

The web has more detail about specific approaches for:

TEACCH: http://www.teacch.com/

SPELL: http://www.autism.org.uk/en-gb/living-with-autism/approaches-therapies-and-interventions/service-based-interventions/spell.aspx

Shoebox tasks: http://www.shoeboxtasks.com

An example of a sensory checklist: http://www.sensory-processing-disorder.com/sensory-processing-disorder-checklist.html

Intensive Interaction: a factsheet from BILD at: http://www.bild.org.uk/pdfs/05faqs/ii.pdf

The UK Autism Strategy: http://www.autism.org.uk/dhstrategy

Section 4

Facilitating transition across the lifespan

Working with people to make choices

21

Simon Duffy

CHAPTER CONTENTS

KEY ISSUES

- People with learning disabilities often find that they are not supported to make choices for themselves
- Even people with profound learning disabilities can be supported in ways which enable them to have choice, control and a life shaped to fit their preferences
- Professionals need to support people with learning disabilities to be full and active citizens
- Citizenship provides a useful framework both for understanding why choice is important and what choices are central to a fulfilling life
- Professionals need to understand the full range of options available to enable people to have authority, direction, money, a home, support and the chance to contribute to the community

Introduction

Choice is important to all of us; and although our own ability to make choices may seem very modest, it is still enough to help us achieve a certain accommodation in the world. We use our choices to find a way of living within the world and have a life worth living. But people with learning disabilities often do not have even this limited power of choice. Too often people find that either they are given no choice or choices that are pre-packaged and highly limited. Moreover, many of the most important kinds of options, the options that will enable someone to build a decent life for themselves, are never explored.

In this chapter I will explore the value of choice, why it is important, how we can help people make choices and describe some of the dimensions of choice that people need to face as they grow into adult life and become full citizens. In the chapters that follow, you can explore these matters in more detail; but in this chapter I hope to explain why these choices are important.

Barriers to choice

Some of the barriers that people face in obtaining choice flow from the real nature of someone's disability: for example, there are real issues of mental capacity. A decision to buy a house is important and it has many long-term consequences. A lawyer will have to be confident that someone making such a decision 'knows what they are doing' and this may require people to think about many different factors and balance them. However, as we will see below, there are also practical solutions to this problem and we can support people with their decisions or get a suitable representative if necessary. Mental capacity is not the most fundamental barrier to enabling people to have choice.

Sometimes it may be fear, ignorance or prejudice that limit choice. Negative stereotypes about people with learning disabilities may lead someone to assume that people don't value making their own decisions or can see no difference between the available options. But this cannot be the main explanation; for anyone who really knows people with learning disabilities will be less likely to have those kinds of prejudices, while strangers, however strong their prejudices, will rarely have much direct influence on someone's ability to make choices.

In fact, it seems that it is often the caring relationship itself that can lead to people being denied choice. This may seem paradoxical and challenging; but there are several reasons why being in a caring relationship with someone else can lead to you limiting their choice or control.

Our thinking about care

The term 'care' is derived from the Norse and Germanic terms for grief and the death bed. Also, when we use 'care' as a verb, it is clear that there is no implication of any activity or consent on the part of the person who is cared for; they are passive. In fact you can 'take care of' a person just as you can 'take care of' a pot plant or a pet. This does not seem helpful language or thinking.

We can usefully contrast the term 'care' with the term 'support'. When we use 'support' we imply that we are there to help someone to do something that they want to do. In fact, the use of 'support' automatically implies the primary importance of the person supported. It is for this reason that the disability movement prefers the use of terms like support or assistance which reinforce the dignity of the person who is being supported (Glasby 2007).

So one factor that may encourage us not to focus on the power and control of the person is the language of care itself and its associated imagery. The idea of caring for someone has associations which are romantic, tragic and heroic. We feel sorrow for carers; we see them as bearing a burden from which only death can relieve them.

It is also noticeable that in contemporary political rhetoric, many families, looking for extra support for their sons or daughters, have found it useful to depict themselves as 'carers'. Quite rightly they have identified that this term wins them public and political support in a way that describing themselves just as a family does not.

None of this implies that someone who uses the language of care will behave inappropriately or will not enable people to have choice; but it is clear that the idea of care can be in conflict with the idea that people with learning disabilities have lives of their own, with all the necessary rights and responsibilities.

The image of infancy

A second factor is the powerful impact of infancy on our imagination. All of us were once infants and most of us will spend some important time in our life taking care of children. And, especially, in the very early years of our life, we know that we must sometimes limit the degree of choice that an infant has over his or her own life. Instead we think that choice is something that children grow into, often quite slowly, and that the responsibility of the adult – especially the parent – is to prepare the child for the full responsibilities of adult life.

This journey of developing responsibility is important and appropriate and many families see their child with a learning disability as being on the same journey to adult responsibility as their other children. However, families are often also told by professionals that their child will not 'develop' or has 'developmental delays' or the 'mental age of a child'. In other words, families find they are often encouraged to see their child as being somehow stuck in childhood and professionals often adopt a language which encourages them, and others, to then treat adults with learning disabilities as if they haven't grown up.

In fact, there is no clear developmental path that everyone must follow into adult life and there are no objective tests for having achieved sufficient mental capacity to be an adult. In the UK, we become an adult when we are 18, whatever our mental capacities, and we will all continue to need help and advice to make decisions through our adult life. So it is unhelpful to use language and ideas, however useful in childhood, which are entirely out of place when supporting adults.

Abuse and the institution

Our images of care and ideas about the role of the child are widespread and rooted in some kind of reality, even if they are capable of distortion. But there are also threats to the dignity of people with learning disabilities which come from the desires which some people have to abuse others. Abuse is a greater risk to people with learning disabilities because it is often harder for them to resist abuse or to report abuse (see Ch. 12 for further coverage of this issue).

Abuse is a risk to people with learning disabilities in any environment and abusers can be found in all walks of life. However, we also know that the risks of abuse increase in institutional environments, for at least three interconnected reasons (Glouberman 1990):

1. Institutions tend to present people in undignified and disrespectful ways and people are more likely to abuse those they think are lacking status.
2. People who want to abuse others may seek to find work in environments where they know there are likely to be people who are vulnerable, unable to communicate, easily intimidated and whose testimony will not be believed.
3. Institutions tend to develop cultures where abuse is tolerated or even seen as normal.

This history of abuse and institutionalisation has also added to society's awareness that people with learning disabilities are more vulnerable to abuse than others. Paradoxically, this also can lead to people finding themselves disempowered for their 'own good'. Even more problematic is the tendency of society to seek to 'protect' people by placing them in environments – like residential care homes – which are inherently more risky. Society's ignorance about the nature of the institution continues to encourage disempowerment. We say we want to make people safer, but end up putting them in inherently unsafe environments.

Convenience and vested interests

A further factor which discourages empowerment is the fact that the interests of the person with a learning disability may often not coincide with those of the person who is supporting them, or with the majority of those being supported. For instance, in institutions, staff would carry out 'necessary' tasks (like cleaning and feeding people) and then would simply place everyone around a television for the rest of the day. The staff team would then sit together, chat and have a drink. Their own interests dominate.

This kind of disempowerment will also tend to grow when people are trying to support larger groups. It is difficult to give detailed attention to one person, or respect their preferences, when you are also trying to think about everyone else. If everyone must attend a day centre and everyone must use the day centre bus then there are real and practical limits to how much control any individual can have over their waking routine, their journey or their destination.

Of course, group activities are something we often choose to do, even if we know that we will have to sacrifice some of our choices in order to do them. But, when you have no meaningful control over when and how you join or opt out of such groups, then such group activities can be very damaging to your ability to shape a life for yourself.

The cognitive challenge

All of these factors help us understand some of the negative reasons why people with learning disabilities cannot take for granted that they will be treated with the same respect as other people or given the same level of choice. They may be seen as:

- not needing to make decisions – because they are being taken care of
- not able to make decisions – because they are not ready to take them.

Or there may be factors that encourage people not to want people to take control or make their own decisions:

- Wanting someone to be vulnerable, weak and powerless in order to abuse them.
- Wanting someone not to disturb their own plans or the needs of the wider group.

However, it is also important to recognise that the task of helping someone with a learning disability to make decisions, even if you are willing to help, is not always easy. There are a number of reasons why this may be the case:

- Problems of understanding – some people may not understand that a decision needs to be made, what that decision is or what the consequences of the decision will be.
- Problems of communication – even if someone has strong preferences, they may still struggle to get others to understand their communications about that preference. Moreover, it is also not always easy to know when a problem is one of communication or understanding.
- Problem of control – sometimes people may understand and be able to communicate their decisions, but they may not want to make the decision on quite the same terms as others may expect.

For example, June knew that she wanted to leave the hostel where she lived and so did the staff who supported her. She was clearly capable enough to live on her own and sometimes she expressed a desire to do so. But whenever she was put on the spot and asked to agree to such a move, she refused. So, after some time, June was offered some independent support to think about her options. She and the people who cared about her identified as many different options as they could and this was written up as a simple book with pictures for her to think about. Some months later June let people know that she was now ready to move; but she wanted to move out with her friend Maureen – someone with higher support needs – and Maureen wanted to move out too. June and Maureen then successfully stuck out for what they wanted. This story tells us that we must be careful not to assume that people will always think about things in the same way as we will. We often need to control how we make our decisions, in our own time – not make decisions to a timetable set by others.

For families and professionals working with people with learning disabilities, these factors reinforce again and again the importance of careful listening and the need to explore the many different forms of possible communication. But, beyond that, we need a positive and respectful attitude at all times.

Understanding choice

Most of us make choices all the time; big choices and small choices. And sometimes these choices seem easy or natural and sometimes they feel big or difficult. But we do not often think about how to make choices and we very rarely think about how to support other people to make choices; but if we are supporting someone with learning disabilities then we need to become much more thoughtful about choice. For choice is not a simple thing, it is complex and it has three essential elements (Lukes 1974):

1. Preferences – what we like or dislike, love or loathe.
2. Options – what is possible or available.
3. Values – what is right or wrong, good or bad, sensible or reckless.

To put this another way, choice is the exercise of human freedom; but it is bound by our knowledge of ourselves, our knowledge of the world and by our values. So it is no wonder that supporting someone to make choices is a complex business.

Although we may not be conscious of these three elements of choice when making choices, they are all necessary to choice. And when we support someone to make choices, we are always having to keep in mind, to some degree, these three elements. For example, if I want to help someone choose a holiday, I must:

- respect their preferences – help them think about what they like to do and particularly help them to avoid holidays that they would not enjoy. I must also avoid imposing my preferences on the other person
- explore possible options – help them find out about different holidays, particularly trying to identify new holidays that will better suit them and their preferences. I must avoid limiting options to only those that I am aware of or which suit me better
- form positive judgements – help them evaluate their options and make a decision, which may mean balancing many different considerations including benefits and costs, risks and opportunities. I must avoid imposing my own particular values.

Reader activity 21.1

Pay attention to any service or environment where people with learning disabilities are supported.

1. Identify what choices people are actually offered.
2. Try and identify all the options that are not made available to people.
3. Think about whose interests are really being served by the organisation of choices in the system.

None of this means that we should become paralysed by attention to choice, or force people to make choices when they are clearly enjoying the natural flow of things. We all go with the flow, sometimes, and let others take some authority. But this must be temporary and negotiated – nobody can pass their choices over to someone else forever. Although some people are sceptical about the value of choice, I think we can see that choice is vitally important to human life.

Reader activity 21.2

Identify someone whose behaviour seems challenging and then begin to treat the behaviour as language meaning 'I am unhappy or angry about something and I want your attention or reaction'. Can you develop any theories about what might be upsetting the person and how might you find out more information to support or falsify your theory?

The value of preferences

It may be tempting to see preferences as unimportant or trivial. But our preferences are essential to defining our individual nature, and if our preferences are ignored or forbidden then we are liable to either become depressed or angry. All of us have preferences which are part of our unique identity. Good support demands that you understand and respect those preferences.

It is particularly important to recognise that preferences are deeply personal – nobody can ever feel quite what we are feeling; and nobody can tell me to like something that I just plain don't like, however good they think it is for me. Preferences should not be treated as trivial or irrational; we each have different patterns of preference and we feel more strongly about some things rather than others.

For instance, one woman hated to have the remains of her finished dinner left in front of her, so she would sweep her plate from her tray with her arm. As she did not use words, her behaviour was taken to be both violent and inappropriate – but more careful listening led people to recognise that the cause of her behaviour was an essential need to have her plate cleared away immediately after she had finished eating and that her environment – in which she had little physical control – had made her action the only way of achieving her goal.

For this reason it is always useful to try and frame any enquiry into someone's negative behaviour as an exploration of the question 'what does this tell us about this person's preferences?' Often this will lead to a vast array of information and this approach is fundamental to the useful person-centred planning tool called Essential Lifestyle Planning (ELP) which is explored in Chapter 9 (Smull & Harrison 1992).

In most situations, identifying a preference will be enough to enable you to help someone to achieve that preferred option. However, sometimes preferences are far more difficult to respect. In the end, other considerations may outweigh the preference (for example, it's too risky, or it's wrong). However, even in those situations, strong preferences will need to be respected and support offered to ensure that the person can cope with not getting their preference.

The need to explore options

It is certainly the case that some people with learning disabilities may have less knowledge and information about their options than some other people (although it is dangerous to assume that is always true; many people with learning disabilities find they have to tell their social worker about new ideas like direct payments or individual budgets). In fact, we all need to ensure that we are making informed decisions and this means both knowing what options are available and what are likely consequences of taking any option.

In fact, if we are offering other people advice on their options then we have an even greater responsibility to provide accurate and well-informed information. Unfortunately it is also rather easy to slip into offering bad advice based on limited or distorted information, particularly given the negative history experienced by people with learning disabilities. For example, until quite recently, the only accommodation option provided by the state for people with learning disabilities was a bed in a ward in an institution. Today this has changed; but our options are still very limited, with the major option being a bedroom in a care home or group home. These are not good options; they are common because in the past the state continued to support the negative view of disabled people which had led to the rapid growth of institutions and other eugenic policies in the 20th century (see Ch. 3 for a more detailed discussion of these events). It is important that advice and information are not based upon this history but, instead, reflect the real housing options available in the whole community, as discussed in Chapter 27.

Reader activity 21.3

Think about the major decisions in your own life. What drove you to choose a particular path? Was it a careful consideration of all options or was it based upon your instinct, dreams or other strong desires?

Exploring options is also not a one-dimensional task. Each option has consequences and those consequences extend over time and can create costs and benefits in the short and long run. And we can never perfectly understand the impact of one decision because there are many things which are outside our control and which are utterly unpredictable. In fact, it is often useful to focus on those options which best reflect the strongest aspirations of the individual. For example, person-centred planning processes like PATH (Planning Alternative Tomorrows with Hope) help people when their lives lack direction, and this then enables the exploration of possible options to become much more focused (Falvey et al 1997).

The role of values

Finally we make choices in the light of their meaning or social value. However, this is complex because there are competing accounts of what is valuable and different factors can seem more important in different situations. There is not one simple system for evaluating options; instead there are many different and competing factors that may frame a decision:

- Happiness – will it make me happier, or help me avoid unhappiness?
- Self-interest – will it serve my interests, make me wealthier, stronger or add advantage in some other way?
- Needs – will it meet needs for health, safety, relationships or meet some other vital human need?
- Legality – will it be legal and am I entitled to do it?
- Morality – will it be right or wrong, ethical or unethical?

This list of competing and complex factors may seem bewildering and there is a long tradition of competition between different theories as to which system is best (Foot 1967). For example, utilitarians argue that we should make decisions which promote our happiness (although even they disagree among themselves as to whether this should be done by seeking our own happiness or everyone's happiness or just by following social rules). However, none of this makes too much difference when we are fully empowered to make our own decisions – for it is up to us to decide how to justify or evaluate those decisions. We do not need a theory to make decisions for ourselves.

However, when supporting someone else to make decisions, this is more complex. If we have a lot of influence over how people make decisions then it is not good enough to impose our own framework of values upon the other person. Yet, if no framework of values is obviously better or fixed and agreed then it can be difficult to know what to think and what to do. It is this problem that I will now address.

The professional and the citizen

There is an approach which might make it easier to think about how to support choice without imposing values on other people. We can begin by recognising that the relationship between the professional and the person they are supporting is a special kind of relationship with three essential properties:

1. Service – the professional must be there to serve the person, and must be able to focus on the person's interests and perspective.
2. Equality – the professional should be in a relationship of equality with the person, not a superior nor an inferior.
3. Community – the professional also has a role which is validated by the wider community and they must also serve the community's interests.

Another way of describing the essential quality of this relationship between the person and the professional is that it must be based on citizenship. That is, it must be a supportive relationship of equals, which is committed to supporting the person's capacity to exercise their own citizenship within the wider community. Citizenship is the name for this respectful living in equality with others. This term 'citizenship' may not be commonly used in English, but it has great value, and as the philosopher Jeremy Waldron suggests, it may be vital to future thinking about the welfare state (Waldron 1993:308):

> Above all, I think the idea of citizenship should remain at the centre of modern political debates about social and economic arrangements. The concept of a citizen is that of a person who can hold [their] head high and participate fully and with dignity in the life of [their] society.

Moreover, if we pay close attention to how to achieve citizenship in practice, we will find that it provides a way of thinking about human life which balances respect for the individual's own interests and the wider perspectives of the whole community. I have argued elsewhere that there are six keys to citizenship (see Fig. 21.1) (Duffy 2003). We can also see that each key to citizenship adds value to the life of the individual, adds value to the community and helps to ensure a relationship of mutual respect between citizens (see Table 21.1).

All of this means that we can use the idea of citizenship to guide how we support people to make choices. First, we can identify the main kinds of choice that citizens need to confront in their lives. We need to support people to have a holistic sense of citizenship. Second, we can offer people some principles by which to make their own choices. This

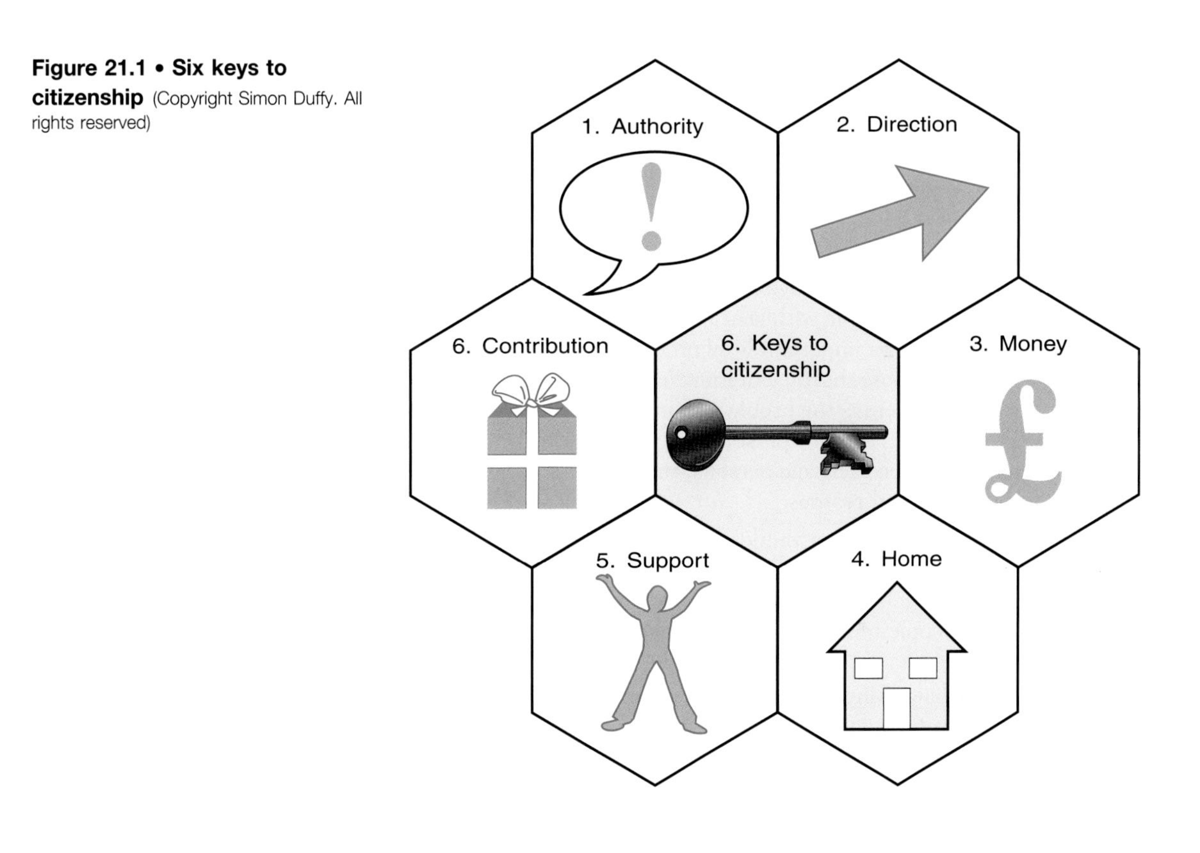

Figure 21.1 • Six keys to citizenship (Copyright Simon Duffy. All rights reserved)

Table 21.1 The meaning of citizenship in practice

Key	Meaning for citizen	Meaning to others
Authority	I am able to make my own decisions.	You have the right to speak and to be listened to.
Direction	I am able to define my own unique role.	Your life makes sense. It has meaning.
Money	I have enough independence to aim for my goals.	You can pay your way and are not unduly dependent on our good will.
Home	I have a safe and private place, where I belong.	You belong with us. You are rooted in our community.
Support	I need other people. I am interdependent, not self-sufficient.	You need us. You provide us with opportunities to give and contribute.
Contribution	I contribute, give to and support my community.	You help us. You make a difference to our community.

will not answer every problem and it will not take away from people their right to make their own decisions, but it will ensure that any support offered is positive and supports increased citizenship and challenges institutionalisation, isolation and powerlessness.

In the following sections I will explore this concept of citizenship in more detail and try to show how it provides a framework for choice which is both positive and flexible enough to help guide professionals and people with learning disabilities in their choices.

Authority

In order to be a citizen, we must have personal authority. This does not just mean being able to make choices, it also means being seen by others as able to make those choices. For people with learning disabilities, this fact raises certain important legal problems that we will go on to explore shortly, but more important than the legal problem is the problem that even those who love or care for the person may have stopped seeing the person as having personal authority; this can be for several reasons:

- We may make the mistake of thinking that some people's views just don't count and that there is some kind of intellectual or communication threshold that people must reach before their choices matter.
- We may think that taking good care of someone, perhaps in the way we take care of our infants, demands that we don't need to help people express their personal authority.
- Or, we may think that it would be dangerous for the person or for others if the person was allowed to make their own choices or be encouraged to express personal authority.

All of these views are understandable and can be rooted in good instincts. But they each share the same error which is to see personal authority as an all or nothing property. But personal authority is never simple and everyone can exercise personal authority, however complex their disability, if they receive the right support.

In fact, if we let them, people with communication difficulties can show us that personal authority – for all of us – is always supported, is always relational. In particular, we will learn that in order to support someone's personal authority, three things are essential:

1. An attitude of respect towards the communication efforts of the person.
2. A system of communication that makes clear the meaning of someone's expressions.
3. An agreement about how decisions are authorised.

It is easy not to notice that these three conditions are essential to the exercise of personal authority for everyone. We expect a certain degree of respect in our interactions with others; we don't expect to be ignored or to have our views discounted. We speak the same language as those around us, we don't expect to be misunderstood or have our expressions discounted as mere noise. We expect our own decisions to count and we don't usually need to involve anyone else in those decisions. But many people with learning disabilities find that their authority is challenged in each of these aspects.

An attitude of respect

Our ability to be understood begins when others begin to treat our expressions as worthy of attention. For young children, this begins in the loving relationship between parent and child; love encourages us to seek meaning in the sounds and noises made by the infant. Our concerns range from ensuring that the infant is not in pain to encouraging self-expression and dialogue.

In adult life, the close relationship between love and communication remains, although it is often unconscious. There is a strong correlation between what we know about someone's preferences and whether we have a positive attitude towards them. For example, Mary lived on a ward in a long-stay institution. She had lived in the institution since being a young child and she used no words to communicate. As part of planning for Mary to leave the institution, an ELP was developed to provide a detailed map of her preferences. However, this task proved nearly impossible, because nobody was able to say anything positive about Mary or to admit to even liking Mary. In the end, Mary left the institution and moved into her own flat; it was only later, after a team of personal assistants were appointed who did come to love and respect Mary, that any useful information could be gathered. Eventually it became clear that Mary really wanted to live as part of a family and so her service was changed to enable this to happen (Duffy & Sanderson 2005).

For professionals working with people with learning disabilities, the importance of love and respect needs to be recognised and built into all our interactions:

- We need to show respect to people at all times and to treat communication as potentially meaningful, even when we do not understand it.
- We need to recognise the importance of those people who do have a positive or loving attitude towards the person. They will be the key to opening up real and meaningful communication and they will have the best understanding of the person's preferences.
- We need to support people to develop and strengthen relationships of mutual respect. This is one reason why people with learning disabilities prefer to get support from people they like and who like them.

In this respect, the role of the professional is particularly complex because there are important pressures that encourage professionals to maintain distance and boundaries. Often, especially for professionals who work with many different people, these boundaries are necessary. But we must also recognise that these kinds of professional relationship are rarely going to be the kind of valued relationships which will open up real channels of communication. At best, the professional is more likely to be helping others, those with real relationships to the person, to improve their communication efforts.

A system of communication

People who share the same language share a system of communication. But where we do not share the same language we need to find a way of translating someone's expressions into a form that we do understand – this is a communication system. And for many people with the most complex communication difficulties, this means attending not just to words but also to movement, sounds, expressions and behaviour (see Ch. 6).

It is also important to see a distinction here between formal systems, like English or Makaton or British Sign Language (BSL), which have their own objective rules and those systems which are developed on an utterly person-centred basis (which are called idiolects) and may be expressed in communication books or other individualised systems. In terms of communicating with the widest group of people, quickly and efficiently, objective systems have many advantages. However, there will also be people where such a system does not seem useful and where it seems more sensible to help them communicate by their own system, one that works best for them.

Reader activity 21.4

Examine the life of someone you work for and the people involved in their life. List all of those who have power or influence over their life. Mark on that list those people who spend a significant amount of time with the person and who have a positive, friendly or loving attitude towards them.

Agreement on decisions

It is worth distinguishing communication and decision making because it does not just take effective communication to enable decisions. Decisions take the agreement of those involved to treat some form of communication as a decision, and this is influenced by both the law and social convention. Overall, the English law takes a very positive approach whose first principle is (HM Government 2005:2):

> A person must be assumed to have capacity unless it is established that he lacks capacity.

For professionals working with adults with learning disabilities, this general approach means that the following principles must be followed:

- You cannot assume because someone has a learning disability that they lack capacity to make their own decisions. For most of the day-to-day decisions that make up ordinary life, you can assume that communication has the authority of the person and can be treated as authoritative.
- You have a general duty to work in ways which support the person's own decision making. You must provide clear information, outline consequences and encourage personal growth.
- If someone really cannot understand a particular kind of decision then you may need to ensure that someone has a suitable representative for that decision – usually this can be done by asking the person to identify who they would like to act on their behalf (this process is discussed in Ch. 7).
- If the person cannot ask someone to act on their behalf then it may be necessary to appoint someone to act on their behalf for a particular decision – this should be someone that there is good reason to believe is capable of determining what decision will be in the person's best interest.

- Very occasionally you or others may seek to get the courts to determine who is the person's representative.

All of this demonstrates the complexity of personal authority. It is not something which simply exists or does not exist; it is something we create, together. For some people with learning disabilities, their personal authority is threatened, but not simply by the fact that their intellectual processes may be different to those of others. Their personal authority is threatened because:

- others may not love or respect them sufficiently
- others may not sufficiently understand their particular form of communication
- others may not acknowledge or support their decisions.

And this means that working to improve someone's personal authority is not a matter of simply asserting it. People need a network of family, friends or supporters so that they can be heard and any communication or decision-making system depends ultimately on the quality of those relationships. For this reason, professionals who work with people with learning disabilities must always understand their wider social role. They must not just serve the person but also support their community of family and friends.

If we support people to exercise personal authority, we will achieve two vital ends. If someone has personal authority, they are in a position to shape their own life, to achieve things they value, to avoid things that they don't. But achieving personal authority also means that other people will see them as citizens, with rights and the ability to act for themselves within the wider community. Authority is the foundation stone of citizenship.

Direction

The second key to citizenship is to have a sense of direction. This is not the same as simply making our own decisions. Instead direction is the authentic meaning that we give to our decisions. For example, if we meet someone on holiday who is visiting a place because they have always wanted to visit it then we would see their visit as having meaning or authenticity for them. If we meet someone who does a job that they love then we recognise that their work has meaning. Two friends, deep in conversation, have a relationship with meaning. It is also easy to see the reverse – people doing things for no reason they value, doing things they hate or spending time with people they don't like, and so on.

This is not the place to explore why some things have meaning for some people but do not have meaning for others. Instead it is important to recognise that the root of meaning is deeply personal. What has meaning for one person may not have meaning for another. This means that we cannot determine what is meaningful from the 'outside' – however much we love or respect someone else, however much we wish that they could experience things which have value to us, they will only have real meaning if they genuinely find meaning in them for themselves. In other words, we can find direction for ourselves. We cannot be given it by another person.

However, we can encourage people to find their own direction. We can listen to people's preferences, dreams and behaviours and we can support people to make decisions which are more consistent with their sense of personal direction. This is the reason why approaches like person-centred planning (see Ch. 9) are so important, for they enable people to set their own personal direction and communicate that direction to others.

While personal authority is conventionally understood to be an aspect of citizenship, it is much less common to see personal direction being understood in this way. However, if we reflect on the nature of human communication, we can see exactly why direction is such an important part of citizenship. For example, we can see the importance of direction in the development of personal profiling, which is a useful tool in supporting someone into employment (see Ch. 26). Personal profiling enables the person to identify the skills they have and that they enjoy using, their aspirations and their hopes for work. If someone begins a job that they want to do or which suits skills that they enjoy using then their motivation will be greater and the chance of success will be greater. But, and this is a vital consideration in most work settings, it will also be clear to their work colleagues why the person is doing that job. For instance, James loves the police, and when he began working for the police, his enthusiasm for his work encouraged others to see him and his work in a new light. If James had been simply been going through the motions and attending a randomly selected work placement, he would not be seen by his colleagues in the same way. James' work with the police has meaning for him, but it also therefore has meaning for those who see him at work (Cowen 2010).

Reader activity 21.5

Can you think through the likely consequences of encouraging people to do activities that they are not motivated to do? How will the person behave? How will their behaviour be understood by others they are with? How will this change their behaviour? What impact will their behaviour then have on the individual?

When we see that someone's actions have meaning and direction then we are more likely to respect those actions. We see them as not just having made a choice, but having made a choice with meaning. Decisions which lack meaning may be formally recognised, but they are not really seen as belonging to the person or adding value to the person.

Respecting direction is therefore valuable not just because it enables the person to have a better or more authentic life – one that suits them; it also helps reinforce the respect in which others hold them. We respect people who act with purpose (even when we don't share the same interests or values). Citizens have lives which are authentic – they are not just swept along by circumstances or placed and controlled by others.

Money

The third key to citizenship is money. Money is a practical medium for achieving our personal goals because it allows us to get vital support, services or resources from other people, even when those people do not have a close personal relationship with us. If there was no money, we would be utterly dependent upon other people. Money gives us independence and lets us exercise choice over:

- what kind of work we do
- how we spend our leisure hours
- where and how we live
- the kinds of personal risks we can take.

If we have insufficient money then is it is harder to shape our life to fit our sense of personal direction. Instead we will need others to make decisions on our behalf, to let us live with them, to offer us work or to have fun. With insufficient money, all our freedoms become utterly private; we can only do what does not require the help or intervention of other people.

But if money is important to achieving citizenship then this demands a number of responses from professionals working with people with learning disabilities; in particular there is a need to ensure that people get every chance to access:

- work, self-employment or other ways of earning money
- benefits, pensions, tax credits and other forms of social security
- individual budgets or other systems of funding support.

We will consider each of these important issues in turn.

Earning money

It is important not to underestimate the value of earning money through employment or self-employment, nor to underestimate the degree to which people, even with the most significant disabilities, can find and keep work (see Ch. 26). The primary advantages of work are:

- extra income, widening other life opportunities
- increased sense of self-worth and inner dignity
- respect from other people
- enjoyment of using and improving skills
- increased social interactions and opportunities for friendship.

It is a mistake to think of work as something passive that is fixed by society or the economy and which is made up of so many empty slots waiting to be filled by someone with the right skills. Work arises out of the social interaction of people's skills and needs. If people have a skill, enthusiasm or interest then there is likely to be someone else who can see a way in which this skill can be used to add further value. This is also why a person-centred approach to finding work can be much more powerful than simply seeking any job (Bolles 1993).

Benefits

People with significant disabilities are entitled to a range of different benefits, some of which are means tested (you need to have a low enough income in order to be entitled to them, for example, income support) and some of which are independent of income (for example, disability living allowance). The current systems of tax and benefits is very complex. There are at least 100 different benefits or benefit rates and there are 27 different forms of taxation (Duffy 2010a). The system also has some damaging side effects or poverty traps:

- You may lose income if you start to work.
- You may lose income if you marry or live with others.
- You may lose income if you save too much.

The system is also so complex that it is hard to feel secure about the impact of any possible change; and this encourages people to rely only on their benefits rather than risk options which may reduce their income or security. All of this means that few professionals are confident about offering any advice about tax or benefits and it is important to help people access real expert advice to ensure that they are getting all they are entitled to and can avoid the worst impact of the poverty traps.

Funding support

Until recently, in England, most people with learning disabilities or their families would not be given any information about what they were entitled to receive as support from their local authority or the NHS. However, since the development of individual budgets in 2003, this is beginning to change (Poll & Duffy 2008). Increasingly, people are being assigned an individual budget after an initial assessment of need and are being supported to determine how this will be used.

The advantages of this approach for people with learning disabilities, families and professionals could be significant, although there is still considerable debate about its consequences. In principle, an individual budget enables people to:

- decide for themselves how they are supported, increasing personal authority
- explore different support options, including developing more flexible personalised support
- better integrate support from their individual budget with support from friends, family or the wider community.

If this model of funding continues to expand then it could have a dramatic impact both on the lives of people with learning disabilities and their relationships with professionals. In particular, some professionals will begin to be commissioned and funded directly by people with disabilities or their representatives.

Money enables us to exercise our citizenship, to direct our life as we see fit. But more than this, having enough money to direct our lives sends a message to other citizens that we are genuinely independent and able to achieve our goals without relying on the good will of others at all times. This kind of respectful independence is also vital to citizenship.

See Reader activity 21.6 on the Evolve website.

Home

The fourth dimension of our citizenship is our home. This raises one of the most controversial areas of concern in the history of disability. For it is only recently that even a very small number of people with learning disabilities have been able to achieve something which is taken for granted by most – having their own home.

Historically, as we saw in early chapters (see Ch. 3), people with learning disabilities either needed to continue to live in the family home or had to live within institutions. The development of different housing and support options only began in the 1970s and it is only in the last few years that the last of the institutions was closed. Today, most people with learning disabilities continue to live in the family home, and there are a limited range of other alternatives, almost all of which rely on making unusually large groups of people live together (Emerson et al 2004):

- 50.4% living with parents.
- 11.7% living with other relatives.
- 4.1% living on their own.
- 2.7% living with a partner.
- 7.6% living with four or less people in supported accommodation.
- 16.4% living with five to ten people in supported accommodation.
- 6.8% living with more than ten people in supported accommodation.

It is useful here to also examine the general statistics for the UK for all households (Communities and Local Government 2010):

- 67.9% owner occupied.
- 14.2% rented privately.
- 17.8% rented from social landlords.

There is no similarity at all between the kinds of homes used by people with learning disabilities and those used by the rest of the population. And the reason for this is not because people with learning disabilities don't aspire to live in the same kinds of housing as other people. The dominance of residential care or group living for people with learning disabilities is caused by the combination of two factors (Glasby 2007).

As institutions were closed, the early alternative models all involved the development of large group homes or residential units. Over time, the average size of these units decreased but providing support to people and finding the housing was treated as the same project, and this led to people being organised into groups that could conveniently be supported by a fixed team of paid staff.

In 1980, the government developed a new funding stream for residential care called Board & Lodging which led to a rapid increase in homes being set up to take advantage of this new funding stream. In 1979, there were 12 000 people using residential care. In 1990, this figure had jumped to 199 000 people living in state-funded residential care homes. Since this funding system, with its incentive towards residential care, was closed down in 1992, this figure has hardly changed.

Interestingly, the rapid growth in these care homes has created a strange twist in meaning so that now, when we say someone has moved into a 'home', we actually mean they have moved out of their own home and moved into something which is not their home, where they are unlikely to have much choice, control or security. In fact, these kinds of homes are often very unsafe: for example, data for older people show that you are 10 times more likely to be subject to abuse in a 'home' than in your own home (Duffy 2010b).

Since that time there has been an increased emphasis on separating housing from support and this idea became known as 'supported living' (Kinsella 1993). Advocates of this approach argued that if people had their own homes, with support organised independently of housing, it would be more likely that:

- people wouldn't need to move house in order to change their support
- people would be seen as independent people with a stake in their own community
- people could tailor the house to their individual needs
- people could better protect themselves from undue intrusions into their privacy
- people could more easily develop new kinds of support.

Supported living has increased for people with learning disabilities and more housing options have opened up. It is also likely that the increased use of individual budgets will open up more housing options as individual budgets gives more flexibility to housing and support options. In fact, some people are now starting to buy their own homes (Duffy 2003). Increasingly, it is recognised that having your own home is an essential part of citizenship and that there can be no one type of home that will suit everyone. Instead people are beginning to realise that finding the right home will be a complex decision which should be made by balancing factors that will have different importance to different people:

- Being close to family, friends or a workplace.
- Being in a neighbourhood you like.
- Being in the right size house for your needs.
- Being with the people you want to share with.
- Being able to change your mind and move on to a different solution.

Today it is possible to support people to explore all their housing options. No longer is it necessary to push people towards narrow and limiting housing options simply because of their disability. This benefits people with learning disabilities by offering them a wider and better set of choices. But it also helps the whole community so that people with learning disabilities are fellow citizens who really do belong in ordinary houses in local communities.

Support

While it may not be surprising to treat having a home as an aspect of citizenship, it may seem much more surprising to argue that the need for support is an aspect of citizenship. Instead there is a tendency to imagine that citizens should be super-independent. But this a fallacy; citizenship only exists because human beings need each other. Without support, and the underlying need for support, citizenship could not exist.

To make this clearer, we can imagine some super-rich inventor of robots living in a private mansion surrounded by his own technology; all of this might mean that he is utterly free from the need for support from other human beings. Whether or not he would be happy may not be certain, but he would not be a citizen in any meaningful way. By not needing anyone else, the inventor has left the human world behind and has become a non-citizen.

On the other hand, Tony needs lots of help. He has a team of support assistants who work with him and help him do the things he wants to do in the community. They support him to get to work, and at work he is supported by his colleagues. His family help him to organise his support and to ensure he is doing the things he wants to do. Tony is a super-citizen; he is animating citizenship for himself at a number of different levels with formal and informal support. Tony's needs give meaning and purpose to a whole range of different people who help him in a range of different ways.

One of the reasons that we tend not to recognise that support is a positive dimension of our citizenship is that we tend to think of needs as a negative aspect of ourselves. In particular, the need for support can create a dependency which then creates further risks for the individual. This is the same issue that we explored at the beginning of the chapter: when we need support we may find that we lose control over our own life. In fact, it is this issue which has led, in recent years, to the development of self-directed support, which is a system for enabling people with disabilities to maintain control over their support. This model of self-directed support provides a framework that shows that people with learning disabilities can still exercise choice even when they need support. The following seven-step process enables support to be designed around the needs and capacities of the individual (Duffy 2010c) (Fig. 21.2):

1. Want support – the person recognises that they need help in some way.
2. Identify resources – the person looks to all the different kinds of resources they can call upon.
3. Make a plan – the person develops their own plan, shaping how they want to be supported.
4. Decide to act – the person decides to act on their plan, and gets the agreement of others if necessary.
5. Organise support – the person organises a suitable system of support, funding and control.
6. Change life – the person uses their support to change and improve their life.
7. Reflect – the person reflects on what they have learned and what needs to change.

Self-directed support means that support no longer needs to be treated as a fixed service that people have to fit into. Instead support is something that people with learning disabilities can design around themselves, their lives and their communities. Even people with the most complex needs and most significant learning disabilities can use this system if they are supported correctly. Some people use their families to act on their behalf, some use advocates, service providers or trusts. In fact, the system was successfully developed and tested with people with the most complex needs before it was extended to other groups by later government reforms (Poll et al 2006).

It is important to recognise that support is a good thing; good for both the person receiving support and good for the person giving it. Support is an essential part of our lives as citizens, creating a community where people need each other and have something to give to each other.

Contribution

We now come to the final aspect of citizenship – contribution. This is an expected part of citizenship. We might even say that the true test of whether someone is a citizen is whether they contribute to the wider community. A citizen who does not actively contribute is not a citizen. In fact, contribution, like support, is part of the glue that makes community happen.

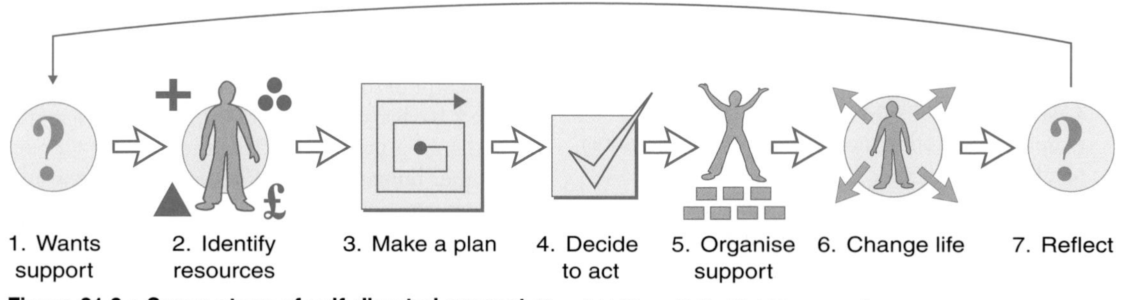

Figure 21.2 • Seven steps of self-directed support (Copyright Simon Duffy. All rights reserved)

There are many aspects to contribution and each brings with it a different kind of community life:

- In love – loving someone, sleeping together, marrying, having a family.
- In family – taking care of someone, baby sitting, spending time together, relaxing.
- In friendship – meeting for a drink, a chat or to play games, watch the football, make dinner.
- In civil society – joining a church, volunteering, hosting a coffee morning, running a club, being a student.
- In business – working, employing, being employed, running a business.
- In political life – voting, doing jury service, advocating for political causes or joining a political party.

It is critical to see that all these forms of community life exist through a process of mutual giving and taking. Community is the fruit of citizen contribution – when people stop contributing, the community diminishes; when nobody contributes then the community is finished.

It is also important to see that there is a complex interplay between these different forms of contribution, so that contribution in one area is often the key to the possibility of further contribution in another area (Messinger & Mills 2005). For example:

- Most friendships that grow outside family life develop from the relationships we form in business or in civil society.
- Most loving relationships start as friendships.
- Families only exist and develop because people fall in love and create new families.

These dynamics are as true for people with learning disabilities as the rest of the population. And this means that we cannot hope to help people strengthen their friendships, love lives or family lives without also paying attention to people's involvement in society through work, faith, leisure or other areas of personal interest. This has not always been fully understood, even by those working hardest to support the inclusion of people with learning disabilities into ordinary life. In the past, well-intentioned professionals, perhaps inspired by theories like normalisation, have tried to achieve a kind of short cut to greater citizenship by making people contribute or get involved in community activities, but not in a way that is real and directed by the person. This can backfire and undermine genuine community building. Meaningful contribution, if it is going to really support citizenship, must be rooted in all the other dimensions of citizenship:

- People must choose to be present and to get involved.
- People's choice must be meaningful to them and to their own identity.
- People must have control over their involvement in community.
- People must belong to the community.
- People must benefit and get support from their community.

Citizenship is not achieved by making people appear, like aliens from another planet, in community places just to carry out acts of kindness. The contribution of citizens to community life is a genuine reflection of the person's own life, story and desire to be in a relationship with others. It is for these reasons that if we want to see people leading full lives where people can love and be loved, we also need to attend to the underpinning issues of authority, direction, money, home and support. There is no reliable short cut to contribution and community life.

Conclusion

This chapter has been a review of how we help people make choices. As we have developed our thinking, we can see that how we support people to make choices goes to the heart of the relationship between the professional and the citizen with learning disabilities. It is not possible to take a paternalistic, patronising or negative view of people with learning disabilities without failing in your role as a professional.

If instead you must work in ways that are respectful then you will want to explore what it means for someone to be a citizen. Citizenship demands that people be in control or their own destiny, and it demands that fellow citizens – including professionals – can engage as equals in helping them express their preferences, explore their options and make positive decisions.

In the following chapters within this section, you will find numerous practical strategies and options that are available to people with learning disabilities. But more important still, than knowing all of these options, is knowing that we know very little about what supports citizenship. This means we have much to learn and that new learning will only come through a genuine partnership with people with learning disabilities, combined with a desire to achieve greater citizenship for all.

References

Bolles, R.N., 1993. What color is your parachute?. Ten Speed Press, Berkeley.

Communities and Local Government, 2010. English Housing Survey. Communities and Local Government, London.

Cowen, A., 2010. Personalised transition. Centre for Welfare Reform, Sheffield.

Duffy, S., 2003. Keys to citizenship. Paradigm, Birkenhead.

Duffy, S., 2010a. Can self-directed support transform the welfare state? In: Gregg, P., Cooke, G. (Eds.), Liberation welfare. Demos, London.

Duffy, S., 2010b. Safety for citizens: personalisation and safeguarding. Centre for Welfare Reform, Sheffield.

Duffy, S., 2010c. Personalisation in mental health. Centre for Welfare Reform, Sheffield.

Duffy, S., Sanderson, H., 2005. Relationships between care management and person centred planning. In: Cambridge, P., Carnaby, S. (Eds.), Person centred planning and care management with people with learning disabilities. JKP, London.

Emerson, E., Malam, S., Davies, I., Spencer, K., 2004. Adults with learning difficulties in England 2003/ 2004. Office for National Statistics, London.

Falvey, M., Forest, M., Pearpoint, J., Rosenberg, R., 1997. All my life's a circle. Using the tools: Circles, MAPS and PATH. Inclusion Press, Toronto.

Foot, P. (Ed.), 1967. Theories of ethics. Oxford University Press, Oxford.

Glasby, J., 2007. Understanding health and social care. Policy Press, Bristol.

Glouberman, S., 1990. Keepers. King's Fund, London.

HM Government, 2005. Mental Capacity Act. .

Kinsella, P., 1993. Supported living: a new paradigm. NDT, Manchester.

Lukes, S., 1974. Power: a radical view. Macmillan, London.

Messinger, G., Mills, L., 2005. Sharing community. Atwood, Madison, WI.

Poll, C., Duffy, S. (Eds.), 2008. A report on In Control's second phase: evaluation and learning 20052007. In Control, London.

Poll, C., Duffy, S., Hatton, C., Sanderson, H., Routledge, M., 2006. A Report on In Control's first phase 20032005. In Control, London.

Smull, M.W., Harrison, S., 1992. Supporting people with severe reputations in the community. National Association of State Mental Retardation Program Directors, Alexandria, VA.

Waldron, J., 1993. Liberal rights. Cambridge University Press, Cambridge.

Further reading

Glasby, J., Littlechild, R., 2009. Direct payments and personal budgets. Policy Press, Bristol.

Mount, B., 1987. Person-centred planning. Graphic Futures, New York.

Snow, J., 1994. What's really worth doing and how to do it. Inclusion Press, Toronto.

Vidyarthi V., Wilson P., 2008. Development from Within, Apex Foundation, Herndon, VA.

Useful addresses

Centre for Welfare Reform is an independent research and development network which works to reform the current welfare state: http://www.centreforwelfarereform.org

Housing Options is a Housing Advisory Service for People with Learning Disabilities: http://www.housingoptions.org.uk

In Control started work in 2003 to change the social care system in England. The old system did not put people in control of their own support or life. In Control designed a new system – Self-Directed Support. The government now wants all local authorities to change their systems to Self-Directed Support: http://www.in-control.org.uk

Ownership Options specialise in the home ownership issues affecting disabled people in Scotland: http://www.ownershipoptions.org.uk

Paradigm's mission is to provide the best range of tailor-made supports in the UK, including consultancy, training, conferences, publications and information; helping people, communities and services build an inclusive future: http://www.paradigm-uk.org

Working with families

Neil James

22

CHAPTER CONTENTS

KEY ISSUES

- Services and professionals need to adapt and deliver effective support that reduces the risk of families experiencing unnecessary hardship and inequality in their caring role
- Services and professionals need to recognise cultural and family diversity so that the experiences and needs of individual family carers are valued
- Providing support needs to be seen as an evolving process as individuals with a learning disability and their carer/s journey through the lifecycle
- Collaborative relationships should be built on an ethos of partnership, involvement and respect
- The experiences of individual family carers needs to be listened to and learnt from so that proactive support can be planned and delivered to meet their specific needs

Acknowledgement

The verbatim quotes that are used within this chapter have been taken from the author's current study into the perceptions of family carers, of adults with a learning disability, about their relationships with professionals. My thanks go to the participants for partaking in the study and for giving me permission to use their words in publications so that others may understand and learn from their lived experience. Pseudonyms are used to ensure confidentiality.

Introduction

> *Ah well at the end of the day um, it come to an end then we couldn't cope no more, you know which it broke our hearts really, because I don't think we had the help we should have been having at that time.*
>
> (John – Father)

It is estimated that about 2% of the population in the United Kingdom have a learning disability (Department of Health (DH) 2001a). By 2021, the number of adults with a learning disability is expected to have increased by 11% of which 36% will be aged over 60 (Foundation for People with Learning Disabilities (FPLD) 2010). Approximately 60% of adults with a learning disability live with their family and about a third of family carers are over the age of 70 (DH 2001b, FPLD 2003). Similar trends have also been identified internationally with Dew et al (2004) reporting that in Australia there are approximately 9000 parents over the age of 65 caring for an adult daughter or son with a learning disability.

Family carers are a valuable commodity to the individual, public, community, services and governments. Without them, the position for services and economic viability would be seriously debilitated. It is important therefore that services and professionals work in ways that complement and enhance their role and capacity to care. By working collaboratively and in partnership with families, their individual needs can be identified so that they are able to support their relative in a way that reduces unnecessary hardship and difficulties.

Who is a family carer?

The conventional view of the family structure, the heterosexual nuclear family, remains powerful and influential in today's society (Giddens 2009, Haralambos et al 2004). However, in reality, families can now adopt many different forms that include heterosexual, gay and lesbian, two parent and single parent (Haralambos et al 2004). Family make up is therefore no longer one that can be seen as having a set structure or formation. This is further demonstrated when cultural diversity is considered and how the rules and norms of family life and relationships can differ across other groups, such as black and minority ethnic families. Within these diverse family structures, the role of care giving is usually taken up by the parent/s, who may be the biological parent/s, adoptive parent/s, step-parent or it may be undertaken by members of the family across different generations, for example siblings or grandparents (Barron et al 2006, Dew et al 2004).

Economic, social and political systems impact significantly on the functioning of families in today's society. Lifestyle factors can result in demographic distancing between extended members of the family group for reasons such as employment opportunities and the cost of housing. As a consequence, care giving responsibility may only be provided by members of the nuclear family as less assistance is available from members of the demographically removed extended family (DH 2008). In most family units, for people with a learning disability, it is usually the mother who assumes the role of primary carer (Dowling & Dolan 2001). Across the UK, it is estimated that about 70% of all informal care givers are women (DH 2008). This may explain why much of the literature exploring the experiences of family care for a person with a learning disability focuses on the experiences of the mother (Barr 2007). In practice, however, it is important that professionals do not automatically assume that the primary care giver is the mother as this role may be one that is adopted by another member of the family, for example the father, brother, sister or grandparent, or is shared within the family. Therefore, what is paramount is that the diversity of a family structure and the function and experiences of all its members are considered (Barr 2007), valued and respected by all professionals and services.

Policies, strategies and legislation

Current policy within the UK demonstrates that there is an increased reliance on informal carers to provide support for individuals who have a learning disability (DH 2001a). Policies, strategies and

Reader activity 22.1

Take some time out to note down your thoughts about family structures and the influence that society has on how families are viewed and function. After you have made your notes, read either the chapters on families by Haralambos et al (2004) and Giddens (2009) or visit:

- http://sixthsense.osfc.ac.uk/sociology/research/approaches.asp and
- http://sixthsense.osfc.ac.uk/sociology/research/family_diversity.asp or
- http://en.wikibooks.org/wiki/Introduction_to_Sociology/Family

Then go back to your notes and think about how your thoughts might have been influenced by some of the issues and theories that these sources discuss.

Table 22.1 Some key provisions from legislation covering the UK and Eire, in respect of family carers of people with a learning disability

Legislation	Covers	Key provisions
Carers (Recognition and Services) Act 1995	England and Wales	• If somebody provides regular and substantial care then they are entitled to request a Carers Assessment. Their abilities to care should be assessed and support to help them in their role as carer identified.
Carers and Disabled Children Act 2000	England and Wales	• Request for an assessment if providing or intending to provide regular and substantial care for someone over age 18. • Right to request an assessment by parents of a child with disabilities. • Provision of services by local authorities to help with caring. • Provision of direct payments. • Vouchers for breaks services.
Adults with Incapacity Act 2000	Scotland	• Involvement of carers in decision making when person lacks capacity.
Carers and Direct Payments (Northern Ireland) Act 2002	Northern Ireland	• Carers have a right to a separate assessment of need. • Health boards have a duty to inform carers of their rights to an assessment. • Reflects similar provisions and rights as those for carers in England and Wales.
Community Care and Health (Scotland) Act 2002	Scotland	• All carers entitled to an assessment even if under 16. • Local authorities have duty to inform carers of right to assessment.
Carers (Equal Opportunities) Act 2004	England and Wales	• Work, life-long learning and leisure are assessed. • Help can be enlisted from housing, health, education and other local authorities to support carers. • Local authorities have duty to inform carers of right to assessment.
Mental Capacity Act 2005	England and Wales	• Involvement of carers in decision making when person lacks capacity.
Disability Act 2005	Eire	• Emphasises an inclusive society. • Support and services should optimise social inclusion and promote participation of carers.
Disability Discrimination Act 1995 and 2005	England and Wales	• Right for people to have equal citizenship and reinforces the rights for carers.

legislation in the UK have also been developed to promote the involvement of people with learning disabilities and their families, as much as possible, in care decisions, the planning of services and making plans for the future (DH 1999, 2001a, 2001b, 2008, 2009, Department of Health, Social Services and Public Safety 2006, Scottish Executive 1999, 2000, Welsh Assembly Government 2007). This process of collaboration with family carers has been advocated within policy and legislation in the UK for several years (for example, Children Act 1989, NHS and Community Care Act 1990). Legislation lays down the rights of carers to an assessment of their needs. However, over half of those providing significant levels of care have been found to be unaware of this (Carers UK 2004). Some of the key provisions from legislation covering the UK and Eire, in respect of family carers of people with a learning disability, are summarised in Table 22.1.

Reader activity 22.2

Consider how policy and legislation supports working between families and services. Identify some of the ethical and moral dilemmas that you have faced or may face in the future when working in line with these frameworks.

Developing understanding of the context of caring

While there is a growing body of literature in respect of people with learning disabilities and their families, a significant proportion of this work focuses on children and the impact that having a child with a learning disability has had on the family (see also Ch. 23). Commonly recurring themes within this literature are stress, burden and psychological distress (Fitzpatrick & Dowling 2007, Hill & Rose 2009). What has been demonstrated within these studies is that parents (primarily the mother) of children with learning disabilities experience higher levels of stress than parents of children without learning disabilities (for example, Esdaile 2003, Hastings 2003, Shin & Nhan 2009). However, the levels of stress vary considerably between these parents and are further influenced by a range of variables, such as the severity of disability; communication skills of the child; lack of information; and behavioural difficulties (Fitzpatrick & Dowling 2007, Hassall et al 2005). Other stressors that have also been identified as part of the caring role include the complex demands of caring; uncertainty surrounding the relative's future when support can no longer be provided; and lack of formal and informal support (Hassall et al 2005, Sardi et al 2008, Todd et al 1993).

The impact and amount of experienced stress therefore depends on whether there are other factors that make the caring role more complex. For example, higher levels of stress and life restrictions were found in parents of children with learning disability and autism than parents of children with Down syndrome (Olsson & Hwang 2003). Also, supporting someone with a profound and multiple learning disability places increased demand on carers as they have to undertake a range of physical caring tasks such as washing; dressing and feeding; dealing with incontinence; physiotherapy; and pressure sore prevention that results in carers spending most of their day providing therapeutic and educational care (Mencap 2001). The role of full-time carer can therefore result in less time being spent actively participating in a social and recreational lifestyle away from caring responsibilities. Personal relationships may also be strained due to the amount of time that other members of the family can find to spend together (Fitzpatrick & Dowling 2007). Rather than being a naturally occurring process, these relationships may need to be carefully negotiated and adapted in order for them to be accommodated. These relationships, along with other lifestyle opportunities, can be further complicated due to having difficulty in finding suitable child care and the need to plan activities well in advance (Todd & Shearn 1996).

Also, the ability to manage and progress with personal development plans, such as career aspirations, can be prohibited due to the difficulty in having to manage multiple time demands (Todd & Shearn 1996). Providing full-time care for a person with a learning disability can adversely influence the socioeconomic position of the family (Emerson et al 2006) leading to financial hardship (Gerstein et al 2009). Lower socioeconomic status has been found to have a negative impact on the wellbeing of carers and their ability to cope resulting in lower levels of happiness and self-esteem (Eisenhower & Blacher 2006, Emerson et al 2006). Exposure to adverse socioeconomic conditions can also increase the risk of experiencing psychological distress and poorer wellbeing (Emerson et al 2006). Lone carers are also more likely to live in poverty; this impacts on their psychological and physical wellbeing making them more vulnerable and in need of support (McConkey 2005).

The diagnosis of additional problems can result in parents re-experiencing the grief and feelings of loss that they may have felt when they were given the diagnosis of learning disability (Faust & Scior 2008) (see also Ch. 23). Also, they may find caring more difficult to manage. For example, in their study of parents of youths with learning disability and psychopathology, Douma et al (2006) found that parents had higher levels of need for support than parents of youths with a learning disability without an emotional or behavioural disorder. They also found that a variety of support needs were reported as frequently unmet. Faust & Scior (2008) found that parents, when inadequately prepared, were often left confused when trying to make sense of changes to their relative's behaviour leading to them being unsure of where to turn for help.

There is an increased risk of psychosocial distress as a result of behavioural disturbance (Bromley et al 2004), which can impact on family life as a consequence of its unfamiliarity; the misunderstanding of its function; its difference to the behaviour displayed by other children/siblings; and the difficulty the care giver may have in being able to manage and/or develop appropriate intervention strategies due to a lack of awareness and/or guidance.

Black and minority ethnic families are reported as having to care in more difficult circumstances than those reported by white families, such as living in poverty; poorer housing; social isolation; a lack of culturally appropriate services; high levels of carer stress; and feelings of isolation (DH 2001b, Mir et al 2001). Also, they are at a substantially higher risk of having poor mental health and wellbeing compared to family carers from white families (Hatton et al 2010). As with other family carers, their situation may be compounded by the additional costs that form part of caring for a child with a disability. They may face substantial inequalities due to racism and discrimination in health and social services, employment and education (Acheson 1998, Hatton et al 2010, Mir et al 2001). This situation is exacerbated by negative stereotypical views that are held about how communities appear to be happy to keep themselves to themselves and care for their own (Ahmad & Atkin 1996).

This overemphasis on stress, burden and other negative factors, however, risks creating a pathological view of the family leading to negative perceptions and expectations that may hide the fact that some families thrive and are resilient despite the challenges they may face (Gerstein et al. 2009). It is important to recognise therefore that not all reports about the impact of caring are negative. There is a growing body of evidence that reports positive aspects from carers such as perceptions of becoming less selfish; developing a greater appreciation for life; achieving personal growth and maturity; and enjoying their relative making progress (Fitzpatrick & Dowling 2007, Hastings et al 2002, Olsson & Hwang 2003). Care giving has also been identified as giving rewards and satisfaction especially when carers are able to cope with difficult behaviours (Grant et al 1998). Other positive aspects identified by carers have been the adoption of a new view to what is important in life; a sense of purpose; being more focused on caring for each other; the development of stronger and more intimate family relationships; and the development of a greater appreciation for things in life (Olsson & Hwang 2003, Todd et al 1993). Also, the caring role has provided mutually beneficial relationships within the family that provide a sense of personal fulfillment (Kenny & McGilloway 2007).

Identifying issues in respect of approaches and support from services

Due to the complexity of situations that family carers may be experiencing, for example poverty, inadequate housing and psychological distress, providing effective support can be very challenging (Wade et al 2007). However, family carers do not always report their role as burdensome but rather the challenge of caring is influenced by external pressures that are not always within their control (Burton-Smith et al 2009, Grant et al 1998). Also, parents have felt that they have lost identity as a 'person' because services fail to distinguish them from their role of 'parent' (Todd & Shearn 1996). Dowling & Dolan (2001) further suggest that the same types of prejudices and social barriers that people with disabilities face are ones that families are disabled by.

Reader activity 22.3

Undertake a critical reflection on a personal experience where a family carer of a person with a learning disability and services have worked together. Consider the following questions:

- What were your initial impressions when you met the family/service provider?
- Did your initial impressions change as you got to know the family/service provider and why?
- What do you think influenced your initial impressions?
- How has the experience influenced you?

In their survey of families caring for a child or adult with profound and multiple learning disabilities across the UK, Mencap found that 48% were either not very satisfied or very dissatisfied with services they received; 80% thought professionals were poorly or very poorly coordinated; 37% had contact with more than eight professionals; nearly 80% had not been able to return to work; and 48% had no outside support for their care tasks (Mencap 2001). It has also been reported that 60% of families that cared for a child or adult with a learning disability either received respite services that did not meet their need or did not receive respite or short break services at all (Mencap 2003). From a review of law, policy and service provision affecting people in Northern Ireland who have mental health needs or learning disability, during 2002–2004, a number of issues were identified that need to be addressed by services (see Table 22.2).

Other issues in respect of support and relationships with services and professionals are that formal support is not always flexible, sufficient, accessible and appropriate for family carers' needs (Walden et al 2000). Mothers have reported being stereotyped, made to feel devalued and have experienced judgemental attitudes (Todd & Jones 2003). Some of the other factors that have been experienced and

Table 22.2 Issues identified during 2002–2004 that need to be addressed by services in Northern Ireland

Breaking the news	• Professionals trained in how to break bad news. • Need for accurate information about condition and support available. • Better communication and coordination of support between professionals. • Speech and language therapy input in the early years.
Support	• Provision of information to help them in their role on issues such as benefits and services. • Flexible respite service provision that can be booked well in advance and as emergency availability. • Input from skilful, sensitive, reliable and well-trained staff. • Timely provision of aids and adaptations to the environment.
Health	• Better preparation of primary and secondary health care professionals in understanding needs of people with a learning disability. • Effective planning for admissions to hospitals. • Involvement and recognition given to the skills and knowledge of carers. • Assessment and support for carers' physical and mental health.
The future	• Support during major transition periods. • Skilful and considerate support for future planning.

(Adapted from Bogues 2004)

reported as negative include a lack of professional sensitivity to the family situation (Knox et al 2000); a lack of psychological support (McGill et al 2006); a lack of flexible and appropriate respite care provision (Mencap 2006, Northway et al 2006); and inequitable access to services (McConkey 2005).

Professionals and services are seen as important sources of information and emotional support, however the responsibility for accessing this generally falls on the carer (Case 2001, Chambers et al 2001) with frequent reports of having to 'fight' for support and services (Case 2001, Redmond & Richardson 2003, Sardi et al 2008). The result of having to constantly search for this information and support increases their feelings of anxiety and frustration (Chambers et al 2001). For example, the transition from child to adult has caused uncertainty and stress due to a lack of efficient planning, support and information (Todd & Jones 2005). Inadequate planning, information and support can result in a state of crisis being reached where more complex resource-intensive interventions are required that may lead to the relative having to be accommodated away from the home and their family (Wodehouse & McGill 2009).

In respect of the experiences of black and minority ethnic communities, they have highlighted experiences of racial discrimination existing within services; negative stereotypes and attitudes; a lack of cultural awareness and understanding; a lack of staff who can converse in the same language as the carer; and culturally inappropriate services in terms of diet, activities and staff provision (Hatton et al 1997, 1998, 2004, 2010). Other areas of concern include having limited awareness of available services; poor standards of communication; delays in diagnosis and treatment; lack of support due to poor access; high levels of unmet need; and low levels of access to benefits and/or receipt of lower amounts of benefits compared to white carers with similar needs (Atkin & Ahmad 2000, Chamba et al 1999, Mir et al 2001).

As has been highlighted, the majority of people with a learning disability live with a member of their family and it is within this environment that a range of support needs, such as physical, emotional and social care are met (Barr 2007). Consequently, a family carer will develop in-depth knowledge and understanding about their relative from these and other experiences across the lifecycle (Mulrooney & Harrold 2004). They can be invaluable sources of knowledge and information regarding the person's history and day-to-day functioning. However, negative views about parents and families being difficult, overprotective, unresourceful and passive are still apparent today (Grant 2005):

> . . . you know, they're not looking at us as though, they're their parents, they're um, they're always saying this you know, how can I put it, um, parents are too protective like you know, or they, they think it's something wrong with him but it's not.
>
> (John – Father)

Box 22.1

Unhelpful approaches to supporting families

- Service led.
- Stereotypical negative view of family.
- Professionals assume the 'expert' position.
- Not listening and identifying what is important to the family.
- Exclusion from decision making.
- Cancelling appointments.
- Being constantly late for appointments.
- Lack of adequate information about services, support and entitlements.
- Lack of awareness and appreciation for cultural diversity.
- Slow to respond to requests for support.
- Disjointed and uncoordinated services.

Box 22.2

Helpful approaches to supporting families and developing effective relationships

- Flexible.
- Consistent.
- Accessible.
- Available.
- Reliable.
- Services that are not imposed.
- Respect.
- Collaboration.
- Effective communication and information sharing.

(Grant & Whittell 1999, Prezant & Marshak 2006, Redmond & Richardson 2003)

Also, carers can be overlooked because they are seen as part of the cause for any problems that their relative may develop (Chapman 2004, Grant 2005). Allied with this, a pathological view of stress whereby it is seen as an inevitable component of the care giving experience, can also create a negative and unhelpful view (Grant & Ramcharan 2001). Feelings of being devalued and stigmatised can be reinforced by poor quality support especially if this is not guided by the needs and agendas of people with learning disabilities and their carers, but rather reflects those of professionals and services (Case 2001; see Box 22.1 for a list of other unhelpful approaches):

> . . . they don't always take on board what you have to say because you're just a mother, and I felt that throughout my life actually. They don't always take on board what you're saying do they because they are, they think that you are emotionally, it's coming from some emotion rather than logic.
>
> (Sally – Mother)

Family carers have reported a number of approaches by services that they have found valuable and useful that also provides the foundations for the development of effective relationships with professionals (see Box 22.2). Other positive components of support reported by families include professionals taking a partnership approach based on careful listening and treating them as equals (Prezant & Marshak 2006); help being provided within the home that supports engagement in wider social activities (Redmond & Richardson 2003); effective communication and joint working between services (Wodehouse & McGill 2009); a key worker; provision of short-term breaks; the active provision of information and advice (Mencap 2001); and a flexible individualised needs-led approach that has empowered carers, valued them as experts and focused on their concerns (Sloper 1999).

Reader activity 22.5

Before you read this section on positive approaches to supporting family carers, take some time out to list the expectations that you would have from professionals in respect of the support you would like to receive if you are or were caring for someone with a learning disability. Also, make a note of what concerns you would have for yourself, other family members and the relative that you are caring for about the type of support you would receive.

Positive approaches to supporting family carers

See Reader activity 22.4 on the Evolve website.

Developing an understanding of influencing systems

When working and planning support for carers, gaining an understanding about how different systems can influence the family can facilitate a more holistic view about the care giving experience. The family

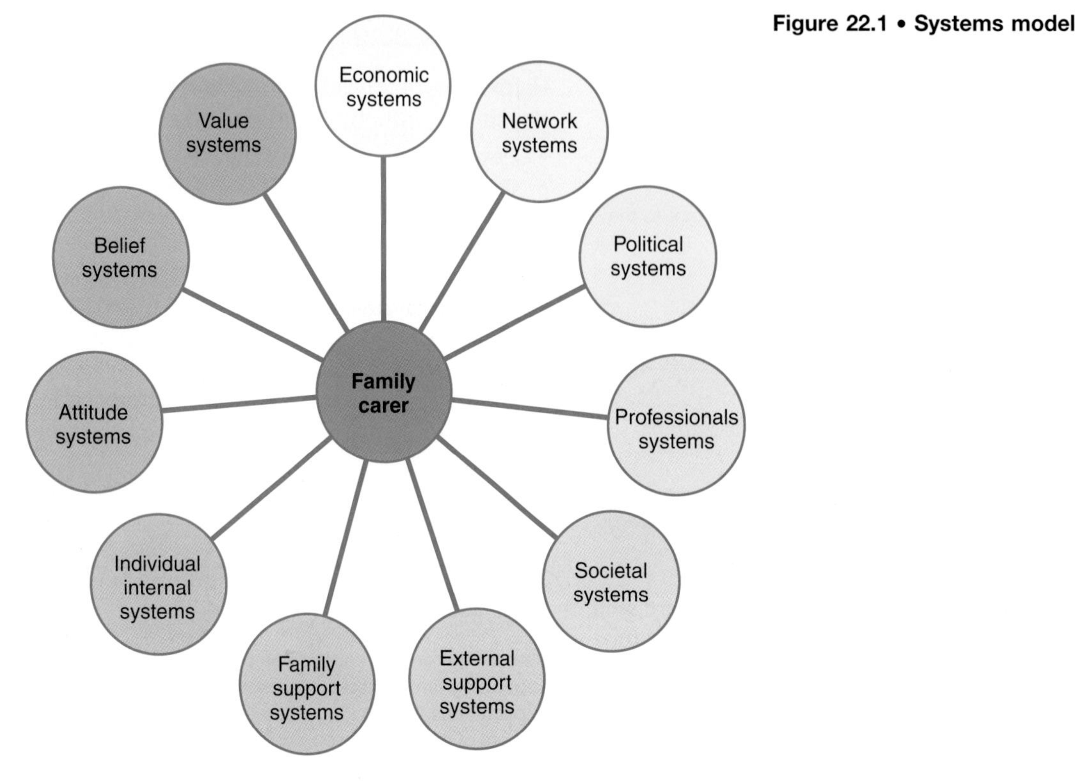

Figure 22.1 • Systems model

should be seen as a complex and dynamic system, with its members having their own characteristics and needs, influenced by a range of systems (see Fig. 22.1 for an example of multiple influencing systems). One of the key systems that can affect how family carers cope and experience the care giving journey is that of service provision and, in particular, its organisation (Knox et al 2000). Therefore, a structured, logical and comprehensive process of assessment, planning, implementation and evaluation of support needs to be facilitated throughout the time of the caring role. Also, continually reviewing and adapting support provisions will give recognition to the changing needs and circumstances as the care giving journey progresses. This individual- and family-centred approach to care is imperative to understand the concerns and needs of the carer and their family (Wong & Wong 2003).

Recognising the role of caring as one that evolves and changes

Life as a carer is not one that stays still but is one that will evolve and progress through a number of different transition periods (see Box 22.3 for examples). Caring therefore involves moving between periods of stability and change (Shearn & Todd 1997) as the needs of their relative fluctuate across the life course. As a consequence, they may need to negotiate a number of different sources of support across education, health and social care services. To help map this journey through the life course of caring, and help to understand the stages and challenges that family carers progress through, different time trajectories have been proposed. These trajectories are identified as 'the caregiving trajectory', 'the development/disability trajectory', 'the family cycle trajectory' and 'the service trajectory' (see Grant et al 2003 and Grant 2005 for a more detailed discussion). In using this as a framework for recognising

> **Reader activity 22.6**
>
> Think about how many different roles you have within your family and in society, for example mother, sister, aunty, niece, granddaughter, neighbour, employee, employer, advocate, friend, etc.
>
> - Is there conflict between these roles?
> - What role/s do you feel is/are more important and why?
> - How do you think others view you in particular roles?

Box 22.3

Examples of transition periods

- Initial diagnosis.
- Birth and the early years.
- Choosing and attending first school.
- Moving to high/comprehensive school.
- The adolescent years.
- Relationship formations.
- Child to adult services.
- Leaving school and going to college/work.
- Moving away from home.
- Experience of health-related problems.
- Ageing.

and developing an understanding of each family's unique journey, professionals can learn key messages about the caring experience and develop support that meets the needs of the family and empowers them as a whole (Grant 2005).

According to Manthorpe (1995:118), the birth of a child with learning disabilities requires families to progress through three separate stages of impact:

1. Re-evaluation and change of expectations for the child.
2. The alteration of future perspectives.
3. Acknowledgement of being a different family.

In practice, it may be beneficial to see these as processes that families go through at other times of their caring journey, for example when there is a change to their relative's behaviour due to physical and/or mental health issues. When dealing with these changes in behaviour, carers require an environment that provides advice and support regarding services available and the different types of interventions that may be utilised to address the concerns they have for their relative. If family care givers and professionals can work within an environment that is both supportive and based on mutual respect then enormous benefits can be gained to reduce the impact of behavioural distress (Marshall & Mirenda 2002). According to Hassall et al (2005), a child's behavioural difficulties are influenced by parenting stress levels and the provision of family support contributes to better coping. Also, a prompt diagnosis of the psychological and/or physical health problems that the relative may be experiencing will help with planning appropriate support and giving advice as well as providing interventions that are aimed at treating the underlying cause and reducing distress.

Valuing the 'expert'

> ... professionals aren't the experts, they have expertise and they have very good skills but they don't have the grounded knowledge that we would have ...
>
> (Mike – Father)

Parents are in the best position to communicate with and understand their child and therefore should be recognised as experts in identifying their needs (Law et al 2003). Viewing carers as experts should not be seen by professionals as threatening but as a way of valuing their input. In utilising the carers' 'local' knowledge, their unique knowledge of the experiential world of their relative, combined with the professionals' 'cosmopolitan' knowledge, technical and general expertise, care can be optimised (Nolan 2001). The development of a relationship based on empowerment and partnership can also be further facilitated by using Nolan's (2001) principles of a 'carers-as-expert' model (see Box 22.4). Within this relationship, professionals and services need to acknowledge and recognise that carers move along a spectrum from novice to expert during their caring journey and have learnt skills by 'trial and error', with a return to a status of novice when faced with new situations, at which time they may need additional help and support (Nolan 2001).

Box 22.4

Carers as expert model

- Provision of support to help carers acquire necessary competencies, skills and resources in order to maintain their own health.
- Value the carers' views about their role.
- Value the carers' willingness to take on the role.
- Undertaking of a comprehensive assessment that includes:
  - identifying the challenges to caring
  - a review of relationships both past and present
  - personal and other social resources
  - coping strategies
  - caring satisfactions.
- Taking a subjective view to understand the carers' perceptions of caring.

(Adapted from Nolan 2001)

Assessing and planning with involvement

The care needs of individuals will vary depending on their level of learning disability and other complex health needs with the structure and function of the family being further influenced by these issues (Barr 1996, Rose et al 2004, Turnbull & Turnbull 1990). Therefore, each individual, their carer/s and family should be assessed by taking into consideration their unique circumstances. What is important during any assessment process is that professionals should not only consider identifying any unmet need/s, but they should also establish the nature of the help that is desired (Prezant & Marshak 2006). Mansell & Morris (2004) highlight the importance of involving parents in the planning and development of services, especially in the assessment and diagnostic process. Families must be seen as wanting to be fully involved in all decisions relating to the care of their relative with a learning disability. If this is neglected and instead professionals focus and place more importance on risk assessments, care plans, rules and regulations, it will make carers feel alienated (Sheard 2004) and devalued.

To avoid imposing services/support that are not wanted, service providers should utilise a 'partnership model' based on the principles of recognition and mutual respect, information and skills sharing, sharing of decisions and feelings (Carpenter 1997). Case (2001) also identifies three important characteristics that can have a positive influence on the relationship that is built between parents and professionals:

1. *Professionals* – approachable; considerate of parental needs and validating of their concerns.
2. *Therapy* – involvement in decisions and intervention implementation; shared responsibility for treatment and decisions.
3. *Advice and Information* – clear and easy to understand; proactive focus rather than waiting to be asked.

Not involving family carers in the planning process will affect the development of a trusting relationship and, as a consequence, the use of negotiation as part of the planning and delivery of services will be affected (Barr 1996). It is important therefore that carers are seen as integral to service planning and delivery and that they are actively and considerately involved in action planning and priority setting, especially given that the outcome of planning may have a significant impact on them and their future. While there may be no blueprint for success, collaboration and cooperation will enhance working relationships and positive outcomes for the person with a learning disability. According to Barr (2007), the starting point for professionals should be to take note of and treat seriously the concerns of carers so they feel they are being listened to. He also says that parents accept that professionals do not have all the answers and that they may need to gather information in order to answer concerns or questions.

When considering involvement and support of the family, it is important that acknowledgement is given to how other members of the family input into the care and support of their relative. Family carers need to be given information about their rights as carers and details of how policy and legislation can support them in their role. In not facilitating this, professionals are doing a disservice to carers and could be subjecting them to managing in situations more demanding than they need to be.

Negotiating the relationship

The parent–professional relationship is integral to the processes of information giving, adaptation and facilitation of effective support. Three models that have been proposed to explain how this relationship can be navigated are the consumer, negotiation and expert models (Case 2001, Cunningham & Davis 1985, Dale 1996; see Box 22.5). For practice based on value, empowerment and inclusion, it is the consumer and negotiation models that need to be used by professionals. The components of these two models should not be seen as mutually exclusive however, but rather ones that can be merged.

Good practice should undoubtedly support the view that the needs of a person with a learning disability cannot be separated from his/her family. However, conflict may occur when sensitive issues and differences of opinion of what is wanted or expected arise between the carer and their relative and/or carer and professional/s. Consequently, these situations will require skills and expertise from professionals that help them to separate the needs of the person with a learning disability from that of their carer, manage the conflict and find a resolution. The use of Henneman et al's (1995) collaborative working framework, although originally developed as a framework for collaborative working for use by nurses, can

Box 22.5

Parent–professional relationship models

Consumer model

- Parents adopt the role of consumer in selecting appropriate services.
- Parents seen as having expert knowledge of their child and family.
- Professional support is via negotiation and bargaining in order to help with appropriate decision making.
- Professionals listen and develop their understanding about parents opinions and resources.
- Professionals still have a crucial role in providing instruction and expertise to help inform parents.

Negotiation model

- Involves dialogue.
- Relationship underpinned by active listening and negotiation by professional.

Expert model

- Professionals seen as the experts.
- Parents are passive recipients of decisions and instructions.

(Adapted from Case 2001, Cunningham & Davis 1985, Dale 1996)

be utilised to help manage conflict by supporting the development of a relationship that shows respect and acknowledgement of concerns (see Henneman et al 1995 for a more in-depth discussion of this framework). The key attributes of this framework include professionals being willing participants contributing their expertise in a joint venture and sharing responsibility with planning and decision making. The relationship is therefore one where power is shared by entering the relationship with a principle of mutual respect and recognition. Some of the benefits in using this collaborative framework approach are highlighted in Box 22.6.

In not conforming to directions by professionals, family carers should not be seen as difficult or obstructive but rather they still need to be viewed as important contributors to the care and support of their relative. It is important therefore that professionals do not see family carers as being involved only if they implement their recommendations for interventions and/or are passive recipients of the decisions made.

Box 22.6

Some benefits of utilising a collaborative approach

- Potential to reduce conflict.
- Values the impact that decisions can have on carers.
- Carers will feel part of the process rather than made to feel like beneficiaries of what is decided.
- Helps to design more carer-centred services.
- Reduces possible stress variables.
- Provides an opportunity to hear how families cope and define their situation.
- Helps to identify key strategies for providing support.
- Removes a 'professional knows best' perception.
- As a forum to identify other support systems.

Recognising and developing services to meet needs

In addressing the inequalities experienced and reported by black and minority ethnic families, services need to ensure that they actively engage with such communities by acknowledging the diversity of need and service requirements rather than choosing to ignore them (Alexander 1999). Also, equity in service delivery can be achieved by providing staff training in implementing anti-racist practice; dealing with racial harassment; increasing local and national policy and legislative awareness; and cultural competence training (Mir et al 2001, Reading & Raj 2000). To help develop cultural competence and remove barriers, services should seek guidance from the *Learning Difficulties and Ethnicity* framework (DH 2004). Also, there is a need to see black and minority ethnic family carers as individually diverse rather than as homogeneous groups (Hubert 2006). In this way, better understanding can be gained of the lived experience of caring within their family settings and cultural environments.

Adopting a flexible and consistent approach

There are a number of factors that can complicate the role of caring and these can include the cost of travel to meetings/appointments; repetition of information to different professionals; pressure of other commitments such as the needs of other members of the family; work commitments; and the number of appointments. Consequently, a more collaborative and synchronous process is required that avoids

Case illustration 22.1

Sunil and Chandrika are married and originate from Sri Lanka. They have two boys and one girl, Saminda who is 7 years old, Priyantha who is 11 and their eldest Athula who is nearly 18. Sunil is employed full time as a senior technician with an international computer company and he regularly needs to travel and stay away from home. Chandrika is the main carer for the children along with her mother-in-law who lives in the family home. Sunil and Chandrika are active members of the local Hindu community group and attend for worship at the local Mandir regularly.

Athula has a diagnosis of epilepsy, autism and learning disability. Until recently, he had been attending a local special educational needs school but this has broken down due to his increasing levels of anxiety and inability to cope within the environment. Saminda has also recently been diagnosed with attention deficit hyperactivity disorder. While Sunil was away working, Chandrika was encouraged to contact the local Community Learning Disability Team (CLDT) by a family friend as Athula's behaviour was getting unpredictable and quite difficult for her to manage. Having contacted her GP, the referral was made. However, at first she was reluctant to do this as her and Sunil's previous experience of professional involvement had resulted in them attending numerous meetings in which they found themselves repeating the same information to different people. This process eventually left them feeling devalued, exhausted and confused by the diverse and sometimes conflicting advice that they were given. They also felt that their family circumstances, knowledge and understanding of Athula were not considered when decisions were being made about support and interventions. This left them with a sense of being stereotyped victims of prejudicial assumptions.

After receiving the referral from the GP, the CLDT appointed a key worker who contacted the family initially by telephone to introduce themselves and to make arrangements to visit and meet with Sunil and Chandrika at a time that was convenient for them. At this initial meeting, the key worker spent time listening to the current concerns of the family and discussed the roles and responsibilities of other members of the CLDT who may be asked to help in undertaking assessments and providing support. Sunil and Chandrika's previous experiences and their feelings about the support they had received were explored and reassurance was given that the cultural and individual needs of the family would be valued and acknowledged. This was further confirmed by explaining that the role of the key worker was to inform and coordinate other professionals during their involvement with the family. Also, they were reassured that as key worker they were the first point of contact should they have any issues or concerns to discuss.

In considering how best to meet the needs of the family and in how to effectively coordinate care, the key worker first established, via discussion with the family and then further research, some of the cultural and religious traditions that needed to be considered. The social networks that the family engaged in were identified and discussion took place as to the support that they gained from these. Advice was given to other networks of support that they could consider accessing and details of these were provided in a booklet that also further exemplified the roles and responsibilities of members of the CLDT to whom they may have contact with.

Initially there was some disagreement between Sunil and Chandrika as to what they felt would be the best way of providing support for Athula. In order to explore, give value and listen to the views and opinions of both Sunil and Chandrika, the key worker arranged, with their agreement, to meet with them individually. After these meetings, the key worker identified the common themes and those issues that would need further discussion and exploration. This was facilitated in a tripartite meeting where the key worker was able to act as negotiator and reflector in order to help Sunil and Chandrika appreciate and understand each other's views and opinions. In mediating this meeting, compromises were made possible and a plan of action agreed.

Other elements to the effective coordination and support of this family included the following:

- Confirmation was sought about which language they would prefer to converse in and the use of a translator was discussed if necessary.
- The cultural, religious and specific needs of Athula and his family were met by continued discussion.
- All referrals were discussed prior to submission.
- Referrals were made for support in respect of meeting the needs of Saminda.
- Referrals were made for support in respect of meeting the needs of Chandrika's mother-in-law.
- Advice was provided about managing Athula's behaviour that was context specific.
- A carers' assessment was undertaken.
- A range of health-related assessments for Athula were identified and any necessary referrals to specialist health care professionals were discussed and sent.
- Views and opinions of both Sunil and Chandrika were continually explored.
- Education and training were provided in respect of autistic spectrum disorder, challenging behaviour and epilepsy.
- Support at home via day service was discussed and facilitated.
- Respite services were identified.
- Relevant legislation and policy were utilised to underpin support.
- The key worker ensured that all those involved in supporting the family understood the cultural and religious needs of the family.
- Advice about a carers' organisation for black and minority ethnic groups was given.

fragmentation and duplication of effort for carers and professionals. Some of these issues can be resolved by the adoption of a flexible approach to the arrangement and time of visits that gives consideration to what is best for the family carer rather than the professional (Dowling & Dolan 2001); the use of a key worker to decrease the amount of appointments, coordinate other professionals, reduce the burden of duplication and to ensure a consistent collective approach to advice and service provision (Limbrick-Spencer 2000).

> . . . if I was really worried about something I would sort of pick up the phone to his care manager and say, look you know is this alright or, and she sometimes would explain things to me as well. So her link was was quite crucial.
>
> (Ann – Mother)

Recognising and enhancing capability

Professionals need to recognise, acknowledge and nurture the diversity of successful coping strategies that have been developed by carers (Grant & Whittell 2000). Examples of these strategies include behavioural, cognitive, problem-solving, solution-focused and stress reduction techniques. Providing support that helps carers to achieve an equilibrium in respect of internal and external emotional and physical demands can help with their ability to cope (Chambers et al 2001). Other effective coping strategies that have been identified include seeking and accessing formal and informal social support; family cohesion; emotion and problem-focused strategies; behavioural and cognitive strategies; seeking information about their relative's condition; marital happiness and social support (Hassall et al 2005, Kenny & McGilloway 2007). The use of greater levels of social support have been found to decrease parenting stress with the perceived helpfulness of these supports being more important than the range of support being provided (Hassall et al 2005). The use of positive perceptions and social support resources has also been identified as helpful in the care giving role with positive development being reported in personal growth and maturity (Hastings et al 2002) (Fig. 22.2).

Figure 22.2 • Positive variables to support

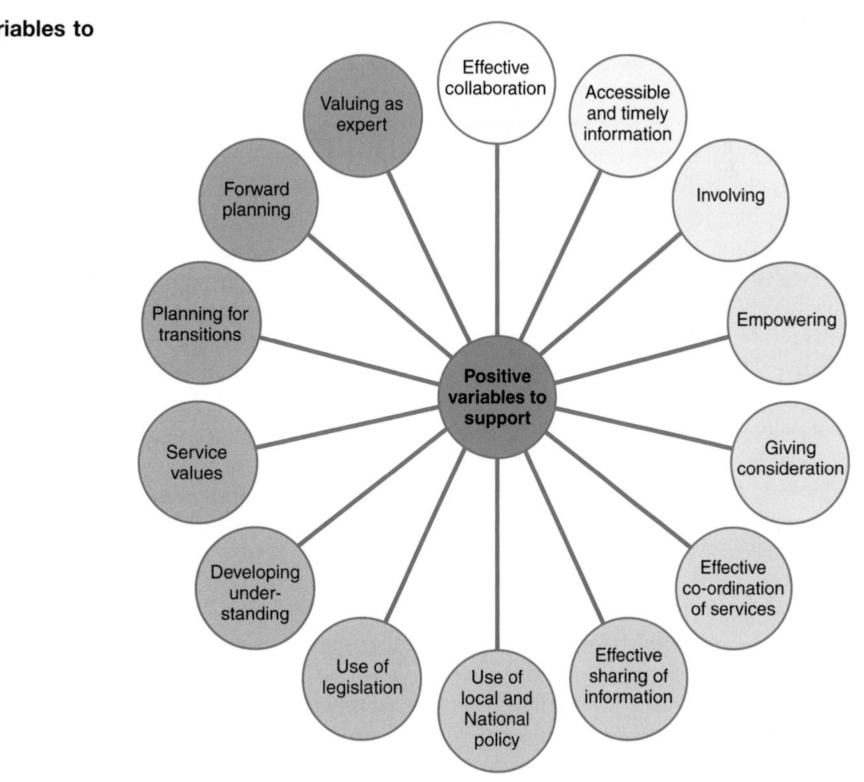

Understanding changing needs

The demand for services and support will vary demographically; however, it is important that services are planned based on the needs of the person with a learning disability, the age of the carers and their capacity to cope. Therefore, unique social and cultural differences need to be accounted for that avoid a 'one size fits all' approach. Informal kinship and access to social support can help to reduce levels of parenting stress dependent on how useful they are found to be (Hill & Rose 2009). Information should be given about local and national social support groups so that decisions can be made regarding their use. Also, the implications of not identifying and planning for future needs will place strain on financial and logistical resources (FPLD 2003) that could leave carers confused, anxious and concerned for the future of their relative.

Given that 25% of people with learning disabilities only become known to specialist services later in life, usually when their carer has become too frail to care for them (DH 2001b, FPLD 2003), the sudden need and involvement of services may lead to carers feeling overwhelmed and disempowered (Grant 2005). Services and professionals, across the arenas of health and social care, therefore need to develop coordinated, collaborative systems and processes that support the identification of older family carers and their relatives. This will help in planning for future need and also in providing services to meet current need by the undertaking of carers' assessments in line with current legislation.

Over time, as parents become older, experience ill health or die, the responsibility for caring for the family member may be taken on by a sibling, or another family member, as they may be the closest relative (Dew et al 2004). However, it is important that services do not assume that this will automatically take place as the relative may be unwilling, or unable, to take on this role. When the role is adopted, there is a need for services to consider the new carer's needs based on their individual circumstances. As a consequence, the support needs may have to be adapted and/or changed dependent on the context in which the family member is providing care as this may be very different to that previously experienced with the parents. The role of care giver may also be one that the family member had not prepared for so providing them with timely information and advice can help to negate some of the stress they may experience at this time of adaption.

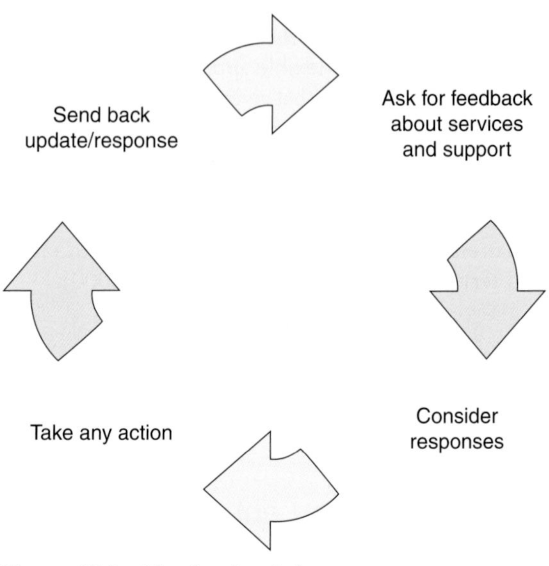

Figure 22.3 • The feedback loop

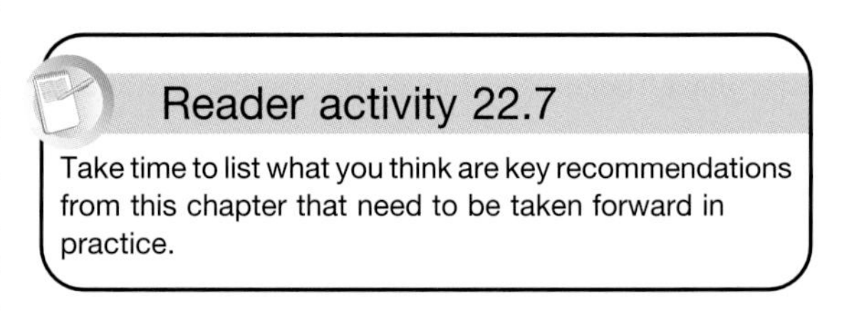

Reader activity 22.7

Take time to list what you think are key recommendations from this chapter that need to be taken forward in practice.

Providing feedback

While good practice should mean that services acquire feedback from people with learning disabilities whenever possible, so it should be that their carers are also given the opportunity to comment on their experiences with services and professionals in order to inform the delivery of services and the development of local and national policies. This gaining of feedback should form part of a feedback loop whereby carers are kept informed of the outcomes of their input (see Fig. 22.3).

Conclusion

It is important that professionals and services acknowledge the important role that families take in caring for people with a learning disability and that they involve carers in delivering high quality, collaborative and effective support and care. Therefore, family carers need to be recognised as the real experts when it comes to their relative. Failing to develop relationships and involve families can contribute to difficulties in developing new policies and ways of working to meet the needs of individuals with a learning disability. It is important to work in collaboration in order to avoid marginalisation, disempowerment and reducing the valuable contribution that family carers can make.

People's situations will inevitably change over time resulting in fluctuating levels of need for support. Caring for a person with a learning disability therefore is not a static state in which professionals can ascribe one mode of working on a long-term basis. Instead, there is a need to re-evaluate and be proactive so that support is provided relevant to the context and particular point in time. Planning and delivery of support to family carers needs to be tailored to individual families rather than a prescribed rigid approach. Services and professionals should be focused on helping the family situation by providing support that helps the family to choose and live life in the best way possible with the person they are caring for.

References

Acheson, D., 1998. Independent inquiry into inequalities in health. The Stationery Office, London.

Ahmad, W., Atkin, K., 1996. 'Race' and community care. Open University Press, Buckingham.

Alexander, Z., 1999. The Department of Health: study of black, asian and ethnic minority issues. Department of Health, London.

Atkin, K., Ahmad, W., 2000. Family caregiving and chronic illness: how parents cope with a child with a sickle cell disorder or thalassaemia. Health and Social Care in the Community 8, 57–69.

Barr, O., 1996. Developing services for people with learning disabilities which actively involve family members: a review of recent literature. Health and Social Care in the Community 4 (2), 103–112.

Barr, O., 2007. Working effectively with families of people with learning disabilities. In: Gates, B. (Ed.), Learning disability: toward inclusion. fifth ed. Churchill Livingstone, Edinburgh, pp. 567–597.

Barron, S., McConkey, R., Mulvany, F., 2006. Family carers of adult persons with intellectual disabilities on the island of Ireland. Journal of Policy and Practice in Intellectual Disabilities 3 (2), 87–94.

Bogues, S., 2004. Focus on families: messages from family carers. Department of Health, Social Services and Public Safety (DHSSPS), Belfast, Northern Ireland.

Bromley, J., Hare, D.J., Davison, K., Emerson, E., 2004. Mothers supporting children with autistic spectrum disorders. Autism 8, 409–423.

Burton-Smith, R., McVilly, K.R., Yazbeck, M., Parementer, T.R., Tsutsui, T., 2009. Quality of life of Australian family carers: implications for research, policy, and practice. Journal of Policy and Practice in Intellectual Disabilities 6 (3), 189–198.

Carers UK, 2004. In poor health: the impact of caring on health. Carers UK, London.

Carpenter, B., 1997. Families in context: emerging trends in family support and early intervention. David Fulton, London.

Case, S., 2001. Learning to partner, disabling conflict: early indications of an improving relationship between parents and professionals with regard to service provision for children with learning disabilities. Disability and Society 16 (6), 837–854.

Chamba, R., Ahmad, W., Hirst, M., Lawton, D., Beresford, B., 1999. On the edge: minority ethnic families caring for a severely disabled child. Policy Press, Bristol.

Chambers, M., Ryan, A.A., Connor, S.L., 2001. Exploring the emotional support needs and coping strategies of family carers. J. Psychiatr. Ment. Health Nurs. 8, 99–106.

Chapman, V., 2004. Carer issues in mental health. In: Kirby, S.D., Hart, D.A., Cross, D., Mitchell, G. (Eds.), Mental health nursing – competencies for practice. Palgrave MacMillan, Basingstoke, pp. 56–65.

Cunningham, C.C., Davis, H., 1985. Working with parents: frameworks for collaboration. Open University Press, Buckingham.

Dale, N., 1996. Working with families of children with special needs: partnership and practice. Routledge, London.

Department of Health, 1999. Caring about carers. Department of Health, London.

Department of Health, 2001a. Valuing people. Department of Health, London.

Department of Health, 2001b. Families matters – counting families in. Department of Health, London.

Department of Health, 2004. Learning difficulties and ethnicity: a framework for action. Department of Health, London.

Department of Health, 2008. Carers at the heart of 21st-century families and communities. Department of Health, London.

Department of Health, 2009. Valuing people now: a new three year strategy for people with learning disabilities. Department of Health, London.

Department of Health, Social Services and Public Safety, 2006. Caring for carers: recognising, valuing and supporting the caring role. Department of Health, Social Services and Public Safety, Belfast.

Dew, A., Llewellyn, G., Balandin, S., 2004. Post-parental care: a new generation of sibling-carers. J. Intellect. Dev. Disabil. 29 (2), 176–179.

Douma, J.C.H., Dekker, M.C., Koot, H.M., 2006. Supporting parents of youths with intellectual disabilities and psychopathology. J. Intellect. Disabil. Res. 50 (8), 570–581.

Dowling, M., Dolan, L., 2001. Families with children with disabilities–inequalities and the social model. Disability and Society 16 (1), 21–35.

Eisenhower, A., Blacher, J., 2006. Mothers of young adults with intellectual disability: multiple roles, ethnicity and well-being. J. Intellect. Disabil. Res. 50 (12), 905–916.

Emerson, E., Hatton, C., Llewellyn, G., Blacker, J., Graham, H., 2006. Socio-economic position, household composition, health status and indicators of the well-being of mothers of children with and without intellectual disabilities [corrected] [published erratum appears in J. Intellect. Disabil. Res. 51 (2): 172]. J. Intellect. Disabil. Res. 50 (12), 862–873.

Esdaile, S.A., 2003. A comparison of mothers' and fathers' experience of parenting stress and attributions for parentchild interaction outcomes. Occup. Ther. Int. 10 (2), 115–126.

Faust, H., Scior, K., 2008. Mental health problems in young people with intellectual disabilities: the impact on parents. J. Appl. Res. Intellect. Disabil. 21, 414–424.

Fitzpatrick, A., Dowling, M., 2007. Supporting parents caring for a child with a learning disability. Nurs. Stand. 22 (14–16), 35–39.

Foundation for People with Learning Disabilities, 2003. Planning for tomorrow – report on the findings of a survey of learning disability partnership boards about meeting the needs of older family carers. Mental Health Foundation, London.

Foundation for People with Learning Disabilities, 2010. Statistics about people with learning disabilities. Available at: http://www.learningdisabilities.org.uk/information/learning-disabilities-statistics/ (accessed 30.04.10.).

Gerstein, E., Crnic, K., Blacher, J., Baker, B., 2009. Resilience and the course of daily parenting stress in families of young children with intellectual disabilities. J. Intellect. Disabil. Res. 53 (12), 981–997.

Giddens, A., 2009. Sociology. Polity Press, Cambridge.

Grant, G., 2005. Experiences of family care – bridging discontinuities over the life course. In: Grant, G., Goward, P., Richardson, M., Ramcharan, P. (Eds.), Learning disability: a life cycle approach to valuing people. Open University Press, Maidenhead, pp. 222–242.

Grant, G., Ramcharan, P., 2001. Views and experiences of people with intellectual disabilities and their families (2). The family perspective. J. Appl. Res. Intellect. Disabil. 14, 364–380.

Grant, G., Whittell, B., 1999. Family care of people with learning disabilities. University of Wales, Cardiff.

Grant, G., Whittell, B., 2000. Differentiated coping strategies in families with children or adults with intellectual disabilities: the relevance of gender, family composition and the life span. J. Appl. Res. Intellect. Disabil. 13, 256–275.

Grant, G., Ramcharan, P., McGrath, M., Nolan, M., Keady, J., 1998. Rewards and gratifications among family caregivers: towards a refined model of caring and coping. J. Intellect. Disabil. Res. 42 (1), 58–71.

Grant, G., Nolan, M., Keady, J., 2003. Supporting families over the life course: mapping temporality. J. Intellect. Disabil. Res. 47 (4/5), 342–351.

Haralambos, M., Holborn, M., Heald, R., 2004. Sociology – themes and perspectives. Collins, London.

Hassall, R., Rose, J., McDonald, J., 2005. Parenting stress in mothers of children with an intellectual disability: the effects of parental cognitions in relation to child characteristics and family support. J. Intellect. Disabil. Res. 49 (6), 405–418.

Hastings, R., 2003. Child behaviour problems and partner mental health as correlates of stress in mothers and fathers of children with autism. J. Intellect. Disabil. Res. 47 (4/5), 231–237.

Hastings, R.P., Allen, R., McDermott, K., Still, D., 2002. Factors related to positive perceptions in mothers of children with intellectual disabilties. J. Appl. Res. Intellect. Disabil. 15, 269–275.

Hatton, C., Azmi, S., Emerson, E., Caine, A., 1997. Researching the needs of South Asian people with learning difficulties and their families. Ment. Health Care 1, 91–94.

Hatton, C., Azmi, S., Caine, A., Emerson, E., 1998. Informal carers of adolescents and adults with learning disabilities from South Asian communities. British Journal of Social Work 28, 821–837.

Hatton, C., Akram, Y., Shah, R., Robertson, J., Emerson, E., 2004. Supporting South Asian families with a child with severe disabilites. Jessica Kingsley, London.

Hatton, C., Emerson, E., Kirby, S., et al., 2010. Majority and minority ethnic family carers of adults with intellectual disabilities: perceptions of challenging behaviour and family impact. J. Appl. Res. Intellect. Disabil. 23, 63–74.

Henneman, E., Lee, J., Cohen, J., 1995. Collaboration: a concept analysis. J. Adv. Nurs. 21 (1), 103–109.

Hill, C., Rose, J., 2009. Parenting stress in mothers of adults with an intellectual disability: parental cognitions in relation to child characteristics and family support. J. Intellect. Disabil. Res. 53 (12), 969–980.

Hubert, J., 2006. Family carers' views of services for people with learning disabilities from Black and minority ethnic groups: a qualitative study of 30 families in a south London borough. Disability and Society 21, 259–272.

Kenny, K., McGilloway, S., 2007. Caring for children with learning disabilities: an exploratory study of parental strain and coping. British Journal of Learning Disabilities 35 (4), 221–228.

Knox, M., Parmenter, T.R., Atkinson, N., Yazbeck, M., 2000. Family control: the views of families who have a child with an intellectual disability. J. Appl. Res. Intellect. Disabil. 13, 17–28.

Law, M., Hanna, S., King, G., et al., 2003. Factors affecting family-centred service delivery for children with disabilities. Child Care Health Dev. 29 (5), 357–366.

Limbrick-Spencer, G., 2000. Parent support needs: the views of parents of children with complex needs. Handsel Trust, Birmingham.

McConkey, R., 2005. Fair shares? Supporting families caring for adults persons with intellectual disabilities. J. Intellect. Disabil. Res. 49 (8), 600–612.

McGill, P., Papachristoforou, E., Cooper, V., 2006. Support for family carers of children and young people with developmental disabilities and challenging behaviour. Child Care Health Dev. 32 (2), 159–165.

Mansell, W., Morris, K., 2004. A survey of parents' reactions to the diagnosis of an autistic spectrum disorder by a local service – access to information and use of services. Autism 8 (4), 387–407.

Manthorpe, J., 1995. Services to families. In: Malin, N. (Ed.), Services for people with learning disabilities. Routledge, London, pp. 111–124.

Marshall, J.K., Mirenda, P., 2002. Parent–professional collaboration for positive behavior support in the home. Focus on Autism and Other Developmental Disabilites 17 (4), 216–228.

Mencap, 2001. No ordinary life: the support needs of families caring for children and adults with profound and multiple learning disabilities. Mencap, London.

Mencap, 2003. Breaking point: a report on caring without a break for children and adults with severe or profound learning disabilities. Mencap, London.

Mencap, 2006. Breaking point – families still need a break. A report on the continuing problem of caring without a break for children and adults with severe and profound learning disability. Mencap, London.

Mir, G., Nocon, A., Ahmad, W., Jones, L., 2001. Learning difficulties and ethnicity – report to the Department of Health. Department of Health, London.

Mulrooney, M., Harrold, M., 2004. Parent's voices. In: Walsh, P.N., Gash, H. (Eds.), Lives and times: practice, policy and people with disabilities. Bray, Ratchdown, pp. 44–62.

Nolan, M., 2001. Working with family carers: towards a partnership approach. Reviews in Clinical Gerontology 11, 91–97.

Northway, R., Sardi, I., Mansell, I., Jenkins, R., 2006. Hopes and fears concerning service developments: a focus group study of parents and carers of people with a learning disability. University of Glamorgan, Pontypridd.

Olsson, M., Hwang, P., 2003. Influence of macrostructure of society on the life situation of families with a child with intellectual disability: Sweden as an example. J. Intellect. Disabil. Res. 47 (4/5), 328–341.

Prezant, F.P., Marshak, L., 2006. Helpful actions seen throughthe eyes of parents of children with disabilities. Disability and Society 21 (1), 31–45.

Reading, J., Raj, M., 2000. Ethnicity and disability: moving towards equity in service provision. CVS Consultants, London.

Redmond, B., Richardson, V., 2003. Just getting on with it: exploring the service needs of mothers who care for young children with severe/profound and life-threatening intellectual disability. J. Appl. Res. Intellect. Disabil. 16 (3), 205–218.

Rose, L.E., Mallinson, R.K., Walton-Moss, B., 2004. Barriers to family care in psychiatric settings. J. Nurs. Scholarsh. 36 (1), 39–47.

Sardi, I., Northway, R., Jenkins, R., Davies, R., Mansell, I., 2008. Family carer's opinions on learning disability services. Nurs. Times 104 (11), 30–31.

Scottish Executive, 1999. Strategy for carers in Scotland. Scotland Executive, Edinburgh.

Scottish Executive, 2000. The same as you? A review of services for people with learning disabilities. The Stationery Office, Edinburgh.

Sheard, D., 2004. Person centred care: the emperor's new clothes? Journal of Dementia Care 12 (2), 22–25.

Shearn, J., Todd, S., 1997. Parental work: an account of the day-to-day activities of parents of adults with learning disabilities. J. Intellect. Disabil. Res. 41 (4), 285–301.

Shin, J.Y., Nhan, N.V., 2009. Predictors of parenting stress among Vietnamese mothers of young children with and without cognitive delay. J. Intellect. Dev. Disabil. 34 (1), 17–26.

Sloper, P., 1999. Models of service support for parents of disabled children. What do we know? What do we need to know? Child Care Health Dev. 25 (2), 85–99.

Todd, S., Jones, S., 2003. Mum's the Word!': maternal accounts of dealings with the professional world. J. Appl. Res. Intellect. Disabil. 16 (3), 229–244.

Todd, S., Jones, S., 2005. Looking at the future and seeing the past: the challenge of the middle years of parenting a child with intellectual disabilities. J. Intellect. Disabil. Res. 49 (6), 389–404.

Todd, S., Shearn, J., 1996. Struggles with time: the careers of parents with adult sons and daughters with learning disabilities. Disability and Society 11 (3), 379–402.

Todd, S., Shearn, J., Beyer, S., Felce, D., 1993. Careers in caring: the changing situations of parents caring for an offspring with learning difficulties. The Irish Journal of Psychology 14 (1), 130–153.

Turnbull, A.P., Turnbull, H.R., 1990. Families, professionals, and exceptionality: collaborating for empowerment. Merrill/Prentice Hall, Englewood Cliffs, NJ.

Wade, C.M., Mildon, R.L., Matthews, J.M., 2007. Service delivery to parents with an intellecutal disability: family-centred or professionally centred. J. Appl. Res. Intellect. Disabil. 20, 87–98.

Walden, S., Pistrang, N., Joyce, T., 2000. Parents of adults with intellectual disabilities: quality of life and experiences of caring. J. Appl. Res. Intellect. Disabil. 13 (2), 62–76.

Welsh Assembly Government, 2007. Carers' strategy for Wales – action plan 2007. Welsh Assembly Government, Cardiff.

Wodehouse, G., McGill, P., 2009. Support for family carers of children and young people with developmental disabilities and challenging behaviour: what stops it being helpful? J. Intellect. Disabil. Res. 53 (7), 664–1653.

Wong, S.Y., Wong, T.K.S., 2003. An exploratory study on needs of parents of adults with a severe learning disability in a residential setting. Issues Ment. Health Nurs. 24, 795–811.

Further reading

Dunhill, A., Elliott, B., Shaw, A., 2009. Effecitve communication and engagement with children and young people, their families and carers. Learning Matters, Exeter.

Holt, G., Gratsa, A., Bouras, N., et al., 2004. Guide to mental health for families and carers of people with intellectual disabilities. Jessica Kingsley, London.

Matthews, J., 2006. The carer's handbook: essential information and support for all those in a caring role. How to Books, Oxford.

Nolan, M., Grant, G., Keady, J., 1996. Understanding family care. Open University Press, Buckingham.

Smith, G., 2007. Families, carers and professionals. John Wiley & Sons, Chichester.

Useful addresses

Carers UK: 20 Great Dover Street, London SE1 4LX, Tel: 020 7378 4999: http://www.carersuk.org/Home

A UK charity that provides a voice for carers.

Carers Northern Ireland: 58 Howard Street, Belfast BT1 6PJ, Tel: 028 9043 9843: http://www.carersni.org/Home

Part of Carers UK and works for a better deal for all carers in Northern Ireland.

Carers Scotland: The Cottage, 21 Pearce Street, Glasgow G51 3UT, Tel: 0141 445 3070: http://www.carersscotland.org/Home

Part of Carers UK and works for a better deal for all carers in Scotland.

Carers Wales: River House, Ynysbridge Court, Gwaelod y Garth, Cardiff CF15 9SS, Tel: 029 2081 1370: http://www.carerswales.org/Home

Part of Carers UK and works for a better deal for all carers in Wales.

The Carers Association: The Carers Association National Office, Market Square, Tullamore, Co. Offaly, Tel: 057 932 2920: http://www.carersireland.com/

Ireland's national voluntary organisation for and of family carers in the home.

Care Information Scotland: Tel: 08456 001 001: http://www.careinfoscotland.co.uk/home.aspx

This is a telephone and website service providing information for people living in Scotland.

British Institute of Learning Disabilities: Campion House, Green Street, Kidderminster, Worcestershire DY10 1JL, Tel: 01562 723 010: http://www.bild.org.uk/

Works to improve the lives of people with a learning disability in the UK.

Mencap

A charity based in the UK that works with people with a learning disability and their families.

Mencap England, 123 Golden Lane, London EC1Y 0RT, Tel: 020 7454 0454: http://www.mencap.org.uk/

Mencap Northern Ireland: Segal House, 4 Annadale Avenue, Belfast BT7 3JH, Tel: 02890 691 351

Mencap Wales: 31 Lambourne Crescent, Cardiff Business Park, Llanishen, Cardiff CF14 5GF, Tel: 02920 747 588

The Joseph Rowntree Foundation: Head Office, The Homestead, 40 Water End, York YO30 6WP, Tel: 01904 629 241: http://www.jrf.org.uk/

A UK- wide social policy research and development charity.

National Family Carer Network: c/o Hft, 5/6 Brook Office Park, Folly Brook Road, Emersons Green, Bristol BS16 7FL, Tel: 01883 722 311 or 07747 460 727: http://www.familycarers.org.uk/

Links groups and organisations that support families.

The Princess Royal Trust for Carers

A provider of comprehensive carers' support services in the UK and provides quality information, advice and support.

London Office: The Princess Royal Trust for Carers, Unit 14, Bourne Court, Southend Road, Woodford Green, Essex IG8 8HD, Tel: 0844 800 4361: http://www.carers.org/

Glasgow Office: The Princess Royal Trust for Carers, Charles Oakley House, 125 West Regent Street, Glasgow G2 2SD, Tel: 0141 221 5066

Wales Office: Victoria House, 250 Cowbridge Road East, Canton, Cardiff CF5 1GZ, Tel: 02920 221 788

Useful websites

Official UK Government website: http://www.direct.gov.uk/en/index.htm

The Government of Ireland: http://www.gov.ie/en/

The Northern Ireland Executive: http://www.northernireland.gov.uk/

The Scottish Government: http://www.scotland.gov.uk/Home

Welsh Assembly Government: http://wales.gov.uk/splash?orig=/

Official website of the Department of Health with links to information, advice and legislation for carers: http://www.dh.gov.uk/en/SocialCare/Carers/index.htm

Every Child Matters: The UK Government's programme for a national framework to support a more joined up approach to the delivery of children's services: http://www.dcsf.gov.uk/everychildmatters/

Information from the National Health Service on conditions, treatments, local services and healthy living: http://www.nhs.uk/Pages/HomePage.aspx

Foundation for People with Learning Disabilities: http://www.learningdisabilities.org.uk/welcome/

NHS website providing up to date evidence about issues to do with learning disabilities: http://www.library.nhs.uk/learningdisabilities/

Childhood

23

Mary Dearing

CHAPTER CONTENTS

KEY ISSUES

- Children with learning disabilities are children first
- Children may be diagnosed at birth or during childhood with a learning disability but this diagnosis will have a lifelong impact on the child and their family
- Children with learning disabilities will achieve some developmental milestones but these may be delayed
- Having a child with a learning disability may impact upon individual family members, for example parents, siblings and grandparents
- Children with a learning disability should be listened to particularly as plans are made to move onto new stages in life
- Children with learning disabilities have an additional risk of harm which should not be underestimated

Introduction

The news of the birth of a baby is generally a joyous event. Mothers and their newborn infant are often showered with gifts to celebrate and mark the significance of this important occasion. New parents have expectations and optimism for their newborn son or daughter but typically their greatest aspiration is that the infant will enjoy good health. For all parents, the birth of their first baby is an important transition. Whatever mothers and fathers expect parenthood to be like, the demands are usually far greater than ever imagined and the birth of a baby not only brings joy but also additional anxieties as new parents attempt to work out how they will make adjustments to their lives. Recent reports suggest that the financial cost of raising a child from birth until the age of 21 is estimated to be £194 000 (Paton 2009), however what is more difficult to estimate is the social and emotional price that parents pay for the happiness and pleasure of having a child. When it becomes apparent that a child has been born with, or is later diagnosed as having, a learning disability, this price may be set even higher, as this generally unexpected and therefore unplanned event may thrust families into a completely new world of professionals and services of which they have no previous knowledge or awareness. They need to adapt to their new situation and may begin to adopt a new set of values, beliefs and expectations.

Learning disability may be diagnosed at any time in childhood or adolescence provided it occurred before the age of 18 (Department of Health (DH) 2001a). In general, the more severe the learning disability, the earlier it becomes apparent and therefore the earlier it is diagnosed (Lindsey 2003). With the advancement of medical technology and ultrasound scans, some parents may already know that their child may have a disabling condition prior to the birth (see Ch. 2). For other families, the news that their son or daughter has a learning disability may imminently follow the birth, while for others, it may be months or years before they are formally told that their child is developmentally delayed or has a specific condition which results in them having a learning disability. However, what is a commonality for these families is the period of readjustment they experience when hopes and aspirations are reassessed (Burke 2004) as they begin to come to terms and adapt to their new situation. It should be stressed that with the right support from their families, friends and professionals, children with learning disabilities can enjoy their childhood, grow up with good self-esteem and make a positive contribution to society (Lindsey 2003).

Given a world population of approximately 6.5 billion, it is estimated that 780 million children between birth and the age of 5 may have a learning disability (Olness 2003). In England, there are an estimated 190 000 children and young people under the age of 20 who have a learning disability (Emerson & Hatton 2004). These statistics differ to those published by the Department of Health (2007) which suggests that there are between 55 000 and 75 000 children with moderate or severe learning disabilities in England. An explanation for the variance in statistics may be found in the Department for Education and Skills (DfES) report *Aiming Higher for Disabled Children* (DES 2007). The report highlights that some local authorities have a good understanding of their local populations and undertake thorough needs assessments, while other authorities still do not have a sufficient understanding of the needs of children in their area or an understanding of their disabled children population. If services for children with disabilities are to be developed then it is vital for local authorities to demonstrate that they have good quality and up-to-date information to plan future provision.

Despite the variance in figures, there is general agreement that the number of children with learning disabilities is set to increase with the advancement of medical technology. A recent longitudinal study revealed that 80% of babies born at 26 weeks... gestation now survive although it is stated that nearly half of these infants will have a moderate to severe disability (Marlow et al 2005). It is important, therefore, that professionals who work with children with learning disabilities and their families not only have sufficient knowledge and skill to meet the changing needs of this group but also consider their own values and attitudes so that positive outcomes can be achieved and an effective parent partnership established.

This chapter focuses on the needs of children with learning disabilities and their families, exploring evidence and best practice to support them to live the most fulfilling lives possible. In order to achieve this, the reader will follow the same journey a family may take following the diagnosis of a learning disability and the effect this may consequently have on the child, their parents, their siblings and other family members as they develop from infancy through to childhood and eventual adulthood.

Defining child

For the purpose of this chapter, the definition of a child has been adopted from the *Family Resource Survey 2008–2009* (National Centre for Social Research 2009) and is used to refer to a dependent individual under the age of 19, living with parents or carers. However, when national and international legislation is reviewed, there are various definitions of 'child' proposed that are dependent on a range of differential factors and which consequently lead to confusion, particularly in transition to adult services when young people can transfer to different services at different ages. The UN Convention on the Rights of the Child, ratified by the UK Government in 1991, states that child "means every human being below the age of 18 years unless, under the law applicable to the child, majority is attained earlier." (United Nations (UN) 1989 Article 1). Although in

England, Wales, Northern Ireland and Scotland definitions of being a child may vary slightly, when keeping children safe is an issue, it is agreed *a child is anyone who has not yet reached their 18th birthday*. There is no single law in the United Kingdom that defines the age of a child, although relevant laws specify age limits; however these can vary between the United Kingdom nations.

Prior to the Warnock Report (Warnock 1978), children with learning disabilities were classified as having mild, moderate or severe difficulties. However, the present United Kingdom classification accepts the advice of the report that the term 'learning difficulties' be applied to all children requiring special educational provision despite the consequences of the nature or severity of their needs (Nabuzoka 2000).

The UK Children Act 2004 provides a strategy to improve the lives of all children. This Act defines a child as a person up to the age of 20 if it is identified that they have a learning disability. However, the *Apprenticeships, Skills, Children and Learning Bill* (Department of Children, Schools and Families 2009) recommends that the responsibility for the funding and organisation of 16–19-year-olds... learning will be reassigned from the Learning and Skills Council to local authorities, hence ensuring that all children up until the age of 19, who are taught in colleges rather than schools, are the responsibility of their local authority. This is to ensure that there will then be a single point of accountability for all 0–19 children's services and that local authorities will be better positioned to plan and coordinate provision across all institutions in their area and able to respond to local situations, local economic demand and learners' individual needs and choices. For children with a learning disability, this age limit is extended to 25. However, these different age limits on when children cease to be children can sometimes obscure what services children and young people are eligible to, particularly in the case of young people with profound and multiple disabilities who may receive services from a range of statutory and voluntary organisations.

The developing child

Child development

All children develop and learn at different rates and in diverse ways but some will develop and learn at a much slower pace than their peers. The diagnosis of a learning disability is most often made by a paediatrician (a doctor specialising in the care of children); however, for this to happen, it first has to be recognised that a delay in development is present. It is important for all who work with infants and young children to understand normal child development to enable them to recognise when a child is not developing as expected. Although every child is unique and no two children will reach their developmental milestones at the same time, for children with learning disabilities early detection is vital so that early intervention programmes can commence. Guralnick (2005) suggests that early interventions will improve the development of young children both by changing their developmental trajectories and by avoiding secondary complications. In some circumstances, a learning disability can be linked to a number of genetic or inherited conditions such as Down syndrome (see Ch. 2), and for parents who already know their child's development will be delayed, there will be moments of pride as their child reaches each new milestone. Other parents may experience growing concern if their child does not appear to be developing at the same rate as others of a similar age; in addition, they may face difficulties and frustration in having professionals acknowledge this and feel they are treated as over-anxious parents. Many parents still experience a long and exhausting diagnostic process as it is not possible to state a definitive diagnosis in 30–50% of children with learning disability (Daily et al 2000). For parents, the recognition that their child has an learning disability is stressful (Case 2001) and it has been established that initial experiences with health professionals have a major, lasting influence on the parents' ability to cope with their child's condition (Davies et al 2003). Professionals should therefore remain acutely aware of how their responses to parental concerns might be interpreted and the manner in which they convey information.

When working with children with learning disabilities, it is imperative to have an understanding of normal child development and the theories that provide an understanding of this process (e.g. Erikson 1950, Piaget 1954). A multitude of terms are used both nationally and internationally that are intended to clarify for parents their child's difficulties but often just add further confusion. The term 'global developmental delay' is generally used to indicate that a child is developing more slowly, in all areas of development, than another child of the same age, while the term 'developmental delay' is used when a child's development is delayed in one or more areas of development (physical, social, cognitive, language and emotional). Adoption of the term 'delay' rather than 'disability' may be more acceptable as some children may match the achievement of their peers once a specific difficulty has been identified and addressed, for example a hearing or visual difficulty. However, for other children, if a significant learning delay persists as the child gets older, and this delay impinges on a number of areas of the child's development, professionals may begin to consider a learning disability. This implies they assume that the child will continue to learn at a slower pace than other children of the same age into adulthood. It is therefore essential for professionals to undertake a holistic assessment before diagnosing a learning disability.

Development is an intricate concept that involves an interaction of biological, cognitive and socio-emotional processes through which we grow and change through our experiences and interaction with the world around us (Santrock 2007). Biological processes refer to the changes which happen to a child's body; cognitive processes relate to the child's thought, intelligence and language development; and socio-emotional processes relate to a child's relationship with other people which may emerge as changes occur in a child's emotions and personality. The development of an infant is usually measured in terms of what is normal and expected at any given age but is influenced by both individual maturation rates and experiences (Empson & Nabuzoka 2004). Simpson & Weiner (1989) offer the definition of the word development as 'a new stage in a changing situation'. Adopting this definition, development starts at the moment of conception and continues until death.

Case illustration 23.1

When Jack was born, his long-awaited arrival was celebrated by his parents and their families. Doting grandparents and aunts and uncles would visit regularly bearing gifts and offering their services as baby sitters. It was not until Jack was 6 months old that his mother began to question his development. She had noticed that other children of the same age were grasping and holding objects as they sat on play mats surrounded by their toys but Jack showed little interest in his toys and was unable to sit unsupported. Initially health professionals tried to reassure his mum that all children are individual and will reach developmental milestones in their own time, but when Jack was a year old they too began to express concern and numerous referrals were made to other professionals to seek their opinion. Jack's mum felt very frustrated as she attempted to juggle her return to full-time employment with a barrage of appointments. Those initial offers of help quickly began to dwindle and Jack's parents began to feel isolated as it slowly dawned on them that their child might be different.

Reader activity 23.1

Consider Jack's story in Case illustration 23.1 and try to answer the following:

- If Jack lived in your area, what professionals might he be referred to for further assessment?
- What emotions might Jack's parents be feeling?
- What additional support might Jack and his family require in the forthcoming months and who might offer this support?

The early years

How children develop is usually measured in milestones; these are skills which children generally acquire within a specific time frame. Child milestones usually develop in a sequential manner, however not all children develop within these specific time frames. If infants have developed in the uterus normally, at birth their senses should be functional although they will still need to fully develop. Over the first few days, the baby's ability to hear should become refined and they become able to recognise differences between almost all speech sounds (Berk 2006). Varendi et al (1998) propose that the smell of the mother's amniotic fluid has been found to comfort distressed babies suggesting that babies respond to smell. The baby's ability to focus and see develops during the first year of life; at birth the infant should be able to track moving objects even though they are unable to fully focus and by 5 months an infant will use shape, colour and texture to identify objects (Cohen & Cashon 2001). A further sense present at this time is touch, hence babies will respond to pain with a stressful cry and a dramatic rise in heart rate and blood pressure (Warnock & Sandrin 2004).

During the first year of life, the baby usually grows and develops rapidly. Within a short period of time (2–3 months), the baby will begin to smile in response to an external stimulus, often referred to as the social smile (Sroufe & Walters 1976). When the baby is 2–3 months old, they are generally able to begin to control their eye muscles by fixating on a face and respond to being touched. Other motor skills such as the baby's ability to lift its head when laid on their stomach also begins to develop. By the time the baby is 4–6 months old, they are beginning to make sounds and have control of their head and arm movements and will generally attempt to roll over. These milestones are examples of gross motor skills, skills that involve large muscle activities such as moving arms and legs (Santrock 2007). Gross motor skills such as crawling, sitting up and walking generally occur between 6 and 18 months and the baby continues to develop socially through play and interaction with others. At this stage, the baby can distinguish between people and recognise who is familiar to them and who is not. During this time, the baby's emotional responses become evident and the baby will protest when separated from its mother or main care provider. At this age, use of the baby's name should elicit a response and interactive games will be enjoyed. As the baby becomes more curious, other emotions are also evident such as affection and anger.

Language development also begins at birth when babies will attract attention from their care givers by actively producing sounds (Lock 2004). Between 8 and 12 months, infants will begin to say their first words. Although parents enthusiastically anticipate this occasion, babies have in fact been communicating with their parents through gestures and sounds, therefore the emergence of first words is just a continuation of this process (Berko Gleason 2005). By 18 months to 2 years, language development should have occurred and a child may have in excess of 200 words in their vocabulary. Fine motor skills are also developing and babies should now be able to build towers of bricks and begin to hold a spoon. Although they are still dependent on others, they are usually beginning to show signs of autonomy (Lissauer & Clayden 2001).

During these first 2 years of a baby's life, GPs (family doctors) and health visitors (HVs) monitor their development (Batchelor 1999). If they are concerned that a child is not developing within an expected range then they are usually referred to a more specialist children's doctor for further investigation into why they may not be developing as anticipated. For some parents, it is at this stage that they are alerted to the fact that their child may be developmentally delayed and subsequently be diagnosed as having a learning disability. As with all children, the developmental profile of a child with a learning disability varies. Global delay is not always present; some children with autistic spectrum conditions and learning disability, for example, may achieve milestones of physical development in line with the norm (National Institute of Mental Health 2004).

As children get older, there is both an expectation and need to complete more complex tasks; it is often at this stage that differences between a child with a learning disability and their peers become more noticeable. Self-care skills may develop at a slower rate and some children will need more support with activities of daily living (for example eating, bathing and dressing). It is vital to not just focus on the physical needs of the developing child but also to place emphasis on the child's emotional development as children with learning disabilities may be aware of being different to their peers and siblings which can then be associated with poor self-esteem. Hence the need to address emotional wellbeing and promote good mental health should be emphasised (Lindsey 2003).

Children with learning disabilities will continue to learn new skills throughout their lives but to assist them to develop to their full potential it is essential to focus on their strengths and assist them. It should be remembered that a child needs to have developed the prerequisite skills before new skills can be learnt, making the old adage true that you really do need to be able to learn to walk before you can run. Careful assessment at this stage is crucial to ensure that the child receives the most appropriate interventions to assist them to develop to their full potential.

Even though there has been a rapid expansion in early intervention services for children with learning disabilities, it has only been in more recent years that a child has been seen in the context of their natural families and communities (Hamilton 2004). More recently, there has been a shift from child-centred interventions to family-centred interventions. This shift in provision is largely based on the principle that children are dependent on their families for survival, growth and development- and as no single agency or discipline can meet all the needs of any one child or family, then the key to any successful intervention programme is collaboration and partnership between families and professionals (Turnbull et al 1999). The starting point for all interventions is a comprehensive assessment and it is at this stage that collaboration between families and professionals should be established.

Common Assessment Framework

The Common Assessment Framework (CAF) is a standard assessment tool originally published by the DES in 2006 to provide guidance to support integrated working. The CAF is acclaimed as a needs-led, evidence-based tool which will promote consistency, ensure appropriate 'early intervention' while simultaneously reducing referral rates to local authority children's services. It is envisaged to promote 'a common language' among professionals working with children in situations where additional needs are observed. The CAF is intended to reduce the number of initial assessments children and their families often have to endure and "avoid children and their families having to re-tell their story" (DES 2006:12). It is envisaged that as children grow and develop, there may be a need for further assessments. These assessments should be conducted in a coordinated manner and, more importantly, be provided in the same place at the same time (DES 2007), to avoid children and families making multiple trips to see multiple professionals from multiple agencies. The challenge to service providers is to identify accurately and sensitively those children who may require services and to ensure appropriate and timely services that result in good outcomes (Cleaver & Walker 2004). The CAF is based on a conceptual framework with three domains:

1. The child's needs.
2. The capacity of parents or carers to respond appropriately to those needs.
3. Family and environmental factors.

The process commences with an initial assessment which is intended to be brief and is designed to determine if a child is in need (as defined by the Children Act 1989). Once the assessment process has been completed, children and families are informed of the support available to them and programmes of intervention can then be offered and planned.

See Reader activity 23.2 on the Evolve website.

Children first

All children should have the opportunity to have the best possible start in life, and the support they need from their families and professionals to encourage them to fulfil their potential. When children with disabilities are considered, it is essential that those supporting them remember that, above all, they are children first; this philosophy was one of the fundamental tenets of the Children Act 1989. In a Commission for Social Care Inspection report (CSCI 2005), it was highlighted that children with complex health and social care needs have the same wishes and aspirations as their peers. They want to live at home, go to school and spend time with their friends and family participating in leisure and community activities. The challenge is to empower children and their families as well as to increase their involvement and inclusion in their communities so that those communities can benefit from the contribution they can make.

The legislative and policy context

Growth over the last two decades of dedicated services challenges any belief that children are 'mini-adults'. This expansion of services can be better understood by a review of legislation and policy that has emerged over this period of time. Historically, there has been legislation relating to children dating as far back as the 1800s (e.g. the Youthful Offenders Act of 1854 and 1870 Education Act). Although this legislation had little relevance at that time to children with severe and profound learning disabilities, those with mild and moderate learning disabilities may have fallen foul of the often harsh law of the time or been sent out to work rather than educated. It was not until 1971 that the statutory right to education for all children with learning disabilities was established and subsequently strengthened by the Education Act 1981.

When the United Nations Convention on the Rights of the Child (UN 1989) was adopted by the UN General Assembly, it became the most widely ratified and complete statement on the international human rights of children ever produced. The Convention protects specific child rights in international law, defining universal principles relating to the status and treatment of children worldwide. In addition, it is the only international human rights treaty which includes civil, political, economic, social and cultural rights, and it sets out in detail what every child needs for a safe, happy and fulfilled childhood. The Convention identifies that human rights are founded on respect for the dignity and worth of each individual, regardless of race, gender, language, religion, opinions, wealth or ability. It sets minimum standards: that every child has the right to survival; the right to the development of their full physical and mental potential; the right to protection from influences that are harmful to their development; and the right to participation in family, cultural and social life (UN 1989).

The existence of separate legislation pertaining to all children, for example the Children Act 2004, suggests acknowledgment both of their vulnerability and rights as individuals and as a group with needs discrete from those of adults. The *National Service Framework for Children, Young People and Maternity Services* (DH 2004) supports the subsequent framework, *Every Child Matters* (DES 2004), both aimed to take forward the government's vision of radical reform for children, young people and families by cross-departmental working with local partners as advocated by *Valuing People* (DH 2001a). This has led in recent years to a surge in the development of joint initiatives, for example Sure Start children's centres, representing collaboration between statutory and non-statutory providers. Originally aimed at children at risk of failing to reach their potential in areas of material deprivation (Sure Start 2005), services are now available to provide a variety of advice and support for all parents and carers from pregnancy to when a child commences primary school. A further example is extended schools which provide a range of services and activities, often beyond the school day, to help meet the needs of children, their families and the wider community.

Every Child Matters

The central precepts of the *Every Child Matters* framework (DES 2004) are to ensure that all children are healthy, safe and happy. To achieve the five outcomes (expanded upon below), there is a need to provide extended services and work with partner agencies, exploring new approaches to multi-agency working. It is envisaged that more cooperative working will ensure better outcomes for children and young people, and more support for parents and carers. The five outcomes, each with further aims, do not stand alone as illustrated in the following exploration and application to children with learning disabilities.

Being healthy

All children should have easy access to the primary, mainstream services provided by GPs, health visiting and school nursing services. Where this is difficult on account of a child's situation, facilitation from a specialist service may be required initially or on a continuing basis, and in some circumstances, a specialist service itself may be indicated. Indeed, children with learning disabilities may often be referred to specialist services when they experience difficulty achieving milestones such as weaning, becoming clean and dry, sleeping through the night and stability of mood, often expressed as 'tantrums'. While in many cases delay is inevitable, approaches useful in the general population of children can be adopted wholesale or adapted where individual need dictates. For example, during the pre- and early school years, dietary and fluid intake and sound routines are often crucial factors in addressing poor bowel function (Clinical Knowledge Summaries 2010) that can become intractable and socially limiting even into adulthood.

Health-promoting initiatives such as 'Five a Day' (DH 2003) and improved school meals are just as important, if not more so, for children with learning disabilities who may run increased risks in adulthood of developing potentially life-limiting conditions such as diabetes linked to obesity (DH 2001b) and coronary heart disease (Merriman et al 2005); issues of access and behavioural expressions of fear can also contribute to poor oral health in adults (Mencap 2004). Translation of health-promoting information and education into easy-read versions and ensuring that screening and preventative measures are routinely offered at an early age can set the future scene more positively.

It is also important that the mental health of children and young people is not overlooked. *New Horizons* (DH 2009) highlights the importance of improving wellbeing and mental health of individuals across the lifespan, laying the foundations for good mental health in childhood. *Every Child Matters* (DES 2004) aims to address the problem of children experiencing gaps in services, a problem which has been clearly evident where children with learning disabilities have been excluded from accessing child and adolescent mental health services because of their primary diagnosis. This disparity exists despite a large body of research showing that there is a much higher prevalence of psychiatric disorders among people with learning disabilities, including children and adolescents (Whitaker & Read 2006).

Staying safe

This section should be read in conjunction with the later section on safeguarding children in need.

Providing care for any child is challenging. Increasingly, the media are highlighting the pitfalls of parenthood as changes in our society occur. Thirty years ago children had more freedom to express their independence. In 1970, the average 9-year-old girl would have been free to wander 840 metres from her front door. By 1997, it was 280 metres (Easton 2007). Children were permitted to play near their home and one of the few distractions was television aimed at children aired after school. Today the picture is very different; parents now feel that they need to supervise the majority of their children's activities as they fear they may be exposed to such dangers as bullying, abduction and the use of illicit substances (Kidscape 2006). Concern over these potential dangers coupled with acquisition of technological 'must haves' such as personal computers and games consoles have resulted in children spending more time at home in sedentary activities and less time engaged in social interaction with their peers (Johnson 2002). Increasing awareness of the benefits of activity in preventing the onset of dementia is of particular interest as it is known that people with learning disabilities are more likely to develop the condition earlier than the general population (Holland & Benton 2004).

Evidence presented to The Children's Society (2007) suggested the number of teenagers who do not have a best friend has risen from one in eight 20 years ago to one in five today; a phenomenon that may be attributed to the advancement of social networking sites. The implications of these statistics for children with learning disabilities are immense and should not be underestimated. Children with learning disabilities probably have fewer opportunities than ever to develop healthy peer relationships within their local communities and limited opportunity and skills to access social networking sites without assistance. Research commissioned by the Department of Health and published in *Valuing People* (DH 2001a) suggests that 30% of people with learning disabilities do not have a friend who does not have a learning disability or is not a family member or paid carer. Children with learning disabilities have limited opportunities to develop real friendships, often accessing specialist leisure services as their carers may feel that they are less vulnerable. However:

> children with learning disabilities want to be treated like other children, not always seen as 'special', and to be included in ordinary services.
>
> (DH 2001a:11)

Enjoying and achieving through learning

This is the outcome that appears to most explicitly exclude many youngsters with a learning disability by incorporating aims stating that children should "achieve stretching national educational standards" (DES 2004:E4) at primary and secondary school. Achieving personal and social development and enjoying recreation clearly impact upon the preceding outcomes, being healthy and staying safe.

Making a positive contribution to society

For decades it has been recognised that making a positive contribution to society is important in preventing the devaluation of adults with learning disabilities (O'Brien & Tyne 1981, Wolfensberger 1998); in the case of children and young people, this is just as important. *Every Child Matters* (DES 2004) details the areas in which this positive contribution can occur. In the 'Children's 2020 goals' (Department for Children, Schools and Families 2007), the intended measure for the development of self-confidence and successfully dealing with significant life changes and challenges is educational attainment, therefore, for children with learning disabilities, this may not easily be achievable. There is a certain irony, a too familiar compounded disadvantage, in potentially excluding children with learning disabilities from evaluating outcomes in areas where they already occupy distinctly weakened positions.

Achieving economic wellbeing

Article 27 of the Convention on the Rights of the Child (UN 1989) declares "the right of every child to a standard of living adequate for the child's physical, mental, spiritual, moral and social wellbeing". However, despite this declaration, evidence accumulated in recent years would suggest that the standard of living of disabled children and their families falls below that essential to fulfill this right (Dobson & Middleton 1998). Poor economic status can result in lost opportunities for children to engage in social activities that may facilitate the development of friendships and relationships.

Aiming higher for disabled children: better support for families

This DES (2007) document builds upon the previous legislation and policy which aims to ensure that all children have the best start in life. It aims to transform services for children with disabilities in England as it recognised that until now they have sometimes been inadequate to enable them to enjoy aspects of life other families take for granted. It recognises the challenges both children and carers face, for example accessing leisure and finding appropriate childcare that will then allow carers to return to employment. The key for this to happen is holistic assessment that considers the needs of the child and family and sets out services available to meet them (see Ch. 22). This document, which has attempted to listen to the views of children and families, recognises important issues that have in the past gone unaddressed, for example the need to provide wheelchairs quickly before the child outgrows the equipment recommended. Table 23.1 summarises the main recommendations of this document

Family experience

Expectant mothers and fathers are often optimistic about their impending role as parents, but for all new parents those early weeks following the birth of their child are fraught with an assortment of challenges including sleep deprivation, learning new skills in caring for their infant and extensive lifestyle changes (Feeney et al 2001). Most parents, siblings, grandparents and members of the extended family will consider how the arrival of this new family member will impact on each of them personally, however when a child is born or is later diagnosed with a learning disability, a different process of adaptation occurs (Kearney & Griffin 2001). The reaction of families will vary but it is not unusual for them to grieve the 'loss' of their 'normal' child while attempting to adjust to their child's disability both emotionally and practically (Lindsey 2003). For some parents

Table 23.1 Main recommendations of *Aiming Higher for Disabled Children: Better Support for Families*

Priority area to improve outcomes	Recommendations
Promoting access and empowerment.	• Information – good information that clearly presents the services children and families can have access to. • Transparency – eligibility criteria that remain consistent and that all can understand. • Participation – children and families to participate and influence the design and delivery of services. • Assessment – Common Assessment Framework (CAF) that properly identifies a child's need and indicates the services they should get and when they should get them. • Feedback – families to be able to complain when things go wrong and get them put right quickly.
Promoting responsive services and timely support.	• Population – local authorities and Primary Care Trusts (PCTs) to improve data collection to enable them to plan appropriately for children with disabilities. • Performance indicators – develop a national performance indicator in addition to benchmarking good practice. • Early interventions – roll out the Early Support Programme (0–5 years) to promote timely provision. • Transition – recognising the critical transition to adulthood, develop a transition support service.
Improving quality and capacity.	• Short breaks – transform services and provide additional funding for children with complex health care needs. • Childcare – enable parents to return to work by improving access to childcare facilities. • Independence – maximise mobility, promote independent living and access to schools, leisure and other services.

(Adapted from DES 2007)

of children with disabilities who initially have difficulties in adjusting, it may be that they are just at the initial stage of a developmental process of coping and adaptation and have not yet reached a stage of adaptation at which point they can accept the child, the disability and themselves.

Parents of children diagnosed with learning disabilities often discuss the impact the birth of their child has had on them personally. The current Prime Minister David Cameron, in recalling the birth of his son Ivan in 2002 (a child who initially appeared healthy but soon after arriving home began to have spasms with subsequent tests indicating he had a severe disability), said that the news hit him "like a freight train . . . you mourn the difference between the child you thought you were going to have and the reality" (Levy 2009:4). However, the family were determined to include him in all family activities up until his death in February 2009 and drew strength from the fact that, despite his complex disabilities, he appeared to respond to their love and care. For other families, this adjustment may be more difficult as they feel they have to fight each step of the way. Research undertaken on behalf of the organisation Contact a Family (Bennett 2009) reveals that the difficulties for these families comes from outside the family circle due to lack of support services, attitudes towards disability and a lack of support from professionals.

Mothers

The majority of children with learning disabilities continue to reside with and be brought up by their birth family (Beresford 1995). Services available to support parents of children with a learning disability are generally aimed at mothers as they continue to be the parent likeliest to be the primary care giver. There have been numerous studies undertaken which relate to the effect that having a child with a learning disability will have on a mother (see Ch. 22) but most emphasise the emotional, financial and physical costs.

Hence the complexities of caring for a child with a disability should not be underestimated. Mothers are required to assume a number of roles from running the family's budget to contributing emotional support to family members and, in some instances, taking on the role of nurse in the administration of medications and the maintenance of technological equipment and procedures (Heaton et al 2003). Combine this role with the intricate tasks of washing, dressing, feeding as well as continuing to provide care for other children, juggling other household duties and personal commitments, then it is no surprise that levels of stress reported in this group are high (Kenny & McGilloway 2007). Factors that create stress or encourage wellbeing are complex; while families do manage to achieve a balance, at times this equilibrium may be delicate and easily disrupted by unpredicted events.

Where mothers choose to return to work after the birth of a child with a disability, they are more likely than mothers of non-disabled children to be in part-time rather than full-time employment (Cuskelly et al 1998). The Childcare Act 2006 has placed a duty on local authorities to secure adequate childcare for working parents of children with disabilities but currently appropriate childcare may not always be available and may prove more expensive than for a non-disabled child.

Fathers

The contribution that fathers of children with disabilities make is reflected in national policy. *The Children's Plan* (Department for Children, Schools and Families 2007) emphasises the need to engage with both fathers as well as mothers to promote their involvement in family life. The adjustment that fathers are required to make often goes unrecognised, but research suggests that men also experience social isolation and other difficulties adjusting to their new role and feel there is a lack of support from employers and social services (Foundation for People with Learning Disabilities 2009), therefore professionals working with the family should make all efforts to listen to both parents and assist them to adapt to their new situation.

In the same study which focused on recognising fathers of children with learning disabilities, nearly half felt they would like to spend more time with their child but work prevented them from doing so. Work commitments also restrict fathers' ability to attend appointments and meetings which results in limited opportunities to have contact with practitioners involved in their child's care. The study emphasised that fathers experience a lack of support at the time of diagnosis which led them to feeling stressed but few had the personal support of friendships that their female partners access, often preferring to engage with friends without the need to discuss their child. It is therefore important that fathers are recognised and respected by practitioners for their contribution in the child's life and that they are included in discussions and decisions.

Siblings' experience

Just as having a child with a learning disability will impact on parents, the presence of a child with a learning disability will affect their brothers and sisters, financially, physically and emotionally. Younger siblings may experience reduced attention from their parents. In addition they may feel isolated and that their health and learning needs come second to those of the child with a disability, as they can appear trivial in comparison.

Children may become involved in providing physical care for their sibling, for example assisting them with personal care. The physical implications of having a sibling with a disability is emphasised in a study by Hill (1999). This study also recognised that siblings often adopt the role of young carers who may be required to become involved in physically caring for a family member without the appropriate health and safety knowledge required to protect them from personal injury. If this is identified, professionals have a duty to raise this issue and request that the child has their own CAF assessment so appropriate help and services can be offered.

Many young siblings can give the appearance of coping during childhood and indeed may seem more mature and stable than their peers. A longitudinal study (Hames 2008) revealed that many siblings develop an early understanding of learning disability; although this may be intangible, they are able to differentiate between disability and illness. In addition, they are able to think about the long-term consequences of learning disability both for themselves and their brothers and sisters.

Some studies highlight the risk of negative psychological effects (Rossiter & Sharpe 2001) as it is not unusual for siblings to believe that they are the only ones coping with a sibling with a disability, as many choose not to disclose this to their friends. Siblings can indeed experience difficulties that other children do not, for example having to deal with other people's responses when their brother or sister becomes distressed. Although some siblings can give the outward appearance they are well adjusted, they may in fact be internalising their feelings.

Much of the work undertaken with siblings accessing groups helps them develop strategies for coping, while simultaneously acknowledging how isolated they may be feeling. Although research by Stalker & Connors (2004) affirms that most children did not see their sibling as intrinsically different from themselves, it is important for siblings to have dedicated time to talk to other children who have a sibling with a disability to reduce their feelings of isolation.

Grandparents

In today's society, grandparents are increasingly adopting a role in their grandchildren's lives. Recent research (Griggs et al 2009) demonstrated that approximately a third of maternal grandmothers provided regular childcare for their grandchildren, with 40% providing occasional help with childcare. This study also revealed that at times of family breakdown and separation, many grandparents played a significant role in bringing stability to their grandchildren. Grandparents are also found to be important in times of difficulty often softening the effects difficulties may have on the family. Although this research refers to the general child population, grandparents often play a significant role when they have a grandchild with a learning disability. Although there remains little research on the role grandparents play with children with disabilities, there is some evidence to suggest they too have a similar initial emotional response to the birth of a child with a learning disability as parents and experience a period of mourning for the loss of the grandchild they expected and also have to adjust (Hastings 1997).

Some grandparents feel that they do not receive support or information regarding the child's disability and therefore this may impact on their relationship with their grandchild (Mitchell 2007). This advice or information may relate to the child's condition or support available. In these situations, grandparents may look to their own children for this support but this may lead to additional burden placed on parents who are already under stress. Similarly to grandparents of non-disabled children, they too frequently provide informal childcare or complement existing childcare during weekends and evenings, however, for these grandparents, there may be additional practical, emotional and financial costs compared to grandparents of non-disabled children (Mitchell 2007).

The role that grandparents of children with disabilities play is very similar to the role of any grandparent; they advise and guide their grandchildren and offer practical, emotional and sometimes financial support to the child's parents. However, research has revealed that those closely committed to looking after their grandchildren could become depressed and have a potential negative effect on the children (Griggs et al 2009). It is therefore vital to consider the support that grandparents may require as parents may reveal their full emotions to them yet they may also be offering assistance in supporting their families.

See Reader activity 23.3 on the Evolve website.

Transition through childhood

It is recognised nationally that too often parents face a postcode lottery in the support available from their school, local authority and health service (DES 2004). *Every Child Matters* (DES 2004) recognised that early intervention is essential to achieving better outcomes for children with special educational needs (SEN) and disabilities. However, poor coordination between health, education and social care for young children with SEN and disabilities leads to gaps in support for parents and limitations in sharing information between professionals.

The promotion of inclusive education has led to an increase in the number of statements (of special educational need) issued in mainstream schools (see also Ch. 25). The emphasis is on establishing and developing coordinated provision planned around the child and family including early support programmes for children with disabilities between the age of 0 and 5, and person-centred planning at the point of transition to adult services (DES 2007). This is a particularly difficult transition period, and at the first annual review of the statement following the child's 14th birthday, a transition plan should be initiated. However, there is presently insufficient consistent multi-agency working to ensure that young people with disabilities are given a real choice about their futures and this is primarily true for children and young people with complex needs who require intricate packages of care (DES 2007). In an attempt to make this transition period smoother, some services have appointed dedicated transition teams or workers (Crickmore 2009).

An example of good practice is offered by Limbrick (2007) who focuses on effective early childhood intervention which requires joint working between all practitioners and parents. This approach, called the *Team Around the Child* (TAC) facilitates the highest degree of joint working for children and families with complex needs enabling collaboration between each child's key practitioners and parents. As part of this process, Limbrick advocates that a key worker is appointed to coordinate and rationalise appointments, meetings and assessments with careful consideration of the family's routines, finances, travel needs and other children.

The transition period to adult services is further complicated for young people who would not have previously been expected to survive to adulthood. Services need to develop swiftly to address their complex needs so they too have the opportunity to fulfil their aspirations. The report *Aiming Higher for Disabled Children* (DES 2007) promotes transition as a way to enable young people to move onto a new stage of life rather than from one service to another. The principles on which this is based are that young people should have choice and control over the support needed in their daily lives, and to allow them to achieve this where appropriate, direct payments should be made available.

See Reader activity 23.4 on the Evolve website.

Safeguarding children in need

The Convention on the Rights of the Child (UN 1989 Article 6) states:

> Parties recognise that every child has the right to life. Parties shall ensure to the maximum extent possible the survival and development of the child.

This article has direct relevance when working to safeguard children as professionals should work together so that children and young people are not at risk of significant harm. However, there continues to be a number of high profile cases which suggest that services are still failing to address the needs of vulnerable children. Following the Care Quality Commission review into the death of Peter Connelly (Baby P) (Laming 2009), Lord Laming was asked by the Secretary of State for Children, Schools and Families to prepare an independent report on progress against the recommendations made after the Victoria Climbié inquiry (Laming 2003). He concluded that child protection issues in England have not had the priority they deserved and many of the changes brought in after Victoria Climbié's death in 2000 had not been properly implemented. Two of the major issues highlighted in this latest report by

Lord Laming (Laming 2009) again identified a lack of communication and joined-up working between agencies.

The Care Quality Commission report (Laming 2009) states that Baby P had been the subject of a multi-agency child protection plan for 8 months, involving social services, health services and the police yet, despite this, he died. It suggests therefore that one of the main challenges is to ensure that leaders of local front-line services effectively translate policy, legislation and guidance into day-to-day practice.

One of these policies, *Every Child Matters* (DES 2004), aimed to reinforce preventative services by focusing on the support families needed before they reached crisis. A further important element was the duty of local authorities and their partner organisations to create a local Safeguarding Children Board to replace the Area Child Protection Committee. The subsequent Children Act 2004 aimed to improve outcomes for all children including those with a disability.

Protection from harm

Although the term 'safeguarding' has not been defined by government guidance or by law, it is a concept that has developed over concern about children and young people nationally (see Ch. 12). The protection from harm of all children and young people has been seen as a fundamental principle of the numerous agencies that work with both children and their families. The Children's Rights Director for England (Morgan 2004) defines 'safeguarding' as keeping children safe from harm, such as illness, abuse or injury. This definition is much broader than the general public's description in that it considers illness in addition to abuse and injury.

Identifying child protection issues for children with learning disabilities reveals specific concerns. This is because of the following:

- Marks or injuries on children are not always recognised as abuse and are sometimes rationalised by other explanations such as self-injury or that the child is particularly clumsy.
- In some circumstances, practitioners may be reluctant to suspect abuse as they see that carers are struggling with the efforts of providing around the clock care.
- There may be communication difficulties between a practitioner and a child. Not all practitioners who come into contact with children with learning disabilities possess the essential skills of communicating, specifically with those who are unable to communicate verbally.
- Even when practitioners do endeavour to listen to the opinions and anxieties of children with learning disabilities, these are sometimes disregarded because inadequate effort is put into overcoming the identified communication, sensory and learning obstacles that exist.
- In situations where children with learning disabilities are interviewed by the police, they may be placed at further risk as the police may not have access to trained professionals who can act as an 'interpreter' for the child.

The National Children's Bureau (2008) has written guidance to ensure that children with disabilities are listened to. In some situations, children and young people have not been given the time or opportunity to discuss what is happening to them or professionals do not ask to see them but rely on information given by parents and carers.

Increased vulnerability to abuse

Although there is still little research in this area, children with learning disabilities are exceptionally vulnerable and the evidence base suggests that they are more likely to experience abuse and neglect than any other children (National Society for the Prevention of Cruelty to Children 2003). Statistics are variable as to the actual number of children subject to child protection processes as not all local authorities record in their systems if the child has a disability (Morris 1998).

The Department of Health (DH 1999) in *Working Together to Safeguard Children* suggests that disabled children are at greater risk of abuse and that the presence of multiple impairments appears to increase the risk of both abuse and neglect. This is because children with disabilities may:

- receive intimate personal care, possibly from a number of carers, which may increase the risk of exposure to abusive behaviour
- have an impaired capacity to resist or avoid abuse
- have communication difficulties or lack of access to an appropriate vocabulary which may make it difficult to tell others what is happening
- not have someone to turn to, may lack the privacy they need to do this, or the person they turn to may not be receptive to the issues being communicated

- be inhibited about complaining because of a fear of losing services
- be especially vulnerable to bullying and intimidation
- be more vulnerable than other children to abuse by their peers.

Helping children protect themselves

In 2006, the Office of Public Sector Information (OPSI) introduced the Safeguarding Vulnerable Groups Act; the focus of this was to strengthen the safeguarding of children insofar as allowing employers a single point of access for checking the names of potential employees who intended to work with children. This subsequently contributed to the establishment of the Criminal Records Bureau (CRB). Although these safeguards exist, families and organisations should not become complacent but, where possible and appropriate, make children aware that they are vulnerable and promote the necessity of children keeping themselves safe. One area that needs to be promoted with all children, but is often overlooked, is educating children and stressing to them that people that they already know may harm them. This was spotlighted following the murders of two 10-year-old girls by a school caretaker, an adult in a position of trust for whom procedure had not been carefully followed in relation to his appointment and to previous concerns (Bichard 2004).

All children, whether they are educated in a mainstream or in a special school, will have a statutory access to Personal, Social and Health Education as part of the National Curriculum from 2011. Although currently this is sometimes inconsistent, this style of education does aspire to make children more aware of topics such as self-harm, bullying, drug awareness, sex education and personal safety. However, policies in schools and other organisations relating to the prevention or disclosure of bullying or harm are not always adapted or accessible to the needs of children with learning disabilities.

All individuals who come into contact with children should be familiar with and follow their organisations' procedures for promoting and safeguarding the welfare of children and know who to contact to express their concerns that a child may be at risk of harm (CSCI 2005). Concerns should be acted upon in the same way as with any other child (DH 1999). A number of stumbling blocks continue to exist within safeguarding systems for children with disabilities and active steps should be taken to minimise these. Those professionals who work specifically with children with learning disabilities should be alert to recognising possible signs and symptoms of abuse such as changes in behaviour, loss of weight and becoming withdrawn. They should always listen to what a child is trying to tell them and allow them the time and opportunity to do so and, in particular, to consider the communication method of the child. In addition, they should remain alert to non-verbal messages, for example reluctance to leave with a particular person which may be an indication that they are at risk of harm from that individual.

Conclusion

The predominant message readers should take from this chapter is that children, despite their disabilities, are children first. Each child will receive a diagnosis of their difficulties at a different time and they and their families will experience a process of adaptation. A permeating theme for all children will be transition; how each child will adapt to new stages in their life will largely depend upon those who support them and the services available. Contemporary policy exists to guide the development of services and to provide a framework for all professionals to respond to specific health, social and educational needs. It has been established that all children are vulnerable but children with learning disabilities are particularly so. The value placed on providing the best possible start in life for children with learning disabilities and their families cannot be overestimated. Only then can a child begin to achieve their full potential and be accepted as a full contributing member of their society.

References

Batchelor, J., 1999. Failure to thrive in young children. The Children Society, London.

Beresford, B., 1995. Expert opinions: a national survey of parents caring for severely disabled children. Policy Press, Bristol.

Bennett, E., 2009. What makes my family stronger: a report into what makes families with disabled children stronger – socially, emotionally and physically. Available at: http://www.cafamily.org.uk/pdfs/wmmfs.pdf (accessed 8.10.10.).

Berk, L.E., 2006. Child development, seventh ed. Pearson Education, Boston.

Berko Gleason, J., 2005. The development of language: an overview and a preview. In: Berko Gleason, J. (Ed.), The development of language. sixth ed. Allyn & Bacon, Boston.

Bichard, 2004. The Bichard inquiry report. The Home Office, London.

Burke, P., 2004. Brothers and sisters of children with disabilities. Jessica Kingsley, London.

Case, S., 2001. Learning to partner disabling conflict: early indications of an improving relationship between parents and professionals with regard to service provision for children with learning disabilities. Disability and Society 16, 837–854.

Cleaver, H., Walker, S., 2004. Assessing children's needs and circumstances: the impact of the assessment framework. Jessica Kingsley, London.

Clinical Knowledge Summaries, 2010. Constipation in children. Available at: http://www.cks.nhs.uk/constipation_in_children (accessed 27.07.10.).

Cohen, L.B., Cashon, C.H., 2001. Infant object segregation implies information integration. J. Exp. Child Psychol. 78, 75–83.

Commission for Social Care Inspection, 2005. Safeguarding children. The second Joint Chief inspections report on arrangements to safeguard children. CSCI, Newcastle.

Crickmore, D., 2009. School-aged children. In: Gates, B., Barr, O. (Eds.), Oxford handbook of intellectual and learning disability nursing. Oxford University Press, Oxford.

Cuskelly, M., Pulman, L., Hayes, A., 1998. Parenting and employment decisions of parents with a pre-school child with a disability. J. Intellect. Dev. Disabil. 23, 319–332.

Daily, D.K., Ardinger, H.H., Holmes, G.E., 2000. Identification and evaluation of mental retardation. Am. Fam. Physician 61, 1059–1067.

Davies, R., Davis, B., Sibertt, J., 2003. Parents' stories of sensitive and insensitive care by paediatricians in the time leading up to and including diagnostic disclosure of a life-limiting condition in their child. Child Care Health Dev. 29, 77–83.

Department for Children, Schools and Families, 2007. The children's plan. OPSI, London.

Department for Children, Schools and Families, 2009. Apprenticeships, skills, children and learning bill. OPSI, London.

Department for Education and Skills, 2004. Every child matters. Change for children. DfES, Nottingham.

Department for Education and Skills, 2006. The common assessment framework for children and young people: practitioners' guide. HM Treasury, London.

Department for Education and Skills, 2007. Aiming higher for disabled children: better support for families. HM Treasury, London.

Department of Health, 1999. Working together to safeguard children. HMSO, London.

Department of Health, 2001a. Valuing people: a new strategy for learning disability for the 21st century. HMSO, London.

Department of Health, 2001b. National service framework for diabetes. DH, London.

Department of Health, 2003. Five a day: just eat more fruit and veg. DH, London.

Department of Health, 2004. National service framework for children, young people and maternity services. HMSO, London.

Department of Health, 2007. Valuing people now: a new strategy for people with learning disabilities. HMSO, London.

Department of Health, 2009. New horizons: a shared vision for mental health. HMSO, London.

Dobson, B., Middleton, S., 1998. Paying to care: the costs of childhood disability. JRF, York.

Easton, M., 2007. Rearing children in captivity. BBC News 4 June.

Emerson, E., Hatton, C., 2004. Estimating future need/demand for support for adults with learning disabilities in England. Institute for Health Research, Lancaster University, Lancaster.

Empson, J., Nabuzoka, D., 2004. Atypical child development in context. Palgrave MacMillan, Hampshire.

Erikson, E.H., 1950. Childhood and society. WW Norton, New York.

Feeney, J.A., Hohaus, L., Noller, P., Alexander, R.P., 2001. Becoming parents: exploring the bonds between mothers fathers and their infants. Cambridge University Press, Cambridge, MA.

Foundation for People with Learning Disabilities, 2009. Recognising fathers. http://www.learningdisabilities.org.uk/publications/?entryid5=32902 (accessed 27.07.10).

Griggs, J., Tan, J.P., Buchanan, A., Attar-Schwartz, S., Flouri, E., 2009. They've always been there for me': Grandparental involvement and child well-being. Child. Soc. 24 (3), 200–214.

Guralnick, M.J., 2005. Early intervention for children with intellectual disabilities: current knowledge and future prospects. J. Appl. Res. Intellect. Disabil. 18, 313–324.

Hames, A., 2008. Siblings' understanding of learning disability: a longitudinal study. J. Appl. Res. Intellect. Disabil. 21 (6), 491–501.

Hamilton, D., 2004. Intervention approaches. In: Empson, J.M., Nabuzoka, D. (Eds.), Atypical child development in context. Palgrave Macmillan, Hampshire.

Hastings, R., 1997. Grandparents of children with disabilities: a review. International Journal of Disability, Development and Education 44, 4.

Heaton, J., Noyes, J., Sloper, P., Shah, R., 2003. Technology-dependent children and family life. SPRU, The University of York, York.

Hill, S., 1999. The physical effect of caring on children. Journal of Young Carers' Work 3 (1), 6–7.

Holland, T., Benton, M., 2004. Ageing and its consequences for people with Down's syndrome. Down's Syndrome Association, Teddington.

Johnson, L.H., 2002. The challenges of modern society. PT, Magazine of Physical Therapy 10 (11), 42–44, 46, 48.

Kearney, P.M., Griffin, T., 2001. Between joy and sorrow: being a parent of a child with developmental disability. J. Adv. Nurs. 34 (5), 582–592.

Kenny, K., McGilloway, S., 2007. Caring for children with learning disabilities: an exploratory study of parental strain and coping. British Journal of Learning Disabilities 35, 221–228.

Kidscape, 2006. Helping teenagers to protect themselves. Available at: http://www.kidscape.org.uk/parents/teenagers.shtml (accessed 27.07.10.).

Laming, H., 2003. The report of the Victoria Climbié inquiry. HMSO, London.

Laming, H., 2009. The protection of children in England: a progress report. The Stationery Office, London.

Levy, G., 2009. Boy who turned a toff into a leader. Daily Mail 26 February, 4–5.

Limbrick, P., 2007. Team around the child (TAC): the small collaborative team in early childhood intervention for children and families who require ongoing multiple interventions. Interconnections, Herefordshire.

Lindsey, M., 2003. Overview of learning disability in children. Psychiatry 2, 9.

Lissauer, T., Clayden, G., 2001. Illustrated textbook of paediatrics. Mosby, London.

Lock, A., 2004. Pre-verbal communication. In: Goswami, U. (Ed.), Blackwell handbook of cognitive childhood development. Blackwell, Malden.

Marlow, N., Wolke, D., Bracewell, M., Samara, M., 2005. Neurological and developmental disability at 6 years of age following extremely premature birth. N. Engl. J. Med. 352 (1), 9–19.

Mencap, 2004. Treat me right: better healthcare for people with a learning disability. Mencap, London.

Merriman, S., Haw, C., Kirk, J., Stubbs, J., 2005. Risk factors for coronary heart disease among inpatients who have mild intellectual disability and mental illness. J. Intellect. Disabil. Res. 49 (5), 309.

Mitchell, W., 2007. Research review: the role of grandparents in intergenerational support for families with disabled children: a review of the literature. Child and Family Social Work 12, 94–101.

Morgan, R., (Children's Rights Director), 2004. Safe from harm: children's views report. Commission for Social Care Inspection, London.

Morris, J., 1998. Still missing disabled children and the Children Act: who cares?. Who Cares Trust, London.

Nabuzoka, D., 2000. Children with learning disabilities: social functioning and adjustment. British Psychological Society, Leicester.

National Centre for Social Research, 2009. Family resource survey 2008–2009. Office for National Statistics, Newport.

National Children's Bureau, 2008. Listening to young disabled children. Available at: http://www.ncb.org.uk/dotpdf/open%20access%20-%20phase%201%20only/revised-listening-disabilities_2008.pdf (accessed 27.07.10.).

National Institute of Mental Health, 2004. Autistic spectrum disorder (pervasive developmental disorders). Available at: http://www.nimh.nih.gov/publicat/autism.cfm (accessed 27.07.10.).

National Society for the Prevention of Cruelty to Children, 2003. It doesn't happen to disabled children. Child protection and disabled children report of the National Working Group on child protection and disability. NSPCC, London.

O'Brien, J., Tyne, A., 1981. The principle of normalisation: a foundation for effective services. CMH, London.

Olness, K., 2003. Effects of brain development leading to cognitive impairment: a worldwide epidemic. J. Dev. Behav. Pediatr. 24, 120–130.

Paton, G., 2009. The cost of raising children soars to £194 000. Telegraph, 23 January.

Piaget, J., 1954. The construction of reality in the child. Basic Books, New York.

Rossiter, L., Sharpe, D., 2001. The siblings of individuals with mental retardation: a quantitative integration of the literature. J. Child Fam. Stud. 10, 65–84.

Santrock, J.W., 2007. Child development, eleventh ed. McGraw-Hill, New York.

Simpson, J.A., Weiner, E.S.C. (Eds.), 1989. Oxford English Dictionary. second ed. Clarendon Press, Oxford.

Sroufe, L.A., Walters, E., 1976. The ontogenesis of smiling and laughter: a perspective on the organisation of development in infancy. Psychol. Rev. 83, 173–189.

Stalker, K., Connors, C., 2004. Children's perceptions of their disabled siblings: 'she's different but it's normal for us'. Child. Soc. 18 (3), 218–230.

Sure Start, 2005. A Sure Start children's centre for every community: phase 2 planning guidance 2006–8. Department for Education and Employment, Nottingham.

The Children's Society, 2007. The good childhood inquiry. The Children's Society, London.

Turnbull, A.P., Blue-Bannin, M., Turbiville, V., Park, J., 1999. From parent education to partnership education: a call for transformed focus. Topics in Early Childhood Special Education 19, 164–172.

United Nations, 1989. Convention on the rights of the child. United Nations, Geneva.

Varendi, H., Christensson, K., Porter, R.H., 1998. Soothing effects of amniotic fluid smell in newborn infants. Early Hum. Dev. 51, 47–55.

Warnock, M., 1978. Special educational needs report of the committee of enquiry into the education of handicapped children and young people. HMSO, London.

Warnock, F., Sandrin, D., 2004. Comprehensive description of newborn distress behaviour in response to acute pain. Pain 107, 242–255.

Whitaker, S., Read, S., 2006. The prevalence of psychiatric disorders among people with intellectual disabilities: an analysis of the literature. J. Appl. Res. Intellect. Disabil. 19, 330–345.

Wolfensberger, W., 1998. A brief introduction to social role valorisation: a higher order concept for addressing the plight of societally devalued people, and for structuring human services, third ed. Training Institute for Human Service Planning, Leadership and Change Agency, Syracuse University, New York.

Further reading

Department for Education and Skills, 2007. Aiming higher for disabled children: better support for families. DfES, Nottingham.

Foundation for People with Learning Disabilities, 2006. Children and young people leaflet. FPLD, London.

Foundation for People with Learning Disabilities, 2005. First impressions: emotional and practical support for families of a young child with learning disability. FPLD, London.

Useful addresses

Contact a Family: www.cafamily.org.uk

Carers UK: www.carersuk.org

Mencap: www.mencap.org.uk

National Portage Association: http://www.portage.org.uk

Leisure and friendships

24

Roy McConkey

CHAPTER CONTENTS

KEY ISSUES

- Friendships and leisure pursuits add to everyone's quality of life yet many people with learning disabilities lead lonely and unfulfilled lives
- Our current models of support service may inhibit people from developing a rich social and leisure life
- A new type of relationship is required between paid staff and the people they support; one that actively promotes the social status of people with learning disabilities, creates opportunities for active participation in community activities and supports the development of social networks and friendships
- A primary aim of modern support services should be to link people into the network of community facilities and services in their locality rather than trying to meet their needs within specialist learning disability provision

Introduction

> *People with learning disabilities want to lead ordinary lives and do the things that most people take for granted. They want to study at college, get a job, have relationships and friendships, and enjoy leisure and social activities. Many people need support to do these things; and some will need high levels of support on an ongoing basis as well as multi-agency investment to have any kind of meaningful life.*
>
> (Department of Health 2009:83)

This chapter is aimed at all staff working in services for people with learning disabilities. It is within their gift to promote an active social and leisure life for the people they support rather than inhibiting or indeed denying them this opportunity, albeit unintentionally.

Leisure and friendships add to the quality of everyone's life yet many people with learning disabilities are lonely and unfulfilled. This lifestyle persists even within modern support services which ostensibly offer much better opportunities than the institutionalised provision of yesteryear. Hence promoting a richer social life for people with learning disabilities has to go beyond the strategies and techniques that have proved effective in other aspects of their lives, such as improving their health, managing behaviours or personal care (McConkey et al 2009).

Fundamental to this new approach is promoting the social status of people with learning disabilities. Engagement in community leisure activities can be an ideal means for doing this and in this respect these activities are a means to an end and not just an end in themselves. This theme is examined in the opening section of the chapter. Here too, the contribution of friendships and active leisure activities to the quality of people's lives is summarised as is the impact on their emotional wellbeing, increased self-reliance and the promotion of positive self-images.

The second section, 'Removing barriers to active leisure', describes the solitary and passive nature of the leisure activities of children and adults with learning disabilities and outlines the main barriers that inhibit the formation and sustaining of friendships and their participation in more active leisure pursuits. These include obvious factors such as a lack of transport and support personnel but also less appreciated influences, including concepts of leisure and staff perceptions of their role. This section challenges the priorities and presumptions that underlie service provision based on a 'deficit' or 'care' model. An alternative approach based around *creating opportunities* is proposed.

'Creating active and social lifestyles', the final section of the chapter, describes the supports (both personal and contextual) that encourage the formation of social networks from which leisure pursuits and friendships can emerge. A particular feature is the mediating role that paid staff can play in supporting friendships and the qualities required to achieve this goal. A major emphasis is on strategies that empower individuals to experience mutual relationships within networks and with partners.

Throughout the chapter, two questions recur on which readers should ponder. Might our current model of support service actually inhibit people from developing a rich social and leisure life? Is a new type of relationship required between paid staff and the people they support to allow this to happen?

The social status of people with learning disabilities

People with learning disabilities do not have a high status within society. First, in part it is because most people have never met a person with this impairment; in fact, three-quarters of the population according to surveys conducted in Ireland (McConkey 2004). Second, the public's image of them – admittedly perceived through the media – is one of helplessness; "people who cannot do things for themselves" said one survey respondent (McConkey 1994). Third, people in local communities are reluctant to have personal contact; fearing that they would not know what to say or how to react. Even nurses and therapists in mainstream health services expressed less confidence in treating patients with learning disabilities than those with physical disabilities (McConkey & Truesdale 2000).

It is clear too that the special services for this client group have done them no favours in raising their status. The era of long-stay institutions may be drawing to a close but the memory lingers on. 'Putting people away' implied worthlessness, even a threat to the wellbeing of others in the family or community. Yet the community services that replaced them – be they group homes or day centres – also have a glass wall around them that keeps them apart from society. Only 1 in 20 householders in the neighbourhood of a Scottish day centre had been inside the building (McConkey 1994).

While the public commonly applaud the patience and dedication of staff working in such services, they frequently go on to add: "I could never do your job". The implicit message is clear – special people need special staff. In fact, the predominant rationale for many of the specialist services for this client group can reinforce negative stereotypes of them. Here are three examples of what this can mean:

1. The 'social care model', as found in residential care homes, nursing homes and day centres, creates and reinforces images of people who need looking after; not just among the general public but with relatives, visitors and even the staff who come to work there.
2. The 'treatment model', as typified by challenging behaviour teams, therapists and admitting people

to 'assessment and treatment' units; implies that these are people who need to be 'fixed' because of some underlying abnormality.

3. The 'training model', represented by special needs courses at further education colleges and vocational training centres can unwittingly reinforce the incompetence of those using services; geared as they are to low-level skills.

Of course, these various models of services may be useful, as other chapters in this book have argued. However, what is especially concerning is when the personnel working in them do little to challenge the negative images created and leave to someone else the task of promoting community integration and social inclusion (see Box 24.1). Engaging people in community-based leisure pursuits is an ideal means for doing this. However, social inclusion will only be achieved when everyone takes responsibility for it, no matter which service they work in and the type of job they do. Hence this chapter is targeted at *all* staff working in services for people with learning disability. Promoting leisure opportunities cannot be left to specialists with new titles such as 'befriender coordinator' or 'community link workers'. While such individuals or services have a contribution to make, their efforts will be considerably enhanced if they perform their roles as part of a partnership with all the other people of influence in the person's life.

Enhancing the social status of marginalised groups

In the last two decades we have attained a better understanding of how the social inclusion of marginalised people, such as those with disabilities, can be enhanced. The foundation stone is to actively enhance the social status of the excluded group. The starting point is being clear about their rights within society.

Box 24.1

If the fish in a stream were dying, we would not assume that we could solve the problem by pulling the fish out of the stream and allowing them to swim in a clean fish tank for 30 minutes each day, and then returning them to the stream for the remainder of the day.
Rather we would begin a systematic search to find out what was causing the fish to die. If the health of the fish was important to us, we would do what was necessary to restore the health of the stream so that the fish could thrive.

(Mary Taylor)

It is a generation since the United Nations (1975) first proclaimed the Rights of Disabled Persons but this has been updated by the Convention on the Rights of Persons with Disabilities (United Nations 2007), Article 19 of which proclaims:

> the equal right of all persons with disabilities to live in the community, with choices equal to others, and [states] shall take effective and appropriate measures to facilitate full enjoyment by persons with disabilities of this right and their full inclusion and participation in the community.

Article 30 goes on to define the participation of disabled persons in cultural life, recreation, leisure and sports.

This thinking is also reflected in recent EU Directives, UK legislation and policy making. For example, Article 26 of the Charter of Fundamental Rights (European Union 2000) states that:

> The Union recognises and respects the right of persons with disabilities to benefit from measures designed to ensure their independence, social and occupational integration and participation in the life of the community.

These statements resulted from many years of lobbying by disabled activists, family carers and professionals to ensure that people with disabilities had access to the same opportunities as other citizens and to put an end to discriminatory practices. What progress has been made in the past 30 years towards attaining these goals for persons with learning disabilities? The answer is probably very little; otherwise why do they still need to be repeated a generation later?

Even the general public acknowledges this to be the case. In an opinion poll in Northern Ireland during the European Year of Persons with Disabilities (McConkey 2004), fewer than one in four people felt that disabled people had the same opportunities in life as non-disabled people. Statements of rights and even specific legislation may set a context for action, but they alone are unlikely to produce changes in people's mind-sets and attitudes.

People with disabilities face the negative consequences of ongoing discrimination. In a national survey in England, about one-third of the nearly 3000 people interviewed stated that someone had been rude or abusive to them in the past year because of their learning disabilities (Emerson et al 2005). Bullying is commonly reported by children and teenagers as well (Mencap 2007), and advocates identify it as one of the most important issues faced by people with a learning disability (Williams et al 2008). There are still many miles to go in the pursuit of full acceptance and respect for all citizens in modern society.

Valued social roles

Wolf Wolfensberger (1972), the Canadian sociologist, has long championed the need to promote the social status of people whom society views as different. To do this, he argued, discriminated groups must be seen to fulfil valued social roles (he coined the term 'social role valorisation' for this). This needs to happen in a diversity of ways, in local communities as well as nationally, and to be sustained over time, rather than as part of isolated campaigns.

Four means for enhancing the social status of devalued groups can be identified – projecting positive images of disability, using ordinary settings, creating social exchanges and expecting achievement.

Projecting positive images of disability

The various talents of people with disabilities need to be promoted, and not just in the media. Too often their failings and incompetences are stressed by service staff. Dunne (personal communication) conducted a literature search of all articles relating to learning disability/mental retardation in psychological journals published between 1996 and 2000. Of 2789 articles found, only 21 – or 0.75% – recounted any positive features of these persons and that was using fairly generous criteria.

This negativity can easily go unnoticed. Perhaps there is a need to rebalance the wording of assessment reports, team briefings, service brochures, fund-raising appeals and be more careful of the images painted through word of mouth.

People with learning disabilities also need to be given opportunities to prove themselves and have their successes applauded. That is how self-confidence and self-esteem can grow. This in turn changes other people's perceptions as well. Ordinary activities of leisure and work provide an ideal context for doing this, such as drama performances and sporting achievements.

Using ordinary settings

People who are different have to be seen in the ordinary settings of shops, bars and buses; in schools, colleges and businesses; and in socially valued settings such as on television programmes, in theatres and concerts. However, community presence may be more easily achieved when it involves individuals or pairs of people rather than larger groups, and when it includes non-disabled peers.

Equally, people's participation in community life requires preparation, as when young people are socialised by their families. Self-discipline may also be required to minimise unusual or challenging behaviours.

Creating social exchanges

People lose some of the stigma of their disability as they meet and mix with others. The public's reaction is often: 'they're not as different as I thought!' However, for people meeting a person with a learning disability for the first time, this needs to happen in a planned and purposeful way, perhaps based around a shared activity in a familiar setting to reduce their apprehensions. There are numerous opportunities for doing this in any community; from schools to sports, and clubs to pubs (McConkey 1994).

Expecting achievement

People with learning disabilities may be slow to learn but they can learn; as numerous studies have shown (Emerson et al 2004). Moreover, their initial attempts are often no predictor of ultimate success in learning, so beware of giving up too soon. If achievement is not expected, there will no perseverance in encouraging people to learn. This in turn will impact upon the individuals' self-confidence and motivation. They may come to feel it is safer not to take on new challenges rather than risk failure.

Service evolution

These four means of promoting the social status of people with learning disabilities have stood the test of time. They were pioneered from the 1950s onwards by family carers who were reluctant to commit their sons or daughters to institutional care even though this was the advice of the 'experts' of the day. From the 1970s, professional thinking started to follow a similar path as people were resettled from long-stay hospitals back into the community and an 'ordinary life' became the slogan for all (Towell 1988).

By the 1990s, concerns were beginning to be expressed about continued social isolation (McConkey 1998). Although people with learning disabilities were now physically present within communities, often they were not part of them. Nor were services making much progress in assisting them in achieving this outcome. The Council on Quality and Leadership in the United States of America has devised a series of personal outcome measures that services can use to judge the impact they have on the lives of the people whom they serve. A review of 552 services across the USA involving over 3600 service users identified three outcomes that services found particularly problematic (Gardner & Carran 2005). They were: people choosing where they work (attained for 34% of all service users reviewed); people exercising their rights (39% attained); and people performing different social roles (44% attained). Moreover, one of the few areas in which services had dis-improved over the period 1997 to 2002 was in the participation of the people they supported in the life of the community (falling from 85% attainment to 65%). These percentages are likely to be overly optimistic outcomes given that the services elected to be evaluated and hence they may be considered among the more progressive.

So what do services need to do in order to ensure that people with learning disabilities take on valued social roles within society? Obviously creating new images of those comprising this group is a crucial first step but in itself is insufficient to ensure their inclusion in society. We might gain some clues by considering how this occurs for others within society. Children are an obvious example as are other marginalised groups such as immigrants.

Promoting social inclusion through leisure

Alongside schools and employment, leisure pursuits are a major means through which individuals are integrated within their communities, not only in childhood but as teenagers, adults and more senior citizens. A brief reflection quickly identifies why this is so and the benefits it can bring:

- Leisure pursuits are usually undertaken in the company of others. It is possible to spend all free time alone, but this is the exception. Shared activities provide opportunities for conversations; for working together to achieve a common outcome and for helping each other out when the need arises.
- Leisure embraces a huge diversity of activities which means that individual preferences and talents can be accommodated. Everyone does not need to do the same thing; people can be directed towards the activities that suit them best.
- Leisure offers opportunities for personal growth and development. Admittedly this happens more so in some situations than in others but people tend to be wise to this and move on when they have exhausted the possibilities and before boredom sets in.
- Through leisure pursuits, people's talents can be demonstrated; a sense of achievement and a more positive self-image gained. The affirmation of others is especially helpful in creating a sense of being needed.
- Participation in active leisure pursuits brings positive benefits to children and adolescents in terms of their overall feelings of happiness and improved self-concept which does not happen with passive activities such as watching television or playing video games (Holder et al 2009).
- Friendship, good social relations and strong supportive networks improve people's health at home, at work and in the community. Although well attested with non-disabled persons (Wilkinson & Marmot 2003), these findings are likely to be just as true, if not more so, for people with learning disabilities.

Processes not products

People do not just engage in leisure for the sake of the activity. Rather it is the processes that are inherent in the activities that humans value and which help to create a sense of worth and togetherness. People may train hard at sports, attend choir practices and frequent clubs, but it is not just the activity that is important. They value the companionship, the sense of achievement and the opportunity to chat with others.

This line of argument gives rise to a variant of the chicken and egg conundrum as to which comes first – do people need talents and competences before they can start to join in leisure pursuits or do they acquire these competences through active participation in leisure pursuits? The answer is likely to be some of both. Individuals probably take part in certain leisure activities because they have some of the required skills but they persist in the hope that their tennis, photography, dancing or whatever can get better.

Strangely, this freedom is often not given to people with learning disabilities. Rather the dominant attitude has tended to stress the need to 'prepare' them to take part in community activities, and for them to prove themselves competent before they are considered 'ready' for leisure pursuits with others. A similar attitude kept many people living in institutions for longer than they needed, as the more competent were selected to leave first. Likewise certain people now living in group homes may not be taken out because they may 'create a scene'.

Such attitudes are doubly disadvantaging. People are not given the opportunity to learn in settings that are supportive of their learning and yet they have to meet the same standards of non-disabled people when they are there. It is rather like saying that a person will never learn to swim and then giving them no opportunity to go to the swimming pool. That is called a self-fulfilling prophecy and people with learning disabilities have no need for prophets of doom.

Failure of opportunities

A radical conclusion also emerges from this debate; could it be that people with learning disabilities are incompetent not because of their impairments but because they have not been given the same opportunities to learn as their non-disabled peers? This view harmonises with the position of disabled activists who promote a social rather than medical model of disability (Oliver 1996). It is also embedded in the International Classification of Functioning promoted by the World Health Organization (2001) which examines the degree of activity and participation experienced by the person in assessing their overall level of functioning.

Reader activity 24.1

Keeping a diary

Select a person with a learning disability who you know well. Keep a diary for 1 week (7 days) of all the activities they do morning, afternoon and evening. Note also the people with whom they did the activities or who were present with them.

Once you have the information, you can identify how many activities were done outside of their home, how many could be classed as active pursuits and how many they did with their friends rather than with staff support.

Certainly there is now a growing appreciation within government of the need to provide equal opportunities. The Northern Ireland Review of Learning Disability Services (Department of Health, Social Services and Public Safety 2005:65) highlighted the contribution of leisure:

> Despite the fact that access to social and leisure opportunities is extremely limited for many men and women with a learning disability, relatively few resources have been expended in this area. Greater attention to developing people's social networks could pay dividends in other ways by reducing the possible consequences of social isolation including challenging behaviours and depression.

The remainder of this chapter examines how these aspirations can be put into practice.

Removing barriers to active leisure

Various research studies have documented the extent of people's lack of access to leisure pursuits and paucity of friendships. Four main conclusions can be identified.

1. Verdonschot et al (2009) reviewed 23 research studies and concluded that people with learning disabilities were less likely to be involved in community groups and their leisure activities were mostly solitary and passive in nature. Most people were accompanied by specialist staff or family members rather than their peers when taking part in activities.
2. The pattern of passivity and isolation seems to be set in childhood. Solish et al (2009) found that children with learning disabilities not only participated in fewer social and recreational activities but did so less often with their peers. Smyth & McConkey (2003) found that three in five of the 52 young people leaving special schools were reported to have no friends of their own. Of those reported to have friends (16 students in all), 12 were from the same school or centre as the young person attended. Only one young person had a weekly meeting with her school/centre friends outside of the school setting; more often it was fortnightly (3), monthly (4) or occasionally (4).
3. People living in community settings participated in more activities than people in segregated accommodation but their participation levels were still much lower than non-disabled and other

disability groups. For example, McConkey et al (2007) reported that people living in dispersed supported housing were nearly six times more likely to make use of community amenities than those living in campus-style accommodation. Even so, 40% of these tenants reported having no friends outside their home whom they saw regularly.

4. Widmer et al (2008) examined connectedness among families of adult persons who had an intellectual disability and found that their extended family networks were less dense and more disconnected with the disabled person being less central in them. They concluded that their families provided them with fewer opportunities to create the social capital required to connect into their local communities.

Aspirations to participation

Perhaps these findings neither shock or surprise. Many will put them down to the person's handicap – "they're disabled, aren't they?" Others will claim "they are happy with the way things are"! Yet a growing body of research challenges both these claims.

Kampert & Gorenczny (2007) found that increased community involvement and more socialisation opportunities were the most common desires expressed by over 250 individuals with learning disabilities in Pennsylvania, USA. Likewise, having meaningful activities and spending time socialising and meeting other people were the dominant themes in interviews undertaken with 87 people from a range of services in England and Scotland (Miller et al 2008). So too in Northern Ireland, social activities were the most commonly selected goals when over 120 people living in a variety of accommodation options were invited to identify three things they would like to try in the coming 6 to 9 months; with entertainment and sporting activities the next most popular (McConkey & Collins 2010a).

Beart et al 2001 organised focus groups of people with learning disabilities attending further education colleges and social education centres. Long lists of activities were generated which they wanted to try including night clubbing, theatre and sports, such as rugby, archery, rock climbing and windsurfing. The researchers noted all of these activities were absent from their current repertoire.

Having friends was just as important as the activities. When Murray (2002:70) sought the views of over 100 young people with a range of disabilities through various participatory methods, she concluded:

> Whilst opportunities to try out a range of leisure activities and pursuits are appreciated, it is the opportunity to be in mutually valued relationships that young disabled people identify as the key to the possibility of their inclusion in mainstream culture.

Barriers to leisure

If the aspiration, motivation and potential competence are there, what is it that stops people with learning disabilities from participating in active leisure pursuits? When asked, they are well aware of the barriers they face. Beart et al (2001) identified two main ones: lack of transport and lack of support from friends and carers. Indeed, having support was the biggest single reason for people attaining their chosen goals in the study by McConkey & Collins (2010a).

In the English national survey, the main barrier to connecting with friends and families was living too far away or problems with transport (Emerson et al 2005). Likewise, with teenagers in Ireland, transport was a major barrier as was the lack of amenities in the local neighbourhood (Buttimer & Tierney 2005), although some informants also identified 'not being allowed' as an inhibitor to doing what they wanted to do.

The informants in the focus groups organised by Abbott & McConkey (2006) also noted the lack of community amenities which was compounded by the location of people's living accommodation but they also highlighted the influence of service staff and management on the options provided for them, as did Miller et al (2008). The participants in this study also recounted further barriers arising from staffing of services; namely continuity of staffing in people's lives and the shortage of staffing.

Finally, barriers exist within community amenities. For example, Brodin (2009) found in a survey of Swedish municipalities that the lack of trained staff and financial constraints were the twin barriers to making outdoor education more accessible to adult persons with learning disabilities.

As significant as these barriers are, perhaps there are more fundamental ones to promoting leisure pursuits for people with learning disabilities. Two are especially significant: our conceptions of leisure and the role of support staff in services.

Definitions of leisure

Leisure is often interpreted as activity undertaken in our 'free time' after work is completed. How meaningful is this for people whose lives consist solely of free time? For them, the description 'pass time' is probably more appropriate in that the goal is to find activities primarily as a means of passing the time for them; hence the dominance of watching television, listening to music or playing computer games in their leisure repertoires. Moreover, these pastimes make little demand on support staff or family carers as, when people are occupied in them, they can get on with their own work. Thus it is easy to convince ourselves that people have a life full of leisure – so what more do they want?

If, however, leisure is viewed in terms of active pursuits in which people invest energy, enthusiasm, effort and enjoyment, it would become clear how bereft of leisure their lives really are. Of course, people themselves realise this as do the family carers of children and teenagers, but it is rare for support services to acknowledge this.

Indeed, it has been argued that an active leisure life is the main means of providing a better quality of life for those people for whom employment and/or independent living is not likely to be an option (Patterson & Pegg 2009). Stebbins (2000:3) coined the phrase 'serious leisure' which he defined as:

> the systematic pursuit of an amateur, hobbyist, or volunteer core activity that is highly substantial, interesting, and fulfilling and where, in the typical case, participants find a career in acquiring and expressing a combination of its special skills, knowledge, and experience.

Enabling people to become leisure activists requires more systematic support strategies around this outcome than happens in services at present. The realisation of this need, only becomes apparent when the meaning of leisure is conceptualised and its importance recognised; two themes we will return to in the final section of the chapter.

Role of services and support staff

A second fundamental barrier is related to concepts of leisure; namely the role of staff in support services. This finds expression in different ways: first, in terms of personal support. McConkey & Collins (2010b) surveyed 245 staff working in either supported living schemes, shared residential and group homes or in day centres. Staff were asked to rate, in terms of priority to their job, 16 tasks that were supportive of social inclusion and a further 16 tasks that related to the care of the person they supported. In addition, staff identified those tasks that they considered were not appropriate to their job. Across all three service settings, staff rated more care tasks as having higher priority than they did the social inclusion tasks. However, staff in supported living schemes rated more social inclusion tasks as having high priority than did staff in the other two service settings. Equally the staff who were most inclined to rate social inclusion tasks as not being applicable to their job were those working in day centres; female rather than male staff; front-line rather than senior staff; and those in part-time or relief positions rather than full-time posts. However, within each service setting, there were wide variations in how staff rated the social inclusion tasks. Thus, there could be sizeable proportions of staff who do little to actively support the social and community engagement of the people in their services. Clement & Bigby (2009) suggest that staff working with individuals who have more severe and profound disabilities view them as so different that terms such as 'inclusion' were not meaningful for them.

Pockney (2006) identified another dilemma for staff. While people receiving support are inclined to name staff as their friends, this is not reciprocated. Staff may be wary of encouraging an over-friendly relationship with individuals particularly through involving them in their own social networks. Activities undertaken in groups rather than pairs provide an additional safeguard for staff even though group outings rarely provide opportunities for people to extend their social networks by meeting and becoming acquainted with others (Lippold & Burns 2009).

At another level, services may fail to maintain or extend the social connectedness of people they have supported over periods of time. Bigby (2008) examined the informal relationships of a randomly selected group of people with learning disability who had been resettled from Australian institutions into community-based accommodation. After 5 years, the residents had not formed any new relationships and the numbers in touch with family members had decreased. Hall & Hewson (2006) reported similar findings for an English sample of people who had moved into group homes with no differences in the time they spent outside of their home or in receiving unpaid visitors after 8 years of living in the community.

When the perennial problems of staff turnover and shortages of staffing are added in, then it is no

Reader activity 24.2

Assessing social inclusion

On the list of activities in Table 24.1 below, tick off those you have done in the past 4 weeks. Then talk to, or think about, one or more people with a learning disability whom you know. Tick off the activities they have done in the past 4 weeks. Put a circle around those the person did on their own or with their friends (rather than with support staff or when attending day centres).

Are there any differences between the listings? Why is this?

How many different activities did the people with learning disabilities do on their own or with friends? What does this activity tell you about their opportunities to have an active social and leisure life?

surprise that there are major failures in supporting people to maintain friendships and preferred activities outside of the home. This is crucial when people move from one service to another, notably young people leaving school or people moving from the family home into supported accommodation.

Taken together, these barriers provide formidable obstacles to creating a more active and social lifestyle for people with learning disabilities, but they can be overcome.

Creating active and social lifestyles

Figure 24.1 summarises the proposals that people with learning disabilities identified for overcoming the four types of barriers they experienced to their

Table 24.1 List of activities for Reader activity 24.2

Activities	I have done	Person 1 has done	Person 2 has done
Out for a walk with one or two others			
Had an outing by car with others			
Gone on a bus, train journey			
Been in a café/restaurant/pub			
Been to shopping centres/supermarkets			
Visited park/beach/outdoor events and places			
Been to cinema, theatre, concerts, museums			
Been to swimming pool, water parks			
Watched sports events – football, rugby, ice-hockey			
Took part in *outdoor* sports/activities with others, e.g. football, cricket, tennis			
Took part in *indoor* sports/activities with others – gym, karate, bowling, darts, snooker			
Had a holiday/weekend break			
Attended church, religious celebrations			
Been to dance/drama/art classes			
Gone to discos/clubbing			
Had a friend to visit at home			
Had a friend to sleep over			

Continued

Table 24.1 List of activities for Reader activity 24.2—cont'd

Activities	I have done	Person 1 has done	Person 2 has done
Visited a friend/relative at his/her house			
Slept over at a friend's house			
Had party/celebration at home			
Please list any other leisure activities not covered by the above			

Personal ability and skills

- Access to appropriate skills training (literacy/numeracy/budgeting/ independent travel).
- Getting to know the neighbourhood.
- Encouragement from staff to socialise.
- Information, access and encouragement towards a healthy lifestyle.

The community

- Education of the community – schools etc.
- Accessible information provided on activities/events.
- Make links with community through Open Days in services
- More advocates and volunteers to accompany individuals
- Increased use of existing (mainstream) facilities and activities.

Staff and management

- Being listened to by staff and managers.
- Support to make your own plans and go out independently.
- More staff available for one-to-one support or better use of available advocacy and volunteer groups to do this.
- Up-to-date information on community opportunities.
- Enabled to live independently.

The home/scheme

- Use of a named driver/known local taxi firm.
- Support to access activities available locally.
- Free/affordable/accessible transport options.
- Taught/allowed to use public transport.

Figure 24.1 • Suggested solutions to the barriers to social inclusion experienced by people with a learning disability

social inclusion (Abbott & McConkey 2006) Person-centred planning events, team meetings of support staff and periodic reviews of services all provide opportunities for changes to be made in the way individuals are supported to overcome the specific barriers they face. Mencap (undated) have a useful guide on how to campaign for improved access to mainstream leisure amenities. However, three broad strategies hold particular promise for most individuals:

1. Creating opportunities that widen people's social networks.
2. Identifying informal supporters to develop active leisure pursuits.

3. Generating opportunities for people to make useful contributions which other people value and from which they benefit.

Although these three dimensions are inter-related, each will be examined in turn. While leisure pursuits, along with having a job, offer all these opportunities, it is not the product of the activity on which its value is judged but rather what the person gains through participating.

Widening social networks

How might people's social networks be widened? Left to their own devices, people with learning disabilities often fail to meet and get on with other people. Many lack the conversational skills and social graces needed to initiate interactions with strangers. They may have even greater difficulties locating opportunities in their neighbourhood for socialising and finding their way to them.

What they need is a matchmaker! Someone who knows the needs, interests and talents of the person with a learning disability but who also knows what is available in the locality or is capable of tracking down possible opportunities, such as social clubs, church groups, yoga classes, educational activities, not forgetting more informal opportunities such as visiting friends. It certainly helps if support staff are from the same neighbourhood and have grown up in it. They will then be very familiar with the people and amenities it has to offer. Staff living elsewhere and coming to work in a different area should make the effort to find out about the community in which their work is based. Sadly, few managers and staff think to do this.

The next step is arguably more difficult. The matchmaker has to ask if people are prepared to welcome new members. Schwartz (1992) identified this simple task as one of the most crucial weapons in the armoury of social connectors. Equally he notes the reluctance there can be on the part of professional staff and carers to ask favours of others. Why?

- Perhaps because they are afraid of being rejected; people may say no? Yet experience and research suggests that the majority of people are disposed to be of assistance and very few would ever be rude and critical in refusing to participate.
- Or maybe staff and carers feel that no one can quite measure up to the task or that there are too many risks involved? So they continue to shoulder the responsibility. Again experience shows that professional staff and carers tend to overestimate risk and they do not consider that the person with the learning disability may respond differently to the 'new' person and setting.
- Or, more worrying, could it be that they feel there is nothing in it for the other person; that there are no benefits to befriending a person with learning disabilities? Yet family carers and voluntary helpers are so much more adapt at naming these benefits than are professional staff (Hastings & Taunt 2002).

Having asked and been accepted, the next crucial role of the matchmaker is that of introducing people to one another. Like a good host or hostess, the matchmaker needs to put the two parties at their ease by facilitating the conversation, modelling interactions, suggesting joint activities and, when the opportunity arises, discretely withdrawing for a time so that they take on the responsibility for maintaining the interaction.

Finally, the matchmaker needs to be supportive of the blooming partnerships by keeping in touch with both parties; checking how things are going; making discrete suggestions and subtly encouraging them in their efforts.

Rarely are these connecting tasks written into the job descriptions of professional workers nor are people recruited to these jobs for their 'matchmaking' skills. Paradoxically though, most of us acquire these skills and utilise them in our personal lives so perhaps their deployment in the service of people with learning disabilities could be readily promoted if only the will to do so was there.

Of course, certain circumstances can make it easier to create and extend people's social networks. Renewing former acquaintances is one strategy that has been used to reconnect people with learning disabilities with their peers they may have known in years gone by at school, day centres or long-stay hospitals. A similar strategy has proved effective for people to reconnect with family members with whom they may have lost touch. Invitations to visit the person with learning disabilities in their home can be a useful starting point. Yet it is surprising how few people are encouraged to use their homes as a place for meeting others (Emerson & McVilly 2004).

Another fruitful strategy can be connecting people with others who have a learning disability, particularly when people have control over the group's activities as happens in advocacy groups (see Ch. 7). Some groups now provide a range of services and supports to their members including educational classes, social events, income generation and holiday breaks. These also provide opportunities for closer and more intimate relationships to develop (see Ch. 28).

Modern technology also offers opportunities for people to keep in touch with their friends. Just as people with learning disabilities have learnt to use mobile phones, so too with some help and practice they could master using e-mail, social networking sites and video links such as Skype on personal computers. As these become cheaper and more portable, they offer new opportunities for people to connect with others provided they have the support to get started (McClimens & Gordon 2009).

Widening access to active leisure pursuits through identifying informal supporters

A similar strategy is commonly used to assist people with learning disabilities to access leisure pursuits of their choosing. This begins with recruiting 'befrienders' or 'buddies' who are of similar age, background and interests to the person needing support and who are willing to share some of their leisure time with a chosen partner (Heslop 2005).

A variety of strategies can be used to recruit them, including newspaper and radio adverts, but the most successful has been through word-of-mouth from people who already have some involvement, such as other staff in the services or through their network of family and friends. People who express an interest need the opportunity to gradually 'opt-in' through a series of meetings so they become fully aware of what is involved. Careful vetting procedures also need to be in place. A contact person needs to be nominated whom befrienders can easily contact at any time if they have queries or if they encounter any problems. They have a vital role in proactively supporting the befrienders, especially in giving them feedback on the importance of their contribution. Many befrienders withdraw because they feel they are not appreciated by service staff. Jameson (1998) identified some further key factors to forming stable relationships: notably strong orientation processes, appropriate matching and a high degree of reciprocity in the experience.

Most befrienders do not receive any payment although their expenses should be reimbursed. Most are offered a time-limited commitment, say for 12 months, which can be renewed if all is going well. Equally they can honourably withdraw when their commitment has been fulfilled.

A survey in Northern Ireland identified befriending as the fifth most popular form of voluntary activity with an estimated 80 000 people involved across a variety of client groups beyond learning disability, such as older people and people with mental health problems (Holloway & Mawhinney 2002). The Special Olympics movement has demonstrated in Ireland and Great Britain, as well as internationally, the latent willingness there can be in communities to befriend people with learning disabilities. Their Unified Sports® initiative is a promising means of furthering social inclusion beyond the sports field (Special Olympics 2010).

Adult placement

In recent years, the befriending idea has evolved into a number of other specialist functions such as citizen advocacy. This entails recruiting a person who is independent of services and families in order to advocate on behalf of a person with learning disabilities (Ward 1988).

Another role for befrienders is in family placement schemes (McConkey et al 2004). Here people with disabilities – adults as well as children – are placed with carefully selected families for daytime breaks or overnight stays in their home. Although initially intended to provide a 'respite' break for family carers, these schemes also provide opportunities for the person with a learning disability to become part of another social network and to experience the leisure pursuits that the host families are involved in. Indeed, some family carers also comment on the relationship they have built up with the host family and how the schemes have widened their social and support networks.

The majority of placement providers in two family placement schemes in Northern Ireland were recruited from the care sector and many had previous experience of people with learning disabilities. Overall they were very satisfied with the way the schemes operated and the support they received. The main complaint was the low level of payments which were pitched so that people in receipt of social security benefits (for example, retirement pensions) would be unaffected. However, the evaluation identified a number of key issues affecting the further development of such services, notably the failure to recruit male providers, training and registration issues of placement providers and the difficulty in meeting the needs of those with multiple disabilities who require special equipment which was not available in the home of the host family (McConkey et al 2004).

Potential drawbacks

Moreover schemes may fail to provide clear information and guidance as to what constitutes good practice within befriending services as they strive to maintain informality and spontaneity (Heslop 2005). This balance is difficult to sustain for people whose main support comes from more formal services. Moreover, these schemes have some conceptual difficulties (McConkey 2010):

- The matching of 'friends' is often made by a professional worker or scheme coordinator; hence the person with a learning disability has very limited scope for choosing and developing their own friendships.
- The 'friendship' that develops runs the risk of being artificial in the sense that the non-disabled person is invariably cast in the role of helper and supervisor. Through time, this can place quite a strain on the relationship.
- If the non-disabled person is no longer able or willing to continue, there is the added problem of finding a replacement while dealing with possible feelings of disappointment and loss in the person left behind.

The befriender approach is an example of adopting a specialist solution to a disability issue. Therein lies the biggest risk of all; a befriender absolves everyone else – busy support staff and social workers for example – from their responsibilities of nurturing friendships and leisure opportunities for the people with whom they work.

Circles of friends

Another approach attracting much interest is that of creating 'circles of support' or 'circles of friends' (Neville & McIver 2000). There is no prescription for the form and format these take, as they will be guided very much by the wishes and needs of the person with learning disability as identified in their person-centred plan. That said, there are some common strands in such circles.

They might include family members – siblings, cousins, aunts and uncles; neighbours and acquaintances; co-workers for people in work settings; members of clubs, churches and such like who know the person. The circle deliberately does not have professional workers as members although they can have a key role as facilitators or 'go-betweens' in starting the circles.

The depth of friendship will vary across the members of the circle. Some may be prepared to be intimately involved; others will continue as acquaintances but they will be better informed than previously. The circle can seek out social, educational, employment as well as leisure opportunities and support people within these pursuits.

Circles Network – a UK-wide organisation – is a charity which promote circles of support through training courses and consultancies (Circles Network 2009).

This same idea can find expression in other ways. For example, KeyRing is a Housing provider for people with a learning disability that works by building up mutually supportive networks among the tenants living within a geographical area as well as linking them into the communities where they live (Simons 1998). Likewise new forms of day provision often operate on the basis of creating social networks for their clients by slotting them into educational, employment and recreational opportunities in the community (Towell 2008). As yet, there have been few formal evaluations of these networks as to whether or not they fulfil their promise but informal feedback from members is very positive.

See Reader activity 24.3 on the Evolve website.

Creating opportunities for contributions

Notions of helplessness pervade many people's perceptions of adults with learning disabilities. Many appeals for donations are based on this premise but this approach further alienates them from society as people in need of charity. In reality, many more people with learning disabilities could be active contributors to society if given the opportunities, preparation and support. Two areas are highlighted in particular.

Household tasks

One area that is easily overlooked is helping people to contribute to household tasks. Skills such as vacuuming and cleaning floors are a necessary part of housekeeping but they can also be deployed in

Bigby, C., 2008. Known well by no-one: trends in the informal social networks of middle-aged and older people with intellectual disability five years after moving to the community. J. Intellect. Dev. Disabil. 33 (2), 148–157.

Brodin, J., 2009. Inclusion through access to outdoor education: Learning in Motion (LIM). Journal of Adventure Education and Outdoor Learning 9 (2), 99–113.

Buttimer, J., Tierney, E., 2005. Patterns of leisure participation among adolescents with a mild intellectual disability. J. Intellect. Disabil. 91 (1), 25–42.

Circles Network, 2009. Available at: http://www.circlesnetwork.org.uk (accessed 10.07.10.).

Clement, T., Bigby, C., 2009. Breaking out of a distinct social space: reflections on supporting community participation for people with severe and profound intellectual disability. J. Appl. Res. Intellect. Disabil. 22, 264–275.

Department of Health, 2009. Valuing people now: a new three-year strategy for people with learning disabilities. DH, London.

Department of Health, Social Services and Public Safety, 2005. Equal lives: review of policy and services for people with a learning disability in Northern Ireland. DHSSPS, Belfast.

Emerson, E., McVilly, K., 2004. Friendship activities of adults with intellectual disabilities in supported accommodation in northern England. J. Appl. Res. Intellect. Disabil. 17, 191–197.

Emerson, E., Hatton, C., Thompson, T., Parmenter, T.R. (Eds.), 2004. The international handbook of applied research in intellectual disabilities. John Wiley & Sons, London.

Emerson, E., Mallam, S., Davies, I., Spencer, K., 2005. Adults with learning difficulties in England 2003/04. National Statistics and Health and Social Care Information Centre, London.

European Union, 2000. The Charter of Fundamental Rights of the European Union. Available at: http://www.europarl.europa.eu/charter/default_en.htm.

Gardner, J.F., Carran, D.T., 2005. Attainment of personal outcomes by people with developmental disabilities. Ment. Retard. 43, 157–174.

Hall, L., Hewson, S., 2006. The community links of a sample of people with intellectual disabilities. J. Appl. Res. Intellect. Disabil. 19 (2), 131–224.

Hastings, R.P., Taunt, H.M., 2002. Positive perceptions in families of children with developmental disabilities. American Journal on Mental Retardation 107, 116–127.

Heslop, P., 2005. Good practice in befriending services for people with learning difficulties. British Journal of Learning Disabilities 33, 27–33.

Holder, M.D., Coleman, B., Sehn, Z.L., 2009. The contribution of active and passive leisure to children's well-being. J. Health Psychol. 14 (3), 378–386.

Holloway, T., Mawhinney, S., 2002. Providing support, reducing exclusion: the extent, nature and value of volunteer befriending in Northern Ireland. Praxis Care Group, Belfast.

Jameson, C., 1998. Promoting long-term relationships between individuals with mental retardation and people in their community: an agency self-evaluation. Ment. Retard. 36 (2), 116–127.

Kampert, A.L., Gorenczny, A.J., 2007. Community involvement and socialization among individuals with mental retardation. Res. Dev. Disabil. 28, 278–286.

Lippold, T., Burns, J., 2009. Social support and intellectual disabilities: a comparison between social networks of adults with intellectual disability and those with physical disability. J. Intellect. Disabil. Res. 53 (5), 463–473.

McClimens, A., Gordon, F., 2009. People with intellectual disabilities as bloggers: what's social capital got to do with it anyway? J. Intellect. Disabil. 13 (1), 19–30.

McConkey, R., 1994. Innovations in educating communities about learning disabilities. Lisieux Hall, Chorley.

McConkey, R., 1998. Community integration. In: Fraser, W., Sines, D., Kerr, M. (Eds.), Hallas' the care of people with intellectual disabilities. Butterworth-Heinemann, Oxford.

McConkey, R., 2004. Northern Ireland Omnibus Survey – European Year of Disabled Persons. EYPD Committee, Belfast.

McConkey, R., 2010. Promoting friendships and developing social networks. In: Grant, G., Ramcharan, P., Flynn, M., Richardson, M. (Eds.), 2010 Learning disability: a life cycle approach to valuing people. second ed. Open University Press, Maidenhead.

McConkey, R., Collins, S., 2010a. Using personal goal-setting to promote the social inclusion of people with intellectual disability living in supported accommodation. J. Intellect. Disabil. Res. 54 (2), 135–143.

McConkey, R., Collins, S., 2010b. The role of support staff in promoting the social inclusion of persons with intellectual disabilities. J. Intellect. Disabil. Res. 54 (8), 691–700.

McConkey, R., Smyth, M., 2003. Parental perceptions of risks with young adults who have severe learning difficulties contrasted with the young people's views and experiences. Child. Soc. 17, 18–31.

McConkey, R., Truesdale, M., 2000. Reactions of nurses and therapists in mainstream health services to contact with people who have learning disabilities. J. Adv. Nurs. 32, 158–163.

McConkey, R., McConaghie, J., Roberts, P., King, D., 2004. Family placement schemes for adult persons with intellectual disabilities living with elderly carers. J. Learn. Disabil. 8, 267–282.

McConkey, R., Sowney, M., Milligan, V., Barr, O., 2005. Views of people with intellectual disabilities of their present and future living arrangements. Journal of Policy and Practice in Intellectual Disabilities 1, 115–125.

McConkey, R., Abbott, S., Noonan-Walsh, P., Linehan, C., Emerson, E., 2007. Variations in the social inclusion of people with intellectual disabilities in supported living schemes and residential settings. J. Intellect. Disabil. Res. 51 (3), 207–217.

McConkey, R., Dunne, J., Blitz, N., 2009. Shared lives: building relationships and community with people who have intellectual disabilities. Sense, Amsterdam.

Mencap, 2007. Bullying wrecks lives: the experiences of children and young people with a learning disability. Mencap, London.

Mencap, (undated). Leisure for everyone: how to campaign to help people with a learning disability take part in leisure activities more easily. Mencap, London.

Miller, E., Cooper, S.A., Cook, C., Petch, A., 2008. Outcomes important to people with intellectual disabilities. Journal of Policy and Practice in Intellectual Disabilities 5 (3), 150–158.

Murray, P., 2002. Hello! Are you listening? Disabled teenagers' experience of access to inclusive leisure. Joseph Rowntree Foundation, York.

Neville, M., McIver, B., 2000. Circles of support. In: Kelly, B., McGinley, P. (Eds.), Intellectual disability: the response of the church. Lisieux Hall, Chorley.

Oliver, M., 1996. Understanding disability: from theory to practice. Macmillan, Basingstoke.

Patterson, I., Pegg, S., 2009. Serious leisure and people with intellectual disabilities: benefits and opportunities. Leisure Studies 28 (4), 387–402.

Pockney, R., 2006. Friendship or facilitation: people with learning disabilities and their paid carers. Sociological Research Online 11 (3) Available at: http://www.socresonline.org.uk/11/3/pockney.html.

Roker, D., Player, K., Coleman, J., 1998. Challenging the image: the involvement of young people with disabilities in volunteering and campaigning. Disability and Society 13 (5), 725–741.

Schwartz, D.B., 1992. Crossing the river: creating a conceptual revolution in community and disability. Brookline Books, Cambridge.

Simons, K., 1998. Living support networks: an evaluation of the services provided by KeyRing. Pavilion, Brighton.

Smyth, M., McConkey, R., 2003. Future aspirations of parents and students with severe learning difficulties on leaving special schooling. British Journal of Learning Disabilities 31, 54–59.

Solish, A., Perry, A., Minnes, P., 2009. Participation of children with and without disabilities in social, recreational and leisure activities. J. Appl. Res. Intellect. Disabil. 23 (3), 226–236.

Special Olympics, 2010. Available at: http://www.specialolympics.org/unified_sports.aspx (accessed 10.07.10.).

Stebbins, R., 2000. Serious leisure for people with disabilities. In: Sivan, A., Ruskin, H. (Eds.), Leisure education, community development and populations with special needs. CABI, Oxon, pp. 101–108.

Towell, D., 1988. An ordinary life in practice: developing comprehensive community-based services for people with learning disabilities. King's Fund, London.

Towell, D., 2008. People with intellectual disabilities: exploring strategies for achieving equal citizenship. Centre for Inclusive Futures, London.

United Nations, 1975. Declaration of the Rights of Disabled Persons. UN, Genev.

United Nations, 2007. Convention on the Rights of Persons with Disabilities. Available at: http://www.un.org/disabilities/.

Verdonschot, M.M.L., de Witte, L.P., Reichrath, et al., 2009. Community participation of people with an intellectual disability: a review of empirical findings. J. Intellect. Disabil. Res. 53 (4), 303–318.

Ward, L., 1988. Innovations in advocacy and empowerment for people with intellectual disabilities. Lisieux Hall, Chorley.

Widmer, E.D., Kempf-Constantin, N., Robert-Tissot, C., et al., 2008. How central and connected am I in my family? Family-based social capital of individuals with intellectual disability. Research in Developmental Disabilities: A Multidisciplinary Journal 29 (2), 176–187.

Wilkinson, R., Marmot, M. (Eds.), 2003. Social determinants of health: the solid facts. second ed. WHO, Denmark.

Williams, V., Marriott, A., Townsley, R., 2008. Shaping our future: a scoping and consultation exercise to establish research priorities in learning disabilities for the next ten years. HMSO, National Co-ordinating Centre for NHS Service Delivery and Organisation R&D (NCCSDO), London.

Wolfensberger, W., 1972. The principle of normalisation in human services. National Institute on Mental Retardation, Toronto.

World Health Organization, 2001. International classification of functioning, disability and health. WHO, Genev.

Further reading

Grant, G., Ramcharan, P., Flynn, M., Richardson, M. (Eds.), 2010. Learning disability: a life cycle approach to valuing people. second ed. Open University Press, Maidenhead.

McConkey, R., Dunne, J., Blitz, N., 2009. Shared lives: building relationships and community with people who have intellectual disabilities. Sense, Amsterdam.

Nind, M., Seale, J., 2010. Understanding and promoting access for people with learning difficulties: seeing the opportunities and challenges of risk. Routledge, Abingdon.

Useful addresses

Down's Syndrome Association: http://www.downs-syndrome.org.uk/

Understanding Intellectual Disability and Health: http://www.intellectualdisability.info/

Foundation for People with Learning Disabilities: http://www.learningdisabilities.org.uk/

Mencap: http://www.mencap.org,uk

Special Olympics: http://www.specialolympics.org/unified_sports.aspx

Education for children and young people with learning disabilities

25

David S. Stewart OBE

CHAPTER CONTENTS

KEY ISSUES

- The Warnock Report and subsequent legislation have had a major impact on education for students with learning disabilities in the UK
- It is important for professionals and parents to understand the process of the Special Educational Needs Code of Practice
- There is still much debate on the issue of inclusion and in what setting children and young people with learning disabilities are taught
- There needs to be clear planning and preparation to ensure smooth transition from school
- Professionals need to ensure a holistic approach when working with parents and families
- The student voice must be developed and heard

Introduction

Education for children and young people with learning disabilities has an interesting history, and it is important at the start of this chapter to review the past provision to make better understanding of the current practices and situations today. The most significant development in the last 40 years was the Warnock Report (1978) and the subsequent Education Act 1981 has had a profound influence on provision made in mainstream and special schools. Understanding the Special Educational Needs (SEN) Code of Practice (Department for Education and Skills (DfES) 2001) is vital to make sense of the procedures and practices in schools and how they affect pupils and their families. No subject is more hotly debated than inclusion and the constant question 'Does it matter where children are taught?' The curriculum for young people with learning disabilities is also discussed: does it fit them for life, does it challenge and does the system ensure entitlement to a full and enriched education?

Moving on from school is potentially a difficult time for all students but for those with learning disabilities it can be particularly traumatic. What is in place to ensure smooth transition and what is available to young people once they have left school? Are colleges of further education (FE) able to provide for all students and what happens once college courses finish? Schools need to work closely with parents, families, other disciplines and services to ensure a holistic approach and these relationships are explored. Strategies for developing the student voice and enabling children and young people with learning disabilities to take their place as citizens are also offered.

A historical overview

The earliest detailed account of an attempt to educate a child with learning disabilities was in France in 1800 when Dr Itard began his work with Victor, or the Wild Boy of Aveyron. While people in the UK took an interest in this work, and later in the 1840s in the work of Guggenbuhl in Switzerland, it was not until 1846 that Charlotte and Harriett White, two young sisters of 26, set up a small school in Bath for children with learning disabilities. Sustained by local donations and fees, they supported around 20 children at any given time from as far north as Scotland. Their work had been inspired by the writings of Dr Twining who had visited Guggenbuhl and, on his return, had urged that similar work might start in Britain.

Further charitable institutions, such as Earslwood, were built but it was not until 1878 that the Metropolitan Asylums Board opened the Darenth Schools near Dartford, Kent, for some 1000 children. This was the first educational establishment for children with learning disabilities to be paid for out of the public purse. Subsequent legislation toward the end of the 19th century enabled authorities to provide for those with moderate and mild learning disabilities. School boards began to provide special classes. As testing of intelligence became more prevalent, further distinctions were made between those who were deemed to be educable and ineducable. Education authorities were keen to know for whom they did *not* have to provide. Indeed, the development of psychological testing by Binet and Simon in France at this period was similarly to assist in the ruling out of those who might receive education. Larger authorities began to provide special schools as well as classes. The London County Council was the first authority to employ an educational psychologist, Cyril Burt, in 1913.

Further legislation in 1914 made the provision of special education for those with moderate learning disabilities mandatory for local education authorities. Toward the end of the First World War (1914–1918), provision of occupation centres for those not eligible for education began to be established though many children still remained in long-stay hospitals.

Even the Education Act 1944, which categorised pupils with special needs into 11 categories (see Box 25.1), failed to make provision for pupils with the more severe and profound needs. The categories now included educationally sub-normal (ESN) which would roughly correspond to mild or moderate learning difficulties in current educational descriptors. It was recognised soon after that some education authorities were using schools for ESN for children who were failing at school for reasons other than low intelligence. Intelligence testing ruled out those with IQs below 50 whose provision was governed by mental deficiency and later mental health legislation. With the onset of the NHS in 1948, many of these children were to be found within a system

Box 25.1

Education Act 1944 categories

1. Educational sub-normality.
2. Blind.
3. Deaf.
4. Epileptic.
5. Partially sighted.
6. Partially deaf.
7. Physically handicapped.
8. Delicate.
9. Diabetic.
10. Speech defects.
11. Maladjusted.

which was not appropriate to the provision of education or indeed the welfare of children with disabilities. Most of the long-stay hospitals until that time had been the responsibility of the local authority.

Campaigning and seminal texts such as Stan Segal's *No Child is Ineducable* in 1967 led to the Education Act 1970 in England and Wales which brought all children within the responsibility of the education authorities. Scotland did the same in 1975 but it was not until 1987 that children in Northern Ireland received the same rights. In April 1971, all children in England and Wales became entitled to education irrespective of their degree of disability. This is a notion not to be taken lightly. When studying comparative information worldwide, practitioners would do well to ascertain the status of all pupils. In many countries, access to education may still mean those who are deemed worthy or educable.

The Warnock Report and beyond

In 1974, a committee was established under the chairmanship of Mary Warnock to review the provision for children with special educational needs. The committee reported in 1978 and one of its main recommendations was to abolish the use of categories, advocating a continuum of special needs. The committee suggested that only 2% of the school population required a separate educational provision but that there was another 18% in mainstream schools that would require special provision. They argued that this group had always been there but there had not been consistent efforts to accommodate their needs.

The report formed the basis of the 1981 Education Act and its policies on special educational needs (SEN) which stated that:

> A child will have a special educational need if she has a learning difficulty requiring special educational provision. The 'learning difficulty' includes not only physical and mental disabilities, but also any kind of learning difficulty experienced by a child provided that it is significantly greater than that of the majority of children of the same age.
>
> (Warnock Report 1978)

The Act promoted the notion that the education of pupils with SEN should be carried out in mainstream schools if possible. This gave an impetus to the inclusion agenda for schools. Before the Act, it could be argued there was a very varied approach as to who received services and who might be sent to a special school.

The Act introduced the 'statementing process' which sought to bring clarity to the process of access to appropriate education and enable a wide range of views and information to be in place before a decision was made. The process has been at the heart of much discussion over the last 30 years. Should a pupil receive appropriate support without the need for a Statement of Special Educational Needs? There is great variation across the country in the numbers of pupils statemented by individual local authorities. It is also worth noting that the Office for Standards in Education, Children's Services and Skills (OFSTED) commented in 2006 that:

> Statements did nothing to determine the quality of provision or outcomes for the pupil in any type of setting.

So a statement might determine need but not what is received in practice.

If a child has a particular condition or health problem which has caused concern from an early age, they may be referred by the parent or a health professional to the local authority for a statutory assessment. If they are under the age of 2, the local authority must carry out the assessment but not necessarily follow the statutory procedures for children over 2. Statements for those under 2 are rare and the local authority would consider individual support based on needs.

The Education Act 1996 defined special educational needs as experienced by children who have considerably greater difficulty in learning than others the same age. It also includes children who cannot use the educational facilities which other children of a similar age use because of their disability. Statutory school age is currently 5–16 years but children under school age, who would normally fall into either category without extra help, are also included. All may need extra or different help in education from that given to other children without SEN.

Some 10 years after the 1981 Act, it was apparent that the process was being focused very heavily on the statementing process rather than targeting the largest proportion of pupils with SEN in school. Parents were often left bewildered by the process. Reform came in the SEN Code of Practice in 1992 which was itself revised in 2001 (DfES).

SEN Code of Practice

Every school has a special educational needs coordinator (SENCO) and, in mainstream schools, that person will establish a register of SEN. Registers vary widely in regard to the pupils. In a recent survey in East Sussex, the numbers on the register in secondary schools varied from 10.4% to 33.1%, and in primary schools from 19.9% to 38.1%. The national average for secondary schools is 21% and for primary schools 19.7%. Sir Alan Steer, in his review on pupil behaviour in 2009, commented:

> Accurate identification of children's special educational needs is essential if those needs are to be met and that a child is to progress. While many schools display exemplary practice there is a lack of consistency of practice in the system as a whole and there are problems both with the over identification and under identification of SEN in individual schools. Some schools identify far higher numbers than found in other schools in a similar context. This might result from a desire to emphasise to the outer world and OFSTED the difficulties the school faces, but over identification as well as under identification can be damaging to the children and to good practice in the school.

The SEN Code of Practice (DfES 2001) establishes a graduated approach to working with pupils with SEN.

School Action

Once a child or young person has been identified as having a SEN which requires extra or different help, strategies are put in place such as different ways of teaching, extra adult support or specialist equipment. This is called *School Action.* Parents will be involved and there will be an individual education plan (IEP) which is reviewed. This applies to pupils in Key Stage (KS)1 (5–7 years old), KS2 (8–11 years old), KS3 (12–14 years old) and KS4 (15–16 years old). For those in pre-statutory early years education, this is called *Early Years Action.*

School Action Plus

If it is felt that the interventions have not provided sufficient support, the school will consult external agents such as a specialist teacher or educational psychologist. A meeting is held with parents. This is then deemed to be *School Action Plus.*

Individual education plan

Strategies used to enable the pupil to progress at School Action and School Action Plus should be recorded in an IEP. This should contain:

- short-term targets for the pupil
- teaching strategies to be used
- provision to be put in place
- when the plan is to be reviewed
- success and/or exit criteria
- outcomes.

The IEP should be reviewed at least twice a year (three times a year for children in early years education). Parents must be kept in touch throughout the process.

Statutory assessments

If interventions at the School Action Plus stage have still not given satisfactory resolution or parents have lost confidence, application can then be made for a *statutory assessment.* This is a multi-professional review of a child or young person's special educational need. A parent or school can request a statutory assessment from the local authority. Other agencies, such as health and social services, can also make a request. Once a request has been made, the local authority considers whether to make a statutory assessment. They may ask for further evidence from the parent to support the request. It is then when access to the Parent Partnership can be invaluable for parents and carers (see p. 457). The local authority must respond with its decision to assess within 6 weeks. An authority can refuse to carry an assessment out if they feel that adequate arrangements are in place, but a parent can appeal. If an assessment is agreed, the local authority will ask for advice from a range of professionals so that a detailed report can be established on which a decision can be made to issue a *Statement of Special Educational Need.*

Statement of Special Educational Need

A statement is made up of six parts:

1. Introduction – the basic details of the child such as name and address.
2. Special educational needs – this is a description of the child's current SEN as identified by the local

authority. It should draw on and refer to the professional advice attached in the appendices.

3. Special educational provision – this will include the objectives of the provision; details of the special educational provision the local authority considers necessary to meet the child's educational needs; and the arrangements for monitoring progress to see if the provision is meeting the objectives.
4. Placement – this is left blank in the proposed statement, but once the parent has agreed the placement with the local authority, the school or other provision will be named. The placement might include a residential school or school outside the local authority. In relation to such placements, it is useful to note that in 2007 the Audit Commission called for a review of the way children with special education needs are placed out of authority after research showed they may not be receiving appropriate or cost-effective education provision. At that time, authorities were spending more than £500 million on such placements, an average of £57 000 per pupil, but little regard was given to pupil progress.
5. Non-educational needs – this contains the child's non-educational needs as agreed between health, social services or other agencies and the local authority.
6. Non-educational provision – this is the provision to meet the needs outlined in part 5. It should include the objectives of the provision, and explain the arrangements agreed between the local authority and the organisation making the provision for ensuring it is delivered. Part 6 does not have any legal force.

Often statements will be couched in quite general terms, stating, for example, that a child requires access to speech and language services but not stating how much and how often. This can often be a cause of tension and may result in the parent asking for reassessment.

Reader activity 25.1

Review the special educational need (SEN) assessment process for an individual pupil. How were they assessed and which staff were involved in the process? Identify ways in which the young person and parents were involved in the process.

Reassessment

A reassessment can be requested if a parent or school thinks that the child's needs have changed since the last statement was issued, or that the child now needs different or more support than that described in the current statement. It might be that it is felt the child needs a different type of school, for example from a mainstream to a special school, and the statement will need to be reviewed and amended. It is a general rule that a child attending a special school would have a statement while a child with a statement could attend either a mainstream or a special school. Some children may be in special schools on assessment placements. This might particularly apply to pupils from abroad for whom the local authority may have little information. The statement is reviewed annually.

Annual reviews

All statements (other than those for children under 2) must be reviewed at least annually. Statements can be reviewed more frequently when needed. The annual review is to discuss with parents the child's progress and whether any changes need to be made to the statement. The views of the parents and child are important and recorded. Practice on the involvement of children and young people with learning disabilities tends to be varied. This should be encouraged at all times (see Developing the pupil voice, below). An example of collection of a young person's views is shown at Figure 25.1.

Arrangements should be in place that make the experience meaningful for the young person. Parents may bring a friend or someone from Parent Partnership (see p. 457) for support. The review should provide a new set of targets which meet the objectives set out in the statement.

A copy of the review is sent to the local authority which will determine whether to amend the statement, leave the statement unchanged or cease to maintain the statement.

Appeals

If a parent is not happy about the process or decisions made about their child with SEN, there are avenues for appeal. Appeals can be made to the Special Educational Needs and Disability Tribunal

Young person's views

This review is all about YOU
Use this form to tell us about yourself and how you think you are doing.

Name: *Paul R*

Form completed by: *Ellis Price* Date: *26/03/2010*

What do you like best about yourself?

I am always happy and willing to try new things.

I like lots of staff in school and I like talking to Phil and Chris.

What do you feel you have done well this year?

I have started to use my voice more.

I have developed my listening skills and I do lots of exercise.

I have enjoyed my work experience this year.

What have you found difficult this year?

I have found it difficult to find my way around the school.

I have found it difficult to be quicker when taking my coat off in class.

I find it difficult to look people in the eye.

Figure 25.1 • Example of collection of young person's views for annual review

Continued

(SENDIST). Appeals need to be made within 2 months of the local authority's decision. An appeal can be made if:

- the local authority refuses to carry out a statutory assessment or reassessment
- the local authority refuses to issue a statement after carrying out an assessment

If the local authority makes a statement, amends an existing statement or refuses to amend a statement after reassessment, an appeal can be made:

- against the description of the child's special educational need in part 2 of the statement
- against the description of the educational provision in part 3 of the statement

What would you like to acheive next year?

I would like to keep doing my work experience.
I would like to do more sport.
I would like to do more cooking.

What help do you think you will need to achieve this?

I need sensitive staff who can help me to start these tasks.

You can use this space to tell us about anything else you think is important, such as what you enjoy most in school:

With the help of photographic prompts and encouragement from Elley and Matthew, Paul said the following:

- He is good at dancing, likes listening to music, (any music) and is involved with the rock band. He also likes wrestling;
- He would like to do music at College with the help of Mary, Sally and Matthew;
- He has a good French accent;
- He is more confident at swimming and has a relaxed body;
- He is very proud of his appearance and is tidy;
- He enjoys Work Experience and does filing and shredding;
- He enjoys the Cyber Cafe and has taken money;
- He is good at fitness with Carol and Amin;
- He could get to class quicker and will continue to use his voice more to say what he would like and what he wants.

Figure 25.1 • Cont'd

- against the name of the school named in part 4 of the statement
- if no school is named in part 4 of the statement
- if the local authority refuses to change the name of the school if the statement is at least a year old
- if the local authority decides not to maintain the child's statement.

A parent cannot appeal to SENDIST:

- if the local authority refuses a request to change the name of the school to an independent or non-maintained school
- about the way the local authority carried out the assessment and/or the length of time it took
- about how the local authority is providing the help specified in the statement

- about the way the school is providing for the child's needs
- about the non-educational needs provision
- if the local authority will not amend the statement after an annual review.

Appeals can be made to SENDIST about disability discrimination if a parent feels that their child has experienced discrimination relating to:

- admissions arrangements
- education and associated services, including school sports, school trips, lunch and break times
- exclusions, whether they are permanent or for a fixed period.

Once SENDIST has made a decision, the local authority must comply within a fixed term, beginning with the date the decision was issued. There are different time frames. For instance, to continue a statement is immediate; to start the statement is 4 weeks. A parent or carer can also make a complaint to the local government ombudsman, seek a judicial review or a direct approach to the Secretary of State.

Transition

In the school life of a young person with learning disabilities, there can be several transitions. This could be between different types of schools and in an all-age school, as in the transition between different Key Stages. All such transitions need to be planned so that the pupil feels confident and safe. The most challenging transition is that of leaving school and moving to adult provision.

Transition planning

In year 9, when the pupil is 14, the school should arrange for the annual review to include other agencies who will be involved in the young person's life after school. This will include Connexions, and other agencies such as health and social services. Connexions provides support and advice for young people aged 13–19, and for those with learning difficulties or disabilities up to the age of 25. The service can support in school, college or work and provide advice and support around personal and family life. The service is able to refer students to specialist support if needed. At the transition stage, the service will be very active with the student planning the next stage after school. The review should focus on the needs of the young person as they move to further education and training, employment or day services. A transition plan should be created which is reviewed annually. In reality, certain services – who feel that for some pupils leaving school may be some time hence – will have little involvement for the next few years. This is not helpful to the young person or their family for whom the whole idea of transition can be fraught as they move from statutory services to permissive ones.

Pupils should be at the forefront of this process, being actively involved in the planning and preparation. The pupil and family will begin to meet a new range of professionals who should help with the process. The Connexions service will have a key role as may social workers. In truth, some of the input comes far too late and many pupils and their families become very anxious.

For those with additional health needs, there should be a great deal of consultation for access to health professionals such as a nurse or physiotherapist. In a school, this access may be every day but will generally be far less in adult provision. Similarly, families who have been used to seeing the school doctor may need to make new relations with their GP. If a young person is going to require health support at college or in adult provision, a transitions nurse will usually be part of the transitions team. Most authorities have transitions teams, comprised of Connexions workers, social workers, therapists and nurses. It is hoped that a more holistic approach will give more stability to the process for the young person and their family.

During their time in years 12, 13 and 14, students should usually have had tasters of further education courses so that they will have some ability to choose what they wish to study at college. Increasingly colleges of further education have raised the bar on admissions particularly in relation to proscribed progression. This means that some students who may have previously had an opportunity at college no longer meet the requirement. With reducing budgets, local authorities are revising the criteria for adults who attend day or social centres. This has meant that there may be increasing numbers of young adults who after 2 or 3 years at college may be sitting at home. So the transition plan which may have been full of hope and expectation is not realised. It should be remembered that the Connexions team can work with young people up to the age of 25.

The world of work is still the dream of many young people and Connexions should be supporting this where identified. This provision varies around the country. For many people, there is the offer of work experience similar to school schemes, but gaining employment is far less a reality (see Ch. 26). Doing voluntary work or working in cooperatives is a much more likely option.

Aiming High for Disabled Children (Department for Children, Schools and Families (DCSF) 2007) was launched as part of the government's transformation programme for disabled children's services. One of the issues raised was transition. There was a National Transition Support Team established to drive the Transition Support Programme as part of this transformation. Their goal is to drive and shape the programme in local areas.

Working with parents and families

Early intervention is clearly vital and once a child is identified as having a SEN, Portage workers and other early years advisers will be working with families and their children. Portage workers are usually employed by the local authority to work with families of very young children with disabilities, advising on suitable programmes of learning and providing individual one-to-one support for the child. They work in the home and the children they work with may be yet to have a statement if indeed they need one. In some areas, voluntary organisations may provide training for parents, as indeed will some schools.

Parents need to feel they can be active in the life of the school. Where possible, a parent room provides possibilities for training, listening and support. A home/school liaison officer within a school can provide a real support to parents and families. Parents are encouraged to become parent governors and become involved in the life of the school.

There are particular issues for siblings. In a mainstream setting, there may be bullying because the pupil has a disabled brother, and if the child comes to a special school, the siblings may have no idea what it looks like. Activities where families can attend with their child are much to be encouraged. For special schools, there is always the issue of distance from the child's home and also the fact that their child cannot communicate about what they have done during the day. Home school diaries and telephone calls help in keeping families in touch. Parent evenings, other meetings and social events are important to ensure parents feel part of their child's education.

Parent Partnerships

It was identified by the Code of Practice (DfES 2001) that parents and families find the whole process of special education daunting and confusing. Parent Partnership Services were established to provide information, advice and support to parents and carers of children and young people with SEN. They can be invaluable in supporting parents, including those with very young children. Parents will be generally completely unaware of what needs to happen. They may still be coming to terms with the child's disability. Having the support of the Parent Partnership gives reassurance and it can often steer the parent through the process. Parents need to be used as a fountain of knowledge for they know their child better than anyone else.

Parent Partnerships have a role in making sure that parents' views are heard and understood and they are active in making these views inform local policy and practice. They are usually based with a voluntary organisation or with the local authority or Children's Trust. All Parent Partnership Services, wherever they are based, are at arm's length from the local authority and the services they provide are confidential and impartial. They can provide information about the following:

- How special educational needs are identified and assessed by schools and the local authority.
- Who parents can talk to in a school or local authority about their concerns.
- The SEN Code of Practice, the statutory assessment process and statements.
- Parents'/carers' rights and responsibilities.
- Meetings and reviews about a child's needs.
- How progress is monitored and reviewed.
- What parents can do if they are not happy about a decision made about their child's special education.

Do not assume that all parents know about Parent Partnerships – they may need guiding to their nearest team. Often within the team of paid and volunteer staff will be parents who have been through a similar process. Professionals should never underestimate how difficult it can be for a parent trying to negotiate the minefield of bureaucracy.

Inclusion

Inclusion is probably one of the most talked about subjects within the area of special education. Should children and young people with learning disabilities be educated alongside their mainstream peers or in separate provision? In 2006, OFSTED commissioned a report *Inclusion: Does it Matter Where Pupils are Taught?* The report was very clear in its findings:

> The most important factor in determining the best outcomes for pupils with learning difficulties and disabilities (LDD) is not the type but the quality of provision. Effective provision was distributed equally in the mainstream and special schools visited, but there was more good and outstanding provision in resourced mainstream schools than elsewhere.

The inspectors were not impressed by the quality of work between special and mainstream schools. Equally they were sceptical about the strategies in place:

> Provision of additional resources to pupils such as support from Teaching Assistants did not ensure good quality intervention or adequate progress by pupils.

What they did identify as positives were the involvement of specialist teachers, good assessment, work which challenged pupils sufficiently and the commitment from school leaders to ensure good progress for all pupils.

It is useful to reflect on these findings rather than see inclusion as just a question of setting. The debate on inclusion for children and young people of school age can also be very school based, rather than thinking of opportunities in the local and wider communities.

Reader activity 25.2

Examine the impact of legislation on the education of pupils with learning disabilities. Highlight the issues in the inclusion debate. Talk with pupils about their experiences.

Every Child Matters and Every Disabled Child Matters

The government published a Green Paper, *Every Child Matters* (DCSF 2003), following which it published *Every Child Matters: the Next Steps* (DCSF 2004) and passed the Children Act 2004. The key aims of the Every Child Matters agenda which should be embedded into the lives of every school are:

- be healthy
- stay safe
- enjoy and achieve
- make a positive contribution
- achieve economic wellbeing.

The challenge for schools is to make this a reality for those with disabilities. For instance, *Healthy Lives, Brighter Futures* (DH 2009a) is extremely important in the education of pupils with learning disabilities. Issues of diet, nutrition and obesity are ever present. If we know the statistics for obesity in adults with learning disabilities are running higher than for the general population (McGuire et al 2007), what is being done in schools to tackle this problem as part of the Be Healthy agenda? What is being done about mental wellbeing when we know that adults with learning disabilities are more likely to experience mental health issues? (See Ch. 17.)

It is important when working with pupils with profound and multiple learning disabilities (PMLD) or complex needs to ensure that all these aims apply to them. Children and young people with complex learning difficulties and disabilities (CLDD) have conditions that coexist with one or more special educational need. The combination of layered needs might include mental health, relationships, behavioural, physical, medical, sensory, communication and cognitive. Their attainments may be inconsistent.

There has been debate about what 'achieve economic wellbeing' means when applied to someone with PMLD. Schools need to decide what they are going to put in place to make this a reality – for either we say every child matters or we don't. Undertaking a quality network review with a group of young people with PMLD, one school found that there were many ways to consider this when looking at outcomes for pupils based on the Every Child Matters agenda (DCSF 2004). It made the whole school consider what it was doing for these pupils.

See Reader activity 25.3 on the Evolve website.

At the time of the launch of *Every Child Matters* (DCSF 2004), there was a feeling that issues for those with disabilities were being ignored. This led in 2006 to the Every Disabled Child Matters (ECDM), a consortium campaign run by Contact a Family, the

Council for Disabled Children, Mencap and the Special Educational Consortium (see Useful addresses). They campaign to give disabled children and their families new rights to the services and support they need to lead ordinary lives.

The curriculum

The National Curriculum sets out the stages and core subjects a child or young person will be taught during their time in school. Children aged 5–16 in maintained or state schools must be taught the National Curriculum. Its framework is intended to ensure that teaching and learning are balanced and consistent. The National Curriculum equally applies to pupils with learning disabilities. Yet it is certainly not the only curriculum which should be offered to pupils who should expect an enriching diet of educational opportunities. There is clearly an issue of entitlement and this must never be lost in the debate on what is appropriate to pupils with a wide range of abilities. A good example of this was the introduction of modern foreign languages in special schools in the early 1990s. 'What's the point of teaching this to these pupils?' some said, yet pupils enjoy the subject and the challenge of learning something new.

The challenge is not therefore how we can limit the curriculum but how we can make the entitlement a reality in an appropriate way. Schools will have worked out a wide range of strategies to ensure that individual pupils have a curriculum appropriate to their particular needs. For instance, with maths, as a young person moves toward independence, so the subject becomes necessarily very practical. Can they tell the time, manage money, budget? Financial competence is high on government agendas for young people and this is particularly so in the case of pupils with moderate and mild disabilities who may be managing their own allowances and services in the future.

Both mainstream and special schools can hold subject and SEN specialisms and this may give a particular focus to the curriculum, though the idea of specialisms is that they drive up progress across all subjects. Pupils with PMLD often pose real challenges for staff and it is important that the curriculum is relevant and that the teaching style reflects their needs. They will need a curriculum which focuses very much on the self and how things and ideas relate to their most immediate needs.

Sex and relationship education

For young people with learning disabilities, sex and relationship education is a vital area of the curriculum, yet its delivery in schools is still very varied. There is national guidance which until the change of government in May 2010 was under review. Sadly is now on hold. It cannot be assumed that pupils have picked up information, knowledge, beliefs and appropriate behaviours. Access to such education will be very diverse. Some schools still do very little in this area, and if getting involved in this work in the role of a nurse, it is important to ascertain what policies are in place.

It is important to remind colleagues that pupils have a right to an education to help them understand themselves, their sexual development and the choices open to them; and to safeguarding from sexual abuse and exploitation. Without education, there is the danger that pupils might find themselves in difficulties because of inappropriate sexualised behaviour or because of a lack of assertiveness training, liable to abuse. Parents are very keen that schools support in this work and schools should be prepared to work closely with parents and families. For instance, if talking about masturbation being a private activity, the school will need to talk with the family about the child's bedroom being the private place.

Pupils will often have difficulties understanding about friendships and relationships. Someone being friendly is not the same as a 'friend' and these are lessons which need to be taught. Pupils will require help understanding their emotions and those of others. As they approach adolescence, some pupils may find the experience very difficult; prophylactic education is important, preparing young girls for periods or boys for wet dreams. Some pupils may become distressed as they begin to have hair on their arms or face and will need to be supported in coming to terms with growing up.

Support for the development of friendships is important. If asked, many pupils will reveal that they are never invited to another pupil's house either for tea or a sleepover. They will often only have friends within the context of school. When they leave school at 19, they may never see those friends again unless plans are in place to keep those friendships in place. There is a real danger then that young people may be friendless and therefore potentially vulnerable. Schools are in a good place to work with families and other agencies to create situations in which young people can develop friendships. These might be through after-school clubs, residential trips and evening and weekend activities. Old student associations can also keep people together.

Young people need to be aware of their sexual health and safety. They need to value themselves. Many of the pupils may not be generalist learners so each situation needs to be explained. If talking about safer sex in relation to using a condom, then this needs to be explained that this is with whomever they are having sex, whether it be a man and woman or two men. To not do so can leave pupils vulnerable to unsafe practices.

Recording and assessment

As all pupils are assessed according to their attainment within the National Curriculum, so those pupils with more complex learning needs are assessed on P Levels. These levels are for those pupils considered to be working below National Curriculum Level 1. All schools must report on pupils who are on P Levels. While aimed at the population with the least skills, the steps are still too wide and schools have sought help from elsewhere. There are published schemes which fill in these gaps such as PIVOTS or BSquared, or a combination of the two.

The Equals Organisation (see Useful addresses) issues an assessment programme called P Scale Assessment of the National Curriculum for Equals (PACE) which enables a clearly managed moderated process within school. Schools can send their end of year data for analysis to the University of Durham, or to Comparison and Analysis of Special Pupil Attainment (CASPA), and this will give some comparative data on pupil progress with like-minded schools. CASPA is a tool to assist with the analysis and evaluation of attainment and progress of pupils with special educational needs. It provides a rich set of comparative data to allow benchmarking and thus allow schools to demonstrate to OFSTED evidence of progress based on national comparators. PACE allows schools to gather summative data from those pupils working on P Levels.

It has already been mentioned that pupils will have individual education plans with targets to be met. It is how those targets are arrived at and how they are subsequently measured in terms of impact on the pupils on which the quality of recording and assessment depends.

As schools and local authorities have striven to determine some structure to attainment and progress of pupils with SEN, so the DCSF in 2009 published its *National Strategies Progression Guidance*. The key principles of the guidance are that:

- high expectations are key to securing good progress
- accurate assessment is essential to securing and measuring pupil progress
- age and prior attainment are the starting point for developing expectations of pupil progress.

The guidance states that in the report *The Children's Plan: One Year On* (DCSF 2008), 20% of parents reported that their school provided little encouragement for them to have high aspirations for their child. Getting good comparative data particularly for those with complex needs can be difficult, but teachers, learners and their parents and carers need to know whether they are making good progress. Schools need to be challenged where learners are not making good progress. Better use of data can raise expectations even for those pupils working at the lower P Levels throughout their school career.

One of the most important purposes of assessment is to inform teaching and learning. Every learner needs to know how they are doing, what they need to do to improve and how to get there. Particularly at the lower P Levels, it is more challenging to make accurate and reliable judgements. Reliability is often based on moderation. Can a child perform the same task at a different time and for a different teacher? The P scale data and lower-level National Curriculum data are based on teacher assessment. Effective procedures for moderation are needed to ensure assessments are sound and consistent across class teams and teaching groups within a school and between clusters of schools.

See Reader activity 25.4 on the Evolve website.

Developing the pupil voice

The Convention on the Rights of the Child (United Nations 1989) states that children who are capable of forming views have a right to receive information, to express an opinion and to have that opinion taken into account in any matters affecting them. The challenge is to ensure that those children and young people with learning disabilities are afforded this right. Giving pupils a voice must start in the early years. Work on self-esteem is crucial for a child or young person to appreciate that she/he is important and that people will listen to her/him. Young people need to be given confidence whatever form of communication they might use.

The SEN Code of Practice (DfES 2001) states that children, where possible, should take part in all decision-making processes in education. This includes setting targets, choosing a school, contributing to the assessment of their needs, annual reviews and the transition process. All children, regardless of whether they attend a special or mainstream school, should be given the same chance to take part in discussions about their education. There will need to be different levels of support provided for individual pupils. Some may need greater time to express their views. A young person may have a different view to the parent and that view should be listened to.

Involving a pupil in the review process can demand some creative thinking and much preparation and planning but the results and the richness of the engagement are always well worth the effort. For instance, person-centred approaches such as graphic facilitation of meetings, Circles of Support and MAPS (see Ch. 9) provide effective ways of ensuring that the student is fully included. A permanent record of this acts as a powerful reminder when being reviewed. Making the young person the centre of that picture is crucial and identifying what needs to happen and who will make it happen is important for all concerned. Preparing the young person beforehand is critical so that he or she is aware of what is going to happen. They have had time to consider what they want to say. There are some important considerations: ensuring that the pupil is comfortable with the meeting room; the length of time the pupil might spend in the meeting; those who need to be in the meeting. Expecting the voice from a young person in a room full of professionals is often unrealistic. There are other opportunities for the professionals to meet. It is important to reflect on how the views of those with PMLD are elicited. Work needs to be done with the pupil and families prior to the meeting.

Involving pupils in their annual reviews as early as possible establishes the fact that there are opportunities for them to voice their hopes and fears. School councils and youth parliaments are useful in focusing on the necessity of speaking in public. Pupils may join other advocacy groups organised by other agencies. In school councils, pupils are given opportunities to speak for themselves or on behalf of their peers. Some pupils may need to have an advocate to support them. In large, all-age special schools, they may have a number of school councils appropriate to the age of the pupils. These supported groups can be very useful to develop skills and confidence. Often the councils will report on issues which are of concern to pupils who are seeking solutions. They may be given a budget to begin the process of having responsibility. This can teach pupils the skills of budgeting and that with a fixed amount of money they will have to prioritise.

It has been found that pupils who attend drama and theatre groups develop a confidence that enables them to take part in debate and discussions. Pupils learn to speak up, project themselves and articulate their thoughts. Posture is also improved as they are taught to raise their head when speaking and direct their voice to the listeners. This may seem very obvious but these are skills that need to be learnt if the young person is to become an effective contributor. In one youth parliament in Nottingham, nearly all the young people with learning disabilities have been members of theatre groups.

For pupils with PMLD, it is important to ensure that they too have a voice. There are many simple switches and devices which have made significant differences to these young people in simple everyday choice making. Being able to ask for a drink or being able to turn on the radio when the young person wants to listen is wonderfully empowering. Staff need to persevere and explore all the new technologies which are now available. Many schools will be working with local colleges and universities to develop improved access for those with disabilities. Portable eye-controlled communication devices such as My Tobii (see Useful addresses) can be very liberating for some students.

Where advocates are used to support pupils, it is important to ensure that this is not just the view of one person. Sometimes it has been found useful to have a small group for one child. In one example, a young man clearly became distressed in shops. In his advocacy group, the female staff tried to think of ways to help. The sole male worker remarked that he hated shopping and that perhaps the young man was no different and this should be taken into account. This led to a much more satisfactory conclusion.

It has also been found useful in working parties of young people to include those without learning disabilities. They are able to bring a broader context. A young person with a disability may feel that they are being disadvantaged by something or their parent does not allow them to do an activity. It may be nothing to do with their disability but their age or safety and this would equally apply to their non-disabled peers.

Citizenship Education forms part of the National Curriculum and there should be an opportunity to inform young people of their rights and responsibilities. While people with learning disabilities have rights, they may not know about them, or if they do, they may not be able to exercise them. The sooner such rights and responsibilities are discussed in school, the more likely that this information will support future learning and behaviours. In both mainstream and special schools, staff need to ensure that those with learning disabilities have access to information and knowledge. Those who have responsibility for timetabling must ensure that there is time for this information to be repeated and reinforced.

Life-long learning

In the past there was a tradition that those who were identified with moderate learning disabilities generally left school at 16 while those with severe or profound learning disabilities had the opportunity to remain at school until 19. This situation is much more diverse now and young people with moderate learning disabilities may be offered the same opportunity to stay on into a sixth form. Whether a young person leaves at 16 or 19, the question of what further education is available is a major consideration.

The White Paper *Valuing People* (DH 2001) and subsequent reviews (DH 2009b) assert that people with learning disabilities should have the same rights and opportunities as everyone else in regards to post-16 education. It enjoins the Learning and Skills Council (LSC), learning disability partnership boards and colleges of further education to support choices and ambitions of people with learning disabilities. In addition, the Learning and Skills Act 2000 asserts that the LSC must have regard to the needs of people with learning disabilities. There must be due regard to promote the equality of opportunity between disabled and non-disabled people.

In 2005, the LSC published *Through Inclusion to Excellence*. It noted that the quality of provision for these learners remains highly variable and a fundamental change in provider capacity and capability is called for. The report highlighted the need for workforce reform and listening to the learners. In regard to funding, the necessity for better struc- [illegible]upport individual need was stressed. There [illegible]l emphasis on progression to employment and the acquisition of skills that enable disabled people to play a full and active part in their communities.

This was followed by a further strategy to implement the vision of *Through Inclusion to Excellence* in 2006 with *Learning for Living and Work* (LSC 2006). This is underpinned by six themes of communication: of priorities, planning, funding, quality, working with partners and learner progression. In this last theme, the LSC returns to the importance of providing for progression in 'work preparation' and 'living skills'. It was stated that, by 2010, the LSC would no longer fund providers who deliver work preparation programmes for learners with learning difficulties and/or disabilities, which were not focused on learning in the workplace and the supported employers model. Whether this target has been met appears to be uncertain and further research is required to assess the national picture.

In April 2010, local authorities in England took over commissioning and funding of training and education for 16–19-year-olds. Their responsibility covers 16–19 participation at schools with sixth forms, at colleges and at private and voluntary sector provision. It also extends to commissioning education and training for young people with learning difficulties up to the age of 25. The main role of the Young People's Learning Agency (YPLA), set up at the same time, is to support and partner local authorities in their new responsibility. It also has responsibility for direct support such as the Education Maintenance Allowance (EMA). Another agency, the Skills Funding Agency, funds and regulates adult further education and skills training in England. This will be particularly relevant for adult learners with learning disabilities over the age of 25.

Traditionally, colleges of further education have offered a variety of courses for students with SEN. These might be on mainstream courses with additional support or on discrete programmes tailored to the needs of individual pupils. The majority of these will be in the young person's locality. For a smaller number of students, funding might be found through the local authority and YPLA to provide a place in one of the independent residential colleges. For such places, a case would need to be made that local provision could not meet the needs of the student.

In a college of further education, 15 hours is considered to be full time and in practical terms this might mean a student attending for 3 days. For some families, this might present a problem so they might not choose this option even if it the most appropriate, opting for a day centre which might offer 5 days. There might also be a package provided which includes time at a college and day centre. At the same time, colleges of further education have become more selective in which students they accept onto courses, wishing to demonstrate certain degrees of progression within an academic year. This had led to fewer students being able to take up this opportunity and being directed immediately to social day care provision.

A review of further education provision by PricewaterhouseCoopers for learners with learning disabilities in the North West reported in 2007. The Manchester focus group reported the significant increase in applications from students with complex needs, with parents demanding more local provision. Providers experiencing an increase of students with profound needs found there was not sufficient funding to support them. The colleges within this group had identified that there was nothing to be gained by every college trying to provide the same when resources were limited and were recommending that particular colleges specialised with students with complex needs. Ironically, this is a return to the situation in the 1970s and 1980s when colleges of further education were controlled by local authorities and designated particular colleges for those with disabilities.

In relation to the learning which is now active in the post-16 education arena is the Foundation Learning Tier. This is predominately for those working at entry level or level 1. Entry level qualifications provide a stepping stone toward nationally recognised qualifications. They are the first level of the National Curriculum framework. There are over 100 entry level certificates to choose from. They enable a student to build skills and increase knowledge. They are made up of a number of units each assessed separately. Learners and practitioners should negotiate and agree an individual personalised learning programme, reflecting the learner's entry point and intended destination. Foundation Learning is about progression, and for people with learning disabilities, this should be about independent living and supported employment.

Courses tend to be vocational with still an emphasis on basic numeracy, literacy and IT. This can often seem to be a repetition of what the young person had at school. There are clearly instances when a young person has the possibility of work and finds that the courses followed have not been relevant to the type of employment offered. Much will depend on the individual college and practice is very diverse around the country. Some colleges will be active in preparing the student for the next stage. There is little longitudinal study to show what becomes of students post college.

As with many adult courses in the UK, there have been major cuts over recent years and the opportunity to follow life-long learning becomes increasingly difficult. It is important that students have courses that are for recreation and pleasure as well as just those for life skills. For example, an evening poetry course has been organised over the last 6 years in an East Midlands city together with the local university. This has enabled the students to not only give reign to their feelings but has given them greater knowledge of poets and poetry styles. Similarly, courses for drama, the arts and dance are run in many parts of the country. These will often be funded by voluntary organisations as access to further education reduces.

Issues for staff in school

There have been particular issues for over 20 years in ensuring an adequate supply of appropriately trained teachers for pupils with severe and profound learning disabilities. In 1989, the specialist training was removed. In 1986, more than 200 teachers qualified at initial teacher level to teach pupils with severe learning disabilities. By 1994, this was reduced to 15. Sixteen years later the situation is not much better. In February 2010, the Salt Review (DCSF 2010) reported on the situation of the supply of teachers for pupils with severe learning difficulties (SLD) and PMLD.

The conclusions of the Salt Review are that there is currently not enough focus on supplying a highly skilled workforce trained to meet the needs of learners with SLD/PMLD. Continuing professional

Reader activity 25.5

Find out what continuing professional development activities are available in your area for staff working in schools and colleges with children and young people with special educational needs. Talk to staff about what they identify as their training needs. This may highlight an opportunity for cross-sector training and/or sharing of expertise. In this way, health and social care staff could be supporting pupils' access to education.

development (CPD) provision to fill the gap varies greatly from area to area and region to region and the systems of developing and disseminating it are largely unstructured.

As the situation of teacher supply has become a pressing issue, so the population among pupils has changed. The number or learners with SLD/PMLD is increasing and, in many cases, individual needs are becoming more complex. This is largely a result of great strides made by the medical profession, with more premature babies being saved than would have been the case even a decade ago and interventions including enteral (tube) feeding becoming common practice.

Multi-agency working

Pupils who are identified with learning disabilities will usually have a number of other additional needs, be they medical, emotional or social. From an early age, many will have contact with a wide range of professionals and this will continue into school life. In special schools in particular, there may be several health professionals on site, and in other schools, there will be many staff visiting.

Colleagues from different agencies will have received a variety of training and education. On some professional training courses, there may be little in the way of input on children and young people with learning disabilities. Often professionals have little idea of the training of others. This can get in the way of working together and there needs to be more cross-sector training.

The relationship between professionals may be dependent on the service level agreements organised by agencies such as primary care trusts (PCTs) and local authorities. This will vary greatly in different parts of the country. For many students, there will be involvement of social care, whether for respite care or for other social needs. Psychologists, mentors, doctors and Connexions workers will also engage with the pupils and their families.

With so many people working on behalf of the pupils it is important that there is good multi-agency working. People need to understand the roles of others and what they can contribute to the lives of the young people. There is a need to be mindful, however, when engaging with pupils and parents at reviews and meetings that there is an optimum number of people if the voice of the pupil or parent is to be heard. Professionals can arrange to share information but they do not necessarily all need to be at a review meeting as this gets in the way of the pupil's confidence to contribute.

The global dimension and the international perspective

As part of social cohesion, all schools are enjoined to consider the global dimension as part of the wider curriculum and this is just as relevant for pupils with SEN. Schools will be working with partner schools in Europe and the rest of the world. To support this work, there is a variety of schemes run under the auspices of the British Council (see Useful addresses). One of the most popular and one that has attracted many special schools is the International School Award. This encourages schools to audit what they are doing in relation to the global dimension and to plan for further action. As part of Citizenship Education, pupils need to have the sense that not only are they local citizens but European and world citizens. What goes on elsewhere does affect their lives. If wars are being fought, there is less money for disability services. Children like themselves in other countries may not have the same entitlements. This is all part of the greater disability agenda.

Some schools may have links through their local twinning associations but generally working with partner schools in Europe is funded by the Comenius Programme and schools can collaborate with a number of European partners on 2-year projects. This enables staff to visit schools in other countries and promotes pupils learning about young people from diverse backgrounds. For schools in the UK, finding a similar school in Europe can be an interesting experience.

It is very clear that the provision for pupils abroad with SEN varies greatly and many of those with severe or profound learning disabilities may not be under the education system. When making a comparative study, always check when countries state 'all children are included' or 'this is provided for all children'. Does this mean all children or those who are deemed worthy of this provision? This can be two very different things. Generally teachers in Europe are civil servants and may change schools more frequently than in the UK. Head teachers may only hold the post for a short number of years. Some teachers may have been sent to a special school but it is not their particular interest. For UK schools working with colleagues in Europe, this can sometimes be a problem as personnel changes make relationships hard to maintain.

eTwinning is a useful way for schools to make contact. Schools can log on and contact similar types of schools or institutions in Europe. This is useful for short projects when a visit would not be possible but pupils can make easy contact via the Internet. The teaching of modern foreign language in school is relevant here – part of the pupils' right – and experience would suggest that this is very popular. Pupils have fun acquiring a new skill and enjoy putting the simple phrases they learn to good use when abroad or entertaining visitors.

The British Council also promotes global partnerships. This enables projects with countries further afield. For instance, one school has a link with the only special school in The Gambia. The partnerships have enabled staff from both countries to meet and develop teaching strategies and resources. Other schools with significant ethnic representation have developed links with schools in Pakistan and The Caribbean.

There is much to be learnt and shared by such international cooperation. Pupils with learning disabilities enjoy visits to schools in other countries. They have also been supported at international conferences, speaking to and learning from others from around the world.

Conclusion

Special education has come a long way since the days of the Wild Boy of Aveyron. The right to an education for children and young people with special educational needs and disabilities has been enshrined in legislation, with education and equality a statutory duty on schools and local authorities. There is a duty for schools and local authorities to identify, assess and make provision for children's special educational needs. These are further reinforced by government initiatives such as *Every Child Matters* (DCSF 2004)

The challenge for the future is the changing nature of the pupils, becoming more complex and with additional health needs. At the same time, there will be the challenge of providing a workforce with the appropriate skills and knowledge to engage with these young people. There is a real need to focus on multi-agency working, with a holistic approach which supports the pupil with learning disabilities wherever they happen to be educated.

References

Audit Commission, 2007. Out of authority placements for special educational needs. Audit Commission, London.

Department for Children, Schools and Families, 2003. Every child matters. DCSF, London.

Department for Children, Schools and Families, 2004. Every child matters: the next steps. DCSF, London.

Department for Children, Schools and Families, 2007. Aiming high for disabled children. DCSF, London.

Department for Children, Schools and Families, 2008. The children's plan: one year on. DCSF, London.

Department for Children, Schools and Families, 2009. The national strategies progression guidance 2009–10: improving data to raise attainment and maximise the progress of learners with special educational needs, learning difficulties and disabilities. DCSF, London.

Department for Children, Schools and Families, 2010. Salt Review: independent review of teacher supply for pupils with severe, profound and multiple learning disabilities (SLD and PMLD). DCSF, London.

Department for Education and Skills, 2001. Special Educational Needs (SEN) Code of Practice. DfES, London. Available at: http://www.teachernet.gov.uk/_doc/3724/SENCodeofPractice.pdf.

Department of Health, 2001. Valuing people. DH, London.

Department of Health, 2009a. Healthy lives, brighter futures: the strategy for children and young people's health. DH, London.

Department of Health, 2009b. Valuing people now: a new three year strategy for people with learning disabilities: making it happen for everyone. DH, London.

Learning and Skills Council, 2005. Through inclusion to excellence: the report of the steering group for the LSC's planning and funding of provision for learners with learning difficulties and/or disabilities across the post-16 learning and skills sector. LSC, London.

Learning and Skills Council, 2006. Learning for living and work: improving education and training opportunities for people with learning difficulties and/or disabilities. LSC, London.

McGuire, B.E., Daly, P., Smyth, F., 2007. Lifestyle and health behaviours of adults with an intellectual disability. J. Intellect. Disabil. Res. 51, 497–510.

Office for Standards in Education, Children's Services and Skills, 2006. Inclusion: does it matter where pupils are taught?. OFSTED, London.

PricewaterhouseCoopers, 2007. Review of further education provision for learners (16–25 year olds) with learning difficulties and/or disabilities in the North West. PWC, London.

Segal, S., 1967. No child is ineducable, first ed. Pergamon Press, Oxford.

Steer Sir, A., 2009. Learning behaviour: lesson learned. DCSF, London.

United Nations, 1989. Convention on the Rights of the Child. United Nations, Geneva.

Warnock Report, 1978. Available at: http://sen.ttrb.ac.uk/attachments/21739b8e-5245-4709-b433-c14b08365634.pdf.

Further reading

Contact a Family, 2008. Special educational needs – England: information for families. Available at: http://www.cafamily.org.uk/pdfs/educatio.pdf.

Qualifications and Curriculum Development Agency, 2009. Foundation Learning Tier: 14–19 delivery guidance. QCDA, London.

Useful addresses

Advisory Centre for Education (ACE): http://www.ace-ed.org.uk

British Council: http://www.britishcouncil.org/new/

Entitlement and Quality Education for pupils with learning difficulties: http://www.equals.co.uk

Mencap: http://www.mencap.org.uk

National Association of Special Educational Needs (NASEN) is the leading organisation in the UK which aims to promote the education, training, advancement and development of all those with special and additional support needs: http://www.nasen.org.uk

National Children's Bureau: http://www.ncb.org.uk

Council for Disabled Children: http://www.ncb.org.uk/cdc

Sex Education Forum: http://www.ncb.org.uk/sef

Special Educational Consortium: http://www.ncb.org.uk/sec.aspx

TeacherNet – Education site for teachers, with Northern Ireland, Scotland and Wales links: http://www.teachernet.gov.uk

Tobii Technology is a world leader in eye tracking and eye control: http://www.tobii.com

Training and Development Agency for Schools: http://www.tda.gov.uk

Employment

26

Julie Ridley Susan Hunter

CHAPTER CONTENTS

KEY ISSUES

- A substantial body of research has shown that given the choice, many people with learning disabilities would prefer a real job to attending a day centre
- Having a real job or paid work is an aspiration that many people with learning disabilities in the UK have been able to realise in the past 30 years through the approach known as 'supported employment'
- 'Supported employment' is a specific approach that involves finding and supporting disabled people in real jobs in ordinary workplaces and providing as much support as needed for as long as necessary
- Support to people with learning disabilities during the day is still predominantly in segregated day centres or sheltered workshops and not all those who want a real job are being encouraged or supported to get one
- Unemployment rates among people with learning disabilities remain high despite policy drives to increase opportunities to participate in ordinary jobs
- Health and social care professionals working with people with learning disabilities need to understand key concepts surrounding employment, the barriers facing people with learning disabilities who want a real job and what support is available to achieve this goal

Introduction

Since the 1980s, having a 'real job' or being employed has become a reality for an increasing number of people with learning disabilities across the world. The right of disabled people generally to participate in the workforce is recognised internationally in policy (United Nations Convention on the Rights of Persons with Disabilities 2008, Article 27, Work and Employment) and practice. National policy statements about services for people with learning disabilities such as *The Same as You?* (Scottish Executive 2000) and *Valuing People* (Department of Health (DH) 2001) underline the need to increase the range of opportunities people with learning disabilities have to be socially integrated, including accessing real jobs in the community. These national policy statements have recognised that paid, integrated employment can be a positive part of people's lives. The 'supported employment' model introduced in the United States in the 1980s has successfully enabled thousands of people with learning disabilities worldwide to enter the labour market and, as a result, to contribute to their communities as valued employees and tax payers. A substantial body of research exists, much of it conducted in the USA, to show employment has the potential to improve quality of life for people with learning disabilities.

Despite this, statistics show that the majority of people with learning disabilities still attend segregated centres or special provision, and that only a minority of people have the opportunity to fulfil their aspiration to be in a real job (Forrester-Jones et al 2010). While there have been improvements in people's lives resulting from the shift in emphasis from institutional to community care (Emerson & Hatton 1995), similar efforts to promote inclusion in the workforce have not been as impressive. An independent national review of services for people with learning disabilities and complex needs concluded that employment opportunities were a distant goal for most people with very few in paid jobs (Commission for Social Care Inspection/Healthcare Commission/Mental Health Act Commission 2009). The historic service solution of bringing people together in protected environments, in places such as occupational centres, adult resource centres and sheltered workshops, has proved resilient. In these segregated places, people with learning disabilities have engaged in industrial contract work and work placements but such settings have provided little opportunity to move to ordinary jobs in the community. At the same time, some families and carers continue to express reservations about the reconfiguration of day services (DH 2009a), which can be a powerful barrier to seeking alternatives.

In Western society, paid work not only represents an important source of income to satisfy basic needs, but also provides other benefits such as status, occupation, purpose and the focus of social relationships, the loss of which can result in poor mental and physical health (Bambra 2010, Bambra & Eikemo 2009, Smith 1985). As such, paid work is a central component in adult identity and people often define themselves, and others, by their occupation. When introduced to a new person, how often is 'what is your job?' or 'what do you do?' asked? As McConkey (2007) stated in an earlier edition of this book, in many cultures, people are defined by their talents or occupation and many societies value people according to their contribution.

Practitioners in health and social care may find themselves at the interface between the wishes of people with learning disabilities, the anxieties of their families, changing policy expectations and the legacy of traditional services. Those supporting people with learning disabilities have a pivotal role to play in helping them achieve employment if that is a desired goal. Professionals may be involved in assessment, person-centred or lifestyle planning, helping people with learning disabilities to identify their needs, aspirations and support requirements. The promotion of employment as an option cannot be left solely to employment specialists. It is important that all those involved with people with learning disabilities understand the key concepts surrounding employment, the barriers facing individuals who want a real job and what support is available to achieve this goal.

This chapter adopts a position that perceives disability as a product of social organisation rather than of individual impairment or personal limitation. In the literature, this is known as the 'social model of disability' (Oliver 1990, 1996) (see also Ch. 1). In terms of the debate around employment, this recognises the importance of examining structural as well as individual barriers to employment, and of adopting a broader approach when identifying where the responsibility for change lies and the kinds of solutions that are effective. The chapter draws on international literature and research evidence to support the presented discussion.

Definition of employment

This chapter is about employment but what is meant by the term? In practice, 'employment' has been used as a rather loose concept that has been variously interpreted and is used synonymously with the term 'work' (Ridley et al 2005). However, while work could be defined as an activity involving the exercise of skills and judgement within set limits prescribed by others, Beyer et al (2004) defined employment as work you get paid for at least at the national minimum wage for working a certain number of hours and completing specified tasks. Employment support covers a wide range of diverse provision, not all of which is about supporting people in real paid jobs. Some of this is illustrated in the account of one individual's employment experience given in Case illustration 26.1.

Research mapping the employment support available to people with learning disabilities and/or

Case illustration 26.1

In the following account, Mary (not her real name), who participated in a study about life-changing jobs, refers to unpaid work placement as 'voluntary work' and distinguishes between this and a real paid job she secured through supported employment:

> *Before this job I helped with the lunches at the sheltered housing complex. I used to set the tables for the older people, get the plates ready, serve their lunches and clear all the tables. It was my job to get their food orders from the menus for the week. I worked 9 hours a week. It was only voluntary work. I was there for 3 years getting £20 a week because that's what you're allowed to earn when you're on benefits. I moved from there onto being in full-time employment and came off my benefits.*

autistic spectrum conditions identified the following types of employment support. Such a list can commonly be found in much of the literature:

- Open competitive employment in the mainstream.
- Work placements or work experience trials or on-the-job placements for a fixed period.
- Work preparation including help with curriculum vitae (CV) and interview.
- Voluntary work for a non-profit-making organisation on an unpaid basis.
- 'Training for Work', a government scheme.
- 'Permitted work' (previously 'therapeutic work').
- WORKSTEP, the government's supported employment programme.
- Unpaid jobs with private or commercial employers.
- Sheltered or non-open employment in segregated workplaces.
- 'Supported employment', real work for 16 hours or more in an integrated setting with ongoing support.
- Cooperatives and social firms that are viable businesses.

(Ridley et al 2005)

Policy context

As is now widely discussed, employment and people with learning disabilities is neither a new idea nor a newcomer to the policy context (Beyer & Robinson 2009, European Union of Supported Employment (EUSE) 2006, Hunter & Ridley 2007). Arguably, the Industrial Revolution and its impact on working patterns, demanding an organised, skilled and ultimately literate workforce, propelled the question onto the policy agenda, where it has remained ever since though with varying degrees of prominence. The prime focus of this chapter is on policies in the UK, which are similar across the four jurisdictions. However, it is worth noting that similar trends are discernible in Europe and in the USA where unique policies have been mandated with the result that developments are more embedded in many states.

In the heyday of institutional provision for people with learning disabilities unable to adjust to new labour conditions, the institutions themselves provided often heavy work associated with self-sufficiency in maintaining buildings, growing food and domestic chores – labour in the true sense (Ingham 2002). Community-based institutions such as day centres developed patterns of contract work; often repetitive, boring jobs that went unremunerated beyond 'pocket money'. Although contract working has survived in the shape of 'sheltered' workshops, more 'enlightened' welfare policies towards the end of the 20th century began to promote personal development and social inclusion within day services. This led to the emergence of work experience or placements, usually unpaid, and volunteering as a means of achieving these objectives. Stalker (2001) provides a detailed account of these historical trends.

As the broad rights, equalities and citizenship agenda has gathered momentum in society in general, so has the concept of an 'ordinary life' for people with learning disabilities. In other words, services should support individuals to have their own homes in the community (see Ch. 27) and indeed to pursue what have been called 'real jobs for real pay' (Wertheimer & Real Jobs Initiative 1992). Whether in housing, leisure or employment, this has led to the concept of the 'support' model as opposed to the more traditional 'readiness' model of service delivery where people pass through a range of preparatory stages before graduating into the 'real world'. One criticism of the readiness model in employment is that individuals rarely move onto paid employment but get stuck as a perpetual trainee (Beyer et al 2004). Supported employment, originally developed to support people with profound disabilities in employment (Gold 1980), is the most significant methodology that has emerged as a way of 'placing, training and maintaining' people in jobs tailored to their strengths and interests while providing on-site support through job coaches in a manner that promotes integration into the workforce.

In terms of learning disabilities policy in the UK, supporting individuals to get jobs is high on the agenda. Typical of these policies, and a particularly well-developed one, is the recent *Valuing Employment Now* (DH 2009b). This sets out a government strategy in England that emphasises paid jobs (16 hours a week plus) for all, irrespective of disability; tackling the barriers to employment; and increasing the provision of specialist supported employment personnel and organisations. More recently, through self-directed support (Carr & Dittrich, 2008) and In Control (Poll et al 2006) initiatives, the policy focus has been on expanding the use of individual budgets to employ personal assistants to support choice and flexibility in employment as well as other aspects of daily living.

A good illustration of how effective supported employment can be even in circumstances of economic restraint is to be found in the development of the North Lanarkshire Employment Service (McInally 2008). North Lanarkshire Council has developed a corporate strategy for supported employment that tackles these barriers by maximising benefits, only supporting jobs of 16 hours plus a week to attract tax credits and increase opportunities for social integration, and offering school leavers employment options as a matter of routine (Joseph Rowntree Foundation 2002). Not all service users will opt for employment, but over time the expectation is one of culture change among service users, their families and staff. Of course, this is not cost free and the council has invested £783 000 a year to meet bridging costs. However, the initiative has not only doubled individuals' disposable income on average but the provision of each job costs half that of a day placement (DH 2009b).

Although the North Lanarkshire Employment Service is an expression of a corporate strategy within the local authority, the main policy driver has come from social work. Historically, it is typical to find the locus of employment policy within welfare though many specialist employment agencies operate in the voluntary sector for a range of reasons, including the possibility of a light-touch bureaucracy and the freedom to innovate quickly and operate a business model including recruitment of staff from business backgrounds whose rapport with employers is more immediate. However, the potential impact of the adoption of a corporate strategy and leadership by public bodies is evident in the example from North Lanarkshire and offers a powerful model to other authorities.

In a parallel set of policy developments called 'welfare to work', the Department for Work and Pensions (DWP)/Workforce Plus, has been developing the concept of 'employability' that focuses on how to enable people who have been long-term unemployed or 'furthest' from the labour market to get back into work with its associated positive impact on health (Black 2008) as well as income. These broader policies, such as the Green Paper *New Deal for Welfare* 2006, the Freud Report 2007, and Workforce Plus 2006, are concerned with reducing unemployment. The Freud Report cites the 'New Deal for Disabled People' as having increased employment for disabled people by 9%.

'Employability' is operationalised through a series of individualised and intensive support arrangements, job brokers and vocational profiling – techniques that are considered best practice in supported employment. Further, throughout the New Deal and associated initiatives, there are echoes of the personalisation agenda promoted by the independent think tank DEMOS (Leadbeater 2004) and being pursued by government in all sectors including health and welfare. The personalisation of service development and provision based on individual funding, choice and participation in decision making (DH 2008) is central to supported employment in relation to vocational profiling, job matching, on-the-job support and career development.

While it would be naïve not to acknowledge that the underlying drivers for change in employability and supported employment, those of reducing welfare dependency on the one hand and promoting social inclusion and social justice on the other, are in potential conflict, the possibility of 'synergy' between them in the interests of disabled people also exists (Ridley & Hunter 2007). This presents not only an important opportunity for the disability lobby to raise the profile of employment within generic national policies, but to lend expertise in the efforts to support those groups who are furthest from the labour market.

Returning briefly to how UK policies sit alongside those of comparator countries, Beyer & Robinson (2009) summarise some information from both the USA and Europe though it is far from comprehensive. Commenting on the limited information available but referring to the study by the Open Institute in 2005, they conclude that despite the trend away from segregated to community-based provision across Europe, the balance of investment is in favour of specialist workshop provision and with limited development of supported employment. The EUSE

(2006) draws attention to a range of factors within various countries that impact differentially on the extent to which supported employment has developed. These include lack of a rights-based approach to disability issues; the absence of a national policy framework for supported employment within an individual country; the lack of dedicated funds to support the implementation of the policy framework; complicated and rigid welfare benefit systems which act as disincentives for people considering full status employment; and the lack of leadership or national strategy regarding mainstreaming supported employment.

In the USA, supported employment has been established for longer and the definition of supported employment is defined in law, with the result that many states have developed comprehensive policies including financial incentives supporting increased numbers of disabled people in employment, up to 50% in some states (Beyer & Robinson 2009). One lesson for the UK seems to be that significant progress, once the model is established, is reliant on embedding of strategic coherent policies for supported employment within wider welfare, employment and funding initiatives.

Key concepts

In discussing employment, it is important to understand the radical shift that occurred during the 1970s and 1980s from a position focusing on getting people 'ready' for real jobs to considering what 'support' someone needs to achieve their individual goals. The 'support model' (Bradley et al 1994) evolved from progressive movements in the field of disability over the past 40 years and has been highly influential in shaping the goals of human services including how employment support is conceptualised. Traditionally, moving into one's own home and/or getting a job was seen as a progression through various stages and the acquisition of skills until the individual reached the point where services or those in authority felt they are *ready* to take on a specific activity or responsibility. In contrast, the support model puts people directly into their own home or job and provides *support* to them where they are; this may be temporary or longer term. In relation to work, it translates into a "presumption of employability for everyone" (Hagner & DiLeo 1993:7).

This change has in no small part been shaped by the concept of community participation and inclusion as expressed by O'Brien's five accomplishments (O'Brien & Tyne 1981) and the principle of normalisation (Wolfensberger 1972). Early ideas around 'normalisation' emerged in Scandinavia where writers such as Nirje (1980) argued that people with learning disabilities were entitled to the same patterns of life as those enjoyed in mainstream society with options for work, leisure and accommodation. Its most extensive articulation can be found in the writings of Wolf Wolfensberger (1972, 1983) who expanded the framework to consider how the historical devaluation of people with learning disabilities in Western society and associated stigma could be counteracted by the creation of positive images and socially valued roles. The 'ordinary life' initiative in the UK (King's Fund Centre 1980, 1984) and most subsequent policy developments, broadly known as deinstitutionalisation and inclusion, can arguably be seen to be direct descendants of normalisation.

While these ideas or concepts have been instrumental in the transformation of service delivery from large, isolated institutions with their eugenic associations (see Ch. 3) into community-based or focused resources that aspire to promote an inclusive and participatory society, they have not been without their critics in terms of social 'conservatism' in the lifestyles being promoted (Brown & Smith 1992, Johnson et al 2010). In theory, as social norms change so do concepts of what is a 'valued lifestyle', but the achievement of what Wolfensberger called 'social integration' has been a more elusive goal. Indeed, research has pointed to less than perfect social integration outcomes in jobs that are few hours and of poor quality (Jahoda et al 2007, Ridley 2001). Other research has shown there is little evidence of the holistic and strategic approach that is needed to

Reader activity 26.1

Check whether your employer and your professional association have explicit policy documents or guidance promoting supported employment. If not, why not?

Reader activity 26.2

Find out about the kinds of work opportunities and settings that were open to people with learning disabilities before the 1980s. Were these options a product of a readiness or support model? Why? What does this say about societal views of learning disability? How has this changed over the past century?

tackle the social exclusion of people with learning disabilities so that they can take advantage of, and benefit from, opportunities such as jobs in ordinary workplaces (Gosling & Cotterill 2000).

The spread of the above ideas has generated many challenges for practitioners and services in the 1990s onwards, demanding new approaches that emphasise individual choice and self-determination, support and guidance, facilitation rather than direction (Bradley et al 1994). The degree of choice exercised by an individual in their daily life is affected by the opportunities and the support available. Despite its lesser impact in the field of learning disabilities, the social model of disability focuses attention on the responsibility of society to ensure that disabled people are not excluded from the workforce for structural reasons. A new type of partnership is needed between people with disabilities, their families and professionals, where professionals more readily accept direction from consumers. This, and the implied shift in the power balance, is captured in the contemporary term, 'co-production' (Hunter & Ritchie 2007). Quality is then defined as conformity with customer requirements, and focusing on outcomes that contribute to improving the individual's quality of life, empowerment and choice.

Meaning of employment

Sociologists and philosophers have identified the basic need to work as being strongly rooted in natural human motivations for survival, desires for pleasure, security and comfort (Baumeister 1991). A recent review of the health of Britain's working age population (Black 2008) stated that for most people, their work is not only a key determinant of material progress but also of self-worth, family esteem, identity and standing within the community, and a means of social participation and fulfilment. The review further asserted that recent evidence suggests that work can be good for health, reversing the harmful effects of long-term unemployment and prolonged sickness absence.

Reader activity 26.3

How might the fundamental ideas behind a co-production approach affect the way that you work with people with learning disabilities? How might services adopting such an approach look and work and how is this different from traditional services?

Some make direct links between employment and happiness (Bauman, 2008), and with quality of life. Indeed, the concept of 'quality of life' frequently appears alongside discussions about work for a variety of reasons, depending on what meanings are attached to work. Kiuranor (1980) argued that work itself can be used as a single indicator of quality of life. Others have discussed the relationship between what people do at work and their overall enjoyment of life (Hedley et al 1980). Positive conceptual links have been made between work and self-worth (Jahoda et al 2007, Ridley 2000). From the 1980s onwards, advocates of an 'ordinary life' (King's Fund Centre 1984) have promoted real jobs as offering a number of positive benefits to people with learning disabilities, summarised as:

- meaningful and valued options in life
- an income/wage
- a purpose or structure to daily life
- social links with the community
- meaningful choices and opportunities
- a sense of personal future.

(Ridley & Hunter 2007)

Research in English day centres (Beyer et al 2004) found that people with learning disabilities who were in paid work identified money, social interaction, making a contribution to society and having something to do as the main benefits. Another UK study found people were more satisfied in supported employment than in their previous day service and reported making new friends at work (Bass 2000).

Case illustration 26.2

Edith works as an events organiser in a nursing home. She plays dominoes and bingo with the residents and makes them cups of tea. Sometimes she goes out with residents. She works four afternoons a week for a total of 16 hours per week. She's been in her job for 8 months. This is her first paid job. She is in her 40s and lives with some other people in accommodation with support. Edith really likes her job because she gets to meet new people and because she gets paid. If she didn't have her job, she would really miss meeting people: the residents, the staff and the visitors: "Without this, I'd be left out – no family, no friends." Edith's pay helps her to manage her bills better (e.g. her telephone bill). She can also go on holiday, which she's never been able to do before: she's going to Spain. She's also doing more line dancing and buying more clothes. She said that the best thing about the job is "I'm happy. Happiness."

(Extract from Ridley et al 2005:69)

Some researchers have been able to show positive effects on undesirable or challenging behaviours (McLoughlin et al 1987) and there is a consistent finding that those in supported employment and their families report higher levels of 'quality of life' and wellbeing (Eggleton et al 1999, Jahoda et al 2007). Some studies have shown workers in supported employment with quality of life levels similar to those of workers without disabilities (Sinnott-Oswald et al 1991). Our understanding of this relationship between supported employment and quality of life is that it is more complex. Research in some European countries, for example, supports linking supported employment and quality of life, but has also shown that there is a greater impact on people's quality of life when aspects of jobs are typical for that workplace, and when there is sufficient support (Verdugo et al 2006).

Alongside such positive claims is a parallel argument that questions the promotion of employment opportunities and an 'ordinary life', favouring instead the concept of quality of life (Redley 2009). This line of argument suggests that the danger of adopting employment as the main source of identity and self-esteem is that it reinforces social exclusion and lack of self-worth associated with unemployment (Johnson et al 2010, Mayo 1996). Nevertheless, while ideas about the place of employment in our lives may seem to be in a state of flux, for the majority of people paid work remains an important determinant of the quality of life and economic status.

People with learning disabilities want real jobs

Radical changes in services have been influenced by the principle of normalisation, especially the work of Wolfensberger and O'Brien, as well as broader civil rights movements, but they have also been influenced by vociferous groups of self-advocates in the US and later in parts of the UK who demanded the right to participate in the ordinary life of their communities (Williams & Shoultz 1982). The consistent message across a number of studies exploring the aspirations of people with learning disabilities is that many people want paid work, to have friends, to live in an ordinary house, to marry or have a partner and, in some cases, to have children (DH 2009b, Stalker 2001). This is, however, sometimes at odds with the views and aspirations of some families and carers (DH 2009a).

> **Reader activity 26.4**
>
> What is the role of employment in your own life and that of your family and friends? Is this any different for adults with learning disabilities? Why? Identify the assumptions behind your answer.

The relevance of the drive towards integrated employment since the 1980s has been evidenced by a substantial body of research and consumer consultation showing that given the choice, people with learning disabilities prefer paid jobs to attendance at day centres (Brandon 1987, King's Fund Centre 1984, Racino & Whittico 1998, Steele 1992). Over 80% of respondents in a large-scale survey of people attending a day centre during 1989–1990 stated that having a paid job was either their first or second most important desire in life (Steele 1991).

More recently, people with learning disabilities attending day centres in England who were interviewed were enthusiastic about work and its benefits and those in part-time work wanted to work more hours as most were only working 5 hours a week (Beyer et al 2004). In this research, just under half of those who had been in work in the past or had never worked wanted a paid job. Similarly, around a third (35%) of people with learning disabilities interviewed in a Scottish study (Curtice 2006) wanted to find a job. Self-advocates now demand not just integrated jobs, but 'good jobs' with good pay and benefits, enjoyable work that enables a contribution, and 'quality' education, career planning and the possibility of advancement (Racino & Whittico 1998).

Potential barriers to employment

People with learning disabilities report they encounter barriers to finding employment (Allen 2006). Some barriers to employment are encountered specifically by individuals with disabilities, while others are experienced by people in general. Reviewing the literature, Ridley (2000) summarised these barriers under three levels: basic or individual; structural; and perceptual or attitudinal barriers.

Basic or individual

At a basic or individual level, adults with learning disabilities may lack skills or qualifications that can be easily matched with the current job market, and have limited experience of workplace culture and the demands of work. They may have difficulties interacting socially with other people and may sometimes challenge others by their behaviour. In many respects, they share many of the problems faced by other long-term unemployed people, particularly young adults who have no experience of the job market.

People with learning disabilities in general receive little encouragement to think of employment as a viable option; there may have been little or no preparation for employment at school; and their experiences will typically be of segregated services received along with other people labelled as 'learning disabled', and of institutionalisation. One woman with learning disabilities who had a job commented:

> I sometimes think of all the people left at the day centres and feel sad for them. Even if people can't read or write they should be encouraged all the time to get jobs. The problem is that people get used to going to the ATC, don't believe in themselves anymore and lose their confidence. Eventually they don't bother trying and give up.
>
> (Demby 1992:6)

Given the lack of opportunity, many people with learning disabilities have little or no experience of the responsibilities and implications of going out to work, such as arriving on time, operating shift systems and so on. In addition to skills and qualifications, many employers expect prospective employees to have prior work experience. They are thus doubly disadvantaged through lack of opportunity to try out their work skills. One strategy for addressing this has been to offer people work experience placements but this has not been without its problems including the length of time some people spend in unpaid work placements without moving onto real jobs (Ridley et al 2005).

It is often assumed that those with more severe disabilities and whose behaviour has been labelled as 'challenging' to others are incapable of employment, but practice has shown this need not be the case. 'Challenging behaviour' might include physical or verbal abuse, involuntary shouting and so on (see also Ch. 18). Campaigners such as Feinmann (1988) have made powerful arguments from experience that employment should not be seen as an unrealistic goal for such individuals.

Reader activity 26.5

When is your earliest memory of having a job? What kind of job? How young were you when you were asked the question by an adult "what do you want to be when you grow up?"

Structural

Taking on paid employment can impact on an individual's welfare benefits (Bewley 1997). Aspects of the UK social security system and other related systems have been identified as causing major problems for individuals as well as for the development of supported employment (O'Bryan et al 2000, Simons 1998). As a result, many people have been advised either to work within the benefits disregard limits, or to aim for the higher amount of 'permitted earnings', or to take unpaid work. Since 1997, however, there have been considerable developments in the benefits system and tax credits, which aim to alter this situation. Evidence supports the view that skilled and knowledgeable professionals who stay well informed of benefit regulations and changes and introduce the income potential of employment from the start can effectively work with such barriers (Hunter & Ridley 2007, McInally 2008, O'Bryan 2002). Financial calculations to find out whether the individual will be worse off in work are therefore a prime consideration for the majority of disabled people contemplating paid employment. Many employment projects consider this a fundamental issue and always include a full welfare benefits check.

A significant factor in considering employment has been found to be housing costs (Simons 1998). Generally, earnings from employment determine the kind of housing an individual can access, while for people with learning disabilities it is the converse: where they live determines whether and how many hours they can work. It is relatively easier for someone with learning disabilities living at home with

Case illustration 26.3

Margaret is 19 years old, has learning disabilities and suffers with depression. She attended mainstream education and on leaving school attended a local college for 2 years. When she was referred to North Lanarkshire Council Supported Employment Service, her sole income consisted of £15 child benefit. An immediate priority for the service was to maximise Margaret's income. With the assistance of the service she was awarded income support and disability living allowance (DLA), increasing her benefit from £15 to £96.85 per week. Margaret started working in a local nursing home in March 2004 (see Table 26.1)

Table 26.1 for Case illustration 26.3

Income prior to employment		Income maximised prior to employment		Income in employment	
Income support	£	Income support	**£66.55**	Earnings	**£161.12**
IB/SDA	£	IB/SDA	£	Tax credits	**£62.71**
DLA (care)	£	DLA (care)	**£15.15**	DLA (care)	**£15.15**
DLA (mobility)	£	DLA (mobility)	**£15.15**	DLA (mobility)	**£15.15**
Other	**£15.00**	Other	£	Other	£
TOTAL	£	TOTAL	£	TOTAL	**£254.13**
Less housing costs	£	Less housing costs	£	Less housing costs	£
TOTAL	£15.00	**TOTAL**	£96.85	**TOTAL**	£254.13
		DIFFERENCE IN INCOME	**£81.85**	**DIFFERENCE IN INCOME**	£157.28

(Extract from Ridley et al 2005:106)

family to take up work, providing they do not want to move to a more independent living situation. The issue is the extent to which means-tested benefits will cover housing costs. It is more challenging for those living in supported living situations or residential care to take up employment. Emerson & Hatton (1998) found that just 5% of people living in residential establishments were in employment.

Other structural issues include the inflexibility of a shrinking employment market, particularly in times of recession. Changing patterns of employment mean that for a significant proportion of the population, full-time work for instance is no longer the norm; job sharing and temporary work have become more commonplace. Teleworking or home-based working are also now more acceptable, and in an increasingly high-tech world there is an expectation that workers will be multi-skilled and will demonstrate a portfolio of skills and experience (Handy 1984). One response to the vagaries of the changing competitive job market has been the development of worker cooperatives and social enterprises, challenging traditional notions of work (Sikking 1986). More recently, there has been increased interest in the notion of self-employment for people with learning disabilities (see websites of Foundation for Learning Disabilities or Virginia Commonwealth University Rehabilitation Research and Training Center on Workplace Supports and Job Retention).

Rates of unemployment can also be seen to impact upon available job opportunities. Some practitioners claim that high rates of unemployment are a major barrier to finding jobs for people with learning disabilities as there is increased competition for fewer positions. However, there is evidence from supported employment research showing that even in areas of traditionally high rates of unemployment, jobs have been secured as long as people get the right support (McInally 2008, Pozner & Hammond 1993).

Perceptual/attitudinal

For most of us, employment is an expected aspiration fostered from an early age, but this is not so for people with learning disabilities. Families are disempowered by professionals discouraging them from holding the idea that one day their son or daughter will be in a job, perceiving this generally as 'unrealistic'. Accepting what professionals offer, parents have continued to demand a service system that perpetuates low expectations of people with learning disabilities (DH 2009a). The King's Fund Centre (1984) concluded that low expectations were possibly the biggest challenge to progress in vocational services. However, although easy to generalise about the overprotectiveness of parents, and the sometimes conflicting interests between people with learning disabilities and their carers, it should be remembered that it was parents, and not professionals, who pioneered the Mencap Pathway Scheme in England and Wales. Parents were also instrumental in many of the changes occurring in the USA and Canada in the 1980s, resulting in a more advanced system of vocational services than in Britain, and more recently in the growth of the service brokerage movement.

Realising the goal of employment for people with learning disabilities depends heavily on an attitudinal shift among employers, as well the general public. It is often assumed that employers can be less than positive. Yet research undertaken in the USA which looked at the subjective judgments of 188 government policy makers, counsellors, supervisors, co-workers and others, of employment training for people with very severe disabilities, found positive reactions, even to the employment of those more severely disabled (Black & Meyer 1992). In light of such findings, Wertheimer & Real Jobs Initiative (1992) concluded that it was time to readjust such negative perceptions.

Research is inconclusive about what determines how sympathetic an employer will be toward employing people with learning disabilities (Unger 2002). What the research does find is that the most positive employers are those who have previously employed people with learning disabilities and/or have experience of support from specialist employment agencies. These employers often emphasise the reliability of employees with learning disabilities, as well as the significance to them in helping them fulfil their duty to implement equal opportunities, and give individuals a valuable role in life (Hanna & McConkey 1992). Luecking et al (2004) asserted that employers with past experience develop more positive views even when these workers have severe disabilities. To an extent, employers have been found to be willing to sacrifice work performance or work quality in exchange for dependable employees (Unger 2002). Research by the Post Office, Bank of England and DuPont (Leslie 1992) showed disabled people took fewer days sick leave, remained with employers longer, were equally productive and had better than average safety records. Similarly, research by Petty & Fussell (1997) found employers viewed people with learning disabilities as reliable, hard-working and effective employees.

A recent survey of people with learning disabilities in Scotland by the Scottish Consortium for Learning Disabilities (Curtice 2006) cited health, disability, not being able to find suitable employment and the benefits trap as common barriers to work. This research found that in order to overcome these barriers, more information and support for employment for people with learning disabilities was needed, and employers needed to be made aware of what people with learning disabilities can offer as employees. Others have provided evidence of the success of pro-active and skilled approaches to addressing structural barriers such as the benefits trap so that this need no longer be the major barrier to employment for people with learning disabilities (Hunter & Ridley 2007, McInally 2008). Given the now vast body of research demonstrating the potential of people with learning disabilities for paid work, the main barriers would appear to reside in the lack of opportunity, low expectations and poor support.

'Supported employment' approach

The model now known as 'supported employment' emerged in the mid-1980s and has become a well-established approach demonstrating success in finding real jobs for a range of disabled people and maintaining them in these jobs (Schneider et al 2002). Founded on the support model, supported employment developed in the US out of dissatisfaction with the outcomes of sheltered workshops (Mank 1994), and from the undeniable reports about the learning capacity of people with severe disabilities to learn skills once considered far too difficult or complex (Gold 1973, 1980). Development of the concept, principles and practices of supported employment owes much to the groundbreaking research of Marc Gold. Through his work, Gold demonstrated, often in a practical way to large audiences, that people with severe learning disabilities can acquire a level of performance comparable with non-disabled workers (McLoughlin et al 1987).

In the UK, the growth of agencies offering supported employment since the 1980s has been associated with the failure of traditional adult training centres and adult resource centres to deliver integrated employment outcomes and a drive to shift from segregated, group-based services to community-based, individualised solutions. One survey (Beyer et al 1996) evidenced the expansion from just five agencies offering supported employment in the UK in 1986, increasing to over 200 by 1995, and an estimated 5000 people nationally, predominantly people with learning disabilities, employed with local employers. This growth was most significant in England and Wales and somewhat slower in Scotland and other parts of Europe (Sutton 1999).

Supported employment, in contrast to what we understand as generic employment support, is a highly structured approach to placing people in jobs, providing individual training on the job and systems for maintaining people in jobs, which, importantly, focuses on 'place-and-train' rather than on getting ready for work or 'train-and-place' (Leach 2002, McLoughlin et al 1987). A key aspect of supported employment is that it is about supporting people in real jobs in integrated settings in the community (Noonan-Walsh et al 1991).

In the USA, supported employment is defined in legislation and supported by a system of federal and state funding. Under the US Rehabilitation Amendments Act 1968, providers are required to target individuals with severe disabilities who require ongoing support in order to perform their work and jobs must be for a minimum of 20 hours per week. No such stipulation exists in the UK and European versions of supported employment. A research study in Scotland adopted the definition that supported employment is real work that is for 16 hours or more in an integrated setting with ongoing support (Ridley et al 2005). However, a key finding of the study was that much that was being offered under the name of supported employment was inconsistent, with only a fifth of supported jobs meeting the criteria (Ridley & Hunter 2006).

Despite a lack of consensus of definition in the UK and Europe, there is agreement internationally across research and policy commentators that supported employment consists of the following three main elements:

1. **Real work**, that is, work that would be done by a typical member of the workforce and is normally paid work.
2. **Work in integrated settings**, that is, where the proportion of disabled workers is roughly equivalent to the proportion of disabled people in the general population.
3. **Flexible, individual support**, which in theory is not time limited.

The Policy Consortium for Supported Employment (O'Bryan et al 2000) defined it as a way of enabling people who need support to obtain and develop their careers in real jobs, with support provided on an individual basis to both employer and employee for as long as necessary. The definition accepted and agreed by the EUSE is "providing support to people with disabilities or other disadvantaged groups to secure and maintain paid employment in the open labour market" (EUSE website). Some authors further distinguish between supported employment and the Department of Employment's 'WORKSTEP Programme' (Stalker 2001), although some suggest the distinction is far from clear cut (Leach 2002). Using the term to describe central government schemes has been found to be contentious as some feel that subsidised employment is entirely different from the original model of supported employment (Weston 2002).

Initially the model embraced four alternatives thought necessary to adapt to local employment situations and individual service requirements. Three were group-based models and it is the 'individual placement model' or 'job coach model' (Tannen 1993) that is generally what is understood as supported employment in the UK and Europe. The process of supported employment can be divided into five sets of core activities as summarised in Box 26.1.

At the heart of this 'place-and-train' approach is the assumption that employment outcomes are maximised when the training of individuals is implemented on site rather than through pre-vocational methods. A key element is the provision of flexible support to an individual, which it is assumed will vary between individuals and may be required at different stages in the process. However, it will typically involve training on the job, usually involving Training in Systematic Instruction (TSI) methods (Leach 2002), presence at the workplace for a period after which support may be faded, and regular monitoring visits and/or telephone calls to the individual and/or the employer. The model presumes that there are some individuals who will require support indefinitely and for whom reduction of support would not be appropriate. The important role of support is illustrated by one woman with learning disabilities

Box 26.1

Five core activities of supported employment

1. **Vocational/Career Planning**. 'Vocational profile' created, including description of ideal job characteristics.

↓

2. **Job finding and matching**. Employers canvassed until job found to suit the individual.

↓

3. **Job analysis**. Job tasks and work culture analysed, a match with worker confirmed and placement agreed.

↓

4. **Place and train**. Individual trained on the job, and support faded until person stable and performing to employer expectation.

↓

5. **Support.** Continued monitoring, problem solving and career development.

Case illustration 26.4

Unpublished project paper

The supported employment team helped me get the job. I wouldn't have moved onto the job without them. It would be kind of difficult to do on your own because not everyone is as nice to you. You can phone anytime you want and once a year she comes up and sees how I'm doing in work. Before I got this job Sam came into the interview with me and showed me some wee techniques, ways of answering questions and how you ask questions at interviews. If you've never had interviews it can be very hard so it prepared me and I got the job. I felt better with Sam being there. The supported employment team helped me find the job and fill in the forms. Now I've got a supervisor at work to support me. The women that you work with as well who've been there longer they help me as well. They're all nice there, it makes a difference.

who gives her account of getting a real job when interviewed for a project about life changing jobs in Case illustration 26.4.

Realities of practice

Employment support covers a vast canvas of activity, not all of which would be considered to be supported employment (Ridley & Hunter 2006). Many of the agencies providing employment support to people with learning disabilities are involved in pre-vocational or work preparation activities. A key finding is that many agencies will say they are supported employment agencies if they are providing job coaching even if the jobs they support are not in ordinary workplaces. There are few dedicated supported employment services, which is significant because research shows better financial outcomes for supported employees in services that have dedicated job finders and staff with qualifications (Beyer 2001).

Many studies conclude that despite the positive outcomes experienced from supported employment, its implementation, not only in the UK but in other European countries such as Spain, as well as the US, has been somewhat disappointing (Beyer & Robinson 2009, Hunter & Ridley 2007, Pallisera et al 2003). A survey of employment options for people with learning disabilities, with responses from 60 countries, showed that despite good practice examples on inclusive employment, the overall picture "remains one of great concern" (Sutton 1999). Participation in inclusive or integrated employment was found to be "very much in the minority". Many countries in the EU invest more resources in segregated or specialist provision than in community employment; supported employment appears to have become part of a continuum of responses rather than an alternative to segregated services. The Policy Consortium on Supported Employment (O'Bryan et al 2000:v) highlighted what it saw as an urgent need to ensure supported employment becomes "much more widely available, with services of consistent quality".

Reader activity 26.6

Find out about the employment support services in your area. How many of these offer supported employment? Would what they offer fit with the definition of supported employment from the literature?

Recent research in Scotland found that many people with learning disabilities who were supported in work were in unpaid or voluntary work, and that of those in paid jobs, half were in jobs for under 10 hours per week, some for as little as 1 or 2 hours a week (Ridley et al 2005). A surprising minority of 14% were reported to have been in unpaid or voluntary work for more than 4 years, which challenges the argument about such placements as ultimately improving people's employment outcomes. A subsequent Scottish survey (Curtice 2006) found only one in three people with learning disabilities to be working and the vast majority were working for less than 16 hours. Similarly, a UK-wide survey of supported employment agencies in the mid-1990s (Beyer & Kilsby 1997) found that almost half of people using supported employment services were working less than 16 hours per week with 42% having total earnings of £15 or less. Working part time for short hours has not significantly increased the incomes of people entering employment from their previous situation (Beyer & Robinson 2009).

Reader activity 26.7

Make a list of what you consider to be quality aspects of a job. What is important? Where does pay and type of job feature in this? Compare your list with the research findings on supported jobs for people with learning disabilities. Discuss.

While supported employment was originally inspired by the needs of people with more severe disabilities, research has consistently found basic inequalities in terms of who has accessed support. Only 7% of supported employees in the Scottish survey were people with severe learning disabilities (Ridley et al 2005). Less well served by existing services were people with autistic spectrum conditions, women with learning disabilities and those from black and minority ethnic communities. A review of supported employment outcomes and practice also noted that outcomes were harder to obtain for people with severe disabilities and there appeared to be gender differences with more men in supported employment than women (Mank et al 1998).

The type and quality of jobs found has tended to vary enormously between supported employment agencies, and this affects the quality of individual outcomes. One of the key issues to emerge from research has been the similarity of treatment of disabled people and non-disabled people in terms of recruitment, compensation and training and this has affected potential for integrating supported employees (Mank et al 1998). Recognising the centrality of these issues can be seen in UK law which has made it illegal for employers to discriminate against disabled people and has introduced the requirement for employers to make 'reasonable adjustments' in the workplace (Disability Discrimination Act (DDA) 1995, 2005, DDA Regulations, 2003).

Although there is increasing interest in supported self-employment opportunities (Callahan et al 2002, Griffin & Hammis 2003), and there are examples of this being used as an option for people with

Box 26.2

Principles for supporting people with learning disabilities in employment

Real jobs/valued roles

There should be a clear focus from the outset on securing the outcome of real paid jobs, providing valued roles for people with learning disabilities in their communities. As an employee, individuals should be paid the going rate for the job and have the same workplace terms and conditions as other employees.

A presumption of employability

Everyone who wants to work should be assumed to be employable with the right support. Employment should be actively considered an option for people with learning disabilities and/or autistic spectrum conditions (ASC).

Learn about work on the job

Individuals with learning disabilities and/or ASC should be trained on the job rather than preparing for future employment.

Flexible support

People with learning disabilities and/or ASC should receive flexible, individualised support that is not time limited and is tailored to meet their individual needs. Follow-on support, and support to develop, progress in or move onto other jobs should be a feature.

Promote early participation in employment

Access to employment support should be at the earliest stage possible, e.g. at school leaving age. If employment is on the curriculum for disabled pupils, progression to employment will increasingly become more of a natural assumption for everyone.

Equality of access

Support to access employment should be available for everyone interested in working regardless of label, support need or perceived level of functioning, including those with more severe learning disabilities and/or ASC.

Personalisation

People with learning disabilities and/or ASC should be treated as individuals and support should be customised for each person. The emphasis should be on finding out what each person wants to do and where his/her skills and aspirations lie and using these in the job finding and development process.

Participation and involvement

Individuals with learning disabilities and/or ASC should be fully involved in all aspects of the process, and have the information and support necessary to enable them to participate.

Self-determination and choice

People with learning disabilities and/or ASC should be asked about the support they need, be encouraged to express individual choice and be involved in deciding what they want. They should be helped to understand their opportunities fully so they can make informed choices.

Social inclusion

People with learning disabilities and/or ASC should be offered real jobs with ordinary or mainstream employers and have the opportunity to work alongside non-disabled co-workers.

learning disabilities, so far in the UK this has only been pursued on a limited scale. Self-employment is seen to provide flexibility and a better adjustment between disability status and working life, and recent European studies have found that people with disabilities generally were more likely to be self-employed than those without disabilities (Pagan 2009). A number of organisations (Foundation for Learning Disabilities and Valuing People/Employment Now) provide useful guides to help people move into self-employment.

See Reader activity 26.8 on the Evolve website.

Key principles for best practice

Clear principles emerge from the increasing body of international research into supported employment and the provider statements about quality standards (EUSE 2006, Scottish Union of Supported Employment 2006) that offer a defining framework for considering how best to support people with learning disabilities to access and sustain real paid jobs (Ridley & Hunter 2007). These principles are derived from research which has sought the opinions of people with learning disabilities and others about best practice and quality in supported employment. They are summarised in Box 26.2.

Conclusion

This chapter has focused on the issue of employment for people with learning disabilities. Some may dismiss the idea of employment as unrealistic, in particular for those considered to have severe disabilities. However, it should be remembered that the 'supported employment' approach was originally developed to help people with more severe disabilities who would not otherwise be able to access the labour market. The fact that they have been failed by supported employment should not be taken as evidence that employment is unsuitable for them, but as an aspect of the limited implementation of this model.

There is great unmet potential in the population of people labelled as having learning disabilities. Many people with learning disabilities who want real jobs are not being supported or encouraged by those working most closely with them and/or their families to realise their vocational aspirations. They are increasingly voicing their desire for real jobs, but not just any job. The shift from supporting jobs to supporting career development in recent years reflects changing expectations (Wehman & Kregel 1998). An emphasis on long-term strategies is favoured on the basis that it better reflects the norm for others in society: for example, the Mental Health Foundation (1996) argued that supported employment jobs should not be assumed to 'be for life' on the supposition that the majority of people take a long time to find the most appropriate job for them.

Presuming that everyone who wants to work is employable with the right support is a radical shift in thinking. Until it becomes the default position to offer people with learning disabilities, regardless of the severity of their disabilities or support needs, the support they need to attain real jobs, they will continue to be in segregated services and on the periphery of their communities. The presumption of employment is the most important underpinning principle of best practice identified by research, and is in line with Government policy.

Dedication

This chapter is dedicated to the memory of George McInally who died suddenly in June 2010. George was the driving force behind the development of the North Lanarkshire Supported Employment Service, and was a vigorous campaigner for the right of people with learning disabilities to have real jobs. He was passionate that people should be significantly better off financially through employment which he showed was not only desirable but possible.

References

Allen, D., 2006. Life better but jobs scarce, say Scottish respondents. Learning Disability Practice 9 (6), 6.

Bambra, C., 2010. Yesterday once more? Unemployment and health in the 21st century. J. Epidemiol. Community Health 64, 213–215. doi:10.1136/jech.2009.090621 (accessed 05.04.10.).

Bambra, C., Eikemo, T.A., 2009. Welfare state regimes, unemployment and health: a comparative study of the relationship between unemployment and self-reported health in

23 European countries. J. Epidemiol. Community Health 63, 92–98. doi:10.1136/jech.2008.077354 (accessed 05.04.10.).

Bass, M., 2000. Supported employment for people with learning difficulties. Joseph Rowntree Foundation, York.

Bauman, Z., 2008. The art of life. Polity Press, Cambridge.

Baumeister, R.F., 1991. Meanings of life. The Guildford Press, New York.

Bewley, C., 1997. Money matters: helping people with learning difficulties have more control over their money. Values Into Action, London.

Beyer, S., 2001. How does agency organisation impact on employment outcomes? Paper presented at 5th EUSE Conference, March 2001, Edinburgh.

Beyer, S., Kilsby, M., 1997. Supported employment in Britain. Tizard Learning Disability Review 2 (2), 6–14.

Beyer, S., Robinson, C., 2009. A review of the research literature on supported employment: a report for the cross-government learning disability employment strategy team. Department of Health, London.

Beyer, S., Goodere, L., Kilsby, M., 1996. The costs and benefits of supported employment agencies. The Stationery Office, London.

Beyer, S., Grove, B., Schneider, et al., 2004. Working lives: the role of day centers in supporting people with learning disabilities into employment. Department of Work and Pensions, Leeds.

Black Dame, C., 2008. Review of the health of Britain's working age population. The Stationery Office, London.

Black, J., Meyer, L.H., 1992. But is it really work? Social validity of employment training for persons with very severe disabilities. American Journal on Mental Retardation 96 (5), 463–474.

Bradley, V.J., Ashbaugh, J.W., Blaney, B. C., 1994. Creating Individual supports for people with developmental disabilities – a mandate for change at many levels. Paul H Brookes, Baltimore.

Brandon, D., 1987. Report of an occupational strategy for people with severe learning difficulties in West Lothian. West Lothian Voluntary Council for Disabled People, Scotland.

Brown, H., Smith, H., 1992. Normalisation. a reader for the nineties. Routledge, London.

Callahan, M., Shumpert, N., Mast, M., 2002. Self-employment, choice and self-determination. Journal of Vocational Rehabilitation 17 (2), 75–85.

Carr, S., Dittrich, R., 2008. Personalisation: a rough guide. Report 20. Social Care Institute for Excellence, London.

Commission for Social Care Inspection (CSCI), Healthcare Commission, Mental Health Act Commission, 2009. Commissioning services and support for people with learning disabilities and complex needs. National report of a joint review. CSCI/Healthcare Commission/ Mental Health Act Commission, London.

Curtice, L., 2006. How is it going? A survey of what matters most to people with learning disabilities in Scotland today. Enable, Glasgow.

Demby, S., 1992. My future is bright. Community Living 6 (2), 6.

Department of Health, 2001. Valuing people. A new strategy for learning disability for the 21st century. White Paper. Department of Health, London.

Department of Health, 2008. Transforming social care. Department of Health, London.

Department of Health, 2009a. Valuing people now: a new three-year strategy for people with learning disabilities. Making it happen for everyone. Department of Health, London.

Department of Health, 2009b. Valuing employment now: valuing real jobs for people with learning disabilities. Department of Health, London.

Eggleton, I., Robertson, S., Ryan, J., Kober, R., 1999. The impact of employment on the quality of life of people with an intellectual disability. Journal of Vocational Rehabilitation 13 (2), 95–107.

Emerson, E., Hatton, C., 1995. Moving out. The impact of relocation from hospital to community on the quality of life of people with learning disabilities. HMSO, London.

Emerson, E., Hatton, C., 1998. Residential provision for people with intellectual disabilities in England and Wales. J. Appl. Res. Intellect. Disabil. 11 (1), 1–14.

European Union of Supported Employment, 2006. Information booklet and quality standards. EUSE, Ireland. Available at: http://www.euse.org.

Feinmann, M., 1988. Project INTOWORK – How Sheffield achieved the impossible. Community Living 1 (5), 12.

Forrester-Jones, R., Gorre, N., Melling, K., 2010. How many people with intellectual disability are employed in the UK? Tizard Learning Disability Review 15 (1), 56–57.

Gold, M., 1973. Research on the vocational habilitation of the retarded: the present, the future. In: Ellis, N.R. (Ed.), International review of research in mental retardation6, Academic Press, New York.

Gold, M., 1980. Try another way – training manual. Research Press, Champaign, IL.

Gosling, V., Cotterill, L., 2000. An employment project as a route to social inclusion for people with learning difficulties? Disability and Society 15 (7), 1001–1018.

Griffin, C., Hammis, D., 2003. Making self employment work for people with disabilities. Paul H Brookes, Baltimore.

Hagner, D.C., DiLeo, D., 1993. Working together: workplace culture, supported employment and persons with disabilities. Brookline Books, Cambridge, USA.

Handy, C., 1984. The Future of work: a guide to a changing society. Blackwell, London.

Hanna, G., McConkey, R., 1992. Employers' attitudes to people with learning difficulties. Scotdat Surveys. Data on Scottish perceptions of mental handicap. Brothers of Charity Press, Scottish Borders.

Hedley, A., Dubin, R., Taveggia, C., 1980. The quality of working life, gender and occupational status: a cross national comparison. In: Szalai, A., Andrews, F.M. (Eds.), The quality of life: comparative studies. Sage, London.

Hunter, S., Ridley, J., 2007. Supported employment in Scotland: some issues from research and implications for development. Tizard Learning Disability Review 12 (2), 3–13.

Hunter, S., Ritchie, P., 2007. Co-production & personalisation in social care: changing relationships in the provision of social care. Jessica Kingsley, London.

Ingham, N., 2002. Gogarburn lives. Living Memory Association, Edinburgh.

Jahoda, A., Kemp, J., Riddell, S., Banks, P., 2007. Feelings about work: a review of the socio-emotional impact of supported employment on people with intellectual disabilities. J. Appl. Res. Intellect. Disabil. 21, 1–18.

Johnson, K., Walmsley, J., Wolfe, M., 2010. People with intellectual disabilities. Towards a good life?. Policy Press, Bristol.

Joseph Rowntree Foundation, 2002. Success in supported employment for people with learning difficulties – findings. Joseph Rowntree Foundation, York.

King's Fund Centre, 1980. An ordinary life: comprehensive locally-based residential services for mentally handicapped people. King's Fund Centre, London.

King's Fund Centre, 1984. An ordinary working life: vocational services for people with mental handicap. King's Fund Centre, London.

Kiuranor, C., 1980. An integral indicator of the quality of work and the quality of life. In: Szalai, A., Andrews, F.M. (Eds.), The quality of life: comparative studies. Sage, London.

Leach, S., 2002. A supported employment workbook. Jessica Kingsley, London.

Leadbeater, C., 2004. Personalisation through participation: a new script for public services. DEMOS, London.

Leslie, H., 1992. Don't handicap the disabled. Sunday Telegraph, June 21.

Luecking, R., Fabian, E.S., Tilson, G.P., 2004. Working relationships. Creating career opportunities for job seekers with disabilities through employer partnerships. Paul H Brookes, Baltimore.

McConkey, R., 2007. Leisure and work. In: Gates, B., Atherton, H. (Eds.), Learning disabilities. Toward inclusion. fifth ed. Elsevier, Edinburgh.

McInally, G., 2008. Supported employment for people with learning disabilities: the case for full time work. Tizard Learning Disability Review 13 (3), 42–46.

McLoughlin, C.S., Garner, J.B., Callahan, M.J., 1987. Getting employed, staying employed. Paul H Brookes, Baltimore.

Mank, D.M., 1994. The underachievement of supported employment: a call for reinvestment. Journal of Disability Policy Studies 5 (2), 1–24.

Mank, D., Cioffi, A., Yovanoff, P., 1998. Employment outcomes for people with severe disabilities: opportunities for improvement. Ment. Retard. 36 (3), 205–216.

Mayo, E., 1996. Dreaming of work. In: Meadows, P. (Ed.), Work out – or work in? Contributions to the debate on the future of work. Joseph Rowntree Foundation, York.

Mental Health Foundation, 1996. Building expectations. Opportunities and services for people with a learning disability. The Mental Health Foundation, London.

Nirje, B., 1980. The normalization principle. In: Flynn, R.J., Nitsch, K.E. (Eds.), Normalisation, social integration and community service. University Park Press, Baltimore.

Noonan-Walsh, P., Rafferty, M., Lynch, C., 1991. The 'Open Road' project: real jobs for people with mental handicaps. Int. J. Rehabil. Res. 14, 155–161.

O'Brien, J., Tyne, A., 1981. The principle of normalisation: a foundation for effective services. The Campaign for Mentally Handicapped People, London.

O'Bryan, A., 2002. Person centred planning and supported employment. In: O'Brien, J., O'Brien, C.L. (Eds.), Implementing person centred planning: voices of experience. Inclusion Press, Toronto.

O'Bryan, A., Simons, K., Beyer, S., Grove, B., for the Policy Consortium of Supported Employment, 2000. A framework for supported employment. York Publishing Services, York.

Oliver, M., 1990. The politics of disablement. MacMillan and St Martin's Press, Basingstoke.

Oliver, M., 1996. Understanding disability. From theory to practice. MacMillan Press, London.

Pagan, R., 2009. Self-employment among people with disabilities: evidence for Europe. Disability & Society 24 (2), 217–229.

Pallisera, M., Vila, M., Valls, M.J., 2003. The current situation of supported employment in Spain: analysis and perspectives based on the perception of professionals. Disability and Society 18 (6), 797–810.

Petty, D.M., Fussell, E.M., 1997. Employer attitudes and satisfaction with supported employment. Focus on Autism and Other Developmental Disabilities 12 (1), 261–295.

Poll, C., Duffy, S., Hatton, C., Sanderson, H., Routedge, M., 2006. A report on In Control's first phase, 20032005. In Control Publications, London.

Pozner, A., Hammond, J., 1993. An evaluation of supported employment initiatives for disabled people. Research Series No 17. Outset, Sheffield.

Racino, J.A., Whittico, P., 1998. The promise of self advocacy and community employment. In: Wehman, P., Kregel, J. (Eds.), More than a job. Securing satisfying careers for people with disabilities. Paul H Brookes, Baltimore.

Redley, M., 2009. Understanding the social exclusion and stalled welfare of citizens with intellectual disabilities. Disability and Society 24 (4), 489–501.

Ridley, J., 2000. Mixed fortunes: a qualitative study of supported employment and quality of life. PhD thesis, University of Edinburgh, Edinburgh.

Ridley, J., 2001. Supported employment and learning disability: a life-changing experience? In: Clark, C. (Ed.), Adult day services and social inclusion. Better days. Jessica Kingsley, London.

Ridley, J., Hunter, S., 2006. The development of supported employment in Scotland. Journal of Vocational Rehabilitation 25 (1), 57–68.

Ridley, J., Hunter, S., 2007. Learning from research about best practice in supporting people with learning disabilities in real jobs: information for commissioners. Workforce Plus, Glasgow.

Ridley, J., Hunter, S., Infusion Co-operative, 2005. 'Go for it!' Supporting people with learning disabilities and/or autistic spectrum disorder in employment. Scottish Executive, Edinburgh.

Schneider, J., Heyman, A., Turton, N., 2002. Occupational outcomes: from evidence to implementation. An expert topic paper commissioned by the Department of Health. Centre for Applied Social Studies. University of Durham, Durham.

Scottish Executive, 2000. The same as you? A review of services for people with learning disabilities. Scottish Executive, Edinburgh.

Scottish Union of Supported Employment, 2006. A blueprint for supported employment in Scotland. Reiver Press, Galashiels.

Sikking, M., 1986. Co-ops with a difference. ICOM Co-Publications, London.

Simons, K., 1998. Home, work and inclusion. The social policy implications of supported living and employment for people with learning disabilities. York Publishing Services for the Joseph Rowntree Foundation, York.

Sinnott-Oswald, M., Gliner, J.A., Spencer, K.C., 1991. Supported and sheltered employment: quality of life issues amoung workers with disability. Education and Training in Mental Retardation December 388–397.

Smith, R., 1985. 'Bitterness, shame, emptiness, waste': an introduction to unemployment and health. Br. Med. J. 291, 1024–1027.

Stalker, K., 2001. Inclusive daytime opportunities for people with learning disabilities. In: Clark, C. (Ed.), Adult day services and social inclusion. Better days. Research highlights in social work, No. 39. Jessica Kingsley, London.

Steele, D., 1991. Survey reveals gulf between work aspirations and success. Community Living 5 (1), 2.

Steele, D., 1992. FLEET – A desperately needed service. Community Living 5 (3), 5.

Sutton, B., 1999. Inclusive employment: international perspectives. In: Stiles, K. (Ed.), Beyond borders: global supported employment and people with disabilities. Training Resource Network, USA.

Tannen, V., 1993. A literature review of supported employment. In: Pozner, A., Hammond, J. (Eds.), An evaluation of supported employment initiatives for disabled people. Research Series No. 17. Outset, Sheffield.

Unger, D.D., 2002. Employers attitudes towards persons with disabilities in the workforce: myths or realities? Focus on Autism and Other Developmental Disabilities 17 (1).

Verdugo, M.A., Jordán de Urríes, J.B., Jenaro, C., et al., 2006. Quality of life of workers with an intellectual disability in supported employment. J. Appl. Res. Intellect. Disabil. 19, 309–316.

Wehman, P., Kregel, J., 1998. More than a job: securing satisfying careers for people with disabilities. Paul H Brookes, Baltimore.

Wertheimer, A., Real Jobs Initiative, 1992. Changing lives: supported employment and people with learning disabilities. National Development Team, Manchester.

Weston, J., 2002. Supported employment and people with complex needs: a review of research literature and ongoing research. Journal of Social Work 2 (1), 83–104.

Williams, P., Shoultz, B., 1982. We can speak for ourselves. Self advocacy by mentally handicapped people. Human horizons series. Souvenir Press, London.

Wolfensberger, W., 1972. The principle of normalisation in human services. National Institute on Mental Retardation, Toronto.

Wolfensberger, W., 1983. Social role valorisation: a proposed new term for the principle of normalisation. Ment. Retard. 21 (6), 234–239.

Further reading

Clark, C. (Ed.), 2001. Adult day services and social inclusion. Research highlights 39. Jessica Kingsley, London.

European Union of Supported Employment, 2006. Information booklet and quality standards. EUSE, Ireland. Available at: http://www.euse.org.

Griffin, C., Hammis, D., 2003. Making self employment work for people with disabilities. Paul H Brookes, Baltimore.

Kregel, J., Dean, D.H., Wehman, P. (Eds.), 2002. Achievements and challenges in employment services for people with disabilities: the longitudinal impact of workplace supports. Virginia Commonwealth University, Virginia.

Leach, S., 2002. A Supported Employment Workbook. Individual Profiling and Job Matching. Jessica Kingsley, London.

McLoughlin, C.S., Garner, J.B., Callahan, M.J., 1987. Getting Employed, Staying Employed. Paul H Brookes, Baltimore.

O'Bryan, A., Simons, K., Beyer, S., Grove, B., for the Policy Consortium of Supported Employment, 2000. A framework for supported employment. York Publishing Services, York.

Wehman, P., 2001. Supported employment in business. Expanding the capacity of workers with disabilities. Training Resource Network, St Augustine, FL.

Useful addresses

Foundation for People with Learning Disabilities, 9th Floor, Sea Captains House, 20 Upper Ground, London, Tel: 020 7803 1100: http://www.learningdisabilities.org.uk

British Association for Supported Employment (BASE), Unit 26, Severnside Trading Estate,

Sindmeadow Road, Hempsted, Gloucester GL2 5HS, Tel: 01452 783596: http://www.afse.org.uk.

Department of Health, http://www.dh.gov.uk.

Department of Work & Pensions, http://www.direct.gov.uk/en/DisabledPeople.

European Union of Supported Employment, http://www.euse.org.

Social Care Online, http://www.scie-socialcareonline.org.uk.

Mencap, http://www.mencap.org.uk/.

Values Into Action Scotland, http://www.viascotland.org.uk/.

Valuing Employment Now Resources, http://valuingpeople.gov.uk/dynamic/valuingpeople371.jsp.

Virginia Commonwealth University Rehabilitation Research and Training Center on Workplace Supports and Job Retention: http://www.worksupport.com/.

A place to live

27

Julia Fitzpatrick

CHAPTER CONTENTS

KEY ISSUES

- People with learning disabilities and their families have a human right to have a place to live which supports their right to citizenship and inclusion
- They can face barriers in finding the right home: poor supply of physically suitable house types; financial and legal hurdles; and the need to secure and organise related support and care
- Access to information and professional support for the purpose of securing suitable housing is often not readily available, and local policies and systems can inadvertently serve to exclude or marginalise
- Housing and support providers and commissioners need to work with people with learning disabilities and families so that they have access to the information and resources to plan for suitable housing with confidence
- New approaches are needed which ensure that adults with learning disabilities have access to the housing and the support they require to live independently of their families when they need or want to do so

Introduction

Having your own home is more than a place to live – being able to choose where to live, how to live and with whom is an essential foundation for inclusion.

The human right to acquire and sustain a secure home in which to live with peace and dignity increases the likelihood that other human rights will be achieved. Shelter is one of the most basic human needs, meeting one's emotional as well as physical needs: lack of the right home can affect ability to play a part in family life, to sustain employment, to make connections and relationships, to participate in community and decision making and to be physically and emotionally healthy. This is as true for someone with learning disabilities as anyone else.

'Adequate' housing in human rights legislation means governments need to pay attention to how they secure for their citizens housing that offers legal security of tenure, affordability and accessibility, among other factors. In the UK, this is generally tackled through housing and building legislation, guidance and funding mechanisms. The Disability Discrimination Act 2005 extended to public service agencies the duty to promote disability equality. *Valuing People* (Department of Health (DH) 2001) in England and *The Same as You?* (Scottish Executive 2000) in Scotland directed local authorities to expand the range and choice of housing for people with learning disabilities, pointing out that people can, and want to, live successfully in many types of housing and tenures. *Valuing People Now* (DH 2009) is launched from a human rights perspective and commits to a strategy and programme of work to ensure that mainstream housing policies include people with learning disabilities.

However, in practice, while some local authorities and housing providers are getting better at developing strategies to increase the availability and accessibility of housing suitable for disabled people, the particular needs of people with learning disabilities or autistic spectrum conditions are frequently overlooked or marginalised. Few local authorities have yet identified the needs of people with learning disabilities or autistic spectrum conditions in their areas and addressed these within their mainstream housing strategies (Harker & King 2004, Mencap 2002, ODS Consulting 2007). Where need is recognised, it has tended to be expressed in term of a need for grouped and 'special' accommodation, with insufficient attention given to the potential for, and value of, making provision within the ordinary and available housing systems. Progress is being made, with government policy explicitly seeking improvements in this area (DH 2009).

Most people get to choose where they live, who they live with and who comes into their home to support or help them. This does not mean that everyone lives in their ideal home – compromises and choices are made, often based on money and availability. Yet where care and support also need to be considered, too often it is the professionals who decide on the compromises to be made and not the people most affected or their families.

This chapter explores aspects of housing for people with learning disabilities: history, policy and reality; housing options; developing personal housing plans and dovetailing these with support plans; housing choices and rights; and common issues for people with learning disabilities and their families.

> **Reader activity 27.1**
>
> What does the word 'home' mean to you and what aspects are most important? Ask yourself this question, and a sample of family members and colleagues. Then, find out about your local authority care needs assessment and housing allocations processes. How well do you think they capture these aspects?

Housing: history, policy and reality

History

In the UK, USA and many European countries, the long-stay institution was the dominant social response to people with a learning disability for all but the last few years of the 20th century. Learning disability hospitals in the UK were built in response to the Mental Deficiency Act 1913, accommodating large numbers and taking people from the Victorian asylums, hospitals and poor houses, as well as from the streets, workplaces and family homes. Some housed well over 1000 people. Driven originally by idealism, then by eugenics and finally by inertia, this shaped society's understanding of disability and difference, and confronted families with the choice between having their family member 'put away' and having no help at all. This choice is less stark today, but as Table 27.1 shows (Emerson & Hatton 2008), we are still in a world where the choice is between living in the parental home or with a relative or living in some form of institutional living, with only 7–17% (depending on definition) owning or renting

Table 27.1 Accommodation arrangements for people with mild/moderate, severe and profound multiple learning disabilities

	Mild or moderate	Severe	Profound multiple	All people with learning disabilities
Private households				
• With parent(s)	48%	61%	60%	55%
• With other relative	14%	11%	4%	12%
• With partner	6%	<1%	<1%	3%
• Alone	7%	2%	0%	4%
Sub-total	75%	75%	65%	74%
Supporting People funded	12%	8%	5%	10%
Residential care home	13%	15%	19%	14%
NHS accommodation	<1%	2%	11%	2%
Total	100%	100%	100%	100%

(Source: People with learning disabilities in England (Emerson & Hatton 2008))

their own home compared with 94% of the general population (Office for National Statistics 2010).

It became increasingly clear that hospitals did not provide a good quality of life for people with learning disabilities, with research pointing to impoverished lives and long-lasting wounds (Howe Report 1969, Wolfensberger 1998). The drive towards 'community care' (Griffiths 1988) became stronger as deadlines for institutional closure were set – but the process of deinstitutionalisation has been painful, lengthy and often compromised by financial arguments, professional protectionism and politics.

Gradually new models developed, some existing alongside and as an alternative to the hospitals. Access to the different models tended to be linked to competency assumptions – the more able or amenable an individual was deemed to be, the fewer unrelated people with whom they had to share their life. Table 27.2 summarises common features of the different models of accommodation today.

Social and community care policy

Valuing People (DH 2001) and its Scottish counterpart, *The Same as You?* (Scottish Executive 2000), reviewed services for people with learning disabilities and set long-term strategies. They found that people wanted access to a full range of housing options, including the option of living with others or on their own with support. *The Same as You?* pointed out that supported individual or joint tenancies and assisted home ownership were popular. It recommended that everyone should be able to have a personal life plan covering, among other things, housing needs and aspirations. *Valuing People* set a target for hospitals to close by April 2004 (later extended to 2006), and *The Same as You?* recommended that all long-stay hospitals should close by 2005. These produced pressure on the statutory agencies and their partners to deliver housing alternatives in communities.

Almost 10 years on, the principles of *Valuing People* (DH 2001) and *The Same as You?* (Scottish Executive 2000) are embedded in national policy drives towards personalisation and the right to control (Scottish Executive 2006, Welfare Reform Act 2009). These include the expectation that people should be supported in the way that makes sense to them, including being supported to have their own home if that is what they want.

Over the last 10 years, a growing number of people with support needs have housing rights that are not tied to decisions about provision and funding of support and care. Most recently, the work of In Control in England and its counterparts in Scotland and Northern Ireland (In Control 2009) encourages people to take control of their support to live the life they want. There is a growing acceptance of the need for transformational change in social services to respond to an expectation that services will be

Table 27.2 Models of accommodation

Common description	Positives	Negatives (present to a greater or lesser degree)
Supported accommodation, hostels/residential care	Own room. Towns or cities rather than isolated from centres of population. Buildings looked more like housing.	No security of tenure. No say in choice of fellow residents. Often no choice of food or meal times. Staff centred, life built around staff rotas. Organisation rules.
Group home	Own room. Smaller place. More integrated into surroundings.	Limited or No statutory security of tenure. '3–6 pack' matching of people, based on compatibility, or lack of obvious incompatibility. Staffing determined by needs of the group. Rules often made by the organisation.
Core and Cluster	Individual flats or houses. Some self-contained, some shared. In communities. Statutory security of tenure for some, i.e. full tenancy rights offered.	Security of tenure or tenancy rights often not understood or respected. Often connected to a group home. Staffing often linked to the group needs. Often owned by the support provider.
Supported living	Own home. Separation of housing and support. Person-centred. Personalised support and staffing. Security of tenure.	Some support providers have limited understanding of tenancy rights, resulting in infringements. Sometimes misused as a term for a 'non-registered' group home: shared living arrangements with no real choice of flat or housemates.

personalised to meet individual needs and aspirations, and that services should be based on strong core values about inclusion and inclusiveness (DH 2009, Scottish Executive 2006).

The reality for people with learning disabilities

There is, however, still a gulf between the experience and situation of people with learning disabilities and government policy aspirations, and between the situation for people with learning disabilities and the rest of the population.

Across the UK, the patterns for individuals with learning disabilities and their families are similar, with some variation in Scotland (Emerson & Hatton 2008, *The Same as You?* implementation group reports 2004–2007). The majority of adults with profound and multiple learning disabilities live with parents; most adults with mild or moderate learning disabilities live with parents or another relative as described above. In Scotland, *The Same as You?* (Scottish Executive 2000) reported that 25% of people with significant disabilities who live with families have a family carer who is aged over 65; Mencap reported on the same issue in 2002, describing a 'housing timebomb' in the UK for people in this situation (Mencap 2002). Similar issues have been identified for people with an autistic spectrum condition, with escalating numbers and inadequate planning for, or understanding of, future housing needs on the part of commissioners and providers (Harker & King 2004). Identifying and acknowledging the issues is of course an essential first step, and awareness raising information and guidance is emerging (Glasgow City Council 2010, King 2003).

Where people are living

Table 27.1 shows where people with learning disabilities in England were living in 2008. The Scottish Government reports that a third of adults with

Reader activity 27.2

Find out about your local or regional authority housing strategy and investment plans. How well do you think they do or will respond to the needs of people with learning disabilities and their families that you know?

learning disabilities known to social services are estimated to be 'living independently' (Scottish Government 2007), gauged by the number of people with tenancies. This is almost twice the number of people in England. However, this is misleading. The term 'tenancy' describes only the legal status of the property occupier and can apply to people living in shared or group homes who have no choice about their co-tenants, as well as those who live in their own self-contained homes. Emerson & Hatton (2008) reported that the majority of people living in supported accommodation had no choice over where or with whom they lived. This was particularly the case for people with more severe disabilities, but also true for a significant minority of those with mild disabilities. Living independently implies choice and control over support arrangements and co-tenants. There is a long way to go before confidence can be expressed that this is happening in a meaningful way for the people now referred to in the statistics.

Changing expectations

There is clear commitment from national governments that long-stay institutions for people with a learning disability need to close, and that a human rights perspective requires the development of strategies for offering people with learning disabilities access to mainstream housing options (DH 2009). However local authorities face the challenge of bringing people back home, from expensive and unsuitable out-of-area placements, people who are now totally disconnected from their original community. As sending people away becomes less and less acceptable, the local housing and support service systems have to gear up to meeting the needs of people who are at risk of exclusion.

Expectations are changing: people with learning disabilities and their families no longer expect that post-school accommodation and support will be based in or part of institutional or quasi-institutional settings. The expectation and aspiration is that people will live as adults in the community they came from. The housing challenge now is to design homes and support services that mean people do not have to leave their community, and can be supported to be part of and to contribute to that community.

The Department of Health and the Scottish Government are also recognising the housing demands arising from an ageing population: people with learning disabilities are living longer, may need to move because of changing needs, and those with Down's syndrome are at a greater risk of developing dementia at a relatively early age (King 2003, Scottish Executive 2002). This is driving work to support best practice in the development of supported housing specifically for older people who have a learning disability (King 2003).

Design for living

The most common housing options are familiar: living in a house or a flat, renting or buying, living with family, alone or with others. A sub-set of possibilities follows: buying a house alone or with someone else, living there together or not; letting out rooms in one's own house; lodging in someone else's home; living in a house owned by a trust – with supporters, or with housemates; renting from the local authority, housing association or from a private landlord; cooperative or community living – living with like-minded people who subscribe to a particular philosophy of life.

When someone has a learning disability, these ordinary choices may be overlooked because assumptions are made that the person's support needs precludes them. Even if they are considered, often a decision is made before any time is spent really thinking with and about the person's needs and aspirations. This is particularly so if the person has no prior experience of being in their own home or even of being listened to; if professional supporters and family members have had little exposure to alternatives to congregate living; or where there is a presumption that people cannot be supported in their home because the associated support will be too expensive to provide.

Where the person with a disability has attended a special school or college, or attends a day centre or activities carried out almost exclusively with other people with disabilities, it becomes extraordinary to think about ordinary. Housing options can therefore become limited, because the starting point is to think about special provision and its availability rather than the kind of life the person wants to live, and how the right housing can enable effective supports for this to happen.

In ordinary living, very few people make an active choice of housing or a lifestyle in inward-looking settlements that have little association with the general community or where they share housing with others long term. Arguments have been put forward in the past for the establishment and maintenance of village or intentional communities for people with learning disabilities (Cox & Pearson 1995). While there is no clear definition of 'village community', these are often in relatively isolated rural locations and are in effect institutional: congregate accommodation and support for large numbers of disabled people on one site with all the attendant risks of exclusion, and limited experiences and choices. Nevertheless they have advantages and disadvantages, and policy makers consider it to be a viable option if actively chosen by the person with a learning disability and their family (Hatton 2001).

Planning for transition and change

There are key points in a person's life where planning well ahead is essential: for example, where transition or change can easily be anticipated such as when leaving school or college, when an institution is closing, when close siblings start to leave home or as family carers get older and less able to care. It is much easier to plan when things are going well, yet too often housing only becomes a priority at a time of crisis.

In any situation where there is a need or aspiration to move home, whether for the person with a learning disability alone or the family, then a personal housing plan can be useful. A housing plan is a way of thinking about an individual's needs and aspirations, about their resources and preferences and then finding out about housing options that could help to meet this vision.

Personal housing plans

Planning starts with asking good questions, listening carefully to the answers and then asking more questions. Everyone's housing plan is unique, reflecting their housing experiences, specific background, family, physical and support needs. Depending on the situation, it can be useful to get help, for example from knowledgeable housing or support advisors or brokers. If there is a significant gap between the minimum requirements and the resources available – in terms of available housing supply or money – then specialist advice may help. Others may have knowledge about new developments, policies, legislation,

Case illustration 27.1

Chris and the art of the possible

Chris has learning disabilities and epilepsy. He lived with his parents and sister, attending a special school and then a day centre. When he was 21, his sister Louise got married and moved to live with her husband on the other side of town. Later that year his mum, Lilian, died. The family was devastated and Chris's father, David, simply could not cope with looking after Chris on his own. Chris started having an increasing number of apparently uncontrollable epileptic fits and was taking his grief and anger about his mother's death out on his father.

After a year of struggling, social services advised David that it would be best if Chris moved into a group home, where support staff could be on hand 24 hours a day. So he moved into a house with eight people in it, about 15 miles away from home. He became increasingly unhappy and unhealthy. He did not like sharing a home with other people and showed this at every opportunity, making it very difficult for the people sharing a home with him. Eventually, after someone was hurt, Chris was admitted to hospital 'for assessment'. Five years later, he was still there, living on a ward with four other men, and visiting his family home at weekends. During this time, no one had been able to come up with a housing option to suit Chris which could also meet his support needs.

A group of people worked with his family and with Chris to think about where and how he wanted to live, and what would be his ideal home. Everyone agreed he needed to have support, during the day and overnight. Chris wanted to live where no one would touch his music tapes, where he could cut the grass and where he could eat dinner in front of the TV. Ideally his family wanted him to live near them so that Chris could come to see them easily. They wanted him to live on a street where he would be safe crossing the road to say hello to neighbours. Chris didn't mind having a support person living in the house providing there was enough space for him to be by himself.

So Chris, his dad, some people from the hospital and the people working out how to support him decided that the ideal was a two or three bedroom house, where he could live with a supportive flatmate and be supported by a small team of people.

The next step was to find out if the ideal existed and, if not, could any compromises be made. This seemed a better way to stay in control than to work backwards from the limited options which had previously been considered and rejected.

(Fitzpatrick 2005)

Reader activity 27.3

Look at the list of questions in Box 27.1. Use these, adapting as necessary, as a base for a conversation with someone with a learning disability or their family or supporters to build up a picture of their ideal home. What different approaches could you use to find out this information?

benefits or sources of finance that can open the door to further options.

A personal housing plan (sometimes called a housing options plan) can:

- provide a useful summary for a person or family and for anybody working to support them in getting or keeping the home of their choice
- help with deciding what is essential and supporting decision making about compromises
- help when looking at available housing options

Box 27.1

Thinking about housing

The starting point for a personal housing plan is thinking, through questions, about who the person wants to live with or near, how and where they want to live, what the property needs to look like in order to meet the person's or family's needs and what is affordable. The questions below are suggested questions for building up a picture about a person's housing needs and aspirations.

Starting points

Before thinking about or researching what options are available, it helps to think about where the person lives now, and about where they have lived before. This can help to build up a picture of what aspects they want to change and what should stay the same: for example, the size of your living room may be ideal but the bathroom is too small to be adapted, or the house is too far from amenities.

- Likes? Dislikes?
- Suitable? Not suitable? Why?
- What needs to change?

Who does the person or family want to live with?

- How many people will live in the house as their main home?
- Will people from different age groups be living in the house, e.g. children?
- Does the person want to share with anyone? If yes, why? What compromises would this mean and are these acceptable or sustainable?
- Will the person need room or space for supporters or carers? What kind of support might be needed and could this affect the size or type of home required?

Where?

- What does the person, and family if relevant, do or would they like to do (or have to do) on a daily, weekly or monthly basis?
- Is it important to live near particular friends or family members?
- What kind of area would suit the person and why?
- Are there any practical considerations? Does the house need to be near public transport or a shop?

What will the person's home look and feel like?

- Does the person or family have particular needs that affect the type of property required, e.g. level or ramped access; good sound insulation; separate dining space?
- What sort of space or design or aids or adaptations might help the person to do (or not do) things in the house or be supported to do them?
- Does the person need help which might affect the size or type of house needed, e.g. with bathing or going to the toilet which may mean a bigger or separate bathroom is needed?
- What elements of a property would be essential, and what would be nice but not necessary? For example, a second bedroom for a supporter might be essential; a garden may be desirable, but not necessary.

What can the person or family afford?

- Where does the person's money come from at the moment and how much do they have?
- Do they, or will they, have to pay any money for care and support?
- What does the person spend their money on now, and would this change if they moved?
- What money is needed in order to get a suitable home, and then to set it up and live in it? Do a budget.
- Can the person get help with any of the costs? Where from and how much?

Any other points which might affect the plan?

- Are there likely to be questions about legal capacity to make decisions?
- Are there local care or housing policies or initiatives which could help, or which might stand in the way?
- Where can you find people or resources that can help to explore options or get more information?
- Does the person or their family need to see or hear from people who have already got their own home? Do they need time to think and reflect before making a decision on how to move forward?

- be used to support an application for rented housing, or when talking to estate agents or new house developers.

Personal housing planning is a process that can support the person to learn about and consider options, and to be, and feel, in control. People can be involved by using graphics, stories, photographs and visits to meet people who have their own home or who live with others.

Any change can be frightening. For people who may have only known institutional living, this may manifest itself in refusal to leave, or deep distress at the suggestion. Family members may feel lonely and unsupported in their concern for the future. Where people have always lived with family members, they may fear isolation or loneliness, and lack of support to build relationships and community connections that keep people safe and secure and make for a good life (Etmanski 2000).

Housing options

An approach based on citizenship and inclusion starts with the underpinning principles that people with learning disabilities should have equal housing opportunities. No one is too difficult or too complex to be supported in their own home if that is what they choose. Some people, like Chris in Case illustration 27.1, may communicate their choices through behaviour. For others, knowledge needs to be solicited from those who know the person well, and then applied to working out what housing environment will best support citizenship. This means people (or those representing them) are likely to need support with information, advice and negotiating housing and support systems. In some situations, new approaches can be created to meet the particular needs of the people involved (Fitzpatrick & Butler 2001).

Living with family can be a clear and valid choice, which includes active plans for how and where the person will live when their parents die.

Reader activity 27.4

Read Tommy's story presented in summary in Case illustration 27.2 or in full in *Home Truths* (Fitzpatrick & Butler 2001 Available at: http://www.altrum.org.uk)

- What were the important factors in helping Tommy decide that it would be acceptable to leave the hospital?
- If you were working on Tommy's housing plan, what features and qualities would be essential for his new home?
- What other information would you need in order to explore his housing options fully?

Case illustration 27.2

Tommy

I am 44, and have lived in hospitals since I was 6 and here since I was 11. Before that I lived in several residential homes. I don't remember much about that. I get on very well with staff at the hospital, especially my best friend Andy, who works on my ward. I go to Andy's house quite often and know his family. My cousin Libby lives in the same town as Andy – she is the only relative I know about. Gerry is my advocate (from an advocacy service) and my friend. I don't want to leave the hospital – this is my home.

Jean from Inclusion Glasgow [prospective support provider] comes to see me and talk to me about leaving the hospital. She's been coming to see me for almost a year now. I didn't want to talk about leaving the hospital for a long time. We are working out where I want to live – I want to live with Andy. Jean and Andy understand this, but Andy says it would not work for him. So if I can't do that, I want to live where I can see him often. I don't want to live with other people from the hospital – none of them are going to live near Andy anyway.

I am a big Celtic fan and I need to be able to watch all the matches on TV when they're not playing at Parkhead. I paint, and one of my pictures has been hung at Parkhead. I like to dance and if I had my own house I would have a party and invite my friends.

I can't speak much and sometimes other people need help to understand what I want to say. I have a club foot, but I manage the stairs to the admin department at the hospital and I get paid from my work there. They wouldn't let me have the money to manage myself at first but Gerry sorted it out and now I have a savings account to put my wages in.

Jean introduced me to Adrian and we decided he could live with me and also be my support worker.
We started looking at houses near Andy. We lost a few houses, but then we saw one near Andy that had green doors.

(This is a summary of a longer story contained in *Home Truths* (Fitzpatrick & Butler 2001))

Reader activity 27.5

Before you read the section on 'Housing options', think of all the different sources of housing you might consider when supporting someone with a learning disability to find a suitable home. Write them down.

Then think about the pros and cons of these different options in general, and then in relation to the particular circumstances of someone you know who has learning disabilities.

However, if this is not the person's (or their family's) active choice, the main options are:

- renting a house from the local authority or a housing association
- renting a house from a private landlord
- renting from a family member, who may buy to let
- home ownership
- ownership by a trust
- supported lodgings or Shared Lives.

Some of these options might involve moving. Others may offer ways of the person staying in their family home, after parents have moved or died. The person's housing tenure should not, in itself, dictate the level of support that is possible. However, house size, design and location can of course influence how support can be designed to suit the person. For example, as a tenant or home-owner, the person may decide to share their home with someone who may offer support, or a lodger.

Renting a house from the local authority (council) or a housing association

Local authorities, or their 'arms length management organisations' (ALMOs) tend to be the largest owners and managers of affordable rented housing in a local area. They offer secure tenancies for people in housing need who do not want or cannot afford the long-term commitments that are associated with buying a house. However, there a limited range of house types and locations on offer. It is a good option if the person can get a suitable property in an area they are happy with and, crucially, within the timescale that they need.

Local authorities have obligations to assist people in certain circumstances to find suitable housing, for example if they are homeless. Even if it seems unlikely that the local authority will be able to help, it is always worth making an application in order to register the unmet need.

Housing associations are also registered, and regulated, social landlords and they offer affordable rented houses. There are hundreds of housing associations across the UK; some are national, some regional, some very local and community based.

An increasing number of local authorities and housing associations are operating a choice-based lettings system. This means that vacancies are advertised and applicants who meet the criteria for the particular vacancy can bid for the property. This is not a financial bid, but simply a bid that they would like the property and it is a good fit for their needs. Many landlords are working to ensure that these schemes offer equal opportunities to people with learning disabilities (Wood & Hall 2008).

Renting a house from a private landlord

Although more expensive than social landlords, private landlords can be a good option if a person needs housing quickly, or if they want to test different housing possibilities. It may be good for a person who is not sure if they want to move permanently, such as a person leaving home for the first time.

Generally, a deposit will be required and a minimum of one month's rent in advance. Some local authorities have 'rent deposit' schemes offering financial assistance to help people access this sector.

Many private landlords say they will not let to people who rely on housing benefit to pay the rent. However, this can sometimes be addressed with reassurances or financial guarantees from the local authority, health service or family. Some landlords may be unsure about the legal position of a proposed tenant with learning disabilities. Without compromising the person's rights not to be discriminated against, it can be helpful to explain how someone with support needs will be supported to sustain their tenancy and meet the tenancy obligations.

Private landlords often offer short leases of 6 months to a year. Such leases can be renewed but this does tend to leave the tenant in a vulnerable position, because if the lease is not renewed they have to move. However, some private landlords let properties as their main business and although the tenancy is 'short' from a contractual point of view, in practice the tenancy can last as long as the person

Box 27.2

Handy tips – local authority and housing association rented housing

- Generally, local authorities and housing associations only have properties in certain areas and so choice of location can be very limited and waiting times long.
- Many local authorities have transferred ownership or management of their homes to registered social landlords (not-for-profit housing providers approved and regulated by government through the Housing Corporation or Scottish Housing Regulator). As a result of this and the right to buy, availability of council houses has reduced.
- People leaving residential care can stay in the same area as their place of care or move to be nearer family in another area. Guidance is available for local authorities on identifying the place of ordinary residence for the purposes of funding care [Dept. of Health, 2010]
- Some housing associations let property to specific groups of people such as young adults, homeless people, people with physical or learning disabilities. Some housing associations also offer supported housing and care – and sometimes as soon as disability is mentioned, the application is diverted to this arm of the organisation. That can be helpful, but it can have the unintended consequence of excluding the person from being considered for ordinary housing opportunities.
- Check that the person is on all the housing lists, and persevere to ensure their housing needs are understood and properly reflected in the priority for housing that they are awarded.
- Social services staff can help people by making a referral, by providing an assessment of the person's housing needs and by active support, particularly if the person has very specific needs in terms of house type or location. This should be carried out in any case as part of a community care assessment.
- New housing association properties should be easier to adapt for wheelchair users. However, there is still a huge shortfall of housing suitable for wheelchair users. Early planning and applications are advised.
- If an application to your local authority or housing association is not going to plan, get independent advice and advocacy if necessary.
- If the council cannot assist directly with housing, it is still obliged to offer advice and assistance to find housing, or with adaptation to the person's current home. This is particularly so if the person is homeless or about to become homeless.

wants to live there. No tenant can be asked to move without having prior notice from the landlord.

Standards vary drastically. Some private landlords are registered with the council and many offer a good service carrying out maintenance whenever needed. Other landlords will try to avoid their obligations and have shoddy work practices within run-down properties. It is worth going to a respected landlord. If this is a possible route to suitable accommodation, talk to local housing and advice services and get advice about the tenancy agreement.

Generally, private rented accommodation is more expensive than social rental options, and housing benefit may not cover the whole rent. Eligible applicants can make the case to housing benefit departments for a 'top up' called discretionary housing benefit. Welfare rights services should be able to provide advice about this.

Renting from a family member, who may buy to let

Where a relative, for example a parent, has or can raise the financial resources, they may decide that the best or indeed only way of securing suitable secure accommodation for their family member is to buy a property and then rent it to them. There are alternative financial approaches depending on the amount of property equity that may be available to give as security and this route can be linked to arrangements for setting up a trust to eventually own and manage the property.

This can be a way for families to help their son or daughter to access suitable housing in the owner-occupied sector. Good legal, financial and welfare rights advice is essential. The housing benefit regulations in this area are complex and it is important that if the tenant would need housing benefit in order to pay rent, that the prospective landlord and tenant approach the transaction carefully.

Home ownership

Around 73% of people in England own their own home and 64% in Scotland (Office for National Statistics 2010, Scottish Government 2009). Local authority housing strategy statistics will provide tenure breakdown for their areas as a whole, and some areas, or communities, will show 85–95% of the homes to be in the owner-occupied sector. Housing

Case illustration 27.3

Suzanne

Suzanne went to residential college away for her family home, learned skills and became more independent. She has learning disabilities and epilepsy, visual and hearing impairments and mobility problems. Her family wanted her to return to her community, but to a place of her own with support. Despite her mother starting to think about her future housing when Suzanne was 16, and asking for help with planning, none was given. At age 21, 3 months before the date she would leave college, the local authority offered a place in a group home (sharing with men) or support back in the family home.

Her mother had taken early action – Suzanne's name was on the council's housing list as well as several housing associations. She was flexible about the area, as long as it was near enough for family to provide help in an emergency and was somewhere she would feel safe. However, even if Suzanne had been offered the perfect rented house, social services were not initially willing to provide the support she would need. Then when the support arrangements had been agreed, no houses were available.

This catch 22 is common and frustrating. Suzanne's mother had heard that some disabled people had been able to buy their own home. She and Suzanne found a flat – two bedrooms, on the ground floor, near the town centre and a reasonable price. Suzanne's mother was able to help with a deposit, which reduced the loan required to a level where a lender agreed in principle to give her a mortgage. Suzanne is on income support and she can get help with the mortgage interest costs as part of her income support, which gets paid direct to the lender.

Suzanne now owns her own home, and has support staff some of the time who have helped her make connections with local people and local amenities. She is part of the community she lives in.

(Fitzpatrick 2005)

currently located within the owner-occupied sector may therefore offer more choice in types and sizes of housing than the rental options in particular localities.

Generally ownership is worth considering if a person wants to put down roots, if they have a preference for ownership, if they have capital or if they have a secure and regular income, or if their needs are not going to be met in the rented housing sector. Many disabled people and their families will fall into the latter category because of the shortage of accessible housing in other sectors, even if home ownership would not be their first tenure choice. However, the credit crunch has made it much more difficult to access mortgage finance, and to become a first-time buyer. The government has developed shared equity models to help free up the market, and while these schemes should also be accessible to people with learning disabilities, they may face legal and financial barriers.

Home ownership is rarely considered as an option for people with learning disabilities. However, King, 2003 states:

- it may be possible for someone on benefits to get help with the costs of a mortgage
- family members may be willing to make a financial investment in the long-term housing security of their relative
- there are a number of ways of supporting someone with learning disabilities to get through the legal processes involved in buying a house
- good planning can protect a family home for the person to inherit or live in.

There is a distinction between owning a house and buying a house. You can own a house outright via inheritance or as a gift. Acquiring property in this way does not require legal capacity as no contract is involved. However, maintaining, managing and insuring the property does need a level of understanding of the responsibility of ownership. Property that is occupied as the principal home by the receiver or inheritor is not considered as an asset for the purpose of welfare benefits. Owning a house in this way should not affect care and support packages as long as the person is living in, and wishes to be supported to live in, the property as their main or principal home.

The other, and most common, route to ownership is through a house purchase involving a mortgage loan agreement. It is possible for some people with learning disabilities to buy a house with a mortgage and to get help with the costs, if they qualify, through the income support system. This can lead to the person having a greater degree of choice and control, but it is crucial to consider the affordability of such a solution in the short and long term. It is equally important to consider what supports the person will require to manage and maintain the property.

Shared equity schemes

Shared equity schemes – some supported by the government in partnership with housing associations (Homebuy in England and Wales, LIFT in Scotland) and others run by private developers aim to improve access to affordable home ownership. There are eligibility criteria for the schemes. A report for the Office of the Deputy Prime Minister (2002) recognised that it offers a solution for disabled people whose needs are otherwise difficult to meet. The purchaser pays a percentage of the house price (usually between 50% and 80%) and the housing association, developer or government holds an equity share (usually 20–50% of the value), which means they get the money back on sale of the property together with a proportion of any increase in the equity of the home.

Shared ownership

Shared ownership is designed to enable people on low incomes to own their home and is usually targeted at first-time buyers and offered by housing associations. Depending upon the occupier's income, they can claim housing benefit for the charge that they have to pay to the housing association. Some housing associations, Advance Housing in England and Link Group in Scotland, have developed shared ownership products that target the needs of people with disabilities, and situations where families can afford to provide financial help.

Ownership by a trust

Parents may set up a trust to come into being on their death, and which manages funds left for the benefit of the disabled person. A trust can be set up at any time to receive and manage funds or assets such as property for the benefit of a disabled person or persons. A trust may also purchase property. This can offer a route to finding a suitable home for a disabled person. A trust can offer a tenancy, and tenants may be eligible for housing benefit towards rent costs, however this all depends on the terms of the trust (King & West 2002). Any legal or financial transactions need to be carefully considered and expert advice should be sought. Further information can be obtained from the references and websites listed at the end of the chapter.

Supported lodgings or Shared Lives

These are schemes which match the needs of someone with support needs to the housing and care or support offered by a 'Shared Lives carer' (Social Care Institute for Excellence 2006). These schemes can offer short- or long-term accommodation and can suit people who want to live as part of a family.

Group homes or residential care

Some care and housing providers offer shared accommodation, sometimes described as supported housing. If three or more unrelated people share a property, it is more likely to be registered by the Care Commission in Scotland, or Care Quality Commission in England, as a care home. This form of registration means the resident does not have access to housing rights under housing legislation, and residents on a low income or who rely on benefits are left with a far more limited personal income, after care and housing costs are covered, than people who do not live in care homes. Sometimes there may be two or more houses next door to one another, with several people sharing each house and one staff team. There may be 24-hour staffing, staff sleepover arrangements or visiting support depending on the needs of the residents. This type of accommodation suits some people very well – they enjoy having companionship available and are not too concerned that a larger staff group provides care and support. A group home may suit a person at a particular point in their life. In general, though, when people are given an active choice, they do not choose to live with unrelated adults. The first phase evaluation of the In Control approach (2006) found that no one who lived in residential care opted to remain in that setting when given an individual budget to make alternative housing, care and support arrangements.

In a group setting, if the person's support needs change, they may be asked to move, whether they want to or not. A support network of people, friends and advocates, whose only interest is the person, is essential to ensure that their needs are uppermost and that their quality of life is maintained (see also Ch. 9 for further discussion on Circles of Support).

Reader activity 27.6

Browse the best source of comprehensive, impartial and accurate information and advice on housing for people with learning disabilities: Housing Options at http://www.housingoptions.org.uk.

Find out what general and specialist housing advice services are available in your local area, and how often they deal with enquiries from people with disabilities, for example Citizens' Advice Bureaux, Shelter, Disabled Persons' Housing Services.

As with all the options, people change and develop, and should have the right to move if their housing needs and aspirations change over time.

Housing rights

This section of the chapter provides a summary of housing rights in different situations.

Staying in the family home

Someone living in a family home may want to continue living there after the death of a parent, or if their parent or other relative moves to alternative accommodation. Legal rights in this situation depend on whether the person's relatives are or were home owners or renters.

Social rented housing

Two rights are of particular interest where a disabled person lives with a relative but does not have their name on the tenancy agreement:

1. The right to succession allows a carer or relative, who has lived in the house for at least a year as their main home, to 'inherit' a tenancy if the tenancy holder dies.
2. The right to assignation means that a tenancy holder in social housing can pass their tenancy over to someone else, with the agreement of the landlord.

Both of these rights can be used to secure a rented property for a person with learning disabilities, where it has been their main home. Sometimes councils or housing associations may raise questions of capacity, and suggest that the person cannot hold a tenancy because they cannot understand the obligations it brings. There are ways round this and the primary objective should be to ensure the person is not treated less favourably than a non-disabled person would be treated in the same circumstances. While local authorities should be clear about this, they can get this wrong and the person may need the support of an advocate, social worker or solicitor to exert their rights.

See Reader activity 27.7 on the Evolve website.

Other tenancy rights in local authority and housing association property

Registered social landlords offer long-term, secure tenancies. In general, this means that the tenant has the right to stay in the house for as long as they want providing they pay the rent, do not cause unreasonable damage to the property and then refuse to fix it or pay for it to be fixed, and do not cause a nuisance, or show anti-social behaviour to their neighbours.

People with learning disabilities also have the right to live in their home in peace and free from harassment. If people are being harassed or have anti-social neighbours then they have a right to complain to the police and the landlord, and to expect help with resolving the problem.

Sometimes a person may have difficulty understanding a tenancy agreement and entering into a legal agreement. Many housing associations and local authorities have a positive approach and will find ways for people with learning disabilities to rent their own house and have maximum security of tenure.

Occupation rights

Rooms in a shared house (or a group home) may be offered on the basis of an 'occupancy agreement'. This is a contract that tries to give the occupier rights by contract, for example that the landlord would not evict unless they had a court order saying this was a reasonable course of action. However, housing and support are often linked together in these arrangements, with associated risks to housing security if support needs change.

Rights in private rented property

A private landlord usually offers a short-term tenancy. A landlord can decide not to renew a tenancy, but they have to give the tenant notice that the contract is not going to be renewed.

Home-owners

Legal provision for inheritance can be made by Will, and family members should be encouraged to take legal advice about arrangements which will support their family member to remain in the family home, or for the asset to be used for their benefit if this is what they wish.

Adapting a home to suit individual needs

Equipment and adaptations and technology can help people to live more independently, improve their quality of life and assist carers. These can range from minor adaptations such as installation of a wetroom shower, to a whole house fire alarm and sprinkler system, or an extension to provide an additional room. The first port of call for advice is an occupational therapist (OT), usually based within social services. The OT should assess needs and discuss options, including rights to disabled facilities grants (England) or adaptations grants (Scotland) to help with the costs of any adaptations work or community equipment.

The procedures for assessment for an adaptation, and for funding, may vary according to local authority, and who owns the property.

Common issues

People with learning disabilities face a number of barriers in exercising housing choice and in finding a home, or moving home.

Reader activity 27.8

Consult your local authority for information and advice about aids and adaptations. Read the reports and toolkits and get a copy of the Telecare DVD from the Telecare Learning and Improvement Network: http://www.dhcarenetworks.org.uk/IndependentLivingChoices/Telecare

Housing market barriers

Some people with learning disabilities prefer, or need, two bedrooms, one for their own use plus one to accommodate overnight supporters, visitors and/or equipment. Many need housing that is designed or adapted for wheelchair use. There are shortfalls of properties designed for wheelchair users or suitable for people with mobility needs and few systematic approaches to addressing this through the planning system or housing grant systems (DTZ Pieda Consulting 2004). In 2007, a third of local housing strategies in Scotland, had no actions in relation to meeting the needs of people with learning disabilities (ODS Consulting 2007).

There is a limited supply of social rented housing in the right location and of a type to suit. Allocations policies rarely give equivalent weight to the need of a single disabled person for a two-bedroom property as is given to households with children.

Few social landlords, or housing strategies, acknowledge the housing needs of those disabled people who live in group homes and seek greater independence. Assumptions are made, reflected in many allocations policies, that people sharing a home with unrelated adults are 'adequately housed', as are disabled adults living with family members, providing they have their own bedroom. People in these situations find they have very low priority to be considered for their own home and can find themselves trapped.

Financial barriers

Property prices and difficulties obtaining mortgage finance are such that people with learning disabilities, their families and housing or support agencies find it difficult to afford the purchase of suitable housing.

The revisions to the local housing allowance scheme for housing benefit in the private sector add a barrier for disabled people seeking affordable housing in the private rented sector. While claimants can apply for discretionary housing benefit, this is not guaranteed. Research shows that disabled people face higher costs and have lower average incomes than non-disabled people (Smith, N et al 2004), with consequent impact on housing and other choices.

The 'inextricable link' between housing and support

Historically, accommodation and support for people with learning disabilities have been linked, with limited housing rights, tied tightly to care and support contractual arrangements. The Supporting People programme was introduced in 2003 on the back of the Local Government Act 2000, and consequent on a judicial review in 1996, which ruled that general counselling and support could no longer be included in rent covered by housing benefit. This provoked a substantial effort to separate housing rights and costs from support arrangements and the start of a consciousness change for support providers and commissioners about the housing rights of people with support needs.

However, in many cases, especially where people live in shared housing, although the person may have a legal contract giving them housing rights, this is seldom matched with the support and advocacy to assert these. Support agencies may lack knowledge or confidence about housing and housing rights. This can make it easy for support and housing agencies – commissioners, care managers or providers – to revert to custom and practice in shared accommodation. This, in effect, limits the person's rights to 'room rights', denies their rights to transfer or exchange home in the social rented sector, and gives them little meaningful control or choice about co-tenants.

Where a person has significant support needs, their ability to exercise housing choice is notional, unless it is accompanied by truly personalised support arrangements, and creative approaches to the funding for these. The absence of this means that, in many or even most cases, social care and support and housing options are still inextricably linked for people with learning disabilities.

Conclusion

The impact of these barriers is that they increase the likelihood that people will be excluded from ordinary housing experiences. The implications include the following:

- The housing needs of people with support needs are frequently only recognised in a crisis situation.
- The lack of planning means quick and sometimes inappropriate or unsustainable solutions are found, leading to further instability and increased support requirements.
- Scarcity of suitable housing in the social rented sector means people languish on housing waiting lists for many years.
- As younger people's aspirations are to live as their peers, traditional group home settings will become less attractive, yet pressure to fill places will increase in order to keep costs low, with a greater risk of ill-matched people trying to live together.
- Some limited innovative and person-centred approaches to meeting housing needs, such as parents or support providers buying to let, emerge in response to a housing system failure rather than an active desire to be a housing provider.

Flexible and responsive housing policies and systems are therefore as important as flexible and responsive support in enabling inclusion. Housing development, planning and funding mechanisms should make better links between bricks and mortar planning and person- or family-centred future needs planning, especially in relation to wheelchair-accessible housing. Allocations policies that do not take into account the particular needs of people with learning disabilities are not currently seen as an infringement of rights. However, equalities impact assessments should lead to more accessible and transparent policies.

Affordable home ownership schemes recognise the problems in supply of housing for disabled people, but they do not always recognise some of the adjustments that need to be made to accommodate legal and financial issues for people with learning disabilities. However, specialist advice is available and some housing providers have developed particular expertise. Resources and professional expertise are available, but scarce. Better housing information and advice is needed for people with learning disabilities and their families, available within mainstream services and from peers. People may need advocacy and support in order to pursue their preferred housing options.

A place to live is only one step to citizenship. People need trusting relationships and networks of support to make sure it is more than bricks and mortar – that it becomes a safe base for a life well lived.

References

Cox, C., Pearson, M., 1995. Made to care. The Rannoch Trust, London.

Department of Health, 2001. Valuing people: a new strategy for the 21st Century. White Paper. HMSO, London.

Department of Health, 2009. Valuing people now: a new three-year strategy for people with learning disabilities. HMSO, London.

Department of Health, 2010. Ordinary Residence: guidance of the identification of the place of ordinary residence of people in need of community care services, England.

DTZ Pieda Consulting, 2004. Mind the gap: an economic evaluation of owner occupation for disabled people in Scotland. Communities Scotland Report 38, Edinburgh.

Emerson, E., Hatton, C., 2008. People with learning difficulties in England. Centre for Disability Research. University of Lancaster, Lancaster.

Etmanski, A., 2000. A good life. Orwell Cove Planned Lifetime Advocacy Network, Canada.

Fitzpatrick, J., 2005. Thinking ahead: a handbook to help families of people with learning difficulties in Glasgow think about planning for the future and keeping control when circumstances change. SHS Trust, Edinburgh.

Fitzpatrick, J., Butler, V., 2001. Home truths: disabled people's stories and strategies for accessing home ownership. SHS Trust, Edinburgh. Available at: http://ownershipoptions.org.uk/.

Glasgow City Council, 2010. Practical guide for registered social landlords (rsls): housing and autism spectrum disorder (ASD). Glasgow City Council, Glasgow.

Griffiths, R., 1988. Community care: agenda for action. Department of Health and Social Security, London.

Harker, M., King, N., 2004. Tomorrow's big problem: housing options for people with autism: a guide for service commissioners, providers and families. National Autistic Society, London.

Hatton, C., 2001. Developing housing and support options: lessons from research. Institute for Health Research. Lancaster University, Lancaster.

Howe Report, 1969. Report of the Committee of Enquiry into allegations of ill treatment of patients and other irregularities at the Ely Hospital, Cardiff. HMSO, London.

In Control, 2006. A report on In Control's first phase evaluation and learning 2003-2005. In Control, London.

In Control, 2009. A report on In Control's third phase evaluation and learning 2008-2009. In Control, London.

King, N., 2003. New provision for older people with learning disabilities. Department of Health, Housing Learning and Improvement Network, London.

King, N., West, S., 2002. Buying, renting and passing on property – a guide to families in arranging housing for disabled relatives. Housing Options, Witney, Oxford.

Mencap, 2002. The housing timebomb. Mencap, London.

ODS Consulting, 2007. Scotland's approach to housing policy and strategy in relation to disability and race. ODS Consulting, Glasgow.

Office of the Deputy Prime Minister, 2002. Evaluation of the low cost home ownership programme. DTLR Publications, Rotherham.

Office for National Statistics, 2010. Social Trends, No. 40. ONS, London.

Scottish Executive, 2000. The same as you? Review of services for people with learning disabilities. Scottish Executive, Edinburgh.

Scottish Executive, 2002. Promoting health, supporting inclusion. Scottish Executive, Edinburgh.

Scottish Executive, 2006. Changing lives: report of the 21st century social work review. Scottish Executive, Edinburgh.

Scottish Government, 2007. Statistical release. Adults with learning disabilities implementation of 'The Same as You?' across Scotland. Scottish Government, Edinburgh.

Scottish Government, 2009. Housing statistics for Scotland web tables. Scottish Government, Edinburgh.

Smith, N., et al., 2004. Disabled people's cost of living. Joseph Rowntree Foundation, York.

Social Care Institute for Excellence, 2006. SCIE Guide 14: improving outcomes for service users in adult placement – Commissioning and care management. SCIE, London.

Welfare Reform Act, 2009. (C 24), HMSO, London.

Wolfensberger, W., 1998. A brief introduction to social role valorisation: a higher order concept for addressing the plight of socially devalued people, and for structuring human services, third ed. Syracuse University Training Institute for Human Service Planning, Leadership and Change Agentry, Syracuse, NY.

Wood, A., Hall, C., 2008. Making choice based lettings work for people with learning disabilities: a guide for choice based lettings schemes and landlords. Department of Health Valuing People Support Team, London.

Further reading

Advance, 2006. Gadgets, gizmos and gaining independence – assistive technology and people with learning disabilities. Department of Health with Advance Housing and Support, Witney, Oxford.

Department of Health, 2010. Valuing people now and PSA housiing delivery plan 2010–11. Department of Health, London.

Duffy, S., 2003. Keys to citizenship. Paradigm, Liverpool.

Housing Learning and Improvement Network (LIN), 2006. Enhancing housing choices for people with a learning disability. Health and Social Care Change Agent Team, Department of Health, London.

Housing LIN Policy Briefing, 2009. Valuing People Now and housing for people with learning disabilities. Health and Social Care Change Agent Team, Department of Health, London.

Both of the above can be downloaded from: http://networks.csip.org.uk/IndependentLivingChoices/Housing/Topics/tags/?tag=learning%20disabilities.

Useful addresses

Advance is a national charity providing housing and support for people with learning disabilities and mental health problems. It is also a registered housing association, and has been at the forefront of developing shared ownership and other low-cost home-ownership initiatives. It mostly operates in central England: http://www.advanceuk.org

Website for the Housing Learning and Improvement Network. Click on topics and browse by topic: learning disabilities: http://www.dhcarenetworks.org.uk/IndependentLivingChoices/Housing/

Housing Options is an advisory service providing advice for people with learning disabilities, their families and organisations on housing and support options. The website has fact sheets, publications for download or purchase and there is a telephone advice line: 0845 456 1497: http://www.housingoptions.org.uk

The Law Society's website lets you search for a locally based solicitor specialising in mental health and capacity issues, trusts, wills and probate or welfare benefits: http://www.lawsociety.org.uk

Mencap provides services for people with learning disabilities but is also the national charity campaigning, researching and providing advice on a range of issues affecting people with learning disabilities and their families. It has a free helpline: 0808 808 111: http://www.mencap.org.uk

Golden Lane Housing Association is part of Mencap and can be contacted on 020 7696 5521 or 0161 888 1203. It provides housing for people with learning disabilities, including shared ownership and is involved in a number of innovative ways of increasing the housing options, and funding for these, for people with learning disabilities: http://www.glh.org.uk

NAPPS represents the interests of those involved in delivering small, individualised community based services such as Shared Lives and Homeshare: http://www.naaps.org.uk

Ownership Options in Scotland provides advice to people with disabilities, their families and organisations on ownership options. The website has information and contact details. It provides specialist advice and a route for accessing grants to enable disabled people in Scotland to become home owners: http://ownershipoptions.org.uk

Sexual and personal relationships

28

Peter Oakes Ros Davies

CHAPTER CONTENTS

KEY ISSUES

- Sexual and personal relationships are fundamental to an ordinary life for everyone
- Some real progress has been made in helping people with learning disabilities to enjoy positive and healthy relationships
- There remain some important challenges if the aim of an ordinary life is to be achieved
- Members of staff and services have a responsibility to help meet these challenges and there are some good examples of practice to learn from
- It is important to reflect on ways of helping people to get out and meet people in their local area

Introduction

In many ways, services for people with learning disabilities across the UK have set themselves a simple task. Perhaps it was best summed up more than 30 years ago by a King's Fund pamphlet that was to influence policy and practice for many years – *An Ordinary Life* (King's Fund Centre 1980). Other titles have reinforced the message: *Valuing People* (Department of Health (DH) 2001), *A Life Like Any Other* (Joint Committee on Human Rights 2008), *The Same As You?* (Scottish Executive 2000), *Valuing People Now* (DH 2009a) and so on. Each returns to the simple task of enabling people with learning disabilities to have the same opportunities to enjoy life as anyone else.

In setting about this task, practitioners, families and communities have not been without guidance. Various people have felt it necessary to define what an ordinary life might look like. For Wolf Wolfensberger, the founder of the normalisation movement, it means a lifestyle that is valued by the rest of society. People might live in a sought after area or choose the same sort of leisure activities as other people (Wolfensberger 1972). In making policy, there has been more of an emphasis on establishing principles or values that are intended to break down the ideas of an ordinary life into its constituent parts. An influential example of this approach in England has been the four principles of *Valuing People* (DH 2001) and subsequently *Valuing People Now* (DH 2009a): choice, rights, inclusion and independence.

People who work in services and other supporters have been given even more assistance. There has been a raft of techniques and approaches designed to help a person set out what an ordinary life might look like for them and put plans in place to make it happen. These have had various titles all of which fall under the overall heading of person-centred planning (Mansell & Beadle-Brown 2005). Person-centred planning has been extensively described and reviewed (Robertson et al 2006). A significant research project found that when it was possible to implement person-centred planning, there were positive effects in respect of health care and choice for individuals who were involved (Robertson et al 2006).

It is very interesting that few of these initiatives have been explicit about the need to think about sexual and personal relationships. There are statements in policy documents that encourage services to recognise the importance of relationships but these are mainly concerned with existing family relationships and the general idea of inclusion and building links in the community. Approaches to person-centred planning have focused on places to live and opportunities for work and leisure. Opportunities to develop community-based relationships are included but again it is rare to read of discussions about sexuality and sexual expression.

Some might suggest that sexual and personal relationships are simply not the appropriate subject for professional involvement and that these should be outside the sphere of policy and professional practice. There are, however, two reasons why such a position is not tenable. First, the nature of learning disability is such that an individual needs support in all parts of life. People need support to meet people and to develop and maintain intimate relationships. The second reason is that in the absence of meaningful and fulfilling personal relationships, people are at risk of personal, emotional and psychological difficulties that will demand and require the attention of a range of different professionals. In the interests of efficiency and prevention of distress, it seems essential to find practical ways of working alongside people to think about their sexual and personal relationships.

This chapter will begin by exploring the progress that has been made in enabling and encouraging people with learning disabilities to express their sexuality and forge intimate relationships with other people. There is much that is positive here although there remain some important challenges. It will then introduce a series of frameworks that are dominating thinking and service provision at the present time. These may assist us in working towards that strangely elusive goal of an ordinary life: an ordinary life that includes and embraces sexual and personal relationships.

The story so far

The nature of learning disability is that people need support in every part of their lives and this includes support to establish and maintain sexual and personal relationships. This is a relatively straightforward statement of the reality of disability but its implications are profound. In his discussion of human sexuality, Foucault describes our sexuality as the 'truth of our being' (Foucault 1982:7). To be involved in the expression of sexuality for another human being is perhaps the most significant involvement that one person can have in another person's life. It is in responding to this challenge over the past 30 years that some important steps forward have been made.

Person-centred planning and self-directed support

Many new ways of supporting people have emerged from the closure of large institutional services. It seems that only a very small number of long-term hospital-based services remain. More people are living as tenants with supports and services where they are also responsible for their own budgets (DH 2009a). Alongside community-based self-directed support, person-centred planning has made a difference in the lives of many individuals. There are numerous anecdotal reports suggesting that where people have embarked on a close personal relationship with another person, opportunities to establish a long-term partnership and to live together have been found through the person-centred planning process. Connected to this have been initiatives to enhance the social networks and support available to people with learning disabilities. For example, Jo Williams (2005) describes some extraordinary work carried out in Bristol where people with profound and multiple disabilities became the focus of a befriending scheme. Young people were invited to spend time with people with complex learning disabilities. There was neither specific technique nor evidence-based protocol adopted here. People were simply given the opportunity to meet each other and spend time together. Positive relationships were seen to grow from this and these relationships were equally valued by both parties.

Specific education and support

There have been examples of specific pieces of work directed at issues related to sexual and personal relationships. There has been widespread use of sexual education and learning programmes – using both published material such as the Living Your Life pack (Bustard 2003) and also locally developed material. For example, Dukes & McGuire (2009) used Living Your Life to encourage knowledge and ability to consent in four adults with learning disabilities. There were some fears among the direct staff team that the programme might encourage people to become promiscuous or inappropriate in their pursuit of intimacy and sexual expression, however these were shown to be unfounded with three of the four people showing a discernible improvement in knowledge and ability to consent over the later follow up. It was also found that a personal approach was needed rather than the strict adherence to a set programme. Published material is helpful as a structure or guide for working alongside individuals or groups. However, it is important to adapt the material for the individual personalities and situations of the people in the group or the individual who is being supported.

There are countless local initiatives in individual services where people with learning disabilities and members of staff have recognised that sexual and personal relationships are fundamentally important to everyone. Support staff may have worked as a team within a service or perhaps linked up with the local community team for people with learning disabilities and worked together.

Reader activity 28.1

There are sure to be examples of good practice in your area. Try to get in touch with people working in the local community team for people with learning disabilities or any other local forum for services for people with learning disabilities. Ask if people are aware of groups or other pieces of work that have been tried in the local area. It might even be possible to set up a small learning event to gather people who use services and people who work in services to share experiences of positive work and learn from each other.

Sexually challenging behaviour

Where there are difficulties and people have strayed into sexually inappropriate behaviour to the point of committing offences, more work has been required to assess and understand their behaviour with a view to treatment or intervention. Lindsay & Taylor (2005) have reviewed this work and describe attempts to understand sexual knowledge and attitudes in a way that helps an assessment of risk of offending or re-offending. They found that interventions are increasingly orientated toward cognitive behavioural approaches. While there remains a lack of appropriately controlled studies, perhaps the most important aspect of this is that people with learning disabilities are receiving the serious attention of professionals and researchers seeking to address needs for sexual and personal relationships.

Staff attitudes

In an excellent paper about nursing practice, sexual and personal relationships are understood in terms of a holistic model of care (Earle 2001). In respect of sexual and personal relationships, holistic care is seen as encapsulating general support and education through to facilitating sexual intercourse. Practitioners are urged to reflect and consider work in this area noting that staff attitudes are open to this conversation. When asked about their attitudes towards the sexuality of people with learning disabilities, people who work in services are increasingly positive.

Abuse

Less positive but every bit as important has been the growing recognition of the sexual abuse of people with learning disabilities that has continued throughout the development of services. Following on from Brown & Turk's (1992) and Brown et al's (1995) work and the key Department of Health paper *No Secrets* (DH 2000), it can be argued that recognition and response to the abuse of people with learning disabilities has made significant progress. Members of staff are trained in the safeguarding of vulnerable adults and a range of systems are in place to ensure that people who have been involved in the abuse of people with disabilities are not free to work with vulnerable people in other settings. In an effort to prevent abuse, there has also been some work to identify the factors in care and support settings that might put the people receiving the service at risk (Marsland et al 2007).

Health action planning

It has become increasingly clear that people with learning disabilities have other challenges in addition to their disabilities. For many years, people with learning disabilities have suffered serious health inequalities in respect of all aspects of physical and indeed mental health (Krahn et al 2006). Supporting people in respect of their physical and mental health is discussed elsewhere in this text (particularly Chs 13 and 17 respectively), however it is important to note here that sexual health has not been neglected in this work and people have increasing access to general health promotion and intervention work in respect of sexual health.

Positive about parenting

One key aspect of the enjoyment of sexual and personal relationships is the possibility and the opportunity of parenthood. There has been some important work in different parts of the country to embrace the possibility and opportunity for parenthood as something hugely positive in the lives of people with learning disabilities and their families. Work has been undertaken to support and empower parents with disabilities

In a detailed review of this issue, Tarleton et al (2006) note that there is a wide range of support available to families where one or both parent has learning disabilities. These supporters are often based in community learning disability teams and offer assessments, help in the home, skills training and emotional support.

To summarise the progress that has been made in supporting people with learning disabilities to make positive personal and sexual relationships, there follows an example of some work carried out in a community service.

Andrew – Time to get a life

Andrew is a young man with learning disabilities who can communicate using just a small number of single words or noises. He requires physical prompting to carry out intimate personal hygiene. He began to reach out and grab at women who were helping him in the bathroom. It was also very clear that he was sexually aroused when he was reaching out and members of his support staff realised that he had never had the opportunity to learn about appropriate touch. Janet, a local community nurse for people with learning disabilities, and Dave, one of the support workers, got together and planned a session using the Living Your Life pack (Bustard 2003). The chapter headings were really useful but they soon realised that they would have to do a lot more thinking before they could get started. The approach had to be personal for Andrew and would involve adapting the material and thinking through a lot of other issues.

The first thing they did was to think about whether Andrew would work best with other people or on his own. It also meant thinking about whether they were the right people to do the work. It was not possible to ask him so they took photos of all the people he spends time with and showed the pictures to him on a board. They recorded whether he used happy sounds when he saw the pictures. Then they waited for a week and asked another member of the support staff to run through the same pictures to see whether he responded in the same way. He made happy noises for Janet and Dave and for three members of staff. He did make a happy response to the pictures of one of the two other people who shared his flat. The responses were the same on both occasions.

Janet and Dave then met to talk about the work so far. Andrew was in the room with them and they referred to him respectfully and used pictures to explain when they could. It seemed important to both of them that even though it was not possible for him to understand the whole discussion, he was there as a reminder about who this was about. They decided that actually Andrew was quite a private person who did not like too many people around him and did not respond well when there were more than two other people with him. It seemed best to start the work with just Janet, Dave and Andrew in the group.

Andrew – Time to get a life—Cont'd

They looked through the Living Your Life pack to get an idea of the ground they needed to cover. As everyone was anxious about the difficulties with female staff in the bathroom, they decided to start on teaching appropriate behaviour. The pack also helped them to see that they could not just leave it there!

The work began with agreeing a shared language and a way of communicating about sex. This step is essential for everyone undertaking work relating to sexuality and sexual expression. It is necessary when people use spoken language for a practitioner to use the language a person is most comfortable with. For Andrew it was a question of pictures and photographs. These were used alongside two faces – one to signify something that is OK and one to signify something that is not OK. The pictures included explicit photographs of people and explicit line drawings. Everyone had to get over their embarrassment and usually did this by laughing. It was important also for the manager of the service to be closely involved to make sure that no one was put in a position of feeling uncomfortable or of acting against their personal ethics.

They covered appropriate behaviour and inappropriate behaviour, and followed this with some sessions designed to help Andrew feel comfortable about his own body. He was encouraged to explore his own body in private. This was important as he seemed to have been taught that masturbation was not OK. The emphasis here was taking time to encourage and understand private behaviour. Each topic took at least three sessions and involved taking many opportunities to check understanding. All sessions involved moving around the house. Where the session talked about behaviour in the bathroom either alone or with a member of staff, the three people went to the bathroom to help explain. Being private also involved moving into Andrew's room and helping Andrew experience time in his room alone.

The final sessions covered all aspects of staying healthy but had a focus on sexual health. Andrew was unable to understand the idea of checking for signs of testicular or prostate cancer and it was agreed to feed this into his health action planning work. Regular checks at his local health centre were set up to cover this and it was felt that a male nurse or doctor would be best placed to carry out these particularly intimate procedures.

During the sessions there was a strong sense that Andrew wished to meet someone and to enjoy an intimate relationship with that person. In talking about this, it was immediately clear that he had no opportunities to do this. It was decided to complete the programme of work and then meet as a team to think about the next steps. Once again they could not just leave it there! Questions to consider included the following:

- Janet remained unsure about whether Andrew was able to masturbate successfully and questioned whether more help would be required and how this might be achieved.
- There had been no further problems in the bathroom, but Dave wondered whether Andrew would be best supported by male staff members in intimate care.
- Notwithstanding all this, the most important question was how can Andrew meet people with a view to exploring sexual and personal relationships in real life? This may lead to supporting Andrew in a long-term relationship.

All is well?

In considering this growth in awareness, positive attitudes, practice and opportunity, it would seem reasonable to suggest that a chapter such as this is no longer necessary in a text book that seeks to introduce practitioners to the needs, hopes and wishes of people with learning disabilities. Andrew's story would seem to reassure us that all is indeed well. Practitioners are now fully engaged in the kind of work that would lead to people with learning disabilities enjoying the same journey through personal and sexual relationships as anyone else. This is far from the case as can be seen from the work that still needs to be done. It seems that we can't just leave it there!

The fall and rise of institutional care

The project to replace large long-stay institutions with small ordinary community-based support seems at first glance to have been a success. In their influential annual review for 2009, Laing & Buisson (2009) report that the number of people with learning disabilities who receive home-based care has more than doubled in the last 7 years – rising from 16 000 to 33 000. The same period has seen the number of NHS placements for people with learning disabilities cut by more than 1000 from 5400 to 4100. This is a substantial reduction from the 65 000 people who were living in long-stay hospitals when the project began. However, the same report points to continued growth in secure provision for people with mental health problems and learning disabilities. Across the NHS and the independent hospital sectors, this has increased by more than 2500 places from 3400 to 6000. There are also some 5000 beds in independent hospitals for people with either mental health problems or learning disabilities. New regulations mean that these settings are increasingly gender segregated yet the length of stay is often measured in years rather than weeks or months. It is unlikely that positive and healthy means of sexual expression will be possible in these settings and it will be a significant challenge to nurses and other professionals to recognise the impact of this lack of opportunity for individuals who find themselves living in this way.

The rise of abuse awareness

Increased understanding and recognition of abuse has been an important and positive step forward for many people with learning disabilities. It has meant that the risks of falling victim to sexual harassment, exploitation and abuse may have reduced and people are safer than they were. At the same time, support staff and services have perhaps become suspicious of close personal relationships and reluctant to take positive risks in the interests of warmth, intimacy and personal fulfilment in relationships. This was seen in the immediate reaction of staff to the sexual education programme discussed earlier (Dukes & McGuire 2009). There is often a raft of policy and protocol designed to protect people and maintain boundaries where the end result is a cold and clinical isolation. The development task for staff and clinicians is surely to enable people to negotiate the various protocols safely and maintain the opportunities for closeness and sexual expression.

Person-centred planning

Person-centred planning received a significant boost through government policy throughout the UK. It remains central to *Valuing People Now* (DH 2009a) and continues to be influential through *The Same as You?* in Scotland (Scottish Executive 2000). It was seen as a means by which services could be organised in the interests of the individuals they are supposed to be supporting. Person-centred planning has two essential elements: first a group of people gather in support of the individual. The person is at the centre of the group or circle of people which might include family and friends working alongside paid workers. The second element is the organising of support and services to respond to the needs, hopes and wishes of the individual. A large study was conducted in the UK to explore the implementation and effectiveness of person-centred planning (Robertson et al 2006). There were important positive results for some people in terms of improved contact with family, choice and the extent of and satisfaction with social networks. These were more likely to occur in places where person-centred approaches and key working practices were already in place. There were also some more challenging findings. Despite involvement of key consultants and a significant amount of extra resource, it was only possible to establish viable person-centred plans for 65 of the 93 people who took part in the study. While there was an increase in social networks, these were not inclusive and tended to remain restricted to members of staff, other people who use the same services and family members. In fact, inclusive social networks where there was the possibility of meeting people and enjoying sexual and personal relationships actually reduced. There was no evidence of an impact of person-centred planning on sexual and personal relationships or indeed whether these issues were addressed at all. In conclusion, the authors of the study report that person-centred planning is helpful but not sufficient to achieve some of the ordinary life goals shared by people regardless of whether they have a learning disability (Robertson et al 2006).

Meeting people and making friends

As part of the development of new services, a number of researchers have studied the relationships that people with learning disabilities are enjoying in new community provision. The results are consistent and they show that people with learning disabilities continue to struggle to establish a positive network of relationships. For example, Forrester-Jones et al (2006) conducted a 12-year follow-up study, exploring the social networks of 213 people with learning disabilities who had moved from long-stay hospitals. They note that there is some improvement on other studies but that two-thirds of all relationships were with people who were in some way connected to learning disability services. Relationships were reported to be close and longstanding but mainly with people with whom sexual and personal relationships would be problematic. The paper calls for services to work to provide opportunities to meet and learn to interact with people. It is interesting that such work continued to be necessary after 12 years of community-based care for people who were seen as relatively able and independent.

Being and becoming parents?

Some of the work to support people with learning disabilities to be parents has been covered as a positive part of the progress made by services in recent years. There is also, however, another side to this work as it has not been possible to provide consistent support to parents with varying disabilities. In 2009, the Commission for Social Care Inspection published a report on the support received by parents with different disabilities and included parents with learning disabilities in their findings (Commission for Social Care Inspection 2009). The report found inconsistency in support across the country and identified a key change that needed to take place if things were to improve. Perhaps because of the separation of adult and child services, it was found that the approach to families with disabled parents was fragmented and unable to see the family as a whole. The paper called for an integrated approach where parents and children are assessed as a family to ensure everyone is kept safe and has the opportunity to receive the support they need.

Contraception

When considering matters of parenthood, it seems that the opportunities for people with learning disabilities to make choices and be in control of their bodies are restricted at an earlier stage. An excellent research paper by Servais et al (2002) explored the use of contraception by women in Belgium. It describes a population-based study of 97% of women with learning disabilities aged between 18 and 46 years attending government-funded facilities in Brussels and a nearby province in Belgium. The researchers compared the use of contraception by women with learning disabilities with a matched group from the general population.

Out of 397 women surveyed, 40.8% did not use any contraceptive method, 22.2% were sterilised, 18.4% used an oral contraceptive agent (OCA), 17.6% used depot medroxyprogesterone acetate (DMPA) and 1% used an intra-uterine device (IUD). It was immediately apparent that this profile of contraceptive use differed widely from the one of the general Belgian population. Women with learning disabilities were:

- less often using contraception (60% versus 68%), with the contraceptive method:
  - less often an OCA (18.5% versus 46%) and
  - more often sterilisation (22.2% versus 7%) or DMPA (17.6% versus <2%).

When the authors of the report explored the differences in more detail, it seemed that decision making with women with learning disabilities was based on institutional factors and protocols rather than individual factors such as personal health status, preferences or lifestyle. It seems that the choice of contraception was simply not driven by personal or medical factors in the same way it is for women who do not have learning disabilities.

The need for a new framework

It seems that that while we have been successful in closing the institutions, there remains a good deal of work to do before the goal of enabling people to live an ordinary life is achieved. It is now possible to explore ways in which modern supporters and services can address issues of sexual and personal relationships for people with learning disabilities. This can best be done using a new framework that has four main elements. Each element is designed to help services and supports build on success up to now and address the challenges that remain. They reflect a modern approach to services where we shift the focus from buildings and structures towards a new relationship between people with learning disabilities and the people who support them (DH 2009a).

Human rights

Services and supports work to ensure that people with learning disabilities have the same protection and opportunity afforded to them as anyone else. This framework has been adopted in a number of modern policies such as *Valuing People Now* (DH 2009a).

Health

This involves seeing health in its widest sense in line with the definition of health given by the World Health Organization (WHO 1948). Sexual and personal relationships are seen as part of a holistic response to health. How can modern supports and services ensure that people stay healthy as they explore new opportunities for sexual and personal relationships?

Power

The idea of power is a more robust idea than that of choice or control. Power speaks of the relationship between people. Foucault defines power as any relationship where the actions of one person influence the range of possible actions of another person (Foucault 1982). It is clear that paid workers and families are in a position of power especially in respect of sexual and personal relationships and the opportunities to pursue those relationships. It will be important to explore ways that professional workers can negotiate that position of power.

Belonging

There are two aspects to this – first, the extent to which people with learning disabilities have the opportunity to be part of a community: be it a community of disabled people, a family community or a local community. Sexual and personal relationships are a key sign that people belong and opposition to sexual and personal relationships between two people is often found where people are not seen as belonging to the same community. The second aspect of this is the need to ensure that specific groups of people are not excluded from mainstream work to enable people to make and maintain close personal relationships. In particular, a theme of valuing people in England (DH 2001) is to ensure that specific groups such as people from ethnic minorities; people with severe and profound learning disabilities; people with severe challenging behaviour; and people on the autistic spectrum are being included in work to support close personal relationships.

These four elements make up a new framework for all modern practice in supporting people with learning disabilities (Fig. 28.1). It has been shown that they have specific relevance when thinking about sexual and personal relationships. The remainder of this chapter deals with each element in more detail and gives some specific ways in which practitioners can understand and apply the framework with a particular focus on health and wellbeing.

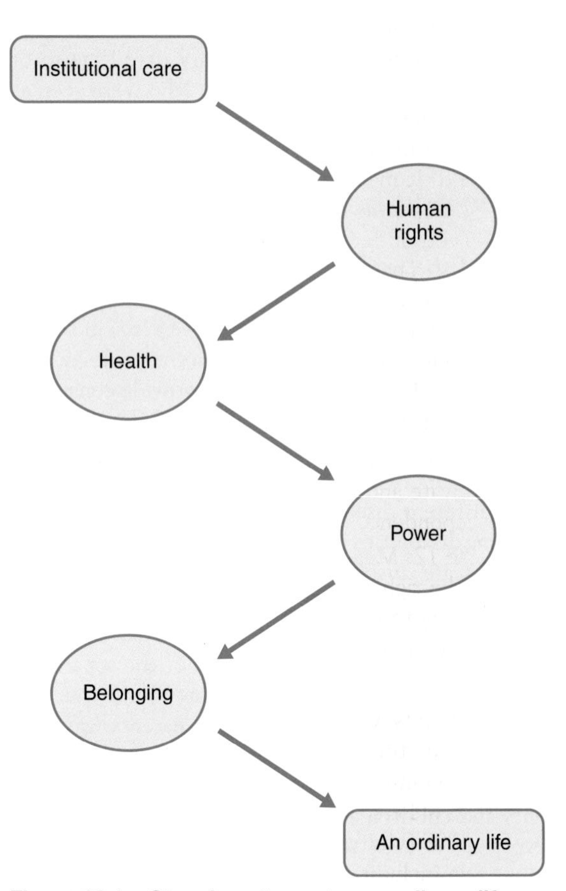

Figure 28.1 • Stepping stones to an ordinary life

Human rights framework

One of the earliest legal cases relating to human rights occurred in the United States and concerned a first-nation American known as Standing Bear. The case of Standing Bear vs. Crook arose because of an attempt to insist that a group of first-nation Americans living in Florida should move to North Dakota. Standing Bear did not wish to move and so returned to his home in Florida. Marshall Crook, who sought to arrest Standing Bear and return him to North Dakota, brought the case. The case turned into an argument about the extent to which Standing Bear was a human being. The conclusion, brimming with irony, was that Standing Bear was indeed fully human, and as such he was subject to the US law, and would therefore have to live where the Marshall directed under the law (Standing Bear vs. Crook, 18 April 1879). Since that time, human rights legislation has moved on to establish an international standard for the treatment of all people. In the UK, the Human Rights Act 1998 came into force in October 2000. Essentially this involved the government adopting all but a small number of the rights contained in the European Convention for the Protection of Human Rights and Fundamental Freedoms

(Council of Europe 1950). It is expected to have a number of implications for people with learning disabilities. This is especially so given that actions can be brought under the Act when services or individuals have not ensured that an individual's human rights are upheld. It may be that failure to provide opportunities for people with learning disabilities will be the subject of legal challenge under the Human Rights Act. The implications of this in the field of sexual and personal relationships remain untested.

This lack of testing cannot be said to arise from a lack of relevance. At least three articles are directly relevant to the support of people with learning disabilities and their sexual and personal relationships:

- Article 8: Everyone has the right to respect for his private and family life, his home and his correspondence.
- Article 12: Men and women of marriageable age have the right to marry and to found a family, according to the national laws governing the exercise of this right.
- Article 14: Prohibition of discrimination.

(Human Rights Act 1998, Ch. 42 Schedules – articles)

Moreover there has been more recent progress from the United Nations where the Convention of the Rights of Persons with Disabilities came into force in May 2008 (United Nations 2008). This convention is clear in including people with learning disabilities and is consistent with the general declarations of human rights. Article 3 sets out the inherent dignity of people with disabilities and article 6 calls for the specific empowerment of women with disabilities. In article 23, however, there are some specific points made about sexual and personal relationships:

> States Parties shall take effective and appropriate measures to eliminate discrimination against persons with disabilities in all matters relating to marriage, family, parenthood and relationships, on an equal basis with others, so as to ensure that:
>
> (a) The right of all persons with disabilities who are of marriageable age to marry and to found a family on the basis of free and full consent of the intending spouses is recognized;
>
> (b) The rights of persons with disabilities to decide freely and responsibly on the number and spacing of their children and to have access to age-appropriate information, reproductive and family planning education are recognized, and the means necessary to enable them to exercise these rights are provided;
>
> (c) Persons with disabilities, including children, retain their fertility on an equal basis with others.
>
> (United Nations 2008:15–16)

What then are the practical implications of working within a human rights framework when thinking about sexual and personal relationships? There are two ways we can practise in respect of human rights. The first is relatively clear cut and deals with practice that denies the human rights of a person. This means reflecting on any aspect of practice that restricts the freedom of a person to exercise their human rights. The second area of practice is where professional staff fail to ensure that the *opportunity* exists for a person to exercise their human rights. This means developing practice that gives people with learning disabilities experiences and opportunities that enable them to exercise their human rights.

Thinking of the need to respect private and family life, there are some important implications here. People who receive services can have every aspect of their lives opened up to the scrutiny of others and this can occur at many different levels. Perhaps a person may enjoy unusual sexual practices or have a secret hope to make a relationship with someone else. It is important for a member of staff who comes across issues such as these to be able to talk them through with someone and perhaps receive guidance and supervision. This would, however, mean seeking permission for such discussion and ensuring that where a person is unable to understand or give permission, great care is taken about how information is shared and recorded. This would include the number of people who have access to personal or private information. Is it really necessary for an entire community team or direct staff team to know every intimate detail about a person's sexual fantasy or yearning to connect with another person?

Turning to the opportunities to exercise human rights, there is a substantial task here. If people are not able to either make or take opportunities to meet people and develop close personal relationships, then it is incumbent on professional staff to help with this. The issues are as practical as knowing about or organising events where people might be able to meet each other – paying attention to the essentials of transport and staff support or personal assistance. In addition to this there may be the need to encourage and support people through teaching and talk about relationships and how they work. This would include the various responsibilities that people have when involved in relationships of a sexual and personal nature. For example, in a study of the sexual knowledge of people with learning disabilities, many people were unaware of consent and other aspects of the law in respect of sexual relationships (O'Callaghan & Murphy 2007).

There remain some excellent resources to support this kind of work including the revised Living Your Life pack (Bustard 2003) while Gardiner & Braddon (2009) describe a more recent and successful teaching programme for adults with learning disabilities in Ireland.

See Reader activity 28.2 on the Evolve website.

In concluding this section about Human Rights there is an approach to making judgements about supporting people in respect of their sexual and personal relationships that can assist us. This comes from the foundations of the Human Rights Act itself. The story of Standing Bear demonstrates that everyone shares a common humanity. This means that we can use our own ideas and experience to assist in some of these judgements. How much information would I want to be shared with other people and who would I want to know about this part of my life?

Health framework

In a superb international review of the health inequalities faced by people with learning disabilities, Krahn et al (2006) remind us that the separation of the concepts of health and disability was not really achieved until relatively recently. Likewise, a review of the role of nursing professionals in respect of sexual and personal relationships adopts the approach of the WHO in promoting the inclusion of sexuality within health care, arguing that all individuals should be able to enjoy and control sexual and reproductive behaviour with freedom from fear, shame, guilt and false beliefs (Earle 2001). This thinking all springs from the idea of health as mental, physical and social wellbeing as opposed to the absence of disease.

There is a range of issues that arise from using a health framework for sexual and personal relationships. These include managing risk and ensuring adequate protection through the maintenance of sexual health to supporting people with learning disabilities who become parents. These issues will be considered in turn and this section includes a practice highlight piece on communicating with people with learning disabilities about sexual health.

Risk and protection

The primary responsibility of professional staff and services remains to protect vulnerable people from harm. It has already been made clear that there is a genuine risk of sexual exploitation or abuse among people with learning disabilities and there are numerous reports to suggest that people continue to experience abuse at the hands of paid workers, other people who use services and members of family and the wider community (see Ch. 12 for a more detailed exploration of these issues).

Here the challenge is to protect but not to overprotect. Perhaps the most important part of positive risk taking is the sharing of risk decisions and ensuring that single professionals or professional groups are not left alone in assessing risk around issues such as these. It is to be hoped that joint working can maintain a sense of positive risk taking in times where ensuring safety can lead to restrictions that are beyond that which other groups are expected to deal with.

A further aspect of risk and protection is supporting people with learning disabilities who have committed sexual offences. This involves the protection of individuals with disabilities and the wider community. At one time it was thought that such protection should be achieved by the incarceration of large numbers of people with learning disabilities in hospital settings. The closure of institutions has been an important step in moving away from such misguided social policy. Likewise there continue to be large numbers of people with learning disability caught up in the prison system where there is no opportunity to access appropriate care and support. This has been addressed in the Bradley Report (DH 2009b). However, for people with learning disabilities who have committed crimes of a sexual nature, there is beginning to be some progress and there are a number of specialist health care services available.

Lindsay & Taylor (2005) review the recent work and describe advances in the assessment of sexual knowledge and attitudes towards different sexual practices. This is mainly in an attempt to understand sexual knowledge and attitudes in a way that helps assessment of risk of offending or re-offending. The paper goes on to evaluate interventions for people with learning disabilities who commit sexual offences. Taken together, this work suggests that members of staff can work to share positive risk taking with the person and with each other. Such work can continue on the basis of robust assessment and an emerging group of evidence-based interventions.

Parenting support

Leading on from the wide ranging issues of sexual health, a recent survey of the lives of adults with learning disabilities in England found that one in

15 adults had a child and that 48% of those parents were no longer caring for their child (Emerson & Hatton 2008). This is a disturbing figure and concern over this issue in recent years has led to a number of research projects and service initiatives. In a comprehensive review of these studies, Tarleton et al (2006) have identified the key issues that need to be addressed in every area, not just the places where professionals have taken an interest. First and foremost, all professionals have a duty to protect children and young people. Given this overriding concern, there remains a good deal that can be done to make systems work for families where a parent has learning disabilities. There are four simple steps to be discerned from research and experience:

1. Values: address prejudice and assumption about the ability of someone with a learning disability to be a parent. It is essential to establish that intellectual ability does not correlate with parenting ability in any meaningful way.
2. Model: research calls for a support model rather than a deficit model to be adopted. This means working with families to identify the kind of support that is needed to ensure that the child grows up in a loving, healthy and stimulating environment.
3. Standards: it continues to be important to establish standards and ideas about what makes up the notion of 'good enough' parenting and to identify the skills and knowledge that are needed to be a parent.
4. Pathways: there is often confusion about care pathways for families where parents with learning disabilities need support. This begins with access to generic services. Families can find it difficult to access voluntary support groups, parenting classes and playgroups. If a referral is made to childcare agencies, they need to be aware of the essentials of communication and support for an adult with learning disabilities who is a parent. If further specialist support is required from people trained in working with people with learning disabilities, it is important to ensure that there is some consistency in this and that evidence-based assessment and intervention are available.

People who are said to be on the autistic spectrum

Before leaving the topic of health, it is important to mention a group of people who may need specific attention. In recent years, the number of people who are identified as being on the autistic spectrum has risen enormously. It includes people with and without learning disabilities and there is a mountain of research and writing about this group of people, the reasons why the numbers are growing and the best ways to support them. This might be seen as thinking and research that is at an earlier stage than for other groups and it seems that issues of sexual and personal relationships are not being addressed very widely. Perhaps the emphasis on 'diagnosis' is leading to the same confusion between health and disability that we have seen in other forms of disability during the earlier stages of research and thinking.

Thankfully, there are some writers who have worked to remind us that people with autism or Asperger syndrome are to be understood as people first and are more than able to experience the same feelings and need for intimacy as anyone else. The desire to enter into the full range of relationships may be hard to uncover sometimes but this is no reason to assume it is not an important issue for the person. The additional difficulties in communication may simply mask the need for closeness and relationship.

Two books have addressed this issue and carry practical and conceptual information. Wendy Lawson is a psychologist who has written from personal experience about sexuality and negotiating sexual relationships. This is a powerful and important book for people with an interest in this area (Lawson 2005). Lynne Moxon has written a chapter in a book about people with Asperger syndrome, also establishing the importance of these issues and giving practical ideas about ways to support people (Moxon 2006).

The message from the limited material available is very clear. We may be overtaken by technical responses to people on the autistic spectrum and ignore the need to think about sexual and personal relationships. Indeed, many of our ideas about the experience of people on the autistic spectrum might promote such an approach. Such a limited, clinical approach would be to deny the essential humanity and relatedness of all people and lead to some serious difficulties in the future.

Power framework

The third framework vital to developing community-based services and addressing fully the challenges of an alternative to institutional support is a framework of power. This is subtly different from ideas of choice and control as it implies that there is an exchange of power rather than a giving of control. Many of the current approaches we adopt as professionals demonstrate this difference. There are examples in day-to-day practice and in the planning of support where people are offered choices and given opportunities to be in control. The words tell the story here. As a person with learning disabilities, I do not have the power to make changes in my life or keep my life as it is. Rather I am given choices by someone more powerful than I am. Those choices tend to be limited by the views and values of the other person or the current policy in my local authority or national government.

There are two ways of understanding this issue further and challenging our practice to reflect this important change in perspective. Both involve listening to the voices of people with learning disabilities. Bramston et al (2005) explored the importance of various elements of quality of life for young people with learning disabilities compared to people who aren't disabled. When asked how satisfied they were with different parts of their lives, intimacy was rated significantly lower in people with learning disabilities than other young people. It would seem reasonable to expect that among those given power to direct the resources available to them, the pursuit of positive intimate relationships might have more prominence in the goals and outcomes that are set. It is important to reflect on how this might influence the content of person-centred planning meetings and other ways in which we work with people to plan support.

It seems that listening to people with learning disabilities reveals the same range of passions and insecurities as are found anywhere else. Some people have got themselves organised. In East Sussex, a group of people with and without disabilities have organised a campaign to play and enjoy live music, meet new people and stay up late (Heavy Load 2009). This is about having fun, enjoying the company of other people, getting close, challenging the middle-aged lifestyle lived by so many people who use services and making the odd mistake. But there is a danger here. In reading this account, it is tempting to assume that the staying up late campaign gives a solution for everyone. This is patently not the case and the challenge is to all services to think about staffing rotas, times and transport – the extent to which it is practically possible for people with learning disabilities to get out, have fun and meet people.

Belonging

In many ways this final framework represents a summary of the other three. The essence of our human nature is that people exist in relationship with other people. A legal and human rights framework is needed to protect and enhance the ways in which people, communities and countries can live and work together. It is clear from research on health and well-being that a sense of belonging in family or other close group and community is an essential part of positive health for people whatever their status, age or disability. Only in communities where issues of power are addressed and, if necessary, kept in check can there be a sense of belonging that in turn enables power to be enjoyed and potential realised.

In respect of people with learning disabilities who use services, the matter of belonging needs to be addressed at different levels. More broadly, this means community and inclusion. There remains a challenge to enhance a sense of belonging in the wider community and it is increasingly being recognised that being part of a community of people with disabilities is not to be devalued. There is no reason whatsoever why having a friend or a lover who is also disabled is in any way inferior to a friend or lover who is not seen as disabled. It is simply a question of there being opportunity to belong.

On a different level, the idea of belonging relates to the sense of belonging that is fundamental to sexual and personal relationships. These relationships carry a unique opportunity to go beyond sexual expression and gratification and reach towards a personal belonging that is perhaps one of the heights of human experience.

Conclusion

This chapter has built on much of the progress that has been made for some people with learning disabilities in respect of sexual and personal relationships. Having taken stock of this progress, a new framework for practice has been introduced. This framework is based on an analysis of what is needed to move away from institutional practice rather than see it perpetuated in community-based buildings. The framework has four elements – human rights, health, power and belonging. If services are able to address the issues raised in each element of the framework, this will lead to truly, personalised support. This, in turn, may bring the simple idea of an ordinary life a little closer.

Practice highlight box

Communicating key sexual health messages to people with learning disabilities

The prospect of talking about sexual matters with others can be daunting, but to avoid the subject when working with people with learning disabilities is not an option. By creating an environment where people feel comfortable in sharing their questions and concerns, a practitioner can enable a person to learn what they need to know and make choices which will keep them physically and emotionally safe.

Setting the scene

A conversation about sex may come about spontaneously as a result of a question or comment, but most of the time there is opportunity for some preparation. Careful preparation can make the difference between an awkward or hurried exchange, and a useful discussion where an individual can question and learn in a safe and relaxed way.

Although this practice highlight focuses on conveying facts and information, a discussion about sex is likely to (and should) include talking about feelings and emotions. Issues of choice, consent or even abuse may arise, so it is important to be prepared for this possibility and to think through what may be of particular concern for any individual or couple.

If working within a team, the first issue to consider is who is the best person to talk through such issues? Is there a staff member whom a person responds particularly well (or badly) to? Is the gender of the person important? A one-to-one conversation can work well but there may be situations when involving a second professional may be appropriate. An observing 'chaperone' may be reassuring to the individual and also the member of staff, especially if there is any risk of discussion around intimate issues being misinterpreted in any way.

It is worth taking time to plan a good time and place to talk, without distractions or interruptions. However, while dedicated time is important, creating anxiety or apprehension about an impending 'big talk' needs to be avoided. It is often better to carefully prepare and plan for an unannounced, 'spontaneous' chat.

When planning the direction of any conversation about sexual issues, the following key questions should be considered:

- What does the individual know already?
- What do they want to know?
- What do they need to know?

Common ground – a shared language and getting the facts right

Even if a person talks with confidence about sex, it is crucial never to assume their knowledge is accurate. Equally, do not assume that a nod or a 'yes' implies understanding of your statements or questions. By gently asking the person to talk to you about what they already know, and by asking them what they mean by the terms you and they are using, you will be able to find out their level of understanding and become aware of any important gaps.

Take time to find out what words and phrases an individual prefers to use when talking about sex, and use them yourself in your conversation. In a topic where words, for example for genitalia, are seemingly endless, it is important to be speaking the same language!

Depending on a person's previous experience of talking about sexual matters, you may find that a discussion produces a range of reactions. One person may be shy or embarrassed while another may find it amusing. It is important to 'roll with' these reactions and not to challenge them. Showing that you are relaxed yourself will be helpful and reassuring.

Starting with the very basic facts is important; it would be meaningless to talk about contraception if a person had no understanding that intercourse could result in pregnancy. There is a wealth of 'sex education' material available and what you choose will depend on the individual. Do not be concerned about making use of books and other resources aimed at children and young people; the simpler messages and more straightforward illustrations in these resources can be more helpful than those in an adult text book.

So then, learning and revising key facts around sexual relationships and reproduction can be a good way of establishing common ground. It is then possible to cover any of the key issues in sexual health. Here we consider two areas that are perhaps the most common topics where effective communication is vital:

Contraception

Although formal contraceptive advice and prescription for such is given by those with specific training, it is useful to be aware of the different choices available. Information given at GP surgeries and family planning clinics can be complicated and prove a lot to remember; the role of the practitioner in explaining this further, and perhaps accompanying an individual or couple to an appointment, is very important.

Once again, be aware of the language when talking about contraception and avoid using medical terms (ovulation, menstruation, ejaculation ...) unless you are certain they will be understood. The physiology and pharmacology involved is complex but does not need to be understood in detail by the contraceptive user. Keep your explanations simple and relate the scientific mechanisms to something a person can relate to. For example, it is easy to see how a woman may have difficulty understanding how an injection or plastic rod in her arm will prevent pregnancy, but she may be familiar with the concept of having a vaccination to prevent a disease.

Choices in contraception have widened greatly in recent years. With such variety it can be tempting to make a choice on behalf of people with learning disabilities, focusing on what we think would be best. While such intentions may be helpful, it is better to provide the individual with a range of choices wherever possible.

Even if hormonal contraception is the preferred choice, it is worth teaching everyone how to use a condom. A condom

Continued

Practice highlight box—Cont'd

is the only form of contraception useful in preventing sexually transmitted infection (STI), so encouraging condom use in addition to another method should be done routinely. As a barrier method, the way in which a condom prevents pregnancy is more easily understood than with other forms of contraception. This in itself is a good reason why teaching condom use is a good place to start. If possible, use a condom demonstrator to teach how to use a condom properly. People often find this an amusing activity, and it is a very useful tool in checking understanding and technique – both crucial for effective condom use.

Contraceptive pills (both combined and progesterone only) are, like the condom, entirely dependent on the user for their effectiveness. For some people, supervision of medication may be an option, but for many it will not be appropriate. If a pill is the preferred choice, the importance of taking it properly must be stressed. Taking a pill every day is not easy. Suggestions to aid memory such as mobile phone alerts and keeping the pills with the toothbrush are simple, and can make the difference between successful pill taking and an unplanned pregnancy.

Long-acting, reversible contraception (LARC) is the new buzzword in contraception. These methods include IUDs and the contraceptive implant and injection. They offer highly effective contraceptive cover for long periods (up to 5 years in some), without being user dependent. For many women these are a very good option. However, the irregular and sometimes prolonged bleeding common in the early use of progesterone-only hormonal methods (used in most LARCs) can be troublesome for many, and this is the most common reason for changing from these methods. Preparation, explanation and reassurance are key to their successful long-term use.

In the past, the permanent option of sterilisation was often the only 'contraceptive choice' offered, and sometimes imposed, on people with learning disabilities. With the advent of newer, effective long-term methods, male and female sterilisation are perhaps considered less often, but should not be forgotten as an option for some. Clearly, as with counselling anyone considering sterilisation, the irreversible nature of the procedure needs to be stressed and the individual's consent very carefully demonstrated.

Prevention and screening

As with contraception, discussion around STIs and other health problems can provide an opportunity to get bogged down in medical terminology and complicated biology. This, combined with a risk of nurturing fear or even guilt, does not always make for the easiest of conversations. While people should be aware that infections can be contracted through sexual activity, information should be given in a way that does not blow the risk out of proportion, or create unnecessary anxiety. For many, the risk of contracting STIs will be low.

Prevention of STIs with condom use as previously discussed is vital to reinforce. People should also be encouraged to discuss any concerns about symptoms such as discharge or dysuria (pain passing urine). The cause of these may not be a sexually transmitted infection, but this may need to be excluded. If a person is felt to be at risk then screening tests should be discussed and offered. Urine testing now offers a quick and easy screen for chlamydia, but other tests will involve taking swabs which for females will require a vaginal speculum examination. For most women, anxiety about the examination itself is the main reason why testing was declined. Once again, preparation and reassurance are crucial if a woman's experience is not to be a negative one. When explaining what the examination involves, it may be helpful to show a woman a vaginal speculum. This can appear a frightening implement (although less so now that the majority are plastic and disposable). Allowing a woman to see the speculum and reassuring her that most of it comprises the handle with only the smaller, smooth end being inserted into the vagina, can relieve anxiety.

Clearly, a similar approach can be used when preparing a woman for a cervical screening test. Cervical screening rates in women with learning disabilities have traditionally been low. As well as increased awareness of the needs of people with learning disabilities among health professionals, women will need careful explanation, support and reassurance if rates are to improve. Human papillomavirus (HPV) infection is one cause of cervical cancer and routine vaccination is now offered to all young women in the UK.

Testing for blood-borne infections including HIV will be appropriate in some cases. Issues around these screening tests are complex and pre- and post-test counselling should be carried out carefully. Consent to testing is essential and the best interests of the individual, bearing in mind the implications of a positive test, should always be considered.

Changing needs, continuing conversation

It will not be the case that 'everything you ever wanted to know about sex' will be imparted during a couple of carefully planned sessions (think for a moment about your own learning of the subject). Of course, if there is an urgent need for a person to have quick information about contraception, for example, then this should be done. However, discussion and learning about sexual issues should be ongoing.

Revisiting conversations and carefully checking understanding will not only help learning, but will also create an environment where questions and concerns can be raised as circumstances and needs change. A woman approaching the menopause will have different needs to a young person discovering their sexuality, but the principles of providing relevant, accessible information while reassuring and listening to concerns remain the same.

References

Bramston, P., Chipuer, H., Pretty, G., 2005. Conceptual principles of quality of life: an empirical exploration. J. Intellect. Disabil. Res. 49 (10), 728–733.

Brown, H., Turk, V., 1992. Defining sexual abuse as it affects adults with learning disabilities. Mental Handicap 20 (2), 44–55.

Brown, H., Stein, J., Turk, V., 1995. The sexual abuse of adults with learning disabilities: report of a second two-year incidence survey. Mental Handicap Research 8 (1), 3–24.

Bustard, S., 2003. Living your life: the sex education and personal development resource for special needs education, revised ed. The Ann Craft Trust UK, Brook Publications, London.

Commission for Social Care Inspection, 2009. Supporting parents with disabilities: a family or fragmented approach. CSCI, London.

Council of Europe, 1950. The European Convention on Human Rights. Council of Europe, Rome.

Department of Health, 2000. No secrets: guidance on developing and implementing multi-agency policies and procedures to protect vulnerable adults from abuse. DH, London.

Department of Health, 2001. Valuing people. CM 5086. HMSO, London.

Department of Health, 2009a. Valuing people now: a new three-year strategy for learning disabilities. HMSO, London.

Department of Health, 2009b. The Bradley Report. DH, London.

Dukes, E., McGuire, B., 2009. Enhancing capacity to make sexuality-related decisions in people with an intellectual disability. J. Intellect. Disabil. Res. 53 (8), 727–734.

Earle, S., 2001. Disability, facilitated sex and the role of the nurse. J. Adv. Nurs. 36 (3), 433–440.

Emerson, E., Hatton, C., 2008. People with learning disabilities in England. CeDR Research Report. CeDR, Lancaster.

Forrester-Jones, R., Carpenter, J., Coolen-Schrijner, P., et al., 2006. The social networks of people with intellectual disability living in the community 12 years after resettlement from long-stay hospitals. J. Appl. Res. Intellect. Disabil. 19 (4), 285–295.

Foucault, M., 1982. The subject and power. In: Dreyfus, H.L., Rabinow, P. (Eds.), Michel Foucault: beyond structuralism and hermeneutics. second ed. University of Chicago Press, Chicago.

Gardiner, T., Braddon, E., 2009. 'A right to know'. Facilitating a relationship and sexuality programme for adults with intellectual disabilities in Donegal. British Journal of Learning Disabilities 37 (4), 327–329.

Heavy Load, 2009. Stay up Late Campaign. Available at: http://stayuplate.org/ (accessed on 14 July 2010).

Human Rights Act, 1998. Elizabeth ll. Chapter 42. (1998). The Stationery Office, London.

Joint Committee on Human Rights, 2008. A life like any other? Human rights of adults with learning disabilities seventh report of session 2007–08, vol. I. The Stationery Office, London.

King's Fund Centre, 1980. An ordinary life: comprehensive locally-based residential services for mentally handicapped people. King's Fund Centre, London.

Krahn, G., Hammond, L., Turner, A., 2006. A cascade of disparities: health and health care access for people with intellectual disabilities. Ment. Retard. Dev. Disabil. Res. Rev. 12, 70–82.

Laing & Buisson, 2009. Mental health and specialist care settings. UK market report 2009. Laing & Buisson, London.

Lawson, W., 2005. Sex, sexuality and the autism spectrum. Jessica Kingsley, London and Philadelphia.

Lindsay, W., Taylor, J., 2005. A selective review of research on offenders with developmental disabilities: assessment and treatment. Clinical Psychology and Psychotherapy 12, 201–214.

Mansell, J., Beadle-Brown, J., 2005. Person centred planning and person centred action: a critical perspective. In: Cambridge, P., Carnaby, S. (Eds.), Person-centred planning and care management with people with learning disabilities. Jessica Kingsley, London, pp. 19–33.

Marsland, D., Oakes, P., White, C., 2007. Abuse in care? The identification of early indicators of the abuse of people with learning disabilities in residential settings. Journal of Adult Protection 9 (4), 6–20.

Moxon, L., 2006. Diagnosis, disclosure and self confidence in sexuality and relationships. In: Murray, D. (Ed.), Coming out asperger. Jessica Kingsley, London and Philadelphia.

O'Callaghan, A., Murphy, G., 2007. Sexual relationships in adults with intellectual disabilities: understanding the law. J. Intellect. Disabil. Res. 51 (3), 197–206.

Robertson, J., Emerson, E., Hatton, C., et al., 2006. Longitudinal analysis of the impact and cost of person-centred planning for people with intellectual disabilities in England. American Journal on Mental Retardation 111 (6), 400–416.

Scottish Executive, 2000. The same as you? A review of services for people with learning disabilities. HMSO, Edinburgh.

Servais, L., Jacques, D., Leach, R., et al., 2002. Contraception of women with intellectual disability: prevalence and determinants. J. Intellect. Disabil. Res. 46 (2), 108–119.

Tarleton, B., Ward, L., Howard, J., 2006. Finding the right support: a review of issues and examples of positive practice in supporting parents with learning difficulties and their children. The Baring Foundation, London.

United Nations, 2008. Convention on the Rights of Persons with Disabilities. United Nations, New York.

Williams, J., 2005. Achieving meaningful inclusion for people with profound and multiple learning disabilities. Tizard Learning Disability Review 10 (1), 52–56.

Wolfensberger, W., 1972. The principle of normalization in human services. National Institute on Mental Retardation, Toronto.

World Health Organization, 1948. The definition of health. WHO, Geneva.

Further reading and resources

There is a wealth of material available to people who wish to read more about these issues or access specific resources. In researching this chapter, however, it has also been very apparent that practitioners in local areas are often carrying out some excellent work that may or may not get published more widely. Perhaps the first thing to do is to find out about such initiatives. People might respond to a simple e-mail or phone call. Others may come to a practice development and learning session. These can be a simple shared lunchtime through to a full day. It is rarely the case that the only good work is being done by published 'experts' in special centres that everyone has heard of!.

Further reading

For a first-hand account of a woman on the autistic spectrum who describes her encounters with issues of sexual and personal relationships, Wendy Lawson's book *Sex, Sexuality and the Autistic Spectrum* is excellent (see Reference list).

The Ann Craft Trust, continues to lead the way in terms of reading and resources that are available from their website: http://www.anncrafttrust.org.

The Norah Fry Research Centre, has also conducted and published some very important research in the area of parenting support, social networks and the experience of people with learning disabilities who are lesbian, gay or trans-sexual: http://www.bristol.ac.uk/norahfry.

Resources

The Living your Life *(Bustard 2003, see References) material continues to prove useful in explaining and exploring sexual and personal relationships.*

Also the Family Planning Association (FPA) has produced a range of material specifically aimed at supporting people with learning disabilities in this area of their lives: http://www.fpa.org.uk.

Finally: don't forget to look in on campaign material produced by people with learning disabilities themselves. The Stay up Late Campaign is a great place to start: http://stayuplate.org.

Growing older: meeting the needs of people with learning disabilities

29

Rob Jenkins Marion Steff

CHAPTER CONTENTS

KEY ISSUES

- The number of older people with learning disabilities is likely to continue to rise
- A range of professionals deal with the growing complexity of need that some older people with learning disabilities may present
- The lifestyle of older people with learning disabilities is often poor with little physical activity and an unbalanced diet
- Healthy living advice and interventions need to start in childhood and across the lifespan into old age
- Currently older people need to be made aware of the benefits of healthy ageing

Introduction

There is little doubt that people generally are now living longer due in part to enhanced social conditions, improved access to health systems and better medical care (World Health Organization 2000). The Office for National Statistics (2009) states that:

> Life expectancy at birth in the UK has reached its highest level on record for both males and females. A newborn baby boy could expect to live 77.4 years and a newborn baby girl 81.6 years if mortality rates remain the same as they were in 2006–08.

This increase in life expectancy is also reflected among people with learning disabilities whose lifespan is now in some instances comparable to the population at large and as such poses new challenges for professionals and services. It has been estimated that the number of people with learning disabilities aged above 60 years will show an increase of 36% between the years 2001 and 2021 (Foundation for People with Learning Disabilities 2010). In the past, people with learning disabilities tended not to survive into older age due to physical ailments and lack of appropriate health and social care (Hubert & Hollins 2000). There is a suggestion that ageing starts earlier in

Table 29.1 Factors which might present a challenge to healthy ageing in people with learning disabilities

Factors	Evidence
Genetic	Down syndrome generally leads to premature ageing and early onset of Alzheimer's disease although not all individuals will be affected (Schupf 2006).
Degree of learning disability	Individuals with severe and profound learning disabilities often do not reach old age due to the presumption that they have more severe associated disorders and neurological deficits (Patja et al 2000).
Health issues	People with learning disabilities generally may be more susceptible to particular health-related problems such as cardiovascular, respiratory, mobility, gastro-intestinal, as well as risks of epilepsy, obesity, mental health, hearing and visual impairment (DH 1995, WHO 2000).
Unhealthy lifestyles	People with learning disabilities often lead unhealthy lifestyles, which contribute to the development of physical ailments in later life (Barr et al 1999). Obesity levels are also higher in this group of people (Rimmer & Yamaki 2006).
Accessing health care	People with learning disabilities have difficulties accessing appropriate health care and can die prematurely (Mencap 2007, Michael 2008).
Employment	Approximately 90% of people with learning disabilities are unable to gain employment (DH 2001a). This may impact on people with learning disabilities being able to enhance their income, skills, social status, activity levels as well as developing friendships (Jenkins 2002).

individuals with learning disabilities as a group of people. The Department of Health (DH 2001a) suggests that ageing should be regarded as starting around 15 years earlier (50 years) compared to that of the general population (60–65 years). Bigby (2004) explains that although people with learning disabilities go through the same ageing process as the general population, they do however experience unique and distinctive challenges. Jenkins (2005a) highlights factors which might present a challenge to healthy ageing in people with learning disabilities (see Table 29.1).

Obviously the specific factors highlighted in Table 29.1 will not concern all people with learning disabilities and they will also not be affected in the same way. Positive ageing in people with learning disabilities is further determined by general factors such as gender, pre-existing health conditions, social class, geographic location, income, poverty, housing, culture, diet, activity level and genetic factors. Any older individual with learning disabilities has the potential to influence some of these factors such as lifestyle choices that can include diet and exercise. There is no specific policy for older people with learning disabilities and much of the implicit policy guidance is contained in documents such as the *National Service Framework for Older People* (DH 2001b) and *Valuing People* (DH 2001a) and the updated version *Valuing People Now* (DH 2009).

Understanding the ageing process among people with learning disabilities

There has been very little research into understanding of the ageing process from the perspective of the older person with learning disabilities. Bigby (2004) argues that this group of individuals age prematurely and their voices are seldom heard. Research which has been carried out to ascertain the views of this group has shown varying results. Erickson et al (1989) found a variety of views from fear of unemployment to fears about dying. There was also some acknowledgement of ageing factors such as loss of mobility and friendships, increasing illness and a decrease in exercise. Other research has tended to focus on mainly health issues (Edgerton et al 1994). Thompson (2002) carried out qualitative research with a group of older adults with learning disabilities (n = 162) on their views regarding ageing and change. He found that participants did not have major concerns regarding the physical changes associated with ageing; however, they did have concerns with issues such as changing family circumstances and service provision. Older people with learning disabilities also have concerns regarding older family carers (Bowey & McGlaughlin 2005).

Case illustration 29.1

David is a 49-year-old man with moderate learning disabilities who has lived with his parents all of his life. He has had to endure a great deal of negativity and discrimination due to the label of learning disability. He has never had a period of paid employment, a partner and his only friendships are those of his parents. He stopped attending a day service when he was 35 years old as he was continually teased about his health problems (poor eyesight, cognition, memory, hearing and mobility). His parents have been very protective of him and have controlled his exposure to experiences, relationships and information which they feel may harm him.

It could be argued that some older people with learning disabilities may not notice the transition into old age as any different from the experience of adulthood. There is an assumption that people with learning disabilities view the world the same as people without a learning disability. In many respects this may well be the case, however, as we can see in Case illustration 29.1, for some the transition may be somewhat tempered or not noticed at all. This is because this group already experience some of the changes and losses associated with older age – negativity, poorer health, lack of friendships, employment, status and cognitive decline. More research is required from the perspective of the older person with learning disabilities in this area to gain a better understanding (Jenkins 2010).

Physical health of older people with learning disabilities

Older people with learning disabilities generally succumb to the same physical deterioration in ageing as the general population (Holland 2000, Janicki et al 2002). However, Holland (2000) states that although there is a levelling out in terms of health and social care needs between the general population and people with learning disabilities in later life, there are still differences in physical health needs. Physical ill health is relatively common among older people with learning disabilities (Cooper & Holland 2007). It has been identified that specific sub-groups of people with learning disabilities have particular health risks. For example, older people with Down syndrome are at increased risk in later years from the early development of visual and hearing disorders, Alzheimer's disease and epilepsy. Older people with Fragile X syndrome have higher rates of epilepsy, visual disorders, mitral valve prolapse, early menopause and musculoskeletal disorders (WHO 2000). Other factors increasing physical health risks include lifestyle, environmental conditions and accessibility to health care and promotion. Jenkins et al (1994) states that people with learning disabilities are more at risk of physical disorders and diseases such as sensory defects, cancer, diabetes and fractures. Older people with learning disabilities are also more susceptible to musculoskeletal, respiratory, cardiovascular and neoplastic illnesses (Day & Jancar 1994). However, it should not be assumed that ill health is inevitable as much can be done to mediate the effects of ageing. In terms of social health, Barr (2001) feels that ageing may well impact on areas such as maintaining social roles and networks, adapting to new roles, managing transitions, exercising rights and social value. Professionals will need to support older people with learning disabilities to deal with changing family dynamics as ageing also impacts on others. The loss of supported employment and day service may impact on the individual's activity level and friendships. Other losses impacting on social health have been given as bereavement and maintaining a sense of independence (Barr 2001).

Reader activity 29.1

Consider the type of life David (Case illustration 29.1) has led in relation to the transition into older age. What would be the difference for him (biologically, psychologically and socially) as he moves from adulthood into old age?

Mental health of older people with learning disabilities

Psychiatric disorders are common among older people with learning disabilities due to additional risk factors stemming from old age and a learning disability (Cooper 1999). The increase in psychiatric disorders in older people with learning disabilities can be attributed to the ageing process and associated social changes (Holland 2000). These added risks arise from vulnerability issues such as neurological changes, sensory impairments, pain, loss of confidence, bereavement, deteriorating physical health and diminishing social networks and activities (Luty

& Cooper 2006). It was reported by Hubert & Hollins (2000) that the higher rates of psychiatric disorders include dementia, anxiety, depression, affective and delusional disorders. However, Cooper (1999) explains these disorders occur at similar rates to those found in younger adults with learning disabilities and calls for more research into differences between older and younger people with learning disabilities. She acknowledges there are difficulties in accurately diagnosing psychiatric disorders in older people with learning disabilities, adding it is necessary for clinicians to have a good understanding of the disorders among older people with learning disability. One such condition is dementia.

Dementia

Dementia in older people with learning disability poses significant challenges to the individual concerned, services and carers. Dementia is four times higher in older people with learning disabilities aged over 65 years compared to similar aged people of the general population (Cooper 1999). However, many symptoms pass unrecognised, especially among people with learning disability without Down syndrome (Strydom et al 2005).

It is well recognised that there is an association between Down syndrome and Alzheimer's disease (Hutchinson 1999) with McCarron (1999) stating that virtually all individuals with Down syndrome aged over 35 years have neuropathological changes characteristic of Alzheimer's disease. Coppus et al (2006) provide dementia prevalence rates for individuals with Down syndrome as:

- 45–49 years: 8.9%
- 50–54 years: 17.7%
- 55–59 years: 32.1%
- 60+ years: 25.6%.

The detection of dementia among people with learning disabilities remains difficult due to a lack of appropriate assessment tools and baseline assessments (Llewellyn et al 2008) as well as few trained staff, poor care continuity and little experience (Watchman 2003). However, resources, while not abundant, are available. For example, Prasher et al (2004) developed criteria for dementia screening in people with Down syndrome while Markar et al (2006) developed a memory clinic to facilitate assessment and diagnosis. They argue that family members and carers need to be involved with professionals in assessing symptoms. Diagnosis, however, may be further compounded if the individual is also suffering from depression, hypothyroidism, sensory impairments, infection and toxic effects of medication (Hutchinson 1999). Regular assessments of the individual's abilities are essential in order to always have a baseline measurement to assist in the detection of conditions such as dementia. Lane (2005) argues that professionals should carry out lifelong physical and psychiatric reviews of people with learning disabilities to make the medical detection of dementia more accurate. As mentioned earlier, parents and carers should be encouraged to keep records of people they care for so that valuable information is not lost if they die or have to give up caring.

Hutchinson (1999) suggests that the clinical features of Alzheimer's-type dementia in individuals with Down syndrome are different compared to the general population. In Down syndrome, there is a decline in personality, behavioural and daily living skills before a decline in cognitive functioning. In some cases, there is also a late onset of epilepsy. Dementia in this client group occurs 30–40 years earlier in life (Holland 2000) and its duration tends to be around 3–6 years when compared to persons in the general population of 2–15 years (Hutchinson 1999). The onset of dementia can bring on feelings of despair and a sense of hopelessness for carers. The challenge facing professionals is to restore a sense of hope and optimism into the lives of those affected through a process of empowering the individual. McCarron (1999) offers nurses specific interventions on communication, which may enhance the quality of life of individuals with dementia. Both Kerr & Wilkinson (2005) and Dodd et al (2009a) offer practical advice to carers and support staff on how to support individuals in areas such as behaviour and emotions, daily living skills and care issues in the later stages of dementia. There is a need for collaboration between services and professionals due to the complexities that mental illness presents in people with learning disabilities (Barlow 1999).

The development of dementia among older people with learning disabilities provides challenges for professionals in terms of housing. For example, their current location may need to be adapted to cater for their changing condition or they may need to be moved to a specialist service. McBrien (2005) provides local data from Plymouth which indicates that most people with Down syndrome over the age of 55 with dementia (95%) are in residential care. While specialist provision may be suitable in dealing with individuals in the terminal stages of ageing or dementia (Cosgrave et al 2000), there is growing support for the concept of 'ageing in place' (Kerr et al 2006). It means that support structures are developed for the ageing individual so they can remain at home. Kerr et al (2006) suggests, for instance, outreach services, better staff training and waking night staff. Janicki et al (2002) discuss the use of a responsive dementia support programme which focuses on service design and agency planning. The ECEPS model has five parts:

E – Early screening and diagnostics
C – Clinical support
E – Environmental modifications
P – Programme adaptations
S – Specialised care.

Kerr et al (2006) report on a study commissioned by the Joseph Rowntree Foundation – *Home for Good* – on three different types of support. The first which has been described earlier is ageing in place. The second is 'in place progression' in which the environment is developed to become specialised in providing care. The third type of support is 'referral out' which involves moving the individual into long-term nursing care usually outside the learning disability service. Due to the complexities presented by people with learning disabilities who develop dementia, it is unlikely that one single model or type of support will be appropriate to all. However, it is likely that learning disabilities services and professionals will play a key role in the care of this client group. To assist this process, a panel of experts wrote a set of principles for people with learning disabilities who have developed dementia to ensure that their rights and needs are addressed (see Box 29.1).

In Wales, Aneurin Bevan (formally Gwent NHS Trust) Health Board developed a dementia care pathway in 2005 to support people with learning disabilities and their carers. The aims were to address areas of diagnosis, coordinated approach to assessment and intervention, planning, monitoring and support. Jenkins et al (2009) undertook a two-phase study exploring aspects of staff training in dementia and carers' experiences of the dementia care pathway. In phase one, training had a positive impact on knowledge, confidence and competence levels of staff and, in most cases, this was maintained in the 6-month follow up. It is reassuring as staff on the front line need this knowledge and confidence in order for the early detection of dementia in older people with learning disabilities. Phase two highlighted that the aims of the care pathway were largely being met. However, carers stressed a lack of clarity regarding which activities relate to the pathway. They also felt they needed to be kept informed, receive flexible services and have their views listened to. The study concluded that in order for the pathway to be effective, more information should be given to carers on the range of interventions available and increasing their contributions to developing the pathway.

Box 29.1

The Edinburgh Principles

1. Adopt an operational philosophy that promotes the utmost quality of life of people with intellectual disability affected by dementia, and whenever possible, base services and support practices on a person-centred approach.
2. Affirm that individual strengths, capabilities, skills and wishes should be the over-riding consideration in any decision making for and by people with intellectual disability affected by dementia.
3. Involve the individual, her or his family and other close supporters in all phases of assessment and services planning and provision for the person with an intellectual disability affected with dementia.
4. Ensure that appropriate diagnostic, assessment and intervention services and resources are available to meet the individual needs and support the healthy ageing of people with intellectual disability affected by dementia.
5. Plan and provide supports and services which optimise remaining in the chosen home and community of adults with intellectual disability affected by dementia.
6. Ensure that people with intellectual disability affected by dementia have the same access to appropriate services and supports as afforded to other people in the general population affected by dementia.
7. Ensure that generic, cooperative and proactive strategic planning across relevant policy, provider and advocacy groups involves consideration of the current and future needs of adults with intellectual disability affected by dementia.

(Wilkinson & Janicki 2002)

Healthy ageing

Healthy ageing is the development and maintenance of optimal mental, social and physical wellbeing in older people. The concept does not differ for people with learning disabilities who experience the same age-related conditions as their counterparts without disabilities such as reduced mobility, sensory loss and falls. The slower functional, motor and cognitive responses found regularly among ageing individuals with learning disabilities can be explained in part by a poor lifestyle with little physical activities and an unbalanced diet (Robertson et al 2000). A poor lifestyle can result in early onset of disease and symptoms linked to ageing, low level of fitness, as well as obesity and its related conditions (e.g. type 2 diabetes, hypertension, heart disease, stroke, arthritis, respiratory diseases and cancer). In general, people with learning disabilities tend to be less physically active, often not achieving the 30 minutes of moderate activity per day that is recommended for individuals of all ages to acquire psychological and physical health benefits (Rimmer 2005). Older adults should do at least 150 minutes of moderate-intensity exercise throughout the week (WHO 2010). Conditions encountered such as fatigue, weight gain and pain are often substantially higher among people with learning disabilities. They have a significant obesity issue with the propensity to be more overweight than individuals without learning disabilities (Rimmer & Yamaki 2006), undoubtedly compounded by the prevalence of poor diets with a high percentage of fat calories (Robertson et al 2000). However, other research has reported lower levels of smoking and alcohol abuse in individuals with learning disabilities compared to the general population (Taylor et al 2004).

Barriers to healthy ageing

In the general population, barriers to healthy ageing are mainly the lack of motivation in being physically active as well as the lack of money and time (Alliance for Aging Research 2010). Steff (2009a, b) interviewed 48 older people with learning disabilities to understand the barriers they encountered in leading an active lifestyle. They identified eight environmental barriers hindering access to the regular practice of a physical activity. These were:

1. distance to travel to physical activities
2. lack of accessibility of sports and leisure centres
3. activities not always offered in winter
4. centres hard to use
5. complexity of the equipment
6. lack of space to practise at home
7. lack of equipment
8. busy schedule.

Psychologically, older people with learning disabilities worried about hurting themselves, were concerned they would be assaulted or have something stolen. They also felt some discomfort being in a sports centre with strangers to practice physical activity and feared looking out of place. In terms of social barriers and self-determination, older people with learning disabilities highlighted the lack of a partner, a model or coach to encourage them and, ultimately, the interest and motivation for the activity. Finlayson et al (2009), in a larger study (n = 433) of adults with learning disabilities of which 34.4% were aged over 55, found some different predictors of low levels of activity. These included faecal incontinence, immobility, epilepsy, living in a residential or nursing home and no daytime opportunities.

Overall, Steff (2009a) explained that older people with learning disabilities had a modest but naïve understanding of what is meant by being active and healthy. They understood the importance of exercising and were active, according to their own standards. However, they believed that if they exercised they will lose weight immediately. They also interpreted being healthy as continuing to work because they did not have to remain in bed. To some degree this is true, but the ability to go to work is a very restricted view of health. Ageing was not a worry as most participants did not grasp its meaning clearly. While some individuals expressed justified concerns (e.g., scared of getting older, pain never experienced before), becoming older did not bring pragmatic changes to their lives. As they aged, their routine stayed identical; they did not retire and were not provided with age adaptations. It is not only older people with learning disabilities who lack knowledge in this area but also carers. Melville et al (2009) found that carers generally had a low level of understanding around the importance of diet and physical activity in health gain. They identified the need for carers supporting adults with learning disabilities to have training in the promotion of healthy lifestyles.

Facilitating healthy ageing among older people with learning disabilities

Recently, there have been attempts to include the views of older people with learning disabilities in regards to what they would like from health care professionals. Fender et al (2007a), in a small-scale study of five older adults with Down syndrome, found that these individuals were capable of communicating what they wanted from their doctor in the GP surgery. Interestingly, they shared their perspective on what being healthy meant to them through their own personal experiences and that of their parents. Participants demonstrated some understanding of areas for health improvement such as healthy eating and exercise. The research conducted by Steff (2009a) in Canada also found that older people with learning disabilities tended to adopt a social model of health when consulted. The 48 participants generally expressed their views of health in functional and social terms such as being able to move about, make a bed and shovel snow. Older people with learning disabilities rated their health as good or excellent although professionals were less optimistic. In terms of exercising, Steff found that older people with learning disabilities recognised the healthy value of exercising. Some participants explained they could not exercise as they had done when they were younger. Professionals indicated that the implications of ageing in older people were not recognised in re-adaptation centers (rehabilitation service providing professional support in areas such as assessment, activity and respite care), let alone the necessity for older people to be physically active (Steff 2009a). User-led approaches have also been developed for older people with learning disabilities when assessing health. A focus group of individuals with learning disabilities (40+ years) influenced the development of a health assessment tool with the inclusion of items reflecting a wider view of health such as hobbies and interests, self-care, participation in activities, diet and being able to do things (Fender et al 2007b). What is emerging from recent research (Starr & Marsden 2008) is that older people with learning disabilities view health as something more than the mere absence of disease and therefore their standpoint is more comprehensive. Future health assessments therefore may need to take a broader view of health to reach older people with learning disabilities: for example, focusing more on what the individual can do for themselves rather than what is beyond them. Health professionals undertaking such assessments need to clearly state how the physical examination links into the overall picture of health.

Presently, it is necessary to address health-related activities to optimise the ageing of people with learning disabilities, to prevent age-related functional impairments and to counteract the adverse effects of risky behaviours. Health reports emphasise the need for more studies about healthy ageing and older adults with learning disabilities. For instance, the World Health Organization (2000:19) advocates an "appropriate and ongoing education regarding healthy living practices in areas such as nutrition, exercise" while Heller et al (2002:10) encourage the development and evaluation of "health promotion programs encompassing health behavior education, nutrition, and physical activity". Empirical research studies (Carmeli et al 2005, Mactavish & Searle 1992, Mann et al 2006, Podgorski et al 2004) strongly suggest older people with learning disabilities benefit physically and psychologically from healthy living interventions and should be made aware of the benefits of healthy living throughout their life. Heller et al (2006) created a successful educative programme promoting the importance of physical activity and good nutrition. While the resource does not focus particularly on older people but for all individuals with learning disabilities, it can be easily implemented and adapted to be used as a guide for professionals. Staff are provided with effective tools to put into practice, including handouts, worksheets, games and newsletters. The results were encouraging with staff becoming more interested in the programme and participants more active and aware of the importance of healthy eating.

Reader activity 29.2

What are the activities that could be implemented with Sarah (Case illustration 29.2) in order to respect her pace and age while still making her aware of the importance of healthy living?

Case illustration 29.2

Sarah is a woman aged 70 years old, with mild learning disabilities. She had been living in an institution but was moved to an adult placement home 10 years ago. Sarah goes every day to a leisure-based centre where she paints. A few years ago, she was offered retirement which would result in her staying at home all day. Sarah refused, worried about being bored. This year, she accepted to be part of a new health programme where she practises physical activity every Tuesday for 2 hours and she learns about a balanced diet every Thursday, also for 2 hours. Sarah does not smoke or drink. She has difficulty walking due to a hip problem. She is also obese and has a tendency to agree to everything in order to please everyone. She has avoided physical activity for most of her life and does not know how to swim.

Quality of life

As people with learning disabilities age, there is a risk that their quality of life may diminish due to reduced mobility, increased health problems and cognitive decline. The definition of quality of life is subjective and depends on the individual's perception, needs, experiences and the knowledge of his/her own possibilities. Mainly, quality of life is an organising concept to guide policy and practice to enhance the life of everyone. It is composed of the following core domains: physical, psychological, level of independence, social relationships, environments, and spirituality/personal beliefs (Schalock et al 2002). The concept of quality of life remains the same for everyone, with or without learning disabilities (Schalock 1996). However, older people with learning disabilities are more likely to be less empowered, poorly self-determined with little decision-making powers or to have control over their lives. Schalock et al (2002) highlight that people with learning disabilities, when supported, can fully become self-advocates and participate in equality, choices and inclusion matters. They can be involved in studies not just as mere subjects but as research participants. To continue improving the quality of life of people with learning disabilities, particularly older individuals who have never been empowered to decide for themselves, Schalock et al (2002) suggest that carers implement programme-based quality techniques related to the core domains highlighted above. This can be achieved in the following ways: emotional wellbeing (provide positive feedback and safe environments), interpersonal relations (facilitate friendships and relationships), material wellbeing (support ownership), personal development (organise stimulating activities), physical wellbeing (assist healthy ageing), self-determination (encourage choices, control and decision) and social inclusion (offer least restrictive environment).

There are a number of advantages to using quality of life as a conceptual framework for determining the needs of older people with learning disabilities. First, the use of the concept of quality of life is growing in importance in both services for older people (Bond & Corner 2004) and learning disabilities (Schalock 1996). Second, Keith & Schalock (2000) state that the concept of quality of life can act as a sensitising notion in giving a sense of reference from the perspective of the individual. There is little reason why this should not be extended to include carers and professionals in determining need. Third, Renwick et al (2000) highlight that the concept of quality of life can be directed in a person-centred fashion. Person-centred planning is seen as a key aim in major policy initiatives for both older people (DH 2001b) and people with learning disabilities (DH 2001a, 2009). Fourth, Northway & Jenkins (2003) argue that the use of quality of life can form the basis for collaborative care planning. Jenkins et al (2006) have developed a model or framework of care which utilises the concept of quality of life in a person-centred manner in residential care settings. It ensures that the voices of the clients, carers and advocates can be heard and acted upon when professionals organise and plan care for people with learning disabilities.

Older carers of people with learning disabilities

Ageing people with a learning disability are likely to outlive their parents who are often their primary carers. The majority of people with a learning disability live in the community with their families and, in later life, usually with one parent – their mother (Hubert & Hollins 2000). It has been estimated that a third of people with learning disabilities who reside in the family home are cared for by a family member who is over 70 years of age (DH 2001a). The health of ageing carers is at risk with higher prevalence of chronic health conditions (e.g. arthritis, high blood pressure, obesity) as well as activity limitations due to a number of factors which include taking care of their health as well as the individual they care for, the length of caring and concerns regarding the future (Yamaki et al 2009). McGrath & Grant (1993) highlight that the level of professional support tends to diminish with ageing; there is also a reduction in family support networks leading to increased household isolation. Life changes and choices by older carers put a strain on their relationship as the individual with learning disability ages (Maggs & Laugharne 1996). Cooper & Holland (2007) state that older people with learning disabilities are unlikely to have close family members care for them once their parents have died. However, research in Australia by Bigby (1997) found that when parents relinquished care, a small informal network of carers supported the older person with learning disability. Often parents would nominate a 'key person' to provide support for their son or daughter when they died. This was necessary because people with learning disabilities seldom marry or have children and consequently lack the two key likely providers of informal care in later life (Bigby 1997).

The loss of parents often results in the loss of vital information about the life of the person with a learning disability as parents seldom make records about their children. Consideration should be given to contingency plans if the key person or networks falter. Health and social services should work together to support and manage the process of ageing of both client and carers (Maggs & Laugharne 1996). The mutual interdependence of families and the individual with learning disabilities they support is now recognised (Walker & Walker 1998). Thompson (2007) argues that there are a number of important factors which need to be addressed in this area such as families ignoring their own health needs and the fact that the level of support from extended family members and others may diminish over time. Thompson (2007) also highlights the poor communication between families and services and the great worries of families about the future care of their relatives. Similar factors were also indicated in Northway et al (2006) in a study exploring the hopes and fears of parents and family carers of people with learning disabilities. They recommend that care managers should provide timely, accessible and accurate information in a pro-active manner to families and carers. Mechanisms for involving parents and carers in planning should be reviewed to improve the consultation process.

Planning with parents regarding their future wishes seems essential in ensuring that major disruption in the lives of their son or daughter is minimised. Parents may wish to keep some control over the future of their sons and daughters even if they move out of the family home (Davys & Haigh 2007). A key ingredient in this process is to encourage parents to maintain and develop records or diaries of their children so that vital information is not lost when they die (Jenkins 2000) (see Ch. 8 on Personal Narrative and Life Story). This is particularly important when assessing the mental health status of people with learning disabilities. Baseline assessments are needed in order to detect changes in areas such as dementia, to know whether there has been a deterioration or improvement in the individual's abilities. Thompson (2007:229) provides an overview of successful interventions which have assisted supporting older family carers. They include:

- a key service person – who the family can keep in contact with and access information from
- emergency planning – if a key carer has to go into hospital or develops a disability/illness
- respite care – when a family requires a break
- future transition – to prepare the individual for possible changes to minimise the impact of potentially losing both parent and home in the same period.

The Growing Older with Learning Disabilities (GOLD) programme was undertaken in the UK in 1998–2002. It developed a number of externally funded projects to help older carers while focusing on in-house service developments and research. Projects were grouped into specific areas which included inclusion, health, supporting people with Down syndrome and dementia, living environments, terminal illness and older family carers. Results found that some parents experienced problems obtaining good quality information, emotional support and respite care. Quality programmes developed from listening to the views of carers brought about positive outcomes for a number of the projects (Foundation for People with Learning Disabilities 2002). It has been acknowledged that care giving for people with learning disabilities can be stressful (McCallion & Kolomer 2003). However, Grant (2001a) highlights some of the reciprocities or rewards that can be gained from this relationship. Financial dependence can develop as carers may become reliant on the income that the person with learning disabilities brings into the household. Older family carers may also become increasingly dependent on their younger sons and daughters to undertake household and shopping chores. Finally, emotional and psychological reliances can develop from lifelong caring which bring intrinsic benefits (Grant 2001a).

Services for older people with learning disabilities

In the UK, Hatzidimitriadou & Milne (2005) suggest that current services are fragmented with limited choice and specialist provision for older people with learning disabilities. In a review of Canadian literature, Salvatori et al (1998:249) argue that "older people with learning disabilities remain largely invisible, undervalued, and rarely the focus of new policy initiatives". Currently, there is no clear policy for providing services for older people with learning

Box 29.2

Service models for older people with learning disabilities

- *Age-integrated*: needs are met by learning disability services throughout the individual's lifespan.
- *Specialist*: needs are met by specialist services developed for older people with learning disability.
- *Generic*: older people with learning disabilities utilise generic older people services for their needs.

Reader activity 29.3

Consider the suitability of each of the service models (see Box 29.2) in your area of practice. Identify strengths and weaknesses of each model. Are all three necessary or should a new all-encompassing model be developed?

disabilities in the UK. Three competing service models appear to be operating for this client group (Grant 2001b; see Box 29.2).

Age-integrated model

As people with learning disabilities grow older, services must change in order to meet age-related needs. For example, 'ageing in place' relates to the person with learning disabilities ageing in their preferred place of residence. This is putting a strain on some social care settings in which they have to cope with the increasing physical health needs of their ageing residents. One study found that some environments and staff seemed ill prepared for this; in one instance, staff were carrying a client up and down stairs (Jenkins 2009a). However, Mirza & Hammel (2009) highlight encouraging results in service-directed use of assistive technology in supporting older people with learning disabilities to remain in the community. Assistive technology and environmental interventions include combinations of any product or items that are used to maintain or increase functional capabilities while also including physical and social environmental changes such as adaptations and training: for example, movement sensors which help to turn on lights or alert carers and computer software programmes which help with exercise. Promising research by Higgins & Mansell (2009) into the quality of life of older people with learning disabilities seems to indicate that this client group would be better served by remaining in learning disability-run services (group homes) compared to generic older people's provision. Quality of life measures indicated positive benefits in areas such as community access and meaningful activity in learning disability homes.

Specialist model

Very few specialist services have been developed for older people with learning disabilities (see Jenkins 2009b for one such example). Jenkins (2009a) explains the importance of specialised intervention when older people with learning disabilities develop dementia, which is frequent among individuals with Down syndrome. Surprisingly, when specialist dementia services are available, very few, if any, older people with learning disabilities with additional dementia needs appear to be referred to them. Chance (2005) highlights that there are still very few professionals who are dually trained in old age and learning disability psychiatry, however there seems to be a willingness to work together in order to meet the clients' complex needs. Making people with learning disabilities and associated mental health needs a specialist group within generic mental health services could be considered (Clark 2007). Dodd et al (2009b) argue that proactive measures are needed to engage older people with learning disabilities in services. A standardised approach is also required to monitor individuals and families refusing such services.

Generic model

This model does not treat people with learning disabilities differently from the general population. However, Hatzidimitriadou & Milne (2005) highlight that older people with learning disabilities and their carers often receive poor quality non-specialist care from inadequately trained staff. When people with learning disabilities utilise residential services for older people, they do encounter difficulties (Thompson et al 2004). For instance, they may not be welcomed by residents in the home, have few activities to undertake and lose contact with family and friends. There also appears to be reluctance by some generic day services to allow access to their provision with the label of learning disability acting as a barrier. Jenkins (2009a) reported similar findings with regards to labelling from community learning disability nurses when he explored their role in meeting the needs of older people with learning disabilities. There still appears to be an expectation that people must fit into a particular service rather than the service being individually tailored to meet the needs of clients and their carers.

Retirement

Retirement usually refers to the formal withdrawal from paid work. However, as the vast majority of people with learning disabilities in the UK never experience paid work, they don't retire in the usual sense. Instead, they are faced with the gradual withdrawal from services such as attending day centres, activity groups or small-scale workshops. It has already been highlighted above that older people with learning disabilities also experience difficulties in accessing generic older people's day services. When they are able to access such services, Walker et al (1996) report that older people with learning disabilities tend to be at a younger age (50–70 years old) when accessing generic services that generally cater for much older individuals. The activities, if they are provided, are usually not suited to the client group. Flexibility and an emphasis on socialising rather than work may make such placements more appealing.

Researchers in two studies (Bigby 1992, Salvatori et al 2003) interviewed carers of older people with learning disabilities. They expressed concern about the lack of leisure activities offered in the community to support healthy ageing for this client group (Bigby 1992) due to funding and resource limitations. They reported that there is often little follow up to support other needs once residential planning is settled (Bigby 1992). Health remains a major concern, especially for family members who are concerned about their own ageing as well as the ageing of their adult children. Parents had a propensity to overprotect their children to ensure that "their ageing adult children will be able to continue the lifestyle that they, as close family members, had fought so hard to achieve for them" (Salvatori et al 2003:6). Overall, it is essential that older people with learning disabilities are surrounded by people who advocate health-promoting activities, as it might be difficult for older people with learning disabilities to initiate them alone. Active strategies need to be developed so that their social networks acknowledge the importance of healthy lifestyles. Activities can only be implemented when it is considered beneficial by both older people with learning disabilities and their support networks, and when it is not seen as burdensome.

Role of professionals in meeting the needs of older people with learning disabilities

An important area which has been overlooked is often the unique relationship between the professional and the people they support and care for. Jenkins (2009a:x) found that professionals such as learning disability nurses do spend a great deal of time with the same clients:

> A lot of us have been in a home for a long time, so we've worked with some people 10–15 years, you know you've been a part of their getting older as we're getting older. So you've been through a lot of triumphs and tragedies together.

One of the challenges as people with learning disabilities age is the increasing complexity of providing appropriate services and professionals for the individual and carers concerned. It is therefore highly unlikely that just one professional or professional group can provide all the support the individual requires (see Case illustration 29.3). Professionals such as social workers, physiotherapists, dieticians, psychologists, speech and language therapists, occupational therapists, drama and music therapists as well as many different types of nurses may be involved in developing packages of care.

Case illustration 29.3

Sahid is a 65-year-old Hindu who has a moderate learning disability. He came to the UK from India when he was 8 years old. He at first found it difficult to settle in the UK and by the age of 15 was placed in the local learning disability hospital where he remained until he was resettled at the age of 50. For the last 15 years he has lived in a flat in the community on his own with daily support from a social care worker. As well as having a learning disability, he also has been diagnosed with paranoid schizophrenia and diabetes. Sahid has been taking medication for both conditions for most of his life. An uncle still keeps in contact with him although his relationship with the rest of his family is rather strained. A community learning disability nurse is in regular contact with Sahid to monitor his health and has recently been helping him to give up smoking. Unfortunately, Sahid has suffered a stroke during an interview with police who were investigating allegations that he had sexually assaulted a former male flatmate.

Reader activity 29.4

Consider the complexities of Case illustration 29.3. What support needs does Sahid require? Which professional groups may be involved in his current and future care?

Professionals have a role in ensuring that older people with learning disabilities have access to appropriate services whether it is in an age-integrated, generic or specialist model. In Wales, there is a move to revamp community services including community learning disability teams. *A Community Nursing Strategy for Wales* (Welsh Assembly Government 2009) document sets out to radically alter the way community learning disability nurses function. In the future, they should become professional nurse clinicians, leading and focusing on priority specialist health needs in areas such as complex physical health, epilepsy, mental health and challenging behaviour. They will have four levels of engagement which include direct intervention, multidisciplinary work, education of clients, carers and generic services and finally an inclusion role in which they will foster greater access to a range of appropriate interventions for people with learning disabilities (Duffin 2009). This new initiative may provide some direction on how learning disability nurses and services can meet the future needs of older people with learning disabilities.

In terms of practice, a number of areas need to be addressed. There needs to be more emphasis and organisation of health-promotion activity for people with learning disabilities across the lifespan. Early interventions with children can help to reinforce healthy behaviour in later life. For example, healthy ageing activities such as exercise are more likely to succeed if service users know the importance of healthy living exercising from their childhood and early youth. Increased exercise has been shown to also improve self-esteem among older people with learning disabilities (Carmeli et al 2008). The client group needs to be prepared to be potential carers for their ageing parents. This will require skills training by a range of professionals in the family home, day services and local colleges. Learning disability nurses should take the lead role in these areas due to their extensive knowledge, skills and values towards people with learning disabilities. However, other nursing specialties also have an important contribution to make (Jenkins 2005b): for example, practice nurses in undertaking annual health assessments, district nurses in ensuring interventions such as percutaneous endoscopic gastrostomy (PEG) feeding and medication are clinically effective and safe. Mental health nurses need to ensure that older people with learning disabilities can access their services particularly in the area of dementia care. All such nurses need to keep themselves regularly updated (Nursing and Midwifery Council (NMC 2008) in areas of knowledge and skills in order to meet the future needs of older people with learning disabilities.

There needs to be much better coordination of services between professionals and agencies in order for effective practice to take place. This requires professionals to embrace team working in their area of practice and link into other specialist support when necessary to focus on the needs of the individual. This is particularly important when dealing with clients who present complex needs. The concept of quality of life should be at the heart of professional practice. The use of models or frameworks which utilise quality of life as a basis for care planning can also act as a sensitising notion for the individual (Northway & Jenkins 2003). By focusing on this concept, professionals will be more likely to enhance the quality of life of older people with learning disabilities by identifying and addressing key areas. This will also ensure that often neglected areas such as spiritual needs are considered and met within this concept. In regards to end of life care, this is covered extensively in Chapter 30. Registered nurses must advocate on behalf of the clients they support in ensuring that they access appropriate health and social care (NMC 2008). Finally and most importantly, older people with learning disabilities and their carers need to feel empowered in order to have real influence and control over the services and support they receive. All professionals and services have a crucial role to play in making this happen.

Conclusion

There is little doubt that the numbers of older people with learning disabilities will continue to increase over the coming years. Research is needed into the perspectives of older people with learning disabilities with regards to their understanding of the ageing process. Individuals with very complex needs will present professionals and services with many challenges that must be resolved. Professionals such as learning disability nurses potentially have a leading role to play in ensuring that the needs of older people with learning disabilities are met. Encouraging healthy lifestyles should be a lifespan approach beginning in childhood. This may go some way to overcoming barriers in later life to engaging in healthy ageing. A wide range of services and approaches will need to be developed in order to ensure that older people with learning disabilities live in the environments of their choice and access the health and social care they require.

References

Alliance for Aging Research, 2010. Advancing science. Enhancing lives. Available at: www.agingresearch.org.

Barlow, C., 1999. Issues in the management of clients with the dual diagnosis of learning disability and mental illness. Journal of Learning Disabilities for Nursing, Health and Social Care 3 (3), 159–162.

Barr, O., 2001. Towards successful ageing: meeting the health and social care needs of older people with learning disabilities. Ment. Health Care 4 (6), 194–198.

Barr, O., Gilgunn, J., Kane, T., Moore, G., 1999. Health screening for people with learning disabilities by a community learning disability nursing service in Northern Ireland. J. Adv. Nurs. 29 (6), 1482–1491.

Bigby, C., 1992. Access and linkage: two critical issues for older people with an intellectual disability in utilizing day activity and leisure services. Australia and New Zealand Journal of Developmental Disabilities 18, 95–109.

Bigby, C., 1997. When parents relinquish care: informal support networks of older people with intellectual disability. J. Appl. Res. Intellect. Disabil. 10 (4), 333–344.

Bigby, C., 2004. Ageing with a lifelong disability. Jessica Kingsley, London.

Bond, J., Corner, L., 2004. Quality of life and older people. Open University Press, Maidenhead.

Bowey, L., McGlaughlin, A., 2005. Adults with a learning disability living with elderly carers talk about planning for the future: aspirations and concerns. Br. J. Soc. Work 35, 1377–1392.

Carmeli, E., Zinger-Vaknin, T., Morad, M., Merrick, J., 2005. Can physical training have an effect on well-being in adults with mild intellectual disability? Mech. Ageing Dev. 126, 299–304.

Carmeli, E., Orbach, I., Zinger-Vaknin, T., Morad, M., Merrick, J., 2008. Physical training and well-being in older adults with mild intellectual disability: a residential care study. J. Appl. Res. Intellect. Disabil. 21 (5), 457–465.

Chance, P.S.G., 2005. The mental health needs of older people with learning disabilities. Reviews in Clinical Gerontology 15, 245–253.

Clark, L.L., 2007. Learning disabilities within mental health services: are we adequately preparing nurses for the future? J. Psychiatr. Ment. Health Nurs. 14, 433–437.

Cooper, S.A., 1999. Psychiatric disorders in elderly people with developmental disabilities. In: Bouras, N. (Ed.), Psychiatric and behavioural disorders in developmental disabilities and mental retardation. Cambridge University Press, Cambridge, pp. 212–225.

Cooper, S.A., Holland, A.J., 2007. Dementia and mental ill-health in older people with intellectual disabilities. In: Bouras, N., Holt, G. (Eds.), Psychiatric and behavioural disorders in intellectual and developmental disabilities. Cambridge University Press, Cambridge.

Coppus, A., Evenhuis, H.G.J., Verberne Visser, F., et al., 2006. Dementia and mortality in persons with Down syndrome. J. Intellect. Disabil. Res. 50 (10), 768–777.

Cosgrave, M., Tyrrell, J., McCarron, M., Gill, M., Lawlor, B.A., 2000. A five year follow-up study of dementia in persons with Down's syndrome: early symptoms and patterns of deterioration. Irish Journal of Psychological Medicine 17 (1), 5–11.

Davys, D., Haigh, C., 2007. Older parents of people who have a learning disability: perceptions of future accommodation needs. British Journal of Learning Disabilities 36, 66–72.

Day, K., Jancar, J., 1994. Mental and physical health in mental handicap: a review. J. Intellect. Disabil. Res. 38, 257–264.

Department of Health, 1995. Learning disability: meeting needs through targeting skills. HMSO, London.

Department of Health, 2001a. Valuing people: a new strategy for learning disability for the 21st century. Cmnd 5086. The Stationery Office, London.

Department of Health, 2001b. Modern standards and service models: national service framework for older people. Department of Health, London.

Department of Health, 2009. Valuing people now: a new three-year strategy for people with learning disabilities. Department of Health, London.

Dodd, K., Turk, V., Christmas, M., 2009a. Down's syndrome and dementia: a resource for carers and support staff, second ed. BILD, Kidderminster.

Dodd, P., Guerin, S., Mulvany, F., Tyrrell, J., Hillery, J., 2009b. Assessment and characteristics of older adults with intellectual disabilities who are not accessing specialist intellectual disability services. J. Appl. Res. Intellect. Disabil. 22, 87–95.

Duffin, C., 2009. Specialist nurses set to lead from the front. Learning Disability Practice 12 (6), 6–7.

Edgerton, R.B., Gaston, M.A., Kelly, H., Ward, T.W., 1994. Health care for ageing people with mental retardation. Ment. Retard. 32 (2), 146–150.

Erickson, M., Krauss, M.W., Seltzer, M.M., 1989. Perceptions of old age among a sample of ageing people with mental retardation. J. Appl. Gerontol. 8 (2), 251–260.

Fender, A., Marsden, L., Starr, J.M., 2007a. What do older adults with Down's syndrome want from their doctor? A preliminary report. British

Journal of Learning Disabilities 35 (1), 19–22.

Fender, A., Marsden, L., Starr, J.M., 2007b. Assessing the health of older adults with intellectual disabilities. J. Intellect. Disabil. 11 (3), 223–239.

Finlayson, J., Jackson, A., Cooper, S.A., et al., 2009. Understanding predictors of low activity in adults with intellectual disabilities. J. Appl. Res. Intellect. Disabil. 22, 236–247.

Foundation for People with Learning Disabilities, 2002. Today and tomorrow. The report of the Growing Older with Learning Disabilities programme. The Mental Health Foundation, London.

Foundation for People with Learning Disabilities, 2010. Statistics about people with learning disabilities. Available at: www.learningdisabilities.org.uk/information/learning-disabilities-statistics/ (accessed on 13 April 2010).

Grant, G., 2001a. Older family carers. Challenges, coping strategies and support. In: May, D. (Ed.), Transition and change in the lives of people with intellectual disabilities. Jessica Kingsley, London, pp. 177–193.

Grant, G., 2001b. Older people with learning disabilities: health, community inclusion and family caregiving. In: Nolan, M., Davies, S., Grant, S. (Eds.), Working with older people and their families. Key issues in policy and practice. Open University Press, Buckingham.

Hatzidimitriadou, E., Milne, A., 2005. Planning ahead: meeting the needs of older people with intellectual disabilities in the United Kingdom. Dementia: The International Journal of Social Research and Practice 4 (3), 341–359.

Heller, T., Janicki, M., Hammel, J., Factor, A., 2002. Promoting healthy aging, family support, and age-friendly communities for persons aging with developmental disabilities: report of the 2001 Invitational Research Symposium on Aging with Developmental Disabilities. The Rehabilitation Research and Training Center On Aging with Developmental Disabilities, Department of Disability and Human Development, University of Illinois at Chicago, Chicago.

Heller, T., Marks, B., Ailey, S., 2006. Exercise and nutrition health education curriculum for adults with developmental disabilities, third ed. Rehabilitation Research and Training Center on Aging with Developmental Disabilities, University of Illinois at Chicago, Chicago.

Higgins, L., Mansell, J., 2009. Quality of life in group homes and older persons' homes. Tizard Learning Disability Review 10 (1), 22–29.

Holland, A.J., 2000. Ageing and learning disability. Br. J. Psychiatry 176, 26–31.

Hubert, J., Hollins, S., 2000. Working with elderly carers of people with learning disabilities and planning for the future. Advances in Psychiatric Treatment 6, 41–48.

Hutchinson, N.J., 1999. Association between Down's syndrome and Alzheimer's disease: review of the literature. Journal of Learning Disabilities for Nursing, Health and Social Care 3 (4), 194–203.

Janicki, M.P., Davidson, P.D., Henderson, C.M., et al., 2002. Health characteristics and health services utilization in older adults with intellectual disability living in community residences. J. Intellect. Disabil. Res. 46 (4), 287–298.

Jenkins, R., 2000. The needs of older people with learning disabilities. Br. J. Nurs. 9 (19), 2080–2089.

Jenkins, R., 2002. Value of employment to people with learning disabilities. Br. J. Nurs. 11 (1), 38–45.

Jenkins, R., 2005a. Older people with learning disabilities. Part 1: individuals, ageing and health. Nurs. Older People 16 (10), 30–33.

Jenkins, R., 2005b. Older people with learning disabilities. Part 2: accessing care and the implications for nursing practice. Nurs. Older People 17 (1), 30–34.

Jenkins, R., 2009a. Nurses' views about services for older people with learning disabilities. Nurs. Older People 21 (3), 23–27.

Jenkins, R., 2009b. Older people with learning disabilities: a quality initiative in caring. In: Froggatt, K., Davies, S., Meyer, J. (Eds), Understanding care homes: a research and development perspective. Jessica Kingsley, London.

Jenkins, R., Brooksbank, D., Miller, E., 1994. Ageing in learning difficulties: the development of health care outcome indicators. J. Intellect. Disabil. Res. 38, 257–264.

Jenkins, R., Wheeler, P., James, N., 2006. Care planning in residential settings. In: Gates, B. (Ed.), Care planning and delivery in intellectual disabilities nursing. Blackwell, Oxford.

Jenkins, R., Davies, R., Sardi, I., et al., 2009. Adults with learning disabilities presenting with dementia. University of Glamorgan, Pontypridd.

Jenkins, R., 2010. How older people with learning disabilities perceive ageing. Nursing Older People 22 (6), 33–37.

Keith, K.D., Schalock, R.L., 2000. Cross-cultural perspectives on quality of life: trends and themes. In: Keith, K.D., Schalock, R.L. (Eds), Cross-cultural perspectives on quality of life. American Association on Mental Retardation, Washington, DC.

Kerr, D., Wilkinson, H., 2005. In the know. Implementing good practice Information and tools for anyone supporting people with learning disability and dementia. Pavillion/ Joseph Rowntree Foundation, Brighton.

Kerr, D., Cunningham, C., Wilkinson, H., 2006. Learning disability and dementia: are we prepared? Journal of Dementia Care May/June, 17–19.

Lane, J., 2005. Down syndrome and Alzheimer's dementia. Frontline Winter, 22–30.

Llewellyn, P., Sardi, I., Davies, R., Northway, R., Jenkins, R., 2008. Learning disability and dementia – a review of the literature. University of Glamorgan, Pontypridd.

Luty, M., Cooper, S.A., 2006. Psychiatric health and older people with intellectual disabilities. In: Roy, A., Roy, M., Clarke, D. (Eds), The psychiatry of intellectual disability. Radcliffe, Oxford.

McBrien, J.A., 2005. Down syndrome and dementia: generating local evidence. Journal of Integrated Care 13 (1), 24–27.

McCallion, P., Kolomer, S.R., 2003. Psychological concerns among ageing family carers of persons with ID. In: Davidson, P.W., Prasher, V.P., Janicki, M.P. (Eds), Mental health, intellectual disabilities and the ageing process. Blackwell, Oxford, pp. 179–195.

McCarron, M., 1999. Some issues in caring for people with the dual disability of Down's syndrome and Alzheimer's dementia. Journal of Learning Disabilities for Nursing, Health and Social Care 3 (3), 123–129.

McGrath, M., Grant, G., 1993. The life cycle and support networks of families with a person with learning difficulty. Disability, Handicap and Society 8 (1), 25–41.

Mactavish, J.B., Searle, M.S., 1992. Older individuals with mental retardation and the effect of a physical activity intervention on selected social psychological variables. Ther. Recreation J. 26, 38–47.

Maggs, C., Laugharne, C., 1996. Relationships between elderly carers and the older adult with learning disabilities: an overview of the literature. J. Adv. Nurs. 23, 243–251.

Markar, T.N., Cruz, H.Y., Elliott, M., 2006. A pilot project on a specialist memory clinic for people with learning disabilities. British Journal of Developmental Disabilities 52 (1), 37–46.

Mann, J.H., Zhou McDermott, S., Poston, M.B., 2006. Healthy behavior change of adults with mental retardation: attendance in a health promotion program. American Journal on Mental Retardation 111 (1), 62–73.

Melville, C.A., Hamilton, S., Miller, S., et al., 2009. Carer knowledge and perceptions of healthy lifestyles for adults with intellectual disabilities. J. Appl. Res. Intellect. Disabil. 22, 298–306.

Mencap, 2007. Death by indifference. Following up the Treat me Right report. Mencap, London.

Michael, J., 2008. Healthcare for all. Report of the independent inquiry into access to healthcare for people with learning disabilities. The Stationery Office, London.

Mirza, M., Hammel, J., 2009. Consumer-directed goal planning in the delivery of assistive technology services for people who are ageing with intellectual disabilities. J. Appl. Res. Intellect. Disabil. 22, 445–457.

Northway, R., Jenkins, R., 2003. Quality of life as a concept for developing learning disability nursing practice? J. Clin. Nurs. 12 (1), 57–66.

Northway, R., Sardi, I., Mansell, I., Jenkins, R., 2006. Hopes and fears concerning service developments: a focus group study of parents and family carers of people with learning disabilities. University of Glamorgan, Pontypridd.

Nursing and Midwifery Council, 2008. The code. Standards of conduct, performance and ethics for nurses and midwives. Nursing and Midwifery Council, London.

Office for National Statistics, 2009. Life expectancy. Life expectancy continues to rise. Available at: www.statistics.gov.uk/cci/nugget.asp?id=168 (accessed on 31 January 2010).

Patja, K., Livanainen, M., Vasala, H., Orksanen, H., Ruoppila, I., 2000. Life expectancy of people with learning disability: a 35 year follow up study. J. Intellect. Disabil. Res. 44 (4), 591–599.

Podgorski, C.A., Kessler, K., Cacia, B., et al., 2004. Physical activity intervention for older adults with intellectual disability: report on a pilot project. Ment. Retard. 42, 272–283.

Prasher, V.P., Farooq, A., Holder, R., 2004. The Adaptive Behaviour Dementia Questionnaire (ABDQ): screening questionnaire for dementia in Alzheimer's disease in adults with Down syndrome. Res. Dev. Disabil. 25 (4), 385–397.

Renwick, R., Brown, I., Raphael, D., 2000. Person-centred quality of life: contributions from Canada to an international understanding. In: Keith, K.D., Schalock, R.L. (Eds.), Cross-cultural perspectives on quality of life. American Association on Mental Retardation, Washington, DC.

Rimmer, J.H., 2005. The conspicuous absence of people with disabilities in public fitness and recreation facilities: lack of interest or lack of access? The Science of Health Promotion 19 (5), 327–329.

Rimmer, J.H., Yamaki, K., 2006. Obesity and intellectual disability. Ment. Retard. Dev. Disabil. Res. Rev. 12 (1), 22–27.

Robertson, J., Emerson, E., Gregory, N., et al., 2000. Lifestyle related risk factors for poor health in residential settings for people with intellectual disabilities. Res. Dev. Disabil. 21, 479–486.

Salvatori, P., Tremblay, M., Sandys, J., Marcaccio, D., 1998. Aging with an intellectual disability: a review of Canadian literature. Canadian Journal on Ageing 17 (3), 249–271.

Salvatori, P., Tremblay, M., Tryssenaar, J., 2003. Living and aging with a developmental disability: perspectives of individuals, family members and service providers. Journal on Developmental Disabilities 10, 1–19.

Schalock, R.L., 1996. Reconsidering the conceptualization and measurement of quality of life. In: Schalock, R. (Ed.), Quality of life: conceptualization and measurement, vol. I. American Association on Mental Retardation, Washington, DC, pp. 123–139.

Schalock, R.L., Brown, I., Brown, R., et al., 2002. Conceptualisation, measurement and application of quality of life for persons with intellectual disabilities: report of an international panel of experts. Ment. Retard. 40 (6), 457–470.

Schupf, N., 2006. Genetics: Alzheimer's disease and Down syndrome. In: Prasher, V. (Ed.), Down syndrome and Alzheimer's disease. Radcliffe, Oxford.

Starr, J.M., Marsden, L., 2008. Characterisation of user-defined health status in older adults with intellectual disabilities. J. Intellect. Disabil. Res. 52 (6), 483–489.

Steff, M., 2009a. Active living and seniors with intellectual disabilities – an ecological perspective. McGill University, Montreal (unpublished PhD thesis).

Steff, M., 2009b. Seniors with intellectual disabilities and physical activity. Intellectual Disability, Pervasive Developmental Disorders, and Intersectorality research team, Montreal. Research News 7. Available at: www.interteddi.ca.

Strydom, A., Hassioti, A., Livingston, G., 2005. Mental health and social care needs of older people with intellectual disabilities. J. Appl. Res. Intellect. Disabil. 18, 229–235.

Taylor, N.S., Standen, P.J., Cutajar, P., Fox, D., Wilson, D.N., 2004. Smoking prevalence and knowledge of associated risks in adult attenders at day centres for people with learning disabilities. J. Intellect. Disabil. Res. 48, 239–244.

Thompson, D., 2002. 'Well, we've all got to get old haven't we?' Reflections of older people with intellectual disabilities on ageing and change. J. Gerontol. Soc. Work 37 (3), 7–23.
Thompson, D., 2007. Older people with learning disabilities. In: Gates, B. (Ed.), Learning disability: toward inclusion. fifth ed. Churchill Livingstone, Edinburgh, pp. 223–241.
Thompson, D., Ryrie, I., Wright, S., 2004. People with intellectual disabilities living in generic residential services for older people in the UK. J. Appl. Res. Intellect. Disabil. 17 (2), 101–107.
Walker, A., Walker, C., 1998. Normalisation and 'normal' ageing: the social construction of dependency among older people with learning difficulties. Disability and Society 13 (1), 125–142.
Walker, A., Walker, C., Ryan, T., 1996. Older people with learning difficulties leaving institutional care – a case of double jeopardy? Ageing and Society 16, 125–150.
Watchman, K., 2003. It's your move. Learning Disability Practice 6 (8), 14–16.
Welsh Assembly Government, 2009. A community nursing strategy for Wales: consultation document. Welsh Assembly Government, Cardiff.
Wilkinson, H., Janicki, M.P., 2002. The Edinburgh Principles with accompanying guidelines and recommendations. J. Intellect. Disabil. Res. 46 (3), 279–284.
World Health Organization, 2000. Ageing and intellectual disabilities – improving longevity and promoting healthy aging: summative report. World Health Organization, Geneva.
World Health Organization, 2010. Global recommendations on physical activity for health. World Health Organization, Geneva.
Yamaki, K., Hseih, K., Heller, T., 2009. Health profile of aging family caregivers supporting adults with intellectual and developmental disabilities at home. Intellectual and Developmental Disabilities 47 (6), 425–435.

Further reading

The Foundation for People with Learning Disabilities (a number of publications regarding older people with learning disabilities are available): www.learningdisabilities.org.uk.

Useful addresses

Alliance for Aging Research (a non-profit organisation dedicated to supporting and increasing the research into ageing and health): www.agingresearch.org

International Association for the Scientific Study of Intellectual Disabilities (IASSID) special interest research group on ageing (a leading ageing group comprising of researchers and practitioners in the area of learning disabilities): www.iassid.org

Rehabilitation Research and Training Center on Aging with Developmental Disabilities: Lifespan Health and Function (RRTCADD) (useful website on ageing issues related to people with learning disabilities in the USA): www.rrtcadd.org

Unit for Development in Intellectual Disabilities (UDID). Research unit based at the University of Glamorgan (useful research reports can be downloaded from this website in areas such as dementia, abuse, carers needs and person-centred planning): udid.research.glam.ac.uk

30

End of life

Sue Read

CHAPTER CONTENTS

KEY ISSUES

- It is important to recognise the range of losses associated with end of life care for individuals with a learning disability, their families and professional carers
- Identifying the inherent and persistent challenges to providing effective support at the end of life from a holistic perspective (with the person at the centre of care and support) is crucial in order for them to be overcome
- People with a learning disability are likely to experience disenfranchised death and disenfranchised grief and carers need to be aware of the implications of this
- Carers need to adopt a creative approach to effective care and support of people with a learning disability when they incur loss
- Carers need to consider the voices of people with a learning disability themselves and their experiences of loss, death and dying and how such experiences can help shape effective care and support (Read & Corcoran 2009)

Acknowledgement

I would like to thank Jacky for sharing her story and giving permission for it to be used within this chapter.

Introduction

The broad aim of this chapter is to consider a range of loss issues surrounding end of life and the persistent and inherent challenges of supporting, empowering and enabling individuals with a learning disability to become actively involved in the decision making processes at this stage of their life. Death never occurs in a vacuum but within a social context (Read 2008) and the nature of that context can influence greatly how the person faces the end of their life and how others accommodate the death of their friend/family member. This chapter will consider the various contexts involved and how such circumstances within these contexts can ultimately affect how individuals with a learning disability are supported with their losses.

As we steer towards the end of this book and come upon this ultimate chapter, it reminds us that we are all travelling along the same route as we age and move towards the end of life. It reminds us all of the persistent challenges involved in that ultimate journey.

This chapter explores the importance of living well until dying; and how people with a learning disability can be best supported as the end of their life approaches and they move towards the dying phase. It also explores the aftermath of death, as those around them cope with losing their loved one in a world that will be fundamentally different forever. These are important journeys; journeys that cannot be rehearsed nor repeated. Sometimes throughout these journeys, for some people who have cognitive impairments, it seems as though they have to try and make sense out of nonsense; trying to truly comprehend what is really happening around them with a limited capacity to understand the complex realities of ill health, death and dying. For those people who simply cannot understand complex abstract concepts such as loss, dying or death, carers need to explore creative approaches to try and engage with people in a simple and meaningful way. We owe it to all people travelling towards the end of life to get this journey right, and to celebrate and delight in the companionship as fellow travel companions along these difficult paths. For people with a learning disability, this journey may be the same as for anyone who is dying, but the routes taken to get there may be different, as carers and people with a learning disability themselves cope with all the challenges that having a learning disability might bring.

This chapter will introduce death within a range of loss experiences; explore end of life and the care required at this intersection; explore the concept of loss particularly in relation to people with a learning disability; and identify the persistent and inherent challenges to effective support from a practical perspective.

Death as loss

Life is characterised by movement, change and development and therefore, by its very nature, by transitions, losses and grief (Thompson 2002); therefore loss and death are omnipresent. Death is often perceived as the ultimate loss and the only certainty within life itself. Death is sometimes a regular companion as, for example, people with life-limiting conditions live with the prospect of an untimely death for many months or even years. Death can be a sudden and unexpected visitor, when it arrives without warning or time to prepare, and is perceived as untimely. Death can be a welcomed friend, after times of enduring pain and no expectation of release. Death can also be a stranger, when, for example, death and loss are shrouded in secrecy and individuals are not allowed to know about death and loss until absolutely necessary, for example when the bereaved person has a learning disability. What is known is that there are a range of responses to the loss of a loved one, and that such reactions can be influenced by many factors including the relationship to the deceased, the nature of the death, previous personal experiences of loss and death and existing coping styles – all of which may influence the true impact of the loss. Whether anticipated, unexpected, welcomed or disguised, death can create a huge chasm in the lives of surviving individuals, as they learn to accommodate their loss and have to relearn their new roles in life in the absence of companions (Attig 1996). Survivors have to reconstruct their lives in an attempt to live in a world that is different, and to continue to remember their loved ones in many different ways in the years to come (Klass et al 1996).

How you might have felt

Work through Reader activity 30.1. You might have noted that you could have felt confused, sad or angry but you couldn't explain or say why this is so. You might have felt frustrated because of feeling all these mixed emotions but not having the ability to find the words to verbalise these thoughts and feelings in a logical and meaningful way. You might have felt lonely because you had no one to share the fears and anxieties with; believing that no one could possibly understand what you are going through or

Reader activity 30.1

For just one moment, imagine if you never got to say a final goodbye to your loved one; imagine if you had no pictures or other mementoes of that person; imagine if no one told you about the funeral; imagine if no one asked you if you wanted to go to the funeral, or take flowers. Imagine living in a world where other people make decisions for you around loss and death, as to whether (for example) you should visit the hospice to visit a dying relative. Imagine not having the voice to articulate your feelings, concerns or questions, or not having anyone who asks you how you are feeling. Make a note of how this might make you feel.

indeed has the time to actively listen to you as you try to express and explain your pain.

Sudden death is recognised as being one of the worse deaths to accommodate, perhaps because survivors are often unprepared, have unfinished business and perhaps because sudden deaths are often tragic and traumatic by their very nature. Whereas anticipatory death is where a person knows that someone is going to die, perhaps because their loved one has an incurable illness. Many people with a learning disability are often exposed to sudden as opposed to anticipatory death because carers may be fearful of exposing them to the stark reality of their loved ones dying or feel that they lack the skills required to support someone at this time. Some carers may want to protect the person from distress; or just don't feel comfortable talking about death themselves. Some professional carers may feel that people with a learning disability simply do not have the capacity to understand loss and grief. Loss can be disempowering for anyone; but for people with a learning disability loss can be *totally* disempowering and often overwhelming.

There is a wealth of literature around loss and death generally, and a developing body of knowledge around this topic, particularly in relation to people with a learning disability. However, there is limited exploration about the personal experiences of loss specifically from a learning disability perspective. Life is fragile, with loss and death often just waiting around the corner, but such concepts become even more complex when the person struggles to make sense of abstract concepts, and is often protected from the stark realities of loss and grief by well-meaning, protective carers. Although loss and death are embedded threads woven into the very fabric of life itself, people with a learning disability rarely get constructive opportunities to learn or talk about such issues. Subsequently, accommodating loss can be difficult for people who have a learning disability, whether the person is accommodating the loss or death of others or is facing their own impending death.

End of life care

The provision of care for dying people in contemporary society is described as end of life care, incorporating palliative and supportive care (National Council for Palliative Care (NCPC) 2007), and embraces all people diagnosed with a life-limiting condition. Palliative care involves the active total care of patients and is defined as being:

> an approach that improves the quality of life for patients and their families facing the problems associated with life-threatening illness, through the prevention and impeccable assessment of pain and other problems, physical, psychosocial and spiritual.
>
> (World Health Organization (WHO) 2003)

Palliative care aims to affirm life and regards dying as a normal process, providing a support system for patients to live as actively as possible until death that:

- provides relief from pain and other distressing symptoms
- affirms life and regards dying as a normal process
- intends neither to hasten or postpone death
- integrates the psychological and spiritual aspects of patient care
- offers a support system to help patients live as actively as possible until death
- offers a support system to help the family cope during the patients' illness and in their own bereavement
- uses a team approach to address the needs of patients and their families, including bereavement counselling, if indicated
- will enhance quality of life, and may also positively influence the course of illness
- is applicable early in the course of illness, in conjunction with other therapies that are intended to prolong life, such as chemotherapy or radiation therapy, and includes those investigations needed to better understand and manage distressing clinical complications.

(WHO 2003)

Palliative care is delivered in various care settings, by a range of health and social care workers, and as such plays an integral part of the nursing role. The social context in which people live (and in some cases the labels which have been ascribed to them) may impact on the end of life care accessed (Oliviére & Monroe 2004) and subsequent care received (Read & Thompson-Hill 2009). While a holistic approach is seen by many professionals as the basis for all high-quality palliative care and support (Department of Health (DH) 2008), some marginalised groups (e.g. people with a low socioeconomic status; people with a learning disability) may struggle to access the appropriate palliative care and support when they need it most, for a plethora of reasons. While it is argued that "... people with a learning disability have poorer health, greater health needs and shorter lives" (Mencap 2004:31), end of life care for this population remains inconsistent across the UK and indeed across the globe (Tuffrey-Wijne et al 2007).

The majority of the general population still die in institutionalised care, whether this be in a private nursing home, hospital or hospice. Places where group dying takes place (such as hospice care and hospitals) can be perceived as creating an 'atypical visibility' which serves to entrench the social devaluation of people who are dying (Sinclair 2007) rather than supporting the individual to die in a familiar place where they have continued to live for all their life. While it is assumed that many people die in hospices, most people actually die in care homes and hospitals (see Box 30.1).

Death and dying have often been called the last taboo within society and only 34% of people are believed to have discussed or shared their end of life wishes with anyone else (NCPC 2009). For people with a learning disability, this figure is likely to be *significantly* lower because of its sensitivity. However, as one person with a learning disability commented in a recent study "You have got to know what I want because it will be down to you to see that it happens". (Todd & Read 2010). Unless we can overcome the uncomfortableness in talking about sensitive topics to the people whom we support, then we can never truly offer them the support they deserve (and indeed need) at the time they need it the most.

Box 30.1

Where people die

503 000 people died in England and Wales in 2006, in the following places:

- 290 000 in hospital
- 95 000 at home
- 47 000 in care homes (nursing care)
- 33 000 in other care homes
- 24 000 in hospices.

(National Council for Palliative Care 2009)

Reader activity 30.2

Think about the last time you talked about death and dying, and under what circumstances. Similarly, think about the last time you talked with a person with a learning disability about loss, death or dying.

End of life care and people with a learning disability

As the previous chapter recognises, as the person ages, loss experiences are likely to increase. One of the many features associated with ageing is that of the person drawing nearer to death, and perceptions of mortality and all this entails becoming more acute as those around them age and die too. While people with learning disabilities are experiencing increased longevity of life (Carter & Jancar 1983, Patja 2001), many more people with learning disabilities will come to have a dying phase in their lives as opposed to dying suddenly. The problems associated with ageing have been well described (e.g. Foundation for People with Learning Disabilities 2002) and in the preceding chapter. For example, people with Down syndrome are living longer, yet the incidence of dementia increases significantly with age for this population (Prasher 2005). Therefore, an ageing population of people with learning disabilities presents two noteworthy corollaries that have not been fully considered by either the research or care communities. That is, as people live longer so too do they die over a longer period of time and most people will enter the dying phase of their lives in some form of service or care setting. This suggests that the professionals working within these care settings should be pro-actively considering the issues associated with caring for dying people as part of their care packages and staff training initiatives. Work through activity 30.2.

Recognising ill health

Professionals rarely talk about death and dying unless prompted to do so because of circumstances (i.e. because an individual is dying) or there is media attention around the death of someone famous. However, some people with a learning disability may have much to contribute to such discussions if given the supportive opportunity to do so. Inherent social problems (including unemployment, limited exercise and restricted social activities), poor diet and additional health problems (such as epilepsy and dementia) compound the general health status of people with learning disabilities (Mencap 2004). Additionally, the *Death by Indifference* report (Mencap 2007) coined the phrase 'institutional discrimination' with regards to health care received by people with learning disabilities in the NHS in the UK. This short but powerful and poignant report tells the stories of six people with learning disabilities, who reportedly died unnecessarily in hospital and Mencap demanded an independent inquiry into these deaths. This resulted initially in an independent inquiry (Michael 2008) and subsequently an Ombudsmen's report which called for an urgent review of health and social care for people with learning disabilities (Parliamentary and Health Service Ombudsman 2009).

While there is a developing research and practice literature base driven by policy around general end of life principles for health care providers (DH 2008), there is relatively little empirical evidence around applying such principles to marginalised groups such as individuals who have various learning disabilities. People with a learning disability may not recognise initial symptoms or changes in their body that indicate ill health and disease, while some people may have had bad experiences of hospitals, doctors and nurses and have a reluctance to follow up any noticeable symptoms. Some may simply be too afraid to follow up changes that are recognised in case it leads to a poor diagnosis (Read & Morris 2009). John Davies (Tuffrey-Wijne & Davies 2007) knew that he was ill (he had penile cancer) but had ignored his illness for many months. He urges everyone to go to the doctor as soon as they notice something out of the ordinary because 'life is precious' (Tuffrey-Wijne & Davies 2007).

Some people with a learning disability may not actively look for signs, symptoms or body changes (Read & Morris 2009), nor easily recognise changes in their bodies that are indicators of potential ill health, so learning disability carers need to remain vigilant in recognising signs of potential ill health that may require further investigations (see Box 30.2).

Box 30.2

Simple things to look out for

- Swellings or lumps.
- Clothes not fitting properly.
- Weight loss or gain.
- Personality changes.
- Changes in eating habits.
- Changes in toilet habits.
- Generally feeling unwell.
- Tiredness or lethargy.
- Changes in behaviour.
- Asking for pain relief more often than usual.

(Read & Morris 2009)

Symptom recognition and identification may be difficult with this population because of communication difficulties and diagnostic overshadowing (Brown et al 2003). Diagnostic overshadowing describes the situation where the label of learning disability overshadows and masks the potential for the recognition of other potentially serious ill-health symptoms. Pain and other symptoms may also be difficult to manage and assess, as the individual with a learning disability struggles to indicate worsening symptoms and carers struggle to understand when to offer, administer or increase prescribed medication.

People with a learning disability may lack the sophisticated language to communicate any concerns they may have in a meaningful way. Macmillan Cancer Support (2003) identified four key barriers restricting access to cancer care services in particular: physical, professional, emotional and social, cultural or religious/spiritual. For people with learning disabilities, knowledge and attitudinal beliefs around the disability itself are also important features that impinge access to, and receipt of, good palliative care (Read & Morris 2009). People with a learning disability are often lost behind barriers that make access to end of life care and support difficult, and these barriers may be compounded if you are an older person with a learning disability (Jenkins 2005) or if you have dementia (Frey 2006).

People with a learning disability remain a vulnerable population generally, but particularly so when it comes to loss, dying, death and bereavement (Read & Elliott 2003), remaining reliant on so many people for so much. They are often actively excluded from the death and dying process, and the more complex their needs, for example if the person has a communication impairment and/or challenging behaviours, the greater the likelihood of this deliberate exclusion (Read & Elliott 2003).

While professional carers of people with learning disabilities remain committed to providing good quality care and support during this time, they may not have all the appropriate knowledge and skills to provide end of life care to their personal satisfaction (Todd 2004). Many face 'role blurring', as they try to move seamlessly between various roles (e.g. carer, advocate or friend) and caring functions. Performing skilled interventions around complex needs (e.g. physical care); simultaneously acting as pseudo families (Brown et al 2003); while also supporting other family members and friends who have a learning disability who live in a care home, as the person approaches death. Many may not be

> **Reader activity 30.3**
>
> Should a person with a learning disability that you support be diagnosed with a life-limiting condition, what might you do to include the person in the choices around their care? How might you prepare him or her for impending death?

familiar with palliative care as a concept, but have had to learn quickly in order to support the people they care for (Read & Morris 2009). Learning disability carers may have to become experts relatively quickly as they learn to provide end of life care for the dying person, but afterwards, as life quickly reverts to a sense of normality, such carers lose their expertise and begin once more to focus on the living well (as opposed to the dying well) aspects of their caring role.

Work through Reader activity 30.3. Initially, you might have considered how able the person is and what he or she already knows and understands about their condition. Even if they have not been told about the severity of the illness, many people often guess that something is wrong already (perhaps because of the number of doctor and hospital appointments recently; or the changes in medications; or the deterioration in health over time; or the simple fact that people are really nice to him or her at the moment). Breaking difficult news is never easy, but practical tips around difficult diagnosis can be found in Chapter 2. The key is to remember that whatever is going to happen, the person who is about to die is the most important person within this care context, and everything that is done is done because it will help them in some way. You might think about the person's circle of support and who is important to that person. You should explore what the person's end of life preferences are (if possible) and whether they have specific ideas about their own funeral. Religious and spiritual belief remain important, and sometimes individuals who may not have been actively practising any religious preferences, as the end of life draws increasingly closer, may turn to their religious leader for help, support and comfort. The amount of active involvement depends entirely on the needs of the person and their ability to understand what is happening to (and around) them, and they have a choice to be involved if they are able and indeed want to be included in this part of their life. No one should be forced to make a Will, or to complete funeral plans, if they do not want to. The carer's role is to help them make choices about their involvement and to treat them sensitively, but with honesty, empathy and compassion. A series of free leaflets and booklets specifically developed to help personal and professional carers and individuals with a learning disability at the end of life can be found in the Further reading and useful addresses section of this chapter.

Hospice professionals need to be aware of the challenges that supporting people with a learning disability may bring to them, and may raise issues such as the importance of being able to access professional (i.e. learning disability) expertise; communicating effectively; and understanding what having a learning disability really means (Cartlidge & Read 2010). How a person with a learning disability dies could be seen as a barometer against which one can measure how the person lived, and the value placed on their lives. Unfortunately, the evidence base against which we can measure a 'good death' of a person with a learning disability is lacking, and more empirical work around this aspect of care is crucial to holistic care and support. *The Best Practice Guide to End of Life Care for People with a Learning Disability* (Read & Morris 2009) is an evidence-based resource that offers a range of practical ideas and more details can be found in the Further reading section at the end of this chapter.

From a pro-active perspective, carers need to ensure that people with learning disabilities access national screening programmes (such as bowel cancer screening) to promote healthier outcomes (Read & Latham 2009), and address the issue of gatekeepers who can facilitate this active involvement. A gatekeeper is someone who controls access to certain people, such as people with a learning disability, and as such can play a pivotal role in orchestrating and coordinating care. An acronym (AWARE) developed to promote health for people with a learning disability is a useful framework for all carers supporting this population (see Box 30.3).

Living with loss

According to Elders (1995), the term loss implies that one has been separated from, is unable to locate or has had something taken from them. Some of the major losses related to death experiences are positively validated by society (such as the death of a parent) but some are not, such as abortion. Loss can be described as a sense of no longer having what you

Box 30.3

AWARE: promoting health for people with a learning disability

A – Alert people to the potential for ill health.

W – Watchful and vigilant: regarding regular personal body checking; carers need to notice any changes in any aspect of the person that might be an indicator of ill health.

A – Attend regular screening programmes: encourage and support individuals to attend for health checks such as mammograms, cervical screening and testicular checking. Identifying disease early can impact on treatment and outcomes.

R – Remember to encourage people to tell someone if they don't feel well or they notice any changes in their body. Talking about such sensitive issues may be difficult, and carers need to give people opportunities to explore how they feel in a way that the person feels most comfortable with (e.g. using pictures, drama, role play).

E – Encourage and enable people to attend appointments and to understand what might happen to them if they don't. Some people may need more time at clinics to help with communication issues; some may need to visit the clinic/hospital prior to the appointment to familiarise themselves with the venue; a familiar carer should accompany the person at appointments to promote consistency of support and minimise distress for the person.

(Read & Morris 2009)

value or losing what you prefer to keep. Evolving literature recognises that grief responses are not solely related to death explicitly, but can relate to other forms of loss. Loss associated with altered body image, disability or some aspect of self; loss related to divorce or separation; material losses (both tangible and intangible); maturational or developmental losses (Hess 1980, Machin 1998) and invisible loss (Machin 2010) all embody feelings of grief reactions as the loss is accommodated into the life of the living (Worden 2001). Machin (2010) identifies and describes invisible grief as that provoked by losses that are not obvious and often lack social and professional recognition such as poverty, old age and cultural identity. Having a learning disability can imply numerous invisible losses, inherent with the label itself: for example, one's social role in society and how devaluing this can be; the stigma associated with the learning disability itself and the inability to find meaningful, valued employment. Each loss carries with it the threat of additional losses and the potential for future associated losses, hence losses are often multiple, complex and successive (Elliott 2003).

Spall & Callis (1997) describe loss through unfulfilled ambitions as 'ought' losses; the perceived loss of things that ought to happen but probably never will, such as childlessness for a couple who always wanted to become parents, or having a child with a disability and the reality of confrontations with expected milestones that are never reached (Babb 2007). While bereavement is perceived as being the most common type of loss, having a child with a learning disability can mean confronting numerous losses, synchronous with hopes, wishes, ideals and expectations. This is echoed poignantly in an article written by a parent of a daughter with Rett syndrome describing a lifetime of disappointment, loss, frustration, sadness and pain as she continually tried to access the appropriate support required for her daughter over more than 30 years of parenting (Babb 2007). This article related explicitly to Ted Bowman's concept of shattered dreams (Bowman 2001, 2004), where a loss (e.g. childlessness, unfulfilled expectations of the self, the role of family and parenting) forces individuals to create new dreams in keeping with their current situations. The challenges inherent in dealing with difficult diagnosis (for example) are echoed in Chapter 2 of this book.

Generally, as people age, their experiences of loss will increase. As parents, their children grow up, move away (temporarily or permanently), find partners and have children themselves. Yet the pride of celebrating successful maturity is often tinged with the sadness of loss; of what's gone before that can never be recaptured, as young children mature into adult children. As people age, changes in the body indicate the need for changes in lifestyles: the regular squash player may not play quite as frequently, and eventually may choose a more sedate activity. The big family house with several bedrooms takes longer to clean and has less frequent visitors; perhaps a move to a smaller, easier to manage home is sought. The older one gets, the more experience of death one is likely to get, as family and friends confront ill health, the associated complexities and subsequent impact. Loss and death are omnipresent, since "death is inevitable and loss universal" (Kellehear 2005:16), yet there is limited research around how people with a learning disability are supported in death and dying and how death is managed from a professional caring perspective (Todd & Blackman 2005). The losses across the life cycle may be entirely different if you are a person with a learning disability.

Loss and learning disability

People with learning disabilities are more likely to "... function on a developmental level that is inconsistent with their chronological age" (Lavin 2002:314), and carry a history of marginalisation, devaluation and stigma. In an evolving society where great esteem is placed on good health, intelligence, independence, wealth, youth and perfection (Blackman 2003), being different is usually negatively perceived. Many people with a learning disability still have limited choices and restricted lifestyles, often living with people they have no choice about being with, as illustrated in the classification of care by Nolan et al (1994) (Table 30.1).

Currently, although much care is provided *in* the community and *by* the community, care *for* the community, where people with learning disabilities are identified as *contributing to* communities is becoming increasingly apparent but still remains the exception rather than the rule. A general pattern of life cycle for a person with a learning disability may involve moving to up to a dozen different care facilities in a lifetime; meeting numerous carers and support staff; changing carers too numerous to mention; having the support of a range of other care professionals to meet various individual (and sometimes complex) needs; and having reams of paperwork and various assessments completed about them by numerous professionals and stored indefinitely. The losses associated with this lifestyle are rarely recognised; barely acknowledged; and are subsequently and inconsistently supported. Change is described as a time of leaving the safe place where 'you know' and entering a strange place where you 'do not know' (Florence 2002), and for many people with a learning disability, they have often been confronted by strange and new experiences which they have neither anticipated, welcomed or been adequately prepared for.

Death never occurs in a vacuum, but from within a social context, and varied social contexts can often impact greatly upon the nature and circumstances surrounding the death itself (Oliviére & Monroe 2004), and the subsequent effects upon those survivors left behind. Loss can impact upon an individual in a physical, emotional, psychosocial and/or spiritual way (Worden 2001). Considering the potential for pain associated with loss, some might think "... loss is hard to bear, but is it worse than having nothing to lose?" (Cordy 2004:258). Yet having a life without companionship, connections, bonds and ties would be perceived to be a barren and unfulfilled existence for many.

Much has been both researched and written about cultural diversity from a loss, death and bereavement perspective, (e.g. Parkes et al 1997), yet for many people, death remains shrouded in mystery, and is often misunderstood (Kellehear 2005). This is particularly the case for those individuals who are perceived as belonging to a marginalised group, a group that has historically been viewed as 'different' from the rest of society. Individuals in this situation may lack the voice to be heard and are often overlooked when psychosocial/emotional support needs are concerned. They may be ignored when issues around loss, dying, death and grief arise, which has been described as disenfranchised death (Read 2006) and grief (Doka 1989, 2002). Disenfranchised death (see Box 30.4) means that the autonomy of the dying person is not

Table 30.1 Classification of care

Perceptions of care outside of hospital	Perceptions of care inside of hospital
Care outside the community.	In long-stay hospitals.
Care in the community by professionals and paid unqualified people.	All care provided in small community. Own homes.
Care by the community.	Care by unpaid family carers and volunteers in local communities. This care mirrors a commitment to ordinary or valued lifestyles.
Care for the community.	Care that is committed to the support of family carers. It also acknowledges that the person with a learning disability can contribute to the community.

(Nolan et al 1994)

Box 30.4

Disenfranchised death

> *... death that is not openly acknowledged with the dying person, where the dying person is socially excluded from the process of dying and deliberately excluded from the decision-making process surrounding the terminal illness.*

(Read 2006:96)

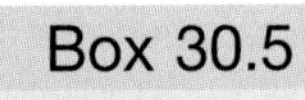

Box 30.5

Disenfranchised grief

> *... the grief that persons experience when they incur a loss that cannot be openly acknowledged, publicly mourned, or socially supported ...*

- The relationship is not recognised.
- The loss is not recognised.
- The griever is not recognised (Doka 1989).
- The circumstances surrounding the death.
- The ways that individuals grieve (Doka 2002).

recognised; the pending death is not recognised or legitimised; and the person's 'rights to know' are overlooked (Read 2006).

Similarly, marginalised groups such as people with mental health challenges, children, older people, people diagnosed with HIV and AIDS and people with learning disabilities may struggle to have their grief needs either acknowledged or responded to in a constructive way and experience disenfranchised grief (Box 30.5). The keys to unlocking disenfranchised grief are to acknowledge the loss and legitimise the emotional pain associated with that loss; active listening (listening with the whole body and not just the ears); empathy (making sense of life experiences by interacting with others, sharing and supporting); and exploring meaning making (finding benefits) throughout the lived experiences of grief (Doka 2002).

Loss is universal and can have a profound impact on individuals throughout life, as Oswin reminds us of its importance when she described loss as if "it sometimes seems as if all our lives we are trying to cope with loss – either the fear of it, or the memory of it or its raw immediate presence" (Oswin 1991:15). Penson (1992) believed that the concept of loss was the key to a genuine understanding of bereavement, and similarly may be the key to understanding how bereaved people with a learning disability learn to live and cope with loss and grief if facilitated appropriately.

Bereavement and people with a learning disability

People with a learning disability do experience grief (Hollins & Esterhuyzen 1997, Oswin 2000), but the impact of grief is varied and often complex (Conboy-Hill 1992, Hollins & Esterhuyzen 1997, MacHale & Carey 2002). While "response to bereavement by adults [with learning disabilities] is similar in type, though not in expression, to that of the general population" (Bonell-Pascual et al 1999:350), they are often neither encouraged nor expected to grieve or express their grief in any way. As some people with learning disabilities experience multiple and successive losses (Oswin 1991, Elliott 2003), suddenly the raw realities of living and the associated losses (not knowing where they might sleep, or whom they might live with or when they may find a permanent home) can temporarily overtake the raw sadness and reality of death. In such circumstances, grief work may be delayed, sometimes indefinitely, as the person is exposed to other successive losses. For the person with a learning disability, as more times passes, the likelihood of their loss being remembered by carers is reduced, and in some cases not recorded at all. Some bereaved individuals with a learning disability may struggle to accept the reality of the loss and accepting the finality and irreversibility of loss may take many months or years, particularly if the person does not receive appropriate support around the time of the death.

Challenges to effective support

The emotional needs of people with learning disabilities are often neglected (Arthur 2003), perhaps because of varied perceptions of their ability to grieve (Elliott 1995, McLoughlin 1986, Read 1996), overprotectiveness by carers (Deutsch 1985), or carers' feelings of fear, inadequacy and uncertainty (Emerson 1976, Oswin 1991, Thurm 1989). Conboy-Hill recognised the role of carers as she argued that:

> failure to recognise the impact of loss on people with learning disabilities arises from our need to see such people as lacking in effective emotional apparatus ... this conveniently feeds our own need to avoid discussion of pain and grief and so the cycle of ignorance and inaction has been perpetuated.
>
> (Conboy-Hill 1992:151)

Such convenience does not help people with a learning disability to learn to cope with loss as it happens around them.

People with a learning disability are vulnerable as many have an external locus of control, remaining reliant on so many people (often professional carers) for so much, and they are actively excluded from responding to death and dying (Read & Elliott 2003). There appears to be an increasing factorial affect with people with a learning disability that precludes active involvement in the sad business of death, where the more complex the needs, such as having communication impairment or challenging behaviours, the less likelihood they have of being involved (Read & Elliott 2003). Additionally, people with a learning disability usually experience sudden as opposed to anticipatory grief (O'Nians 1993), which reduces any opportunity for care givers, staff or counsellors to work towards the death with the dying person, thus minimising any opportunity to say their goodbyes in any meaningful fashion.

This range of issues potentially makes grief support complicated or hard to access, and many people with a learning disability may not receive the support they need following bereavement, and consequently many experience disenfranchised grief (Doka 1989, 2002) as previously described in Box 30.5. Those experiencing disenfranchised grief may have intensified emotional responses to loss (feelings of anger, guilt or powerlessness); they may experience ambivalent relationships and concurrent life crises, which can complicate grief, or the factors that facilitate mourning may be missing (e.g. grief rituals). Ultimately, the very nature of disenfranchised grief precludes social support, at the time when such support is seen as crucial (Doka 2002).

Case illustration 30.1 (A story of loss: Part one) describes the personal experiences of a woman with a learning disability who, following the loss of her son due to a termination, experienced multiple losses. Now work through Reader activity 30.4.

You might have listed Jacky's losses as including her potential to becoming a parent again; her daughter removed into care; her loss of independence; her changed identity; her dreams of parenting and family; the loss of her unborn child; the loss of her daughter; the loss of her partner; the loss of her self-esteem; the loss of her freedom. This example illustrates well how disenfranchised grief impacted significantly upon her life. She was not offered any support or counselling to help her cope with her losses at the time or anytime afterwards, and eventually asked for this herself some 12 years after the loss. Although being admitted to several medium secure environments over a 12-year period, and the myriad of professionals inevitable involved in her care, her loss issues were never addressed in any constructive way. Such disenfranchised grief led to unresolved grief, which needed to be recognised, acknowledged and sensitively supported.

Case illustration 30.1

A story of loss: part one

Jacky was 36 and lived in a medium secure unit for people with learning disabilities. Twelve years ago, Jacky had a termination of her pregnancy. Prior to this, Jackie had a daughter and lived independently with support from her partner, family and social workers. Following the termination, Jackie became withdrawn, her partner left and she began to steal from local shops. She never told her parents about the termination because she felt guilty both about being pregnant again and having the abortion.

Eventually, just 12 months following the termination, she was placed in medium secure care because of her behaviours, depression and self-harm. Her young daughter was taken into a different children's care facility. Jacky never received any help and support for her loss, and at certain key times (namely when the anniversary of the due date of her son was approaching), her challenging behaviours increased both in frequency and intensity. She asked her carers if it was possible to talk with someone about her loss.

Reader activity 30.4

Read Case illustration 30.1 and consider the losses that Jacky experienced as a result of having her termination.

Responding to loss and grief

A continuum of bereavement support is a useful framework to provide holistic support and to minimise disenfranchised grief (Read 2005, Read & Elliott 2007). This involves a broad range of support strategies that are available at many different levels and subsequently provided by a range of different people (see Fig. 30.1). These strategies range from general preparation *before* loss or death has occurred (education) to portraying loss and death as *natural*

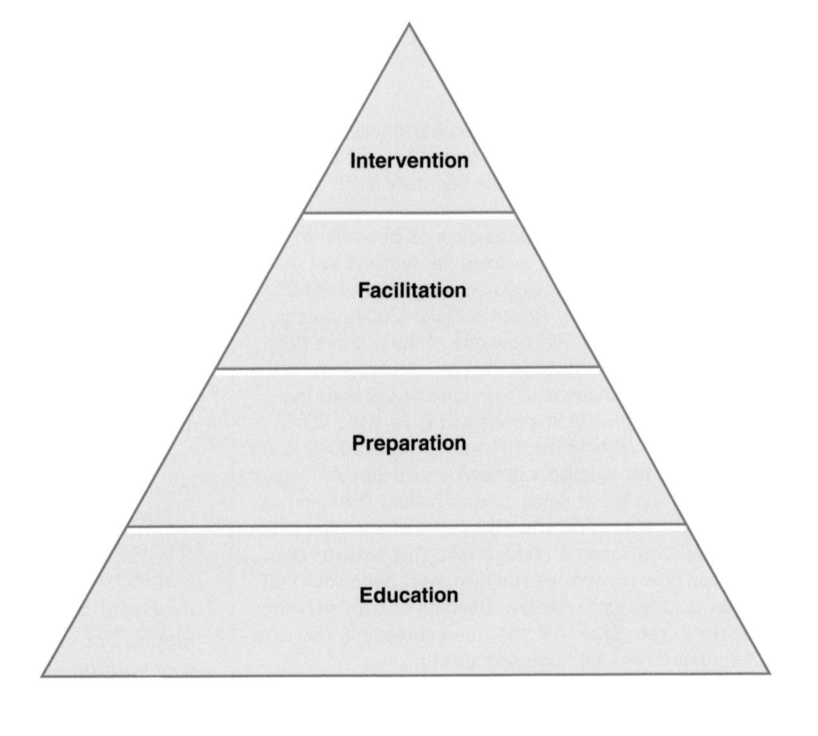

Figure 30.1 • A continuum of bereavement support (Read 2005. Reproduced by kind permission of RCN publishing)

life events (participation) or providing consistent support *after* the death has occurred (facilitation) and identifying the need for *specific help* (therapeutic interventions). Using everyday, natural opportunities to talk, explore and express feelings in a broader context, rather than relying on a reactive approach, involves developing and using a range of resources (e.g. Hollins & Sireling 2004a, b) and utilising a variety of media to communicate effectively, including pictures, books, videos and DVDs, television and radio. While such resources can help in various constructive ways, there is no empirical evidence of what works and why, with respect to bereaved people with a learning disability. Those who support bereaved people with a learning disability need to embrace the challenges inherent in creative support for this population by talking with those bereaved people, listening to their voices and hearing their pain.

Work through Reader activity 30.5. You might have considered the fact that Jacky had no ending for her loss, she never really said goodbye to her son, and often peri-natal loss is ignored and not acknowledged (Chan et al 2003). If Jacky had received adequate preparation and support at the time of her loss; if she had been encouraged to actively mourn the loss of her son; if she had been supported to say goodbye to her son in a way of her choosing; perhaps the need for specialist counselling and support could have been avoided some 12 years later. See Case illustration 30.2 (A story of loss: part two) to see how Jackie was helped to deal with her loss.

> **Reader activity 30.5**
>
> Consider again the story of Jacky introduced in Case illustration 30.1. What might help her to accommodate the death of her son? Considering it was 12 years ago, and the disenfranchised nature of her grief, what might be the impact of this and can she still be helped with her loss and grief?

Creative approaches

Jennings (2005) reminds us of the importance of storytelling because of their healing nature (through listening); explaining how different spaces (as in different places) are conducive to different story telling opportunities. In other words, the stories that you hear in a doctor's waiting room may be significantly different from the stories in a maternity waiting room, or while waiting at a train station or being

Case illustration 30.2

A story of loss: part two

A bereavement counsellor worked with Jacky to help her tell her story which she wrote over 12 typed pages. Jacky liked to write, and wrote her story using a laptop computer.

The counsellor introduced a series of books to help Jacky to recognise and express her feelings in constructive ways. Jacky particularly liked *Michael Rosen's Sad Book* by Rosen & Blake (2004), a very powerful book that tells how one of the authors dealt with the tumult of emotions and behaviours following the death of his teenage son. She specifically liked the following quotes: "Sometimes sad is very big. It's everywhere. All over me." (Rosen & Blake 2004), since this helped her to talk about how overwhelmed with grief and loss she felt at times. She also liked "Sometimes because I'm sad I do crazy things – like shouting in the shower . . ." (Rosen & Blake 2004). This helped her to explain how sometimes she displayed behaviour that she could not quite explain. Reading about this helped Jacky to recognise that she was not alone in how she felt; that others felt huge sadness too.

stranded in an airport lounge. Stories are concrete and can be permanent when written down using paper or on a computer. Recounting stories in grief work can be particularly helpful with people with a learning disability (Read & Bowler 2007), and whether as life story work (see Ch. 8) or memory work, can be cathartic in the bereavement context (Read & Bowler 2007). Many people with a learning disability lack personal heritage and history, and stories of life (and death) can help to construct a meaningful, visible and valued identity for the person. Such stories can also be shared, with consent, by others and help to accentuate the uniqueness of the individual and their life experiences.

Since "... the less articulate client with mental retardation [sic.] may feel uncomfortable in verbally orientated session . . ."' (Prout & Strohmer1994:7), it may mean providing the bereaved person with a language or way to communicate thoughts, feelings and concerns; provide avenues and activities to encourage self-expression; by directly altering techniques that would be used with other people without a disability of the same age; and using child- and adolescent-focused approaches delivered in an age-appropriate way (Prout & Strohmer 1994). Creative approaches include drama, picture books, life story work, memory books, visiting old haunts, drawing and painting (Read 1999). They can be used in the bereavement process

Reader activity 30.6

Think about how you might help a person with a learning disability to attend the funeral of one of his relatives. What might you do to prepare him for this event? How might you involve him in the ritual surrounding the funeral?

by helping carers to access the inner, dynamic world of the bereaved person and help to develop a therapeutic relationship by helping to reduce the client's uncomfortableness; provide concrete, visual aids that develop a sense of identity, history and heritage; promote understanding of personal state; enhance holistic care; and are enjoyable (Read 1999).

Now work through Reader activity 30.6. We need to remember that no one prescription fits all bereaved people, so in answer to the questions, there are a range of helpful activities that can be very useful to some people, but unhelpful in many ways to others. However, you might have considered finding out what previous experience the person had had of death, dying and funerals. You need to establish what the person understands about death and this might be done by using simple questions or by using books from the *Books Beyond Words* series (see Further reading and useful addresses section). Checking previous case notes and life story books might be a way of ascertaining this involvement. Exploring if the person wants to attend the funeral is crucial to this work and no one should ever be forced to attend if they choose not to, despite what other people believe is the right and proper thing to do. You might use a video to explain the difference between burial and cremation (see Further reading and useful addresses section). Taking the person to where the service will take place before the day of the funeral might help to allay fears and anxieties. With regards to active involvement, the bereaved person could be encouraged to select special clothes to go to the funeral and perhaps personally selecting flowers to send. The person might want to write or draw something that could be put with the flowers. They could choose who they would like to go with them (e.g. a special key worker or friend). They might even want to say a few words themselves at the ceremony, and you can help them to prepare for this in advance. Taking pictures after the ceremony of the flowers or place of rest might help to affirm the death to the bereaved person, and can be really useful afterwards when constructing life story or memory books with the bereaved person.

Case illustration 30.3

A story of loss: part three

After much discussion and preparation, Jacky selected and decorated a large stone pebble with her son's name, birth date and colourful flowers. The counsellor arranged for Jacky to take this pebble to the Stillbirth and Neonatal Death Society (SANDS) garden at the National Memorial Arboretum at Alrewas, Staffordshire, providing a memorial of her son. It was a very emotional visit, and it took Jacky a while to find the right place to leave her precious pebble.

Endings are really important in loss work, as Jacky recalled: "When I had the abortion I never had a chance to say goodbye to my baby". Her counsellor explored with her what sort of ending might help her so long after the loss. Jacky said that she wanted somewhere that she could visit and take flowers when she felt like it (see Case illustration 30.3 (A story of loss: part three)).

Rituals that recognise and commemorate loved ones are an important part of grief work. The constructive use of ritual is a powerful therapeutic tool, which can involve funerals; rituals of continuity (e.g. lighting candles on certain days); rituals of transition (e.g. marking the change or transition stage); rituals of reconciliation which allow the person to offer or accept forgiveness or to complete some degree of unfinished business; and rituals of affirmation which allow individuals to affirm the loss and recognise any good things that have come out of the loss experience (Doka 2002). Rituals play an important role in the lives of people with a learning disability too, as Jacky described in her story (see Case illustration 30.3).

The National Memorial Arboretum at Alrewas, Staffordshire remains a poignant reminder of the number of people who have died (and continue to die) in the armed forces and other professional groups and agencies. There are many pebbles in the SANDS garden, all decorated differently and personally, in memory of lost children (see Fig. 30.2).

Jacky recognised the need to say goodbye so that she could move on, and she chose a memorial that she could visit in the future and would always know where her pebble would be. The memory of her son would live on forever. However, she would never have independently selected this ending if someone hadn't known about the memorial and was able to offer the suggestion as one of several potential endings in this case.

"Loss is not just an individual experience. Political and economic disadvantage, conflict and prejudice have a collective impact upon communities" (Machin 2010:31) and, as such, can impact upon marginalised groups such as people with a learning disability. Personal and professional carers can play a crucial role in supporting bereaved people with a learning disability by reinforcing the normality of grief (James 1995); expecting grief reactions; actively looking for grief responses (Kitching 1987); and adopting a pro-active approach to loss through person-centred planning and collaborative working with other specialist practitioners. However, carers need to feel comfortable talking about such sensitive issues, so training and educational opportunities will form the basis of effective immediate and long-term support.

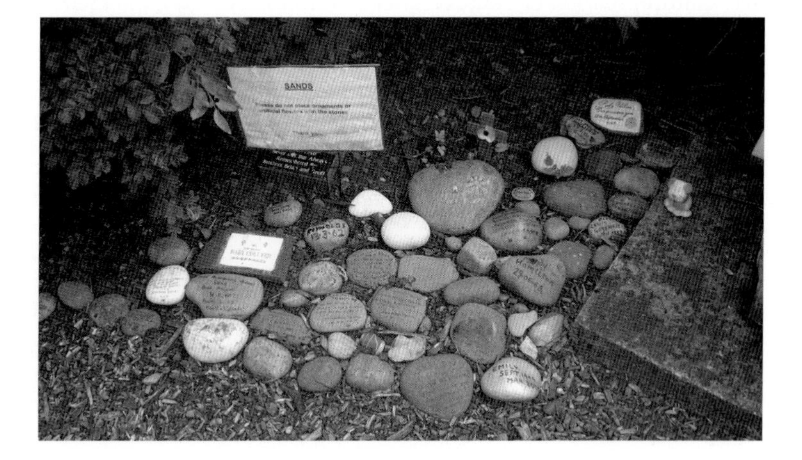

Figure 30.2 • Pebbles at the SANDS garden

Conclusion and recommendations

Case studies (see Box 30.6) provide a rich source of data that can illustrate phenomena within their own particular contexts (Yin 2009), and the case study within this chapter has been used to illustrate the complexities of peri-natal loss within a learning disability context, resulting in disenfranchised grief (Doka 2002).

While counselling and support can never undo the pain and sadness experienced, it can help individuals to accept the reality of the loss; explore the feelings surrounding the loss and the pain of grief; to reflect on, and adjust to, a world that is different; and to emotionally relocate the dead person, integrating their memory into the world of the living (Worden 2001). Such approaches can also help the person to learn how to cope with loss so that when they experience loss again in the future, they are better placed to deal with it. The case study illustrates well the importance of ritual when facilitating grief work with people with a learning disability. It also demonstrates the reality of practice and helps the reader to link theory to practice in a meaningful and constructive way.

This chapter has explored and addressed issues around end of life, loss and bereavement for one particular marginalised population. The author has deliberately woven the issues inherent to effective support for people with a learning disability within the general grief literature, since people with a learning disability have more similarities *to us* than differences *from us* (Read 2006), particularly in relation to death and dying. Carers need to utilise what is available to support the general grief world and explore its potential in relation to this marginalised population. Regardless of age, culture, religion or context, grief is a necessary process and carers need to be mindful of this as they support the individual with a learning disability.

Box 30.6

Defining case studies

A case study is an empirical enquiry that investigates a contemporary phenomenon in depth and within its real-life context, specifically when the boundaries between phenomenon and context are not clearly evident.

(Yin 2009:18)

More research is needed around mortality and morbidity of people with a learning disability and whether care staff are fully prepared and conversant with the holistic nature of end of life care and the type of support needed by the people they care for and what skills are necessary functions within this role. Practical issues surrounding accessibility to, for example, hospice care needs critically exploring, to ensure the key factors to fully accessible services are recognised and go on to provide an evidence base for developing future services. The Palliative Care for People with a Learning Disability network is a useful resource for carers and has a website incorporating resources and research around end of life care (see Further reading and useful addresses section).

Similarly, many research questions remain unanswered in the loss and bereavement arena involving people with a learning disability. While there are a variety of bereavement resources available, we have no evidence as to which are useful and which bereavement interventions work better than others. Sensitively supporting people with more severe, complex needs remains challenging. Collaborative education across generic and specialist palliative services (involving both learning disability and palliative care professionals) is the key to effective palliative care and support (Read 2006), and should include focused discussions around topics such as communication; management of conditions; and knowledge of the learning disability itself (Cartlidge & Read 2010). Many of the skills required to support a person with a learning disability in these sensitive areas of care are useful skills and approaches that can be translated across and generalised to other people under similar circumstances (see Box 30.7). Subsequently, there is much learning still to be done, and we need to remain open and receptive to those who can teach us so

Box 30.7

Learning from learning disability experiences

If palliative care services get it right for people with a learning disability, then they are highly likely to get it right for all of their patients.

(Cartlidge & Read 2010:98)

Reader activity 30.7

Think about the issues raised in this chapter and consider how you can make a difference to the lives of people with a learning disability when experiencing loss.

much, including people with a learning disability themselves. Work through activity 30.2. Having reflected on the variety of losses introduced within this chapter you might consider how loss is a focus in the lives of people you care for and how many of these losses are acknowledged or overlooked. You might think about how you could pro-actively talk about loss to people with a learning disability, by making use of naturally occurring events on the TV or other media.

References

Arthur, A.R., 2003. The emotional lives of people with learning disability. British Journal of Learning Disabilities 31, 25–30.

Attig, T., 1996. How we grieve: relearning the world. Oxford University Press, New York.

Babb, C., 2007. Living with shattered dreams: a parent's perspective of living with learning disability. Learning Disability Practice 10 (5), 14–18.

Blackman, N., 2003. Loss and learning disability. Worth, London.

Bonell-Pascual, E., Huline-Dickens, S., Hollins, S., et al., 1999. Bereavement and grief in adults with learning disabilities. Br. J. Psychiatry 175, 348–350.

Bowman, T., 2001. Finding hope when dreams have shattered. Bowman, Minneapolis, St Paul.

Bowman, T., 2004. Loss of dreams: a special kind of grief, eighth ed. Bowman, Minneapolis, St Paul.

Brown, H., Burns, S., Flynn, M., 2003. Please don't let it happen on my shift! Supporting staff who are caring for people with learning disabilities who are dying. Tizard Learning Disability Review 8 (2), 32–41.

Carter, G., Jancar, J., 1983. Mortality in the mentally handicapped: a fifty year study at the Stoke Park group of hospitals (1930–1980). J. Ment. Defic. Res. 27, 143–156.

Cartlidge, D., Read, S., 2010. Exploring the needs of hospice staff supporting people with an intellectual disability: a UK perspective. Int. J. Palliat. Nurs. 16 (2), 93–98.

Chan, M.F., Chan, S.H., Day, M.C., 2003. Nurses attitudes towards perinatal bereavement support in Hong Kong: a pilot study. J. Clin. Nurs. 12 (4), 536–543.

Conboy-Hill, S., 1992. Grief, loss and people with learning disabilities. In: Waitman, A., Conboy-Hill, S. (Eds.), Psychotherapy and mental handicap. Sage, London, pp. 150–170.

Cordy, M., 2004. The venus conspiracy. Corgi, London.

Department of Health, 2008. End of life care strategy. DH, London.

Doka, K.J., 1989. Disenfranchised grief: recognising hidden sorrow. Lexington Books, Toronto.

Doka, K.J. (Ed.), 2002. Disenfranchised grief: new directions, challenges and strategies for practice. Research Press, Illinois.

Deutsch, H., 1985. Grief counselling with mentally retarded clients. Psychiatric Aspects of Mental Retardation Reviews 4 (5), 17–20.

Elders, M.A., 1995. Theory and present thinking in bereavement. Issues in Psychoanalytic Psychology 17 (1), 67–83.

Emerson, P., 1976. Covert grief reactions in mentally retarded clients. Ment. Retard. 15 (6), 27–29.

Elliott, D., 1995. Helping people with learning disabilities to handle grief. Nurs. Times 91 (43), 27–29.

Elliott, D., 2003. Loss and bereavement. In: Jukes, M., Bollard, M. (Eds), Contemporary learning disability practice. Quay Books, Wiltshire.

Frey, M., 2006. Special needs require special measures. Community Living 20 (2), 22–23.

Florence, S.S., 2002. Change ... is a place where new journeys begin. Helen Exley, UK.

Foundation for People with Learning Disabilities, 2002. Today and tomorrow – the report of the Growing Older with Learning Disabilities programme. Foundation for People with Learning Disabilities, London.

Hess, P., 1980. Nursing and the concept of loss. John Wiley & Sons, London.

Hollins, S., Esterhuyzen, A., 1997. Bereavement and grief in adults with learning disabilities. Br. J. Psychiatry 170, 497–501.

Hollins, S., Sireling, L., 2004a. When dad died. St George's Hospital Medical School, London.

Hollins, S., Sireling, L., 2004b. When mum died. St George's Hospital Medical School, London.

James, I.A., 1995. Helping people with learning disabilities to cope with bereavement. British Journal of Learning Disabilities 23, 74–78.

Jenkins, R., 2005. Older people with learning disabilities: Part 2. Accessing care and the implications for nursing practice. Nurs. Older People 17 (1), 32–35.

Jennings, S., 2005. Creative storytelling with adults at risk. Speechmark, Bicester, Oxon.

Kellehear, A., 2005. Compassionate cities: public health and end of life care. Routledge, London.

Kitching, N., 1987. Helping people with mental handicaps cope with bereavement: a case study with discussion. Mental Handicap 15, 61–63.

Klass, D., Silverman, P.R., Nickman, S.L. (Eds), 1996. Continuing Bonds: new understandings of grief. Taylor & Francis, Washington, DC.

Lavin, C., 2002. Disenfranchised grief and individuals with developmental disabilities. In: Doka, K.J. (Ed.), Disenfranchised grief: new directions, challenges and strategies for practice. Research Press, Illinois, pp. 307–322.

Macmillan Cancer Support, 2003. Barriers to accessing cancer services. The report of the Barriers to Access Project Steering Group (Nov. 2002–2003). Macmillan Cancer Support, London.

MacHale, R., Carey, S., 2002. An investigation into the effects of bereavement on mental health and challenging behaviour in adults with learning disability. British Journal of Learning Disabilities 30, 113–117.

Machin, L., 1998. Looking at loss: bereavement counselling pack, second ed. Pavilion, Brighton.

Machin, L., 2010. Working with loss and grief: a new model for practitioners. Sage, London.

McLoughlin, I.J., 1986. Care of the dying: bereavement in the mentally handicapped. Br. J. Hosp. Med. October, 256–260.

Mencap, 2004. Treat me right!. Mencap, London.

Mencap, 2007. Death by indifference. Mencap, London.

Michael, J., 2008. Healthcare for all: independent inquiry into access to healthcare for people with learning disabilities. Aldrick Press, London.

National Council for Palliative Care, 2007. Palliative care explained. Available at: http://www.ncpc.org.uk/palliative_care.html (accessed on 4 January 2010).

National Council for Palliative Care, 2009. End of life care manifesto for 2010. The National Council for Palliative Care, London.

Nolan, M., Grant, G., Caldock, K., Keady, J., 1994. A framework for assessing the needs of family carers: a multidisciplinary guide. Base Publications, Rapport Publications, University of Wales, Bangor.

Oliviére, D., Monroe, B., 2004. Death, dying and social differences. Oxford University Press, Oxford.

O'Nians, R., 1993. Support in grief. Nurs. Times 89 (50), 62–64.

Oswin, M., 1991. Am I allowed to cry?. Souvenir Press, London.

Oswin, M., 2000. Am I allowed to cry?, second ed. Souvenir Press, London.

Parkes, C.M., Laungani, P., Young, B., 1997. Death and bereavement across cultures. Routledge, London.

Parliamentary and Health Service Ombudsman, 2009. 6 lives: the provision of public services to people with learning disabilities. The Stationery Office, London.

Patja, K., 2001. Life expectancy and mortality in intellectual disability. FAMR, Helsinki.

Penson, J., 1992. Bereavement: a guide for nurses. Chapman & Hall, London.

Prasher, V.P., 2005. Alzheimer's disease and dementia in Down syndrome and intellectual disabilities. Radcliffe, Oxford.

Prout, H.T., Strohmer, D.C., 1994. Individual counselling. In: Strohmer, D.C., Prout, H.T. (Eds.), Counselling and psychotherapy with persons with mental retardation and borderline intelligence. Clinical Psychology, Vermont, pp. 103–142.

Read, S., 1996. How counselling services can help deal with loss and change. Nurs. Times 92 (38), 40–41.

Read, S., 1999. Creative ways of working when exploring the bereavement counselling process. In: Blackman, N. (Ed.), Living with loss: helping people with learning disabilities cope with loss and bereavement. Pavillion, Brighton, pp. 9–13.

Read, S., 2005. Loss, bereavement and learning disability: providing a continuum of support. Learning Disability Practice 8 (1), 31–37.

Read, S., 2006. Palliative care for people with learning disabilities. Quay Books, London.

Read, S., 2008. Loss, bereavement, counselling and support: an intellectual disability perspective. Grief Matters: The Australian Journal of Grief and Bereavement 11 (2), 54–59.

Read, S., Bowler, C., 2007. Life story work and bereavement: shared reflections on its usefulness. Learning Disability Practice 10 (4), 10–15.

Read, S., Corcoran, P., 2009. Research: a vehicle for listening and promoting meaningful consultation with people with an intellectual disability. The British Psychological Society: Qualitative Methods in Psychology Section 8, 29–37.

Read, S., Elliot, D., 2003. Death and learning disability: a vulnerability perspective. Journal of Adult Protection 5 (1), 5–14.

Read, S., Elliott, D., 2007. Exploring a continuum of support for bereaved people with intellectual disabilities. J. Intellect. Disabil. 11 (2), 167–182.

Read, S., Latham, D., 2009. Bowel cancer screening: involving people with learning disabilities. Journal of Gastrointestinal Nursing 7 (7), 10–16.

Read, S., Morris, H., 2009. Living and dying with dignity: the best practice guide for end of life care for people with learning disability. Mencap, London.

Read, S., Thompson-Hilll, J., 2009. Palliative care nursing in relation to people with intellectual disabilities. Int. J. Palliat. Nurs. 15 (5), 226–232.

Rosen, M., Blake, Q., 2004. Michael Rosen's sad book. Walker Book, London.

Sinclair, P., 2007. Rethinking palliative care: a social role volarisation approach. Policy Press, Bristol.

Spall, B., Callis, S., 1997. Loss, bereavement and grief: a guide to effective caring. Stanley Thornes, Cheltenham.

Thurm, A., 1989. I've lost a good friend. Nurs. Times 85 (32), 66–68.

Thompson, N., 2002. Loss and grief: a guide for human services practitioners. Palgrave Macmillan, London.

Todd, S., 2004. Death counts: the challenge of death and dying in learning disability services. Learning Disability Practice 7 (10), 12–15.

Todd, S., Blackman, N., 2005. Reconnecting death and intellectual disability. European Journal of Palliative Care 12 (1), 32–34.

Todd, S., Read, S., 2010. Thinking about death and what it means: the perspectives of people with intellectual disability. International Journal of Child Health and Human Development 3, 87–92.

Tuffrey-Wijne, I., Davies, J., 2007. This is my story: I've got cancer. 'The Veronica Project': an ethnographic study of experiences of people with learning disabilities who have cancer. British Journal of Learning Disabilities 35, 7–11.

Tuffrey-Wijne, I., Hogg, J., Curfs, L., 2007. End of life and palliative care for people with intellectual disabilities who have cancer or other life-limiting illness: a review of the literature and available resources. J. Appl. Res. Intellect. Disabil. 20 (4), 331–344.

Worden, J.W., 2001. Grief and grief therapy: a handbook for mental health practitioners, third ed. Routledge, London.

World Health Organization, 2003. WHO definition of palliative care. Available at: http://www.who.int/cancer/palliative/definition/en/ (accessed on 4 January 2010).

Yin, R.K., 2009. Case study research: design and methods, fouth ed. Sage, London.

Further reading and useful addresses

Bereavement support: a series of leaflets around bereavement support for individuals, parents and professional carers (e-mail: s.c.read@nur.keele.ac.uk).

When someone you know has died....

When someone you know has died ... A guide for carers offering support.

When someone you know has died ... A guide for professionals offering support.

Books Beyond Words series includes a range of books to support people with learning disabilities in a range of sensitive areas. Examples include (all accessible from: http://www.rcpsych.ac.uk/publications/booksbeyondwords.aspx):.

Hollins, S., Downer, J., 2000. Keeping healthy 'down below'. Gaskell and St George's Hospital Medical School, London.

Hollins, S., Perez, W., 2000. Looking after my breasts. Gaskell and St George's Hospital Medical School, London.

Hollins, S., Wilson, J., 2004. Looking after my balls. Gaskell and St George's Hospital Medical School, London.

Hollins, S., Dowling, S., Blackman, N., 2003. When somebody dies. Gaskell and St George's Hospital Medical School, London.

The following book is an evidence-based resource developed specifically for those carers who support people with a learning disability diagnosed with a palliative condition, from within a variety of caring contexts. It is also available as an easy-read version and as a 12-point summary card. These resources can all be freely downloaded from the UK Mencap website: http://www.mencap.org.uk/endoflifecare.

Read, S., Morris, H., 2009. Living and dying with dignity: the best practice guide to end of life care for people with a learning disability. Mencap, London.

Palliative Care for People with Learning Disabilities network. On this website you can find information about the network, news, real life stories, resources and membership forms to join: http://www.pcpld.org.

Support at the end of life: a series of six leaflets and booklets for individuals, parents and professional carers (e-mail: s.c.read@nur.keele.ac.uk):.

Living with an illness that I will die from: the puzzle of palliative care (parts 1–4 series)..

Living with an illness that I will die from: the puzzle of palliative care – a carer's guide..

Living with an illness that I will die from: the puzzle of palliative care – a guide for professionals offering palliative care and support..

A toolkit to support health care professionals caring for people with a learning disability in acute hospitals. Available to download from: http://www.keele.ac.uk/nursingandmidwifery/mnphald/. Alternatively e-mail s.c.read@nur.keele.ac.uk

Index

Note: Page numbers followed by *b* indicate boxes, *f* indicate figures and *t* indicate tables.

A

B

C

E

F

G

H

I

J

K

L

M

N

O

P

Q

R

S

X

Y

Z